The Social Medicine
社 会 医 学

主 编　　郭继志　　汪　洋
Editor-in-Chief　Guo Jizhi　Wang Yang

中国海洋大学出版社
China Ocean University Press
青岛·Qingdao

图书在版编目(CIP)数据

社会医学 ＝ The Social Medicine / 郭继志,汪洋主编．—青岛：中国海洋大学出版社,2004.6 （2019.1重印）

ISBN 978-7-81067-603-8

Ⅰ.社… Ⅱ.①郭…②汪… Ⅲ.社会医学－医学院校－教材－英、汉 Ⅳ.R1

中国版本图书馆 CIP 数据核字(2004)第 049942 号

中国海洋大学出版社出版发行
（青岛市香港东路23号　邮政编码：266071）
出版人：王曙光
日照日报印务中心印刷
新华书店经销
＊
开本：787mm×1 092mm　1/16　印张：32.5　字数：750千字
2004年6月第1版　2019年1月第3次印刷
印数：3801~4300　定价：68.00元

编 委 会

主编
  郭继志 潍坊医学院   汪　洋 重庆医科大学

副主编
  刘达伟 重庆医科大学   张拓红 北京大学
  李宁秀 四川大学   尹文强 潍坊医学院
  朱亚南 潍坊医学院

编委（以姓氏笔画为序）
  王　净 重庆医科大学   邓　冰 贵阳医学院
  李　敏 第三军医大学   陈祥华 潍坊医学院
  苗　菁 重庆医科大学   阎瑞雪 潍坊医学院

主审
  王润华 重庆医科大学

顾问
  Paul Garner 利物浦大学热带医学院
  汤胜蓝 利物浦大学热带医学院

英文审校
  Peter Buggy，Kanchan Dahal，陈庆，李颖，李代昆，汪洋，王曰雷，许艳，刘琴

参加编写或翻译人员
  第一章 郭继志，朱亚南
  第二章 邓冰，王慧勤，蒋莉
  第三章 王净，陈治宇，李颖，龙倩
  第四章 刘达伟，苗菁，帅平
  第五章 李星明，任杰，刁玉涛
  第六章 冯国双
  第七章 李宁秀，岳勇
  第八章 张拓红，李爱兰
  第九章 阎瑞雪，邢建民，邢玉芳
  第十章 李敏，汪洋，陈静，李颖
  第十一章 周春莲，李秀燕，张国英
  第十二章 郭继志，郭继勇
  第十三章 尹文强，周春莲，李秀燕
  第十四章 陈祥华，王红妹，于贞杰
  第十五章 李秀燕

Editorial Board

Editors-in-Chief
    Guo Jizhi   Weifang Medical College
    Wang Yang   Chongqing Medical University

Associate Editors-in-Chief
    Liu Dawei   Chongqing Medical University
    Zhang Tuohong Beijing University
    Li Ningxiu   Sichuan University
    Yin Wenqiang   Weifang Medical College
    Zhu Yanan   Weifang Medical College

Compile Commission (In the order of number of strokes in surnames)
    Wang Jing   Chongqing Medical University
    Deng Bing   Guiyang Medical College
    Li Min   The Third Military Medical University
    Chen Xianghua Weifang Medical College
    Miao Jing   Chongqing Medical University
    Yan Ruixue   Weifang Medical College

Chief Umpire
    Wang Runhua   Chongqing Medical University

Consultants
    Paul Garner   The Tropic Medical College of Liverpool University
    Tang Shenglan The Tropic Medical College of Liverpool University

English Proofreaders
    Peter Buggy, Kanchan Dahal, Chen Qing, Li Ying, Li Daikun, Wang Yang, Wang Yuelei, Xu Yan, Liu Qin

Authors and English Translators
    Chapter 1   Guo Jizhi, Zhu Yanan
    Chapter 2   Deng Bing, Wang Huiqin, Jiang Li
    Chapter 3   Wang Jing, Chen Zhiyu, Li Ying, Long Qian
    Chapter 4   Liu Dawei, Miao Jing, Shuai Ping
    Chapter 5   Li Xingming, Ren Jie, Diao Yutao
    Chapter 6   Feng Guoshuang
    Chapter 7   Li Ningxiu, Yue Yong
    Chapter 8   Zhang Tuohong, Li Ailan
    Chapter 9   Yan Ruixue, Xing Jianmin, Xing Yufang
    Chapter 10 Li Min, Wang Yang, Chen Jing, Li Ying
    Chapter 11 Zhou Chunlian, Li Xiuyan, Zhang Guoying
    Chapter 12 Guo Jizhi, Guo Jiyong
    Chapter 13 Yin Wenqiang, Zhou Chunlian, Li Xiuyan
    Chapter 14 Chen Xianghua, Wang Hongmei, Yu Zhenjie
    Chapter 15 Li Xiuyan

序

我国社会医学经过26年创业,90%以上医学院校已经开设了社会医学课程。卫生部已将《社会医学》列为全国高等医学院校教材,供预防医学专业使用。在卫生管理专业、护理专业和部分院校医学生中也开设了社会医学课程,社会医学已经呈现了一派学术繁荣的景象。社会在前进,学科在发展,教材需要不断更新以适应新形势的需要。潍坊医学院、重庆医科大学等社会医学教研室中的中青年教授们结合多年来积累的经验,总结了近年来社会医学科学发展的最新成就,编写了《社会医学》双语教材,供全国社会医学领域的同道们学习参考。该书具有下列三个特色:

第一,贯彻创新精神。该教材以社会医学理论、社会病理现象、社会卫生诊断和社会卫生处方四篇为框架,将十五章内容网络之上述框架结构之内,在教材体系构思上具有创新精神。上述构思在学术界认识可能并不完全趋同,但是它的基本构思与社会医学的三个基本内容,即研究社会卫生状况、影响卫生状况的社会因素和提出社会卫生状况的策略及措施,是异曲同工的。该教材内容的创新精神还体现在增加了"非典"、艾滋病群防群治、社会心理研究方法、社会保障制度等,都是新世纪初期社会医学学术领域关心的重大课题,这本教材都及时加以总结形成系统的理论。

第二,该书每一章都附有案例。通过案例可以激发教师进一步理论联系实际,提高学生分析问题、解决问题的能力。在社会医学学术界已经酝酿多年要编写一本适合社会医学实习指导的手册,但至今未能付诸行动。该教材采用案例的形式,已经在这一领域做出了尝试,为编写一本通用的实习指导手册提供了成功经验。

第三,国内还没有一本《社会医学》双语教材,该书出版填补了这一领域的空白,并为在改革开放条件下加强国际学术交流,提供一种重要交流手段。

故该书的出版能对提高社会医学学术水平发挥推动作用。

中华预防医学会社会医学学会主任
复旦大学公共卫生学院教授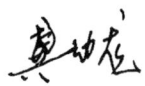

2004年2月

Preface

Having gone through 26 years, social medicine course has been started in more than 90 percent of medical universities and colleges in China. It has been schemed by Ministry of Health into the teaching material of higher medical universities and colleges, for preventive medicine students. It is also open to the students who major in health management, nursing and medical cure. Social medicine has been in her academic glory. With the development of society and the subject, the teaching material needs renovation to meet the demand of the new situation. This bilingual social medical textbook is a good reference in this field, compiled by the youthful and middle-aged professors of social medical teaching office of Weifang Medical College and Chongqing Medical University, summing up much experience in teaching for years and the up-to-date achievement in this field. This book has three features as follows:

First, innovation reflectes itself in the system of this book. We introduce four parts as its frame, namely, the theory of social medicine, social pathologic phenomena, social diagnosis and social prescription, in which there are 15 chapters. Above-mentioned conception is not concordant in the academic circle, but its basic conception is equal, despite different approaches to three basic contents of social medicine, namely, studying social health conditions, the social factors that affect health conditions and bringing up the strategy and measures of social health conditions. The innovation spirit in the content of this teaching material is embodied on adding the contents of SARS, the prevention and cure of AIDS in-group, the research method of social mentality and the social insurance system, etc. These contents are important subjects in the field of social medicine at the prime of new century and they are summarized timely in this teaching material and form systematic theory.

Second, there are some cases in every chapter. These cases can inspire teachers to connect reality further with theory and improve students' ability to analyze and resolve problems. One practical manual instruction that fit social medicine was attempted to be compiled in the academic circle of social medicine during many years, but failed. This teaching material represents the first attempt in this field by the form of cases, and offers the successful experiences to further compile a universal practical manual instruction on the basis of it.

Third, there is not a domestic bilingual teaching material, so this book fills up the blank of this field and provides a cardinal exchanges means to enhance the international academic exchanges under condition of reform and open.

Therefore, the publication of this book can enhance the scientific level of social medicine.

Director of Social Medicine Branch of Chinese Preventive Medicine Institute
Professor of Public Hygiene Academy, Fudan University

Gong Youlong

February, 2004

前言

社会医学在我国已经走过了20多个年头,从一棵稚嫩的小苗,发展到枝繁叶茂的参天大树。迄今为止全国出版了几十种不同版本的《社会医学》教材,最近由复旦大学龚幼龙教授主审、浙江大学李鲁教授主编的卫生部规划教材代表了近年来社会医学研究的最新成就。尽管如此,社会医学的教育和教材发展尚远远跟不上高等教育发展的需要。比如,我国不少医科大学已经招收了五年制医学本科外国留学生班,研究生教育在这些学校也都有了很大的发展,并且业已开始了中外联合培养社区卫生专业硕士研究生。这些都对社会医学教材的语言和内容方面提出了新的要求。并且随着社会的发展,对教材理论联系实际的要求更高,需要在教学改革方面有所创新,如潍坊医学院进行的案例教学模式、探究式教学模式、讨论式教学模式等方面的探索取得了较好的教学效果,并获得了山东省教育厅的教学优秀成果奖。不断提高本科教学质量是时代赋予社会医学工作者的历史重任。编写具有创新性、双语特点,能够引导中外学员探究和解决实际问题的教材便成了当务之急。

基于此,我们组织了部分中青年学者和博士、硕士研究生共同编写了这本汉英双语《社会医学》教材,本教材主要突出以下几个特点:一是英语与汉语对照的双语特色,这是在国内社会医学界进行的首次尝试,对本专业的双语教学和全英语教学提供了一本重要的参考书。二是理论联系实际,在每一章的最后都附有案例,这些案例都是经过反复挑选出来的,力求充分反映当前的社会卫生实践和卫生改革中新的社会医学问题,具有一定的代表性,在案例后附有讨论题,以便在课堂内外开展讨论分析。三是对教材的体系重新进行思考,从创立者讲了什么、现实提出了什么、未来的发展趋势是什么着眼,站在历史、现实、未来的高度,将社会医学分为社会医学理论、社会病理现象、社会卫生诊断、社会卫生处方4篇,在继承儒勒·盖林社会医学体系划分的思想基础上,进行了新的体系划分,同时避免将社会医学分为社会生理学、社会病理学、社会卫生学、社会治疗学,容易使人们认为这是一系列分支学科的误会。四是力求反映当代社会卫生的最新成就和认识,如疾病流行中的社会医学问题,对SARS等新的传染性疾病的认识。又如特殊人群社会医学、农村城市社会医学等内容。

仅此成书之际，编者对潍坊医学院领导和重庆医科大学领导的大力支持，潍坊医学院秦玉明副院长、教务处井西学处长，重庆医科大学董志副校长、预防医学系王润华主任的关心和支持表示由衷的感谢！

中华预防医学会社会医学学会主任、复旦大学龚幼龙教授亲自审阅本书部分书稿，提出了很好的意见和建议，并为之作序，对书稿作了很高的评价，这是老一辈社会医学家对我们的鼓励，坚定了大家的写作信心，我们表示诚挚的感谢！同时对支持我们出版本书的中国海洋大学出版社表示真挚的谢忱！对为本书出版给予帮助的姜维茂教授表示诚挚的谢意！对其他关心和支持本书写作和出版的各位同人致以衷心的感谢！

由于作者知识和水平所限，不妥之处在所难免，特别在英文方面，尽管有外籍专家把关，但限于我们的水平，在中译英的过程中仍然存在不少问题。恳请读者不吝赐教，提出宝贵意见，以便将来进一步修订和改进。

潍坊医学院　郭继志
重庆医科大学　汪　洋
2004 年 2 月

Introduction

Social medicine has already gone through more than 20 years in China, from a small delicate seedling to the big opulent tree. Up to the present, dozens of different editions have been printed throughout the country, in which the teaching material recently planned by Ministry of Health and edited chiefly by Professor Gong Youlong in Fudan University, and Professor Li Lu in Zhejiang University reflects the current topmost success on the research of social medicine. However, social medical education and teaching material still falls far behind the development of higher education. For example, first, some of the medical universities in China have already recruited foreign students class to teach five-year-system medicine undergraduate course, and there postgraduate education has also achieved great development, the cooperation project having started to cultivate professional master of community health, united by China and foreign countries. All mentioned above brings forward the new request on contents and language of the teaching material. Secondly, along with the social development, teaching material needs more to integrate theory with practice. Currently, reforms in higher education constantly come forth and some innovation is requested in it to keep pace with the social development. For example, Weifang Medical College developed example-teaching mode, exploratory teaching mode, discussion-teaching mode and so on and gained wonderful teaching effect and was awarded the outstanding teaching effect by the Educational Department of Shandong Province. The historic task of continuously increasing the teaching quantity of undergraduate course is set by the times to the social medicine worker. Therefore, it becomes urgent affairs to compile such a teaching material that possesses innovation, has theory integrated with practice, bilingual, and can induct Chinese and foreign students to explore and solve the current practical problems.

Based on that we united some young scholars, doctors and masters to compile together this bilingual teaching material of social medicine. This teaching material highlights some characters as follows: first, standing out the characters of bilingual, English and Chinese, it is the first attempt in the field of domestic social medicine and offers an important reference to the bilingual teaching and full-English teaching in the social medical majors; second, standing out the connection of reality and practice. There are cases at the end of every chapter. These choice and representative cases reflect the new social medical problems in the current social health practice and health reforms. Some discussion topics are at the end of these cases, which can be discussed and analyzed in or after class; third, rethinking the system of teaching material, social medicine is divided into several parts such as social medical theory, social pathology phenomena, social health diagnosis and social health prescription at the height of history, reality and future from what the founder said, what the reality ordered and what the future develop. The system is newly divided on the basis of Ruler Gaulin's division to social medical system, which avoids making people mistake that they are a series of branch sciences by reason of dividing the social medicine into social physiology, social pathology, social health and social therapeutics. In addition, this teaching material adds some new chapter that reflects the achievement and acquaintanceship up to the minute in the field of social health. For example, the social medical problems during the prevalence of diseases was added to reflect the understanding of some new infectious diseases such as SARS, and the social medicine about special population, city and village social medicine was added to this teaching material.

Now when this book turns out, we editors thank the leaders of Weifang Medical College such as vice dean Qin Yuming, chief of dean's office Jing Xixue, the leaders of Chongqing Medical University such as the vice dean Dong Zhi, and Wang Runhua, director of Preventive Medicine Department heartily for their strong supports.

Gong Youlong, professor of Fudan University and chief commissioner of social medicine branch of Preventive Medicine Association of China, checked in person some parts of this book, put forward good opinion and suggestion and prefaced it. This is encouragement by old-timers to us and we get firm faith from it. Thanks for it! At the same time, we heartily thank all of the leaders and editors of China Ocean University Press! Thanks go to professor Jiang Weimao, who helped to contact the press! Thanks also go to others who offered supports to compose and publish this book!

Because of the limit to the authors' knowledge and level, problem is unavoidable, especially in the English parts, despite the careful check by foreign experts. Plead for your opinion and suggestion to further improvement.

Guo Jizhi　Weifang Medical College
Wang Yang　Chongqing Medical University
February, 2004

目 录

第一篇　社会医学理论
Part 1　The Theory of Social Medicine

第一章　社会医学绪论 ··· (3)
 第一节　社会医学的对象、内容、性质及任务 ····················· (3)
 第二节　社会医学借鉴的主要学科 ····································· (6)
 第三节　社会医学的发展历史与发展趋势 ···························· (8)

Chapter 1　An Introduction to Social Medicine ····················· (14)
 Section 1　The Object, Content, Nature and Task of Social Medicine ····· (14)
 Section 2　Using the Experience of Other Major Subjects for Reference ···· (18)
 Section 3　The History and the Trend of Social Medicine ·········· (21)

第二章　医学模式 ·· (28)
 第一节　医学模式概念 ·· (28)
 第二节　历史上的主要医学模式 ·· (29)
 第三节　医学模式演变的规律 ··· (32)
 第四节　现代医学模式 ·· (34)

Chapter 2　Medical Model ··· (41)
 Section 1　Medical Model Concept ···································· (41)
 Section 2　Historical Main Medical Model ·························· (42)
 Section 3　The Evolution Law of Medical Model ·················· (47)
 Section 4　Modern Medical Models ··································· (51)

第三章　社会因素与健康 ··· (61)
 第一节　社会制度与健康 ·· (61)
 第二节　社会经济与健康 ·· (62)
 第三节　社会文化与健康 ·· (64)
 第四节　社会心理、行为与健康 ·· (67)
 案例 ··· (69)

Chapter 3　Social Factors and Health ······························· (70)

Section 1　Social System and Health …………………………………………… (70)
   Section 2　Social Economy and Health ………………………………………… (72)
   Section 3　Social Culture and Health …………………………………………… (75)
   Section 4　Social Psychology, Behavior and Health …………………………… (79)
   Case Example ………………………………………………………………………… (82)

第四章　社会卫生状况 ……………………………………………………………… (84)
   第一节　社会卫生状况评价 ………………………………………………………… (84)
   第二节　全球社会卫生状况 ………………………………………………………… (88)
   第三节　中国社会卫生状况 ………………………………………………………… (91)

Chapter 4　Social Health Condition ………………………………………………… (94)
   Section 1　Evaluation of Social Health Condition ……………………………… (94)
   Section 2　The Global Social Health Status …………………………………… (100)
   Section 3　The Social Health Status in China ………………………………… (104)

第二篇　社会病理现象
Part 2　Social Pathologic Phenomena

第五章　疾病流行中的社会医学问题 …………………………………………… (111)
   第一节　传染病流行中的社会因素 ……………………………………………… (111)
   第二节　传染病控制的社会医学策略 …………………………………………… (114)
   第三节　慢性病流行中的社会因素 ……………………………………………… (116)
   第四节　慢性病控制的社会医学策略 …………………………………………… (119)
   案例 ………………………………………………………………………………… (121)

Chapter 5　Social Medicine Problems of Disease Prevalence ……………… (122)
   Section 1　Social Factors of Infectious Diseases Prevalence ………………… (122)
   Section 2　Social Medical Strategies on Preventing Infectious Diseases …… (126)
   Section 3　Social Factors in Chronic Diseases' Prevalence ………………… (129)
   Section 4　Social Medical Strategies in Prevention of Chronic Disease …… (133)
   Case Example …………………………………………………………………… (135)

第六章　社会病 …………………………………………………………………… (137)
   第一节　社会病概述 ……………………………………………………………… (137)
   第二节　自杀 ……………………………………………………………………… (139)
   第三节　车祸 ……………………………………………………………………… (142)

第四节　性传播疾病……………………………………………………………(144)
　　第五节　成瘾性社会病…………………………………………………………(146)
　　案例………………………………………………………………………………(151)
Chapter 6　Sociopathy ………………………………………………………………(153)
　　Section 1　The Summary of Sociopathy ……………………………………(153)
　　Section 2　Suicide ……………………………………………………………(156)
　　Section 3　Traffic Accidents …………………………………………………(160)
　　Section 4　Sexually Transmitted Diseases …………………………………(163)
　　Section 5　Addictive Sociopathy ……………………………………………(167)
　　Case Example …………………………………………………………………(175)

第七章　特殊人群社会医学………………………………………………………(177)
　　第一节　儿童和青少年社会医学………………………………………………(177)
　　第二节　妇女社会医学…………………………………………………………(180)
　　第三节　老年社会医学…………………………………………………………(183)
Chapter 7　Social Medicine of Special Population …………………………………(186)
　　Section 1　Social Medicine of Children and Adolescent ……………………(186)
　　Section 2　Social Medicine of Women ………………………………………(191)
　　Section 3　Social Medicine of the Aged ……………………………………(195)

第三篇　社会卫生诊断
Part 3　Social Health Diagnosis

第八章　社会医学研究方法………………………………………………………(203)
　　第一节　社会医学研究原理……………………………………………………(203)
　　第二节　调查研究的设计和结构………………………………………………(209)
　　第三节　数据收集方法…………………………………………………………(211)
Chapter 8　Research Methods in Social Medicine …………………………………(216)
　　Section 1　Principle Foundations of Research ………………………………(216)
　　Section 2　Design and Structure of Research ………………………………(224)
　　Section 3　Methods of Data Collection ………………………………………(227)
第九章　健康危险因素评价………………………………………………………(235)
　　第一节　概述……………………………………………………………………(235)
　　第二节　健康危险因素与慢性病的演变过程…………………………………(236)

第三节　健康危险因素评价的计算步骤 ……………………………………… (239)

第四节　健康危险因素评价 …………………………………………………… (246)

Chapter 9　Health Risk Factors Appraisal …………………………………… (255)

 Section 1　Summary ………………………………………………………… (255)

 Section 2　The Evolving Process of Health Risk Factors and Chronic Diseases … (257)

 Section 3　The Calculation Stages of HRFA ……………………………… (260)

 Section 4　Health Risk Factors Appraisal ………………………………… (273)

第十章　生命质量评价 ………………………………………………………………… (280)

 第一节　生命质量评价的发展 ………………………………………………… (280)

 第二节　生命质量评价的主要指标 …………………………………………… (283)

 第三节　生命质量评价的相关工具 …………………………………………… (283)

 第四节　生命质量评价量表的设计 …………………………………………… (286)

 第五节　生命质量评价在卫生领域中的应用 ………………………………… (291)

Chapter 10　The Evaluation of Quality of Life ……………………………… (294)

 Section 1　Development of Quality of Life Evaluation ………………… (294)

 Section 2　Indicator for HRQOL …………………………………………… (299)

 Section 3　The Relative Instruments of QOL Evaluation ……………… (299)

 Section 4　Design for Profile of QOL ……………………………………… (303)

 Section 5　The Application of QOL Evaluation in Health Domain …… (311)

第四篇　社会卫生处方
Part 4　Social Health Prescription

第十一章　社会卫生策略 ……………………………………………………………… (317)

 第一节　初级卫生保健 ………………………………………………………… (317)

 第二节　健康教育与健康促进 ………………………………………………… (320)

 第三节　全球卫生策略 ………………………………………………………… (324)

 第四节　中国卫生策略 ………………………………………………………… (327)

 案例 ……………………………………………………………………………… (330)

Chapter 11　The Social Health Strategy ……………………………………… (333)

 Section 1　Primary Health Care …………………………………………… (333)

 Section 2　Health Education and Health Promotion …………………… (337)

 Section 3　The Global Health Strategy …………………………………… (343)

Section 4　Health Strategy of China ……………………………………… (347)

　　Case Example ……………………………………………………………… (352)

第十二章　城市与农村社会医学 …………………………………………… (358)

　第一节　城乡社会结构对卫生发展的影响 ………………………………… (358)

　第二节　城市和农村的主要社会卫生问题 ………………………………… (359)

　第三节　城乡居民保健的社会医学措施 …………………………………… (364)

　案例 …………………………………………………………………………… (366)

Chapter 12　Urban and Rural Social Medicine ……………………………… (368)

　Section 1　The Influence of the Urban and Rural Social Structure on
　　　　　　　Health Development ………………………………………… (368)

　Section 2　The Major Problems of Urban and Rural Social Health ……… (370)

　Section 3　The Social Medical Measurement on Health Care for Urban
　　　　　　　and Rural Residents ………………………………………… (378)

　　Case Example ……………………………………………………………… (382)

第十三章　卫生服务研究 …………………………………………………… (386)

　第一节　概述 ………………………………………………………………… (386)

　第二节　卫生服务需要、需求与利用 ……………………………………… (393)

　第三节　卫生资源 …………………………………………………………… (399)

　第四节　卫生服务的综合评价 ……………………………………………… (403)

　案例 …………………………………………………………………………… (404)

Chapter 13　Health Services Research ……………………………………… (406)

　Section 1　Summary ………………………………………………………… (406)

　Section 2　Need, Demand and Utilization of Health Services …………… (417)

　Section 3　Health Resources ……………………………………………… (427)

　Section 4　The Synthetic Evaluation of Health Service ………………… (433)

　　Case Example ……………………………………………………………… (435)

第十四章　社区卫生服务 …………………………………………………… (437)

　第一节　社区卫生服务的概念与特点 ……………………………………… (437)

　第二节　社区卫生服务的功能 ……………………………………………… (439)

　第三节　社区卫生服务的组织与运作 ……………………………………… (441)

　第四节　社区卫生服务的可持续发展 ……………………………………… (443)

　案例 …………………………………………………………………………… (446)

Chapter 14　Community Health Services …………………………………… (448)

　Section 1　Concept and Characteristics of Community Health Services ……… (449)

Section 2　The Function of Community Health Services ……………（452）
Section 3　The Organization and Operation of Community Health Services
　　　　　………………………………………………………………（456）
Section 4　The Sustainable Development of Community Health Services ……（459）
Case Example ………………………………………………………………（464）

第十五章　社会保障制度………………………………………………（467）
　第一节　社会保障制度概述……………………………………………（467）
　第二节　中国城镇职工医疗保险制度改革……………………………（469）
　第三节　中国农村合作医疗制度………………………………………（473）
　第四节　工伤和生育保险制度…………………………………………（475）
　案例………………………………………………………………………（478）

Chapter 15　The Social Security System ……………………………（479）
Section 1　The Outline of a Social Security System …………………（479）
Section 2　The Reform of the Medical Insurance System
　　　　　for Urban Workers in China ………………………………（483）
Section 3　The Rural Cooperative Medical Care in China …………（488）
Section 4　Industrial Injury and Maternity Insurance System ……（493）
Case Example ………………………………………………………………（497）

参考文献　References …………………………………………………（499）

第一篇 社会医学理论

Part 1　The Theory of Social Medicine

第一章 社会医学绪论

第一节 社会医学的对象、内容、性质及任务

一、概述

社会医学是一门交叉学科,从名称上看,由社会和医学两个部分构成,指社会学与医学交叉而形成的新的学科。社会学的创始人孔德将社会学分为社会静力学和社会动力学,认为前者是研究社会结构,后者是研究社会功能的。我国社会学家郑杭生教授认为社会学是研究社会运行的,认为社会运行分良性运行、中性运行与恶性运行。目前社会学已有70多个分支。

医学,也是一个庞大的学科体系,系统繁多,包括传统医学与现代医学。传统医学包括传统中医、印度阿育吠陀医学和阿拉伯尤纳尼医学,以及许多民族传统医学系统。这些传统医学系统是不同历史时期在世界各洲或国家发展起来的,例如在亚洲、非洲、阿拉伯国家、美国本土、大洋洲、中美洲、南美洲以及其他地区。另一方面是现代医学,可分为基础医学、应用医学和理论医学。应用医学又分为临床医学、预防医学、康复医学、航海医学、航空医学等。

社会医学是社会学与现代医学及传统医学相互交叉、渗透形成的一门相对独立的学科。其学科基础是医学与社会学。其学科性质更倾向于医学的范畴,《内科学》统编教材第三版绪论中指出:生物医学、医学心理学、社会医学已经成为现代医学的三大支柱。社会医学是一门内涵丰富、内容广泛的学科。

二、社会医学的对象、内容

(一)社会医学的研究对象

社会医学的研究对象尽管受不同地区卫生、社会、经济、文化等方面的影响,有一定的差别,但是,目前比较一致的观点是,社会医学是一门独立的学科,是研究社会因素与人群健康的相互作用及其规律,研究社会卫生状况,制定社会卫生策略,提高人群生活质量的科学。换言之,它是一门关于人群的社会生理现象和社会病理现象,对人群进行社会医学"诊断",开出社会医学"处方"的科学。

(二)社会医学的研究内容

我国社会医学经过了几十年的发展,关于社会医学的内容还有很大的争议,特别是20世纪70年代以来,社会医学已经形成了不同学术流派。这些流派相辅相成,对我国的社会医学发展是有益的。

1. 宏观上,社会医学研究社会因素与健康的相互作用。从个体到群体,人的健康受各种社会因素,诸如个人所扮演的社会角色、个人的行为、生活方式、个人所处的家庭环境、所处的工作环境、政治、经济、科技文化、人口、卫生服务等因素都对个体乃至群体健康产生一定的影响。社会医学研究这些社会因素对人群健康的影响,同时研究健康问题对社会的影响、社会因素之间的交互影响等。我国正处在社会转型时期,社会变化日新月异,如职工下岗问题,社会分化问题,青少年压力过大问题,青少年上网中的成瘾问题,自杀与吸毒问题,卫生服务中的欠公平问题,生殖性克隆的发展对人类自身的生存带来的挑战,食品、药品安全问题,生态环境的破坏引发的传染病爆发流行问题等。通过对这些社会病因的分析,进行社会医学"诊断"。

2. 研究社会卫生状况。社会医学像社会学一样具有"群学"的性质,关注的是人群的健康状况,通过社会调查方法,找出主要的社会卫生问题,研究影响这些问题的健康危险因素,发现重点保护的人群,提高人群的生活质量。

3. 研究社会卫生策略或措施,开出社会医学"处方"。通过对上述问题的研究,有针对性地提出改善社会卫生状况的政策和措施,包括发展初级卫生保健,实行医疗保险,推进社区卫生服务,合理实施区域卫生规划,制定适应社会卫生状况的策略、政策、法规和措施。

在组织卫生工作时倡导社会大卫生观,即卫生工作是一项系统工程,社会系统是一个大系统,卫生是其中的一个子系统,政府必须加强对卫生事业的领导,各部门进行协调,配合卫生部门进行工作,群众人人参与卫生工作。

4. 微观上,研究临床、预防、康复、健康教育中的社会医学问题,指导医务人员改变思维模式,真正做到卫生服务过程中以人为本,从以疾病为中心转变到以人为中心上来,从生物医学模式转变到生物-心理-社会医学模式。实现由医疗服务扩大到预防服务,由单纯的生理服务扩大到心理服务,由单纯技术服务扩大到社会服务,由院内服务扩大到院外服务。提高预防、诊断、治疗、康复水平,提高卫生服务的效率与效益。目前,研究方向是社区卫生服务,社区医学是社会医学思想的发展和应用。

社会医学的研究对象与内容不是一成不变,而是随着世界各国社会卫生状况和社会经济发展水平的不同而在变化和发展的。我国在卫生方面经历了三次革命。第一次卫生革命是以传染病、寄生虫病和地方病为主要防治对象,主要采取了国家卫生措施、环境卫生措施和生物医学措施,实行全民免疫接种计划,推行消毒、杀虫、灭鼠计划,通过综合性卫生措施,使得对传染病的控制取得了很好的效果。但是,应当清醒地看到,我国第一次卫生革命的任务还没有完成,传染病和寄生虫病有时还在局部地区出现爆发流行。"非典"和艾滋病在我国的流行说明了这一点。这些疾病应当引起我们高度的警觉。因此,我们同传染性疾病斗争的路子还很长。

随着我国人民生活水平的不断提高,人口寿命的延长,出现了许多慢性病、退行性疾病,如心、脑血管疾病,恶性肿瘤,意外伤害,糖尿病等。第二次卫生革命主要是针对这些慢性病、非传染性疾病而展开的。慢性病主要与不良的行为生活方式、环境因素有关。采取的主要措施是通过综合卫生措施,即通过社会医学措施、生物医学措施、行为医学措施、环境医学措施,重视三级预防,发展早期诊断技术,改善生态环境、生产、生活和人际环境,进行健康促进和健康教育,对不良行为、生活方式进行干预,建立良好的行为、生活方式方式。倡导合理的营养和适当的体育锻炼,降低慢性病、非传染性疾病的发病率与死亡率。

第三次卫生革命的任务是促进全人类的健康长寿和提高人们的生活质量,实现人人享有卫生保健的目标,第三次卫生革命是以健康观念的更新为先导,以人的健康、长寿、全面发展和生活的高质量为目标,倡导自我保健、家庭保健和社区保健。

现阶段,我国三次卫生革命的任务都十分艰巨。三次卫生革命的任务不是孤立的,也不是隔裂开的。需要树立社会大卫生观念,运用社会卫生措施、行为医学措施、环境医学措施、生物医学措施,注意对疾病的监控。注意新的社会卫生特点,包括传染病发生的新特点,总结经验教训。对疾病的控制进行全面规划,在某一个时期内,可能工作的重心不同,但是,人类每一次与疾病的较量,都使自己在认识上产生一定的飞跃。

三、社会医学的性质与任务

(一)社会医学的性质

1. 社会医学学科的交叉性,充分体现了人的生物性与社会性的统一。人既是生物的人,又是社会的人。生育过程表面上看是生物性的,个体从受精到分娩是一个生物过程,但生育在本质上是社会性的。费孝通教授在《生育制度》一书中指出,生育是为了社会的绵延。人的生物过程与社会过程得到了很好的统一,人的社会性使得人的生物性按照一定的规则进行,使社会和谐发展。生物医学模式比较注重人的生物属性的研究,往往忽略对人的社会属性的观察和分析,忽视人的社会心理需要。社会医学要从社会整体出发研究人的社会属性,其他的医学门类也应重视人的社会属性的研究。卫生作为一种公益性社会事业,属于公共事业,其社会性很强。政府对卫生事业的领导不同于一般的工作,关系群众的健康、安全、生命。卫生资源的分配也是政策性很强的工作。在当前,医学的社会化程度越来越高,重视卫生的社会性是必然的。另一方面,从疾病的病因上看,许多疾病虽然生物因素扮演了重要的角色,而社会因素在许多慢性病的致病过程中往往起到主要作用。

2. 研究方法的综合性。社会医学的学科交叉性,决定了研究方法的综合性。作为社会学与医学相交的学科,既要运用自然科学的方法,又要运用社会科学的方法,如社会调查方法、人类学方法、心理学方法等,但同时要运用实验的方法,运用流行病学方法、统计学方法等。还应当熟悉经济学、管理学的方法。在研究不同的社会卫生问题时,其方法的侧重是不同的。如在重点研究病人的行为、人群的生活质量时,更多地运用社会调查方法、心理学的方法;在研究卫生服务的效率时,更多地运用经济学、管理学方法。在一些综合性研究中,往往需要多种方法的配合。总的看来,离不开哲学方法的指导,特别是正确的自然观和科学的方法论,这是指导我们研究的根本大法。

3. 社会医学的实践性。社会医学从产生的那天起,就直接指导社会卫生实践。首先,社会医学并没有像有些学科那样发展了自己的学科语言,而是借用了其他学科的一些理论,针对卫生实践中提出的问题,以解决社会卫生问题为己任,增强了社会医学研究的实践性。其次,社会医学没有固定的研究范式,这使得社会医学的研究范围广阔,不容易陷入教条主义。当然,从另一方面看,社会医学也应当进一步学术化、理论化、专业化。这是学科发展的必由之路。

(二)社会医学的主要任务

1. 为卫生决策者提供社会卫生信息,为卫生决策服务。国家卫生方针政策的制定,卫生策略的规划,都依赖于对社会卫生状况的了解。社会医学为卫生决策提供咨询服务。我国20世纪80年代初,在部分医学院校成立了卫生管理干部学院或卫生管理系,为社会培养了大批科学管理、科学决策的卫生管理人才。正是从那时起,我国的社会医学得到了长足的发展。我国社会医学的发展,与卫生管理教育的发展是分不开的。社会医学的首要任务,就是要通过社会调查的方法,摸清社会卫生状况,找出存在的社会卫生问题,为政府制定卫生事业计划与规划提供信息支持。

2. 提高人群的健康水平和生命质量。通过对人群的健康状况评价,对人群的健康危险因素评价,对人群的生命质量评价、健康行为调查,对人群的健康状况做出社会医学"诊断",开出社会医学"处方",促进个体乃至群体改变自己的不良行为和生活方式,主动改变或调适不良的社会环境,从而达到提高公众健康水平和生命质量的任务和目标。

3. 社会医学的教育与传播。通过社会医学的教育和传播,使社会人群,特别是医务人员和卫生管理干部,树立科学的疾病观、健康观,将社会医学的知识渗透到临床医学、预防医学、康复医学、健康教育学、社区医学和卫生管理学等学科中去。用现代医学模式指导卫生实践与卫生管理工作。通过教育,培养适应现代医学模式的卫生人才和卫生管理人才。社会医学在现代社会中扮演着越来越重要的角色。

第二节 社会医学借鉴的主要学科

社会医学的交叉性,决定社会医学需要从相关学科中广泛借鉴,他山之石可以攻玉。

一、预防医学

一般认为,社会医学是从预防医学中分化而来的。预防医学是在基础科学(生物学、物理学、化学)、医学和环境医学的基础上,应用并发展环境与健康(效应)的基本理论,研究环境中自然因素和社会因素对机体健康的作用机理和疾病发生及分布规律的科学。预防医学的指导思想是预防为主,研究对象主要是人群,研究方法多采用宏观和微观相结合的方法,主要目的是为制定保护人群和促进健康的措施、提高群体生命质量的三级预防措施提供科学依据。新的预防医学的定义提出了将社会因素作为自己的研究对象,这正是社会医学研究的成果。社会医学也要不断地从预防医学中吸收有益的东西,如疾病病因的研究方法,对健康问题的系统分析方法,注意非传染性、慢性病研究的多因素分析等等。当然,社会医学的使命还是主要针对社会因素的研究,其学科的社会性质比较强,而预防医学则重点是针对生物因素。因此,两门学科需要相互结合,相互借鉴,共同发展,促进人类生命质量的提高。

二、社会学

社会学是法国社会学家孔德（August Comte）首先提出来,最初称为社会物理学。社会学与社会医学几乎同一个时代产生,其学科的发祥地都在法国,绝不是偶然的,是社会政治、经济、文化和社会卫生发展状况的必然结果。

对社会学的研究对象目前还有一些争议,有的认为是研究社会结构和社会功能的,也有的认为是研究社会运行规律的,还有的认为是研究社会问题的。社会学在研究上注重实证研究,善于运用实地调查研究的方法。社会学也较注重理论研究,善于提出假说,来推断一些社会现象,比如老年社会学中的活动理论、脱离理论等,都是关于成功老龄化的理论依据。社会学还重视发展了一套学科语言,诸如社会角色、社会阶层、社会分化、社会流动等,筑起了专业人员与非专业人员之间的一道屏障。医学社会学是社会学的一个分支学科,主要运用社会学的理论对卫生领域中的社会运行规律和社会问题进行研究,诸如医院的社会结构与功能、卫生技术人员的社会流动、医生护士角色、医患关系等。我们认为社会医学虽然更倾向于医学的性质,但社会医学与医学社会学很难区分。在德国以发展社会医学为主,在美国则以发展医学社会学为主。在我国,社会医学与医学社会学有融合的趋势。因此,社会医学要不断从社会学和医学社会学中汲取营养,不以门户所限,才能更快、更好地发展自己。

三、社区医学

社区医学是根据社区特点,运用社会医学理论指导,以社区为范围,以家庭为单位,以病人为中心,开展医疗、预防、保健、康复、健康教育、计划生育六位一体的卫生服务。社区是社会的缩影,社会医学为社区医学提供了理论上的指导,同时社区医学实践了社会医学从治疗服务扩大到预防服务、从院内服务扩大到院外服务、从生理服务扩大到心理服务、从技术服务扩大到社会服务的思想,社区医学的实践丰富了社会医学的学科内涵,使社会医学更加理论联系实际,社区医学实践也为社会医学提出了许多新的课题,如社区卫生服务可持续发展问题。因此,社会医学应当深入社区实践,从丰富的社区卫生实践中不断汲取营养。

社会医学与社区医学不论在理论上,还是在实践上都有一致性,英国干脆把社会医学的方向定位为社区医学上。因此,社会医学与社区医学的结合,使宏观研究和微观研究很好地统一起来。

四、医学伦理学

一般认为,医学伦理学是一般伦理学原理在医学实践中的具体应用,是用一般伦理学的道德原则来解决医疗实践和医学科学发展中人们相互之间、医学与社会之间的关系问题而形成的一门科学,研究医疗、预防实践中的道德规范等。现在已经将医学伦理学发展到生命伦理学。生命伦理学已经将道德关系不仅定位为医务人员同患者的关系,而扩展到人与动物的关系;不仅涉及生命神圣论,也研究生命价值论和公益论。社会医学研究卫生政策和策略,制定区域卫生规划,研究卫生服务,必然涉及一定的价值取向,受价值理论和公益理论的影响。在卫生资源的分配中,谁优先得到这些资源?卫生资源应该优先配置到哪些地区、哪些人群?这些都需要医学伦理学和生命伦理学的指导。学习和借鉴伦理学,运用价值分析的方法,使资源的配置更加合理,更加公正、公平。特别是研究宏观社会医学,努力用伦理学的知识丰富自己,掌握医学伦理学、生命伦理学以及生态伦理学的知识尤为重要。

五、医学哲学

医学哲学是关于医学主体、客体的本质及其相互作用的一般规律、一般方法及医学发展观的科学,它是以辩证唯物主义的观点对医学科学成果的概括和总结、对总体发展规律性的探索,是随着科学技术和保健实践的发展而不断丰富的理论体系。医学哲学对社会卫生的指导具有方法论意义。它与社会医学都具有宏观思维的特点。医学模式的演变过程从本质上是一种哲学观的演变。疾病的因果关系分析,危险因素导致疾病的量变质变规律研究,都需要在医学哲学的理论指导下进行。因此,社会医学离不开医学哲学的指导。作为一个社会医学工作者,应当用医学哲学的理论充实自己,善于运用哲学思维去概括和总结社会卫生问题。

六、卫生事业管理学

卫生事业管理学与社会医学是很难分开的两个学科,我国在20世纪80年代是社会医学与卫生事业管理不分的。在研究生专业目录中列有"社会医学与卫生事业管理"这一专业称谓。社会医学与卫生事业管理的基本任务是相同的,都是根据人群的健康需求,合理配置和利用卫生资源,组织卫生服务,提高卫生事业的科学管理水平和卫生事业的社会效益与经济效益。社会医学要更多地从卫生事业管理中借鉴管理学的基本原理与方法,运用计划、组织、协调与控制手段,对卫生事业进行规划。

第三节 社会医学的发展历史与发展趋势

一、西方社会医学的发展

社会医学作为一个活跃的学科得以形成和发展的原因是多方面的。社会医学作为一种科学理论的形成,是近代工业革命和资本主义发展的结果,并非工业革命和资本主义本身促进了学科的产生,而是社会的工业化和资本主义社会所带来的严重的社会卫生问题,诸如贫困、失业、环境卫生问题和职业卫生问题产生了对控制这些问题的社会需求。

社会医学的产生,还与19世纪发生在法国的政治大革命有着一定的渊源。当时社会改良思想、空想社会主义思想等产生了广泛的影响,这对于卫生界和社会学界对社会卫生进行深刻的思考、推动社会卫生改革有很大的关系。西方社会医学的发展一般可以分为三个阶段,即萌芽阶段、形成阶段和发展阶段。

(一)社会医学的萌芽时期

自古以来,人类疾病的发生是生物遗传、理化因素和社会因素等因素共同作用的结果。在对疾病的认识方面,古希腊医学家希波克拉底(公元前450～公元前377年)就在《空气、水、地域》一书提出环境及生活习惯对健康的作用,提出医生要掌握城市的风向、阳光、水质和植物的生长状况,注意居民的生活方式。在医疗过程中,提出认病人比认识疾病更重要。古罗马医师盖伦(约130～200年)重视心理因素对健康的作用。阿维森那(980～1037年)认为土壤和水都可以传播疾病,精神情感影响健康。巴拉塞尔萨斯(1493～1541年)观察到铜矿山工人的疾病,于1534年写了有名的《水银病》一文。意大利的拉马兹尼(1669～1714年)在《论手工业疾病》中描述了52种职业工人的健康状况,分析了职业因素对人健康的影响,被后人称为劳动医学之父。由于当时社会的工业化程度不高、医学科学不发达,加上神学的禁锢,对社会医学的认识只停留在一些现象的描述上。谈论社会医学的发展必然涉及文艺复兴运动,各种思潮冲击着当时的欧洲。早期的产业革命,血腥的资本原始积累,带来的是社会卫生状况恶化,工人贫困,社会发展很不和谐。这个时期,德国社会卫生学家彼得·弗兰克(1745～1821年)指出:悲惨生活是疾病的温床,并在其名著《全国医学监督体制》中提出用医学监督计划使政府采取措施来保护公众的健康。首次采用了疾病控制的社会卫生措施,对公共卫生和社会医学的发展有很大的贡献。资本主义的发展带来了社会的工业化和城市化,出现了一些社会卫生问题,城市环境卫生问题,工人恶劣的劳动条件、食品卫生问题等。当时恩格斯在《英国工人阶级状况》一书中指出,英国的工业是在破坏工人健康的基础上发展起来的。工人运动促进了社会卫生组织的建立和社会卫生措施的逐步完善。

在萌芽阶段,社会医学的思想非常丰富,但尚未形成社会医学的学科和理论体系。

(二)社会医学的创立与发展期

1784年英国人瓦特发明了蒸汽机,以蒸汽机的广泛使用为主要标志的第一次技术革命使社会生产力空前提高,带动人类从农业和手工业时代进入以大机器生产为特征的工业化时代。1789年法国爆发了大革命。在资产阶级的压力下,从中世纪早期延续至当时的封建社会制度被荡涤。资产阶级民主革命派促进了政治民主化,提出了社会救济问题,改组现行医疗系统,对19世纪上半叶产业革命而引起工人健康恶化开始重视,同时法国社会哲学界与医学界互相呼应,促进社会改革,重视健康疾病社会问题的调查研究,并改进卫生措施。

1848年法国医生儒勒·盖林(1801～1886年)第一次提出社会医学的概念,倡导把分散的、不协调的医学监督、公共卫生、法医学等构成一个整体的学科,统称为"社会医学"。并将社会医学分为四个部分:社会生理学研究人群的身体和精神状态与社会制度、法律及风俗习惯的关系;社会病理学研究疾病发生、发展与社会问题的联系;社会卫生学研究各种增进健康、预防疾病的措施;社会治疗学研究对付社会发生异常情况的治疗措施,包括提供各种卫生措施。

到了19世纪后期,细菌学有了很大的发展,还原论的思想也很盛行,但许多医学家非常重视社会因素对健康的作用。德国医学家诺尔曼(1813～1908年)与病理学家魏尔啸都强调社会经济对健康的重要作用,魏尔啸提出"医学科学的核心是社会科学,而政治从广义上来讲,就是医学罢了",在对伤寒的研究中他得出了一个结论:"我们可以把一个相当普遍的结果归纳为:越贫困,食物越单调,居住条件越恶劣,伤寒的发作越频繁。""如果医学要真正实现它的伟大使命,就要参加到伟大的政治和社会生活中去。"法国的社会医学家格罗蒂杨(1869~1931)在《社会病理学》一书中,提出用社会观点研究疾病的原则,指出疾病的社会意义取决于疾病发生的频率,社会状况恶化有助于直接引起疾病,影响病情的发展,社会发展产生反作用,医疗能否成功取决于社会因素。他主张应用统计方法、人口学方法、经济学和社会学方法,并强调优生学以防止身体和社会的退化,提出采用社会措施来治疗和预防疾病。并于1920年,首次在柏林大学开设社会卫生学课程。当时的欧洲社会医学与社会卫生学的名称交互使用。

社会医学在英美的发展比较晚。19世纪末叶英国许多政府官员、医生、慈善家注意到疾病的流行同社会经济因素有密切的关系,采用统计方法和统计资料就可以了解这些问题。19世纪末英国就开设了公共卫生学课程,20世纪40年代开设了社会医学课程。在牛津大学成立了社会医学研究院。英国的社会医学比较强调实用性,牛津大学赖尔教授的观点颇具代表性,他认为公共卫生、工业卫生、社会卫生服务及公共医疗卫生事业都属于社会医学的范畴。20世纪60年代以来,为了适应英国国家卫生服务制度改革的需要,将社会医学改称为社区医学,内容囊括了社区卫生服务中的理论与实践,涉及人口学、社会卫生状况、健康教育保健组织、妇幼保健、传染病防治等。

在美国,由于社会经济、文化的特点,医学社会学和家庭医学不断地得到发展,不开设综合性的社会医学课程,重视社会学、管理学、经济学等。美国社会学家史特劳斯于1957年划分出医学中的社会学和医学的社会学,前者相当于社会医学的内容,后者相当于医学社会学的内容。美国的社会学非常发达,学派林立,医学社会学是一个重要的分支,其研究人员不断增加。而社会医学放在卫生管理与卫生政策中讲授。

前苏联1922年在莫斯科大学医学院成立了社会医学教研室,由当时的保健部长谢马什珂和索洛维也夫任教,1923年成立了国立社会卫生学研究所,后改称为社会卫生与保健组织学研究所。社会卫生研究所的任务是研究社会与环境因素对人群健康的影响,以及消除这些有害的因素所采取的综合性卫生措施。20世纪40年代初改为保健组织学,重点研究保健史、保健理论、卫生统计与保健组织等内容。60年代中期改为社会卫生学。

各国社会医学的发展适应了本国的社会经济发展、文化传统和卫生发展的需要。因此,我国不能一味地模仿,应当根据国情建立适合本国特点的学科体系。

二、中国社会医学的发展

在古代,中国的社会医学思想非常丰富,我国传统医学中就有"天人合一"的思想,这是一种朴素的环境与人的健康相互和谐的社会医学观。"上医治未病"的观点,体现了重视疾病预防的社会医学理念。由于我国古代经历了漫长的封建制度,只有朝廷才有专门的医事组织,在民间都是坐堂的个体医生为群众服务。在我国古代小农经济的社会经济环境中,生产手工化,医学的社会化程度低,使得社会医学未能得到重视。

近代中国,西方医学和社会学的传入,对我国社会卫生事业产生了一定的影响,一些知识分子试图寻求教育救国、卫生强国的路子。从1928年起,陆续在上海吴淞区、高桥区建立农村卫生示范区。1931年后又在河北定县、山东邹平县、南京晓庄乡、江苏江宁县等建立乡村卫生实验区,开展医疗、防疫、卫生宣传、学校卫生、助产与妇婴卫生、劳动卫生、生命统计和卫生人员培训等。1939年成立中央卫生设施实验处,1941年改为中央卫生实验院。还设立了社会医事处,主要负责社会医务人员登记及考试。在1949年以前,一些卫生专家曾倡导过"公医制度",试图建立社会卫生组织,受当时的政治、经济条件的制约,收效不大。

1949年新中国诞生,建立了从中央到地方的全国性卫生行政组织和卫生服务机构,发展社会卫生事业,保障人民的健康成了政府的重要责任。在党和政府的领导下,确定了预防为主的卫生工作方针,在不长的时间内,控制了性病、血吸虫等疾病的流行,大搞群众卫生运动,使得社会卫生状况发生了很大的变化。1949年,中国医科大学建立了公共卫生学院,设立了卫生行政学科,开设了卫生行政学课程。1952年引进前苏联的《保健组织学》作为医学生的必修课,1954年,先后在一些医学院校举办卫生行政进修班、保健组织专修科和工农干部卫生系,培训卫生管理干部。20世纪50年代中期,各医学院校普遍成立保健组织教研组,开展工作。1956年卫生部成立了中央卫生干部进修学院,负责培训省市卫生管理干部,1965年保健组织学科被取消。

党的十一届三中全会以来,我国的社会经济有了长足的发展,卫生高度社会化,政治氛围较为宽松,使得社会医学进入了快速发展的快车道。1978年钱信忠主编的《中国医学百科全书》中有《社会医学与卫生管理学》分卷。1980年卫生部发文要求有条件的医学院校成立社会医学与卫生管理学教研室。在20世纪80年代初期,卫生部在6所医学院校成立卫生管理干部培训中心,并将社会医学作为卫生管理干部培训的主干课程。80年代初我国兴办的《医学与哲学》杂志、《中国社会医学杂志》、《国外医学》社会医学分册,以及80年代后期创刊的《医学与社会》等杂志,对推动社会医学的学术研究、学术交流起到了重要的作用。1988年9月在西安成立了中华社会医学会,社会医学学人有了自己的学术组织。社会医学会是一个非常活跃的学术组织,在师资培训、学术交流、政策咨询、凝聚学术精英等方面都发挥着特殊的作用。目前90%以上的医学院校开设了社会医学课程,社会医学已有博士生培养点多个、硕士生培养点数十个。社会医学在卫生改革和实践中正扮演着越来越重要的角色,在为政府提供决策咨询、进行区域卫生规划、实施社区卫生服务、医院体制改革、慢性病控制、初级卫生保健、社会病防治等领域进行了大量的研究,承担了大量的课题,与国际卫生组织和科研机构进行了广泛的合作,社会医学的研究在国际上也产生了很大的影响。

社会医学的学科体系在我国20多年的发展中从争论逐步趋于同化。20世纪80年代以来,社会医学的教材出版较多,有10余本,关于社会医学的研究对象有一定的争议,大体经历了这样一个过程:一是认为社会医学属于人文社会医学的范畴,一些边缘的医学人文、社会科学学科都属于社会医学的研究对象。医学伦理学、卫生法学、医学社会学、卫生政策学、卫生管理学等都属于社会医学的研究范畴。在学科的发展初期这种意见有一定的市场,但随着学科的分化和这些学科自身的建设,这种意见逐步被否定。二是认为社会医学是一门卫生政策学科,社会医学通过调查研究提供卫生情报支持,然后进行卫生规划,进而为政府提供决策依据。三是认为社会医学主要是研究社会心理因素对健康的影响,认为这是真正的社会医学的研究对象。目前,后两种意见有融合的趋势,认为二者都是社会医学的研究对象,是社会医学的宏观和微观不同的研究侧面,其目标有的可能为卫生管理服务,有的可能为临床、预防、康复、健康教育服务。因此,社会医学在不同的领域都发挥着重要作用。复旦大学龚幼龙教授主编的卫生部规划教材,是老一辈社会医学家对社会医学研究的趋同性总结。此后,李鲁、卢祖洵教授分别主编了卫生部规划教材和教育部面向21世纪教材,对社会医学的发展和体系创新都作出了重要的贡献。

我国的社会医学的快速发展,有着深刻的社会经济基础;政府的及时组织引导起到了关键性的作用;学会的建立和发展促进了学术的繁荣;杂志的创立为学者提供了广阔的用武之地;社会医学课程的建立是学科稳定发展的必要条件。

三、中国社会医学与国外社会医学发展的比较

中国社会医学思想在古代也比较丰富,受传统医学的影响,早期的医学家比较注重人的整体性,重视人与自然、人与人、人与社会的和谐统一,重视情志对疾病的作用,重视治病过程中人的社会因素。在《针灸大成》中,对劳力者和劳心者针灸的深度、手法都有不同的要求。在此阶段,中国的社会医学思想比起西方来毫不逊色。

到了近代,社会医学在我国建树不多。在此时期,中西方在科技、经济方面的差距拉大,19世纪西方经历了工业革命,西方资本主义的发展,法国政治大革命的浪潮,使得中西方文明的差距拉大。中国经历了漫长的封建统治,未经历西方那样的工业文明。中国当时还处在列强的侵略和瓜分之中。在此时期,一是近代中国不具备西方社会那样的政治、经济、文化和社会卫生背景;二是当时的政府无心也无力改良社会卫生问题;三是一个饱经战乱的民族,很难将公众健康放在重要的地位去讨论。这使得中西方社会医学的差距拉大。

1949年中华人民共和国建立后,社会卫生工作有了很大的发展,通过建立农村三级卫生服务网和乡村医生队伍,推行农村合作医疗制度,用有限的卫生资源承担了占我国人口大多数的农村居民的基本医疗卫生服务,农村缺医少药的状况得到较大改善,广大农村居民的健康水平有了较大提高。从20世纪五六十年代起,我国就有效地控制了霍乱、鼠疫、天花等严重危害人民健康的烈性传染病。在城镇,发展公费医疗和劳保医疗,重视疾病预防,注意发动群众,人人参与卫生工作,卫生工作取得了世人瞩目的成就。用较少的投入,取得了较大的收益。但这个时期是国际上社会医学理论发展的重要时期,在这个时期,由于受政治运动的影响,我国理论研究缺乏,有些经验未能很好地进行总结。

改革开放以来,特别是进入20世纪90年代,通过实施农村初级卫生保健,加强农村卫生机构"三项建设",广泛开展爱国卫生运动,我国消灭了脊髓灰质炎,基本控制了大多数地方病和寄生虫病,基本实现了消除碘缺乏病的阶段目标。在城市进行了卫生体制改革,对医疗机构进行分类管理,在职工中推行医疗保险制度,推行卫生单位人事制度改革和医院产权制度的改革。这些社会卫生实践的发展,对社会医学产生很大的需求,用了仅仅20多年的时间,社会医学实现了跨越式的发展。我国在许多领域缩小了与西方的差距,有的甚至赶上或超过了西方的研究水平。在卫生服务研究方面,我国已经取得了重大的进展。在生命质量评价、健康危险因素评价方面,结合我国的实际进行了创新性的探索,出现了诸多新的修订量表和自行设计的量表。在社会病方面的研究也突出了中国的特点,创造出了有价值的成果。社会医学与临床、预防、社区卫生实践结合上进行了有益的尝试,并取得了一定的成绩。对医学科学技术发展带动社会医学问题的探讨,在学术界产生了一定的影响。社会医学在理论的发展上也取得了一定的进展,社会大卫生观理论的提出,为卫生事业的发展提供了重要的理论依据,产生了重大的影响。我们认为,和谐的社会医学观将对卫生事业发展具有重要的指导作用。和谐社会医学观的主要内涵是:卫生事业的协调、平衡、有序、良性运行与发展。探讨和宣传和谐社会医学观,用和谐社会医学观促进我国卫生事业的改革,促进我卫生事业的良性运行和发展。

社会的改革开放,经济全球化,为我们带来了新的历史机遇与挑战。我们应当抓住机遇,迎头赶超西方社会医学,为我国的卫生事业和全人类的卫生事业和谐发展作出更大贡献。

Chapter 1　An Introduction to Social Medicine

Section 1　The Object, Content, Nature and Task of Social Medicine

1. Concept

Social medicine is a newly developed overlapping course of study composed of sociology and medical science. August Comte, the founder of sociology, divided sociology into two parts, social statics and social dynamics. The former studies the structure of society and the latter researches social functions. The Chinese Sociologist, Professor Zheng Hangsheng, considers that sociology should research the way in which society functions. In his opinion, there are three kinds of situations, virtuous, neutral and vicious. At present there have been more than seventy branches of sociology.

As another important branch of the learning, medical science is very complicated as well as systematic. It is composed of traditional and modern medicine. The former includes traditional Chinese medicine and many kinds of other folk medicines. These different traditional medical systems were developed over different periods of time all over the world. Modern medicine can be divided into preclinical medicine, preventive medicine, sports medicine, environmental medicine, aviation medicine and clinical medicine, etc. Because of being composed of sociology and medical science, social medicine contains substantial content. And sociology and medical science overlap and influence each other.

Though the basis is medical science and sociology, the nature of social medicine makes it inclined to medical science. The introduction in the textbook *Internal Medicine* (third edition) tells us that the three pillars of modern medical science are biologic medicine, medicopsychology medicine and social medicine.

2. The objectives and contents of the research of social medicine

(1) The objectives

Although concrete study objectives differ because of the various hygiene conditions, society, economy and culture in different regions in the world, the following is agreed: as an independent branch of learning the research objectives of social medicine include the mutual action and its laws between social factors and people's health, social hygienic situations, understanding tactics of social hygiene and improving the living quality of people. In other words, social medicine is a subject about people's social physiological phenomenon, social pathological phenomenon, and undertakes diagnoses of social medical problems of people in order to prescribe for them.

(2) The contents

Social medicine has developed for decades in our country. However, there is still huge controversy over what is its exact content. Since the 1970's, different schools of thoughts have developed which complement each other and are beneficial to the development of social medicine in China.

①Macroscopically, social medicine researches into the interaction between the social factors and the state of health. Various social factors, such as one's social role, individual behavior, life-style, family circumstances, working conditions, political and economic situation, science and technology, culture, population and health services certainly affect every person's health. Social medicine also studies how health problems affect society and how social factors act and react upon one another among themselves. We live in a period full of social change. New things are emerging one after another. Unemployment has become a grave problem facing the nation. And there exists a wide gap between the rich and the poor. A number of people are unaccustomed to the pressure of modern life. Many are addicted to work, which is particularly harmful. In addition, there are problems of taking addictive drugs, food safety, suicide, unfair phenomena in health services, sexual reproduction, and of epidemic infectious disease caused by destroying the ecological balance. Only by analyzing these social phenomena can we give a complete diagnosis of social problems.

②Study social hygienic conditions

Social medicine, like sociology, is of a mass character and its focus is the public health condition. It determines the major problems and the dangerous factors that affect public health and identifies those people who should be protected. Its emphasis is social investigations. The aim is to improve the quality of people's lives.

③Tactics for the improvement of social hygiene

Measures that can resolve the problems of social medical insurance give impetus to community health services and implementing an appropriate area health plan. All these are based on the above-mentioned study.

Social systems consist of many subsystems and the health care sector is one of them. The government must pay more attention to the operation of the health care system and organize extensive cooperation between different sectors to help health sectors. We hope that everyone takes part in health-promoting activities.

④One of the tasks of social medicine is to conduct a scientific study and resolve questions that arise in clinical medicine, preventive medicine, and rehabilitation medicine and health education, thus making medical staff change their mode of thinking. In order to meet medical consumers' demands, improve service quality and raise efficiency in providing medical care services, the following changes are needed, namely, the change from biomedicine model to bio-psychology-sociology model, the change from medical care services to preventive services, the change from physiological care to psychological care, the change from providing only technical service to social service and the change from inside hospitals to outside of hospitals.

How do social medicine studies keep changeable along with the development of the local economy? Our country has experienced a great revolution on three occasions in the field of health care system since 1949. First, when infectious diseases, endemic disease and parasitic disease were the main problems, a series of measures, which included carrying out a protective inoculation plan, sterilizing, killing rats and insecticide plan, were taken to control the spread of those diseases, and achieved good results. However, the appearance and spread of AIDS and SARS shows that far from having completed our work on fighting against infectious disease, we still have a long way to go.

The second health revolution was directed to the rapidly increasing problems of noncommunicable diseases, which were related to unhealthy behaviors and the pollution of the environment, and injuries.

The measures that were taken focused on the training of health workers, behavior risk factor surveillance and intervention, health education and other health promotion measures, which involved social medicine, environmental medicine, biomedicine and behavior medicine.

The task during the third health revolution which emphasized updating people's concept of health is to promote human health, raise people's living standards and spread the idea of self-care, family health care and community health care.

From the first health revolution till the third we have faced many arduous tasks, which were indivisible and had relationships with one another. We have made tremendous efforts to do all that we can do and have been rewarded with great success. But we must be prepared to meet the challenge of new types of infectious disease. On the basis of summing up our experience, we need to find out the characteristics of social health care and how to control the spread of new infectious diseases. Though we have different focal points of our work during different periods, every time we fight against the disease, we always make a leap in the process of cognition.

3. The nature and tasks of social medicine

(1) The nature of social medicine

①Overlapping of the social medicine

Sociology and medicine overlap, which clearly shows that between them (social properties and biological properties of human beings) there is a unity, an indissoluble connection. Man has sociality as well as biotic properties. On the surface giving birth to children, from insemination to parturition, is a biotic process, but it is essentially a social one. Professor Fei Xiaotong, in his book *Childbearing Institution*, said, "Childbearing is for the continuity of society". It is man's sociality that makes the biological properties of human beings to be under the control of certain regulations, which harmonize society. Biotic medicine model emphasizes the study of man's biotic properties, but often overlooks man's psychological needs socially. Social medicine proceeds from social whole, studies man's sociality which other medical subjects concerned should also pay great attention to. Health care system, as a public welfare, has a strong sociality. The management of health care service that is related to people's health, safety and even life is different from other sectors. The distribution of health resources is a work that has strong politics character. At present, medicine is becoming more and more socialized. And the sociality of health will inevitably be given more attention. Though some biotic factors are playing important roles in causing disease, the social factors are also considered to be important causes of many chromic diseases.

②Synthetic research method

It is the overlapping of subjects within social medicine that determines the researching methods that are synthetic. Being an overlapped subject between sociology and medicine, it needs to use the methods of physical science and social science which include making social investigation, psychology method, anthropology method, epidemiological method, statistics method, economics method and management method. When researching different social health problems, the choice of methods is very important.

For example, when we study patients' behavior and people's life style quality, we prefer to use social investigation and psychology methods. But when our goal is to study health service efficiency we always choose economic and management methods. In some synthetic research work, many kinds of methods are used together. In short, a philosophic approach is essential.

③The practicality of social medicine

From the day social medicine emerged, it has begun to guide social health practice. Unlike other sciences, social medicine has not developed its own language. And many words and theories have been borrowed from other branches of learning. Solving actual problems that emerged from health practice enlightens the practice of social medicine research. Other basic features of social medicine are that there are no regular patterns of research, which gives an even wider scope to our study, and it does not easily degenerate into dogmatism. Of course, social medicine needs to take further steps to be specialized and theorized, which is also the only road to the development of social medicine.

(2) The principal tasks of social medicine

①Providing social health information for policy makers

Formulating general and specific health policies and working out tactics of health depend on the understanding of the national social health situation. And social medicine can provide useful information that will help policy maker's work efficiently. In the early 1980's, many Health Care Management Departments were established in some medical colleges in China. And lots of health management personnel and cadres have been trained. Since then China's social medicine has developed rapidly, which surely is related to the development of health care management education. The most important task of social medicine is to get a clear understanding of the social health situation, find out major problems through social investigation, and provide information for the Chinese government's health programs.

②Raise people's health level and life quality

After evaluating people's health status, health risk factors, life quality and investigations of people's behaviors, a complete diagnosis of people's health problems will be made and a recipe for efficient health care will also be given. Our goal is to make people change unhealthy behavior and harmful life-styles, to improve the social environment, and to raise people's health level and life quality.

③The education and propagation of social medicine

Medical workers and health management cadres set up a scientific and correct understanding of health and disease through education and propagation. Knowledge of social medicine is infiltrated into clinical medicine, preventive medicine, rehabilitation medicine, health education, and community medicine and health care management. It is quite clear that a modern medical model should assist health practice and management. Trained health and management personnel who will be able to keep abreast of the modern medical model are needed. Social medicine is playing an increasingly important role in modern society.

Section 2 Using the Experience of Other Major Subjects for Reference

The overlapping of social medicine determines that social medicine must use the experience of other subjects that are relevant to social medicine for reference.

1. Preventive medicine

Social medicine is generally considered to be separate from preventive medicine. Preventive medicine, based on basic sciences (physics, biology and chemistry), clinical medicine and environmental medicine, uses and develops basic theory of environment and health. Preventive medicine studies how natural and social factors affect people's health and how diseases occur and spread. The guiding ideology of preventive medicine is to put prevention first. And the main objects of study are large groups of people with a goal to provide a scientific basis for the formulation of three-stage preventive measures to protect and promote health and raise people's life style quality.

From the new definition of preventive medicine, we can see that social factors have become the objects of its study, which is similar to social medicine. Many useful things in preventive medicine, such as the special research for pathogenesis, the systems analysis for health problems, and the multivariate statistical analysis for noncommunicable and chronic disease, are of great value to social medicine. Social medicine that mainly researches social factors has a strong social character, while preventive medicine aims at biological factors. So social medicine and preventive medicine have issues of common interest, need to support each other, learn from each other and make joint efforts to raise people's life style quality.

2. Sociology

August Comte first advanced sociology that was called social-physics at that time. Sociology and social medicine emerged almost from the same time and in the same place, which is not accidental. It is an inevitable outcome of the development of social politics, economy, culture and social hygiene.

There is some controversy over the question of what sociology should research, or its social function. Some consider it is a science about the functioning laws of society. Some think it is about social problems. First, sociology lays stress on the on-the-spot investigation and the need to gain substantial evidence. Secondly, sociology also emphasizes theoretical research deductions using some social phenomena from advanced hypotheses. Finally, sociology attaches great importance to the development of sociological language, such as social role, social stratum, social division and social flow. Medical sociology is a branch of sociology, mainly using the theory of sociology to study the social problems in the domain of public health, such as the structure of hospitals, the flow of trained medical personnel, the role of doctors and nurses and the relationship between health workers and patients. We think that social medicine is inclined to medicine in its nature. In fact, it is difficult to differentiate social medicine from medical sociology. China's trend is towards combining social medicine with medical sociology. Germany gives priority to developing social medicine while America gives priority to medical sociology. However, social medicine ought to continually absorb useful things from sociology, medical sociology and other related sciences to make unceasing progress.

3. Community medicine

Community medicine provides health care services, which include medical treatment, prevention, health care, rehabilitation, health education and birth control for people who live locally. Social medicine provides a theoretical foundation for the community health services. Similarly, the application of community health care realises the expansion from treatment only to prevention, from inside the hospital to outside the hospital, from physiological care to psychological care, from the technical service to social service. The implementation of community health care enriches social medicine and makes it much more inclined to combine theory with practice. Many new questions have been put before the social medicine, such as how community health service will develop continually.

Social medicine is partially consistent with community medicine both in theory and in implementation. In Britain, the social medicine orients its development toward community medicine. The combination of social medicine and community medicine forms macroscopic and submicroscopic research.

4. Medical ethics

Generally speaking medical ethics is the concrete application of general ethics in medical practice. Ethics is a doctrine of the study of the origin and the development of morals, the standards of behavior and the obligations among humans. Now medical ethics has developed into bioethics. Bioethics involves the relationship between humans and animals and the doctor-patient relationship; it also studies life style values. When studying health policy, health strategy, health services and formulating area health programs, social medicine inevitably will be influenced by theories in both values and public benefit. Care should be exercised in distributing health care resources. Which area or target population will have priority for resources over others? All these questions need the guidance of medical ethics and bioethics. So we must master the knowledge of medical ethics, bioethics and ecologicalethics, use the method of value analysis and make the distribution of health resources more rational and fair.

5. Medical philosophy

Medical philosophy is about the essence of the subject, the object and the general law of the interaction between them. It is the generalization and summarization of the achievements in medical scientific research from the dialectical materialist point of view. It is a theoretical system that probes into the regularity of overall development and that will enrich continually along with the development of scientific technique and health practice. Medical philosophy has methodological significance for social health. The essence of the change of medical mode is the change of the modes of thought. Medical philosophic theories are being used to analyze disease causal relationships and to research the law of the qualitative and quantitative changes of diseases caused by risk factors.

So social medicine needs the guidance of medical philosophy. A social medicine worker should enrich himself with the theory of medical philosophy using philosophical thought to summarize social health problems.

6. Health care administration

Health care administration is inseparable from social medicine. They have the same basic tasks that distribute and use health resources rationally, organize health service, raise administrative levels, social benefits and economic benefits of health care. Social medicine should make reference to health care administration that has very important basic principles and methods, such as planning, organizing, coordinating and controlling, so that an overall plan can be made for providing health services more effectively.

Section 3 The History and the Trend of Social Medicine

1. The development of western social medicine

Social medicine, as a brisk branch of learning, came into being and developed after the emergence of the Industrial Revolution and the development of capitalism which brought grave social health problems, such as poverty, unemployment, environmental health problems and occupational health problems. It is not the Industrial Revolution but the social needs that brought about the emergence of social medicine. That is, there is a need to tackle the above-mentioned problems. The emergence of social medicine was also connected with the political evolution that occurred in France in the 19th century when utopianism was current. Because of the influence on the whole society, social health reform therefore was propelled forward. The development of western social medicine is generally divided into three stages, the embryonic stage, the forming stage and the developing stage.

(1) The embryonic stage of social medicine

Since ancient times the occurrence of disease is the result of the action of a number of factors that include biological hereditary, chemical, physical and social factors. In understanding disease, an ancient medical worker Hippocrates (450 – 377B. C.), who was Greek, said in his book *Air, Water and Region*, the environment and life-style had effects on people's health. He considered that doctors should pay attention to the city's natural environment, such as wind direction, sunlight, and water quality, local plants' growth and to the citizen's life-style. He thought that it was more important to understand patients than patients' disease during medical practice. Galen (about A. D. 130 – 200), an ancient doctor in Rome, attached great importance to psychological factors upon health. Vienna (A. D. 980 – 1037) thought that soil and water would spread diseases and that a person's emotions or spirit would affect one's health. Paracelsus (A. D. 1493

– 1541) observed that copper miners suffered from a peculiar disease, and wrote a book called *Mercury Disease*. The Italian Ramazzini (A. D. 1669 – 1714) in his famous book *Disease in Handicraft Industry* described the health status of workers from 52 different occupations and the effects these factors have on people's health; he is called the father of labor medicine by posterity. Since society did not reach intense industrialization at that time, and because of the underdeveloped stage of medical science, man's understanding to social medicine remained only describing some phenomena. The Renaissance was also connected with the development of social medicine. Various trends of thought were being expounded in Europe. During the early Industrial Revolution the primitive accumulation of capital and workers' poverty worsened social health conditions. German social hygienist Johann Peter Frank (A. D. 1745 – 1821) pointed out that miserable life was a hotbed of diseases. In his famous book *The National Medical Supervision System* he suggested that a medical supervision plan could be used to make the government take measures to protect public health. He was the first man who used social health measures to control disease, and made a great contribution to the development of public health and social medicine. New social health problems arose along with industrialization and urbanization, such as urban environment, workers' adverse working conditions and food hygiene problems. Friedrich Engels in his book *British Working Class Situation* said British industry had been built up from the workers' breakdown in health. And the workers' movement promoted the establishment of the social health organization and social health measures were improved step by step. At the embryonic stage, the theoretical system of the social medicine had not formed.

(2) The forming and developing stage

In 1784 the Englishman James Watt invented the steam engine. The first technological revolution that was marked with the wide use of the steam engine made the productive forces stronger and brought about change from the era of agriculture and handicraft to the era of industrialization, which featured machine building. In 1789, the French Revolution brought an end to the feudal society system, which had existed from the Middle Ages. The people who belonged to the bourgeois democratic revolution promoted the realization of political democracy. The people who belonged to this political group suggested the social relief facilities, reorganized medical care systems, paying attention to workers' health and medical research, and improved health measures. In 1848, Frenchman Jules Guerin (A. D. 1801 – 1886) advanced for the first time the concept of social medicine. He considered that scattered medical supervision, public health and legal medicine should be collected and combined to form an entire branch of the school of social medicine which was divided into four parts: Social physiology researching the relationship between people's health status and the social system; law, customs and habits; social pathology researching the relationship between diseases and social problems; social hygiene researching how to promote health and protect disease; and social therapeutics researching how to cure diseases when there was an abnormal social situation.

By the late 19th century bacteriology had developed greatly and many medical workers still paid great attention to the effects of social factors on health. German pathologist Rudolf Virchow said that the kernel of medical science is social science, while politics is just medicine in a broad sense. From his research on typhoid he concluded that the more people lived in straitened conditions, the more monotonous the food was, the worse the housing conditions were, the more frequently typhoid occurred. He also said that the best method to achieve the goals of medical science is to combine medicine with social life and political activities. The Frenchman A. Grotjahn who was an expert at social medicine pointed out in his book *Social Pathology* that diseases should be studied from the standpoint of social view. The social meaning of diseases depended on their frequency. The worse the social status then would directly cause diseases and affect development. Medical success depends on social factors. Social measures should be used to cure and prevent diseases. He also advocated the use of statistics, economics, demography and sociology. In 1920 the social hygiene course was given in Berlin University and in those days the names of social medicine and social hygiene were mutually used.

Social medicine developed late in Britain and America. In the late 19th century many British officers, doctors and philanthropists noticed that the spread of disease was connected with social economic factors and statistics could be used to determine the problems. In the late 19th century a course in public hygiene was given and in the 1940's a course in social medicine was offered. A social medicine research institute was established in Oxford University. British social medicine was very practical and Professor John A. Ryle's view was quite representative of it. He considered that all public health, industrial health, social health and medical care belonged to social medicine. Since the 1960's, in order to adapt to the reforms in the British National Health Service System, social medicine has been changed into community medicine, which includes the theories and practice of community health care which includes demography, social health status, health education and health care organization, maternal and child health care and the prevention and treatment of infectious diseases.

In America, because of the features of its economy and culture, medical sociology and family medicine have developed continually with the emphasis on sociology, management and economics. American sociologist R. Strause in 1957 advanced the division of social medicine and medical sociology. There is a school of thought in the field of sociology in America and medical sociology is an important branch. Social medicine is included and taught in the course of health management and health policy. In 1922, a social medicine teaching and research department was established in the Medical College of

Moscow University in the former Soviet Union. In 1923 the National Social Health Institute was set up which was later renamed Social Hygiene and Health Organization Institute. Its task was to research how social and environmental factors affected people's health and how to take synthetical measures to remove harmful factors.

The development of social medicine adapted to the needs of each country's economy, culture and health development. Similarly, we should set up our own school of thought instead of blindly imitating others'.

2. The development of social medicine in China

In China there have been ideas, which were in fact a naive social medicine view about a harmonious relationship between environment and health. Since ancient times China has been through long years of the feudal system. It was in the royal court where medical organizations existed and the doctors who usually were self-employed set up a pharmacy to practice medicine and to provide medical services for the people. In the environment of small-scale peasant economy, and because of the manual operations, socialization of medicine was at a very low level and was paid no attention to.

In modern times western medicine and sociology were introduced into China, influencing China's health services. Some intellectuals tried to seek ways to save our country and believed that the well-developed education and health systems might solve the problems. Since 1928, many rural health demonstration or experimental areas were set up in Shanghai, Hebei, Shandong and Jiangsu one after another, spreading health knowledge, providing medical care and preventive services, and training in school hygiene, maternal and child health (MCH), labor hygiene, life statistics and medical care. And the Central Health Facilities Experimental Office (later renamed Central Health Experimental Institute) and Social Medical Office were established in 1939, in charge of the registration of the social medical workers and giving them examinations. Before 1949, some health experts proposed public health service systems, trying to set up a social health organization but produced very little effect because of the restrictions due to the political and economic conditions in those days.

Since the birth of New China in 1949, many national administration health organizations and health service institutions have been set up all over the country. In addition, it has been the government's responsibility to improve social health services and protect people's health. Under the leadership of the Party and the government, the policy of putting prevention in first place in medical work was determined and within a short time the spread of venereal disease and snail fever was controlled and mass health campaigns brought about great changes of social health conditions. A Public Health College was set up in the China Medical University in 1949 and the college offered a course in health administration. The course health organization was introduced from the former Soviet

Union, being an obligatory course. One after another some medical colleges ran the advanced study classes of health administration, health organization and established Health Departments of Worker and Peasant Cadres. In the middle 1950s all medical colleges set up health organization teaching and research groups and set to work. In 1956, the Ministry of Health established Central Health Cadres College, training health administrative cadres for the local governments. And in 1965, the health organization school of branch was called off in China.

Since the Third Plenary Session of the Eleventh Central Committee of the Chinese Communist Party, our country has had great economic development and social medicine has been rapidly developed because of the high degree of socialization of health and because of the easy political atmosphere. *China Medical Encyclopedia* edited by Qian Xinzhong in 1978 includes the part or fascicle (FASCICLE) of social medicine and health management. In 1980 official documents were dispatched from the Ministry of Health to medical colleges, demanding that if there is a permitting condition, social medicine and health care management departments should be established. In the early 1980s the Health Managements Cadre Training Centres were set up separately in six medical colleges with social medicine being the main course. At the same time many informative journals such as *Medicine and Philosophy*, *China Social Medicine Magazine*, *Foreign Medicine's Social Medicine* fascicle (FASCICLE) and *Medicine and Society*, started publication. All these magazines have played an important role in pushing academic research and exchanges forward. The China Social Medicine Society was set up in Xi'an, Shanxi Province in September, 1988. From then on social medicine scholars have their own academic organization, which has been playing an important and specific role in teacher training, academic exchanges, and policy consultation. At present 90% of the medical colleges have offered courses in social medicine and there are more than 10 Masters degree training bases and several PhD training bases. There have been many important problems such as helping government make policy, area health programmes, community health services, reforms in the hospital system, primary health care, treatment and prevention of social diseases into which social medicine workers have researched. In addition we have undertaken a lot of research projects and have wide cooperation with some international health organizations and scientific institutes, making a great impact around the world.

Social medicine, after developing for more than 20 years, has gradually matured into an important and independent branch of learning. Since the 1980s many teaching materials have been published, but there is still controversy over the objectives of study. Three different views are taken. First, it is considered that social medicine belongs to the field of humanities and its objectives of study should include medical ethics, hygiene jurisprudence, medical sociology, health policy, and health management. In the earlier days of the development, this point of view had much been support from the people. But along with the growth of branch of social medicine it has been gradually neglected. Second, it is thought that social medicine is the branch of health policy and what should be done is provide health information through investigation for government. Third, it is regarded that the real objective for study of social medicine is how social psychological factors affect health. And today's trend is towards combining the latter two together, being macroscopic and microscopic objectives of study, serving for health management or for clinical core, prevention, rehabilitation and health education. So social medicine is playing an important role in different fields.

The rapid development of social medicine in China should be attributed to good economic foundation and the government's direction and organization and establishment of the social medicine society promoting academic research. Informative journals give scholars the opportunity for academic exchanges and the courses in social medicine offered in medical colleges are the necessary conditions of academic development.

3. A comparison between China's social medicine development and foreign social medicine development

In ancient times there were rich social medicine ideas in China. Being influenced by traditional Chinese medicine the medical workers in those days paid great attention to the concept that viewed the human body as a whole and attached great importance to the harmony of human and society. They devoted much attention to the action of emotions on diseases and to the action of social factors on treatment. Ideas about social medicine in China at this period were in no way inferior to western social medicine.

In modern times, the gap in science and technology and economy between China and Western countries has become wider and Industrial Revolutions has also widened the gap in civilization between China and Western countries. So one of the reasons that there were great gaps between the East and the West was lack of policy, economic, culture and social health background as there was in western society. The second reason was that the Chinese government in those days was unable and in no mood to solve the social health problems. And the third reason was that a country, which had repeatedly experienced the chaos caused by war, would not put public health in an important place.

After the People's Republic of China was founded on October 1st, 1949, social health has developed rapidly. Through establishing rural three-level health care networks and teams of village doctors, introducing rural cooperative medical systems, using the limited health resources, the problems in providing primary medical health services for the rural residents who shared most of China's population, were solved. The health status of these people has been improved greatly. Since the 1950s some severe infectious diseases such as cholera, plague, and smallpox, which were detrimental to Chinese health, were controlled effectively in China. In cities and towns, labor insurance medical care and free medical care were provided for residents. The government paid attention to the prevention of diseases, aroused masses to take part in the medical and health work and had succeeded in inputting less and yielding more. But during this important period when social medicine was developing rapidly in the western countries, because of the domestic political effects, we did not research social medicine theoretically and sum up our experience which was very valuable. Since China's reforms and opening to the outside world, especially since the 1990s, carrying on primary health care in rural areas, strengthening the construction of health facilities, developing the patriotic health campaign widely, polio has been wiped out, most endemic diseases and parasitic diseases have been basically controlled, and the process objective of eliminating iod-basedow has been basically reached. In cities many reforms in the health system were made, classification management of medical institutions has been done very well and a new health-insurance plan was introduced among workers and staff members. All these social health practices have made great and new demands on social medicine. That is why in only a 20-year period, social medicine has developed so rapidly in China. The distinction between China's social medicine and that of Western countries has been gradually reduced and some research has even surpassed that of Western countries.

The main achievements of social medicine are as follows: Significant progress has been made in the study of health services. Being bold in putting things into practice and blazing new trails, we have in the light of the specific conditions of our country designed several new scales of health risk factor evaluation and life quality evaluation and social diseases have also been very well researched and good results obtained. We have been successful in combining social medicine with clinical medicine, preventive medicine and community health.

A new theory of the macroscopic view of social medicine has been advanced, providing an important theoretical basis for developing the cause of health care, producing a great impact.

We consider that the leading action of the harmonious views of social medicine on the development of China's health system will manifest its importance. The main connotations of the harmonious views of social medicine are that there is harmony and balance in health work, and keeping it in perfect order, virtuously functioning and developing.

The open policy and the globalization of the economy present new opportunities for developing social medicine in our country. We should seize the opportunities with both hands, meet the new challenges, propagandize the harmonious views of social medicine and promote reforms in the health system in China. Our goal is to try hard to catch up and surpass the advanced western social medicine and to make a greater contribution to the development of the cause of health care both in China and throughout the whole world.

第二章 医学模式

第一节 医学模式概念

模式(model)最初是一个数理逻辑概念,即用系统中的一系列公式来表达形式逻辑理论。哲学学科引进并延伸了模式的概念,用作分析或阐明事物的关系与本质,并运用到人文社会科学和自然科学领域,成为总结各种学科世界观和方法论的核心。建立模式是科学研究的一种方法,人们通过建立模式来分析和表达事物间的关系与本质,对人们观察、思考和解决问题起着指导作用,因此模式也可理解为人们认识和解决问题的思想和方式。

医学模式(medical model)是在医学实践的基础上产生的,是人类从与疾病抗争和认识自身生命过程的无数实践中得出的对医学的总体认识。这种高度概括、抽象的思想观念和思维方法既表现了医学的总体结构特征,又是指导医学实践的基本观点。医学模式属于自然辩证法领域,是以医学为对象的自然观和方法论,即人们按照唯物论和辩证法的观点和方法去观察、分析和处理有关人类的健康和疾病问题,是对健康和疾病现象的科学观。医学模式的核心是医学观,它研究医学的属性、职能、结构和发展规律。

医学科学研究和医疗实践活动,无一不是在一定的医学观及认识论的指导下进行的。如人类健康是从单一的生物学角度去观察,还是从生物学、心理学与社会学全方位去认识;人类疾病的防治、健康促进是单纯从生物学角度来处理,还是从生物学、心理学和社会学多维角度综合地研究。这种观念、认识及方法上的区别,主要起因于不同医学模式的影响,实质上也就是不同医学观的反映。医学模式,既体现医学观,也体现方法论。医学理论是通过总结医学实践而产生的,而医学实践又是在特定的医学思维指导下产生的医学行为来完成的。因此,医学观不仅影响医学思维和行为,也关系到医学行为所产生的结果。医学模式对于保护人类健康和疾病防治及其效果,起着重要作用。

1977年,美国纽约州罗彻斯特大学精神病和内科教授恩格尔指出:"生物医学模式逐渐演变为生物-心理-社会医学模式是医学发展的必然。"这一观点在1981年第一次全国医学辩证法讨论会上被介绍到中国,开始为我国医药卫生界所关注。

无论如何,医学模式的演变是客观存在的历史潮流,从医学发展的历程看,曾产生希波克拉底为代表的古希腊医学和中医《内经》等完整的理论体系及阴阳五行学说为理论基础的整体医学模式。随着医学科学的进步、医学社会化的进程和人类对健康需求的提高和变化,医学模式经历了多次转变。回顾医学模式的转变过程,将有利于人们更好地理解当代医学理论和实践正面临着从单一的生物学角度去观察和处理医学问题的生物医学模式,向由多元的生物、心理和社会学角度综合去观察和处理医学问题的现代医学模式转变。认清医学模式转变的概念有利于解决个体医学与群体医学的关系,生物医学与社会医学的关系,临床医学与预防医学的关系,微观医学与宏观医学的关系,防治疾病与增进健康的关系,医学进步与社会发展的关系。

第二节 历史上的主要医学模式

一、神灵主义的医学模式

原始医学(确切地讲还不能算作一门科学)与原始宗教结缘,是因为人类祖先无法解释疾病、死亡、梦等现象。受梦中景象的影响,产生一种观念,即思维和感觉不是人类的自身活动,而是独立寓于身体之中的灵魂活动。梦是灵魂活动的反映;死亡是灵魂离开肉体,肉体死亡而灵魂不死;造成疾病看不见摸不着的原因是魔鬼幽灵或逝者游魂的侵入。先民们认为人类的生命与健康是上帝神灵所赐,疾病和灾祸是天谴神罚。这就是神灵主义的医学模式(spiritualism medical model)。因此,人们对健康的保护和疾病的防治主要依赖求神问卜,祈祷神灵的宽恕与保佑。也采用一些自然界中有效的植物和矿物作为药物使用,但大多为催吐或导泻等猛烈的方法,主导思想仍然是驱除瘟神疫鬼。神灵主义的医学模式,在当时社会条件下其职责和文字上都达到了统一,醫(medicine)即巫医(medicine-man)。

二、自然哲学的医学模式

宗教是对自然力的屈服,并将其神秘化的结果;医学则是对自然力的征服,并将其明朗化的过程。随着生产力的提高,人类终于从主客浑然一体的自然界中脱颖而出,产生了自我意识,成为能认识客体的自主体。

古希腊兴盛的哲学思想与当时医学对人之本体及疾病本原的认识是一致的。那时的哲学家常常也是医生。西医学鼻祖——希波克拉底深受阿尔克迈翁(Alcmaeom)和恩培多克勒(Empedocles)的影响,这两位先哲都是希腊著名的自然哲学家和名医。希波克拉底在《人和自然》(*About the Nature of Man*)一书中提出了万物之源的水、火、土、气的元素和人体的黏液、血液、黑胆汁和黄胆汁相对应。人的健康、疾病和性格是四种体液混合比例变化的结果。因此,医生的职责不过是维持人的机体的自然本性。由此逐渐形成米利都学派的医学体液学派,以后又发展为德漠克利等原子论的医学固体学派,初步建立了人体不是体液就是躯体结构的认识。这些自然哲学的思想和理论,起到驱逐神灵医学,发挥启蒙医学科学的作用。

表 2-1　希波克拉底 4 种体液的比较

体液	来源	特性	季节	疾病	治疗	气质
黏液	脑	冷	冬	伤风/肺炎、头痛、胸膜炎、中风、尿痛	热水浴、热稀粥、利尿剂、催吐剂	黏液质
血液	心	热	春	咽痛、关节炎、痢疾、麻风	放血、退热药、催吐剂	多血质
黑胆汁	脾和胃	干	秋	水肿、肝炎、坐骨神经痛、斑疹伤寒/疟疾、溃疡	催吐剂、热水浴	抑郁质
黄胆汁	肝	湿	夏	霍乱、口腔溃疡、黄疸、胃病	放血、退热药、灌肠、流食、止痛药	胆汁质

中医学通常被认为是以儒学、道学的认识论和方法学为基础构筑起来的医学，而"易"为医理之母。"易"有三项基本原理：易简、变易和不易。《内经》及其以后的中医学理论，继承并发展了阴阳学说，建立了阴阳五行病理学说及外因（风、寒、暑、湿、燥、火）、内因（喜、怒、忧、思、悲、恐、惊）等病因学说。

无论古希腊医学，还是中医学说，这种把健康、疾病与人类生活的自然环境与社会环境联系起来观察与思考的朴素、辩证、整体的医学观念，称为自然哲学的医学模式（nature philosophical medical model）。

三、生物医学模式

15 世纪以后，欧洲文艺复兴推动了自然科学技术的进步，带来了工业革命的高潮和实验科学的兴起。著名的实验科学家培根提出要"用实验方法研究自然"。在实验思想的影响下，机械学与物理学有了长足的进步。代表机械思想的著作有笛卡儿的《动物是机器》、拉美特利的《人是机器》。他们把人当做自己发动的机器，而疾病则是机器出现故障和失灵，因此，需要修补和完善，这就是机械论的医学模式（mechanistic medical model）。在这种思想影响下，医学取得了一定进步，如机械观点影响到生理学，促使哈维发现了血液循环。细胞的发现，产生了维尔啸的细胞病理学，提出"一切疾病都是由细胞发生"，"细胞的不正常活动是各种疾病的根源"。机械论解释生命活动是机械运动，保护健康就是保护机器，机械论的医学模式可被看做现代生物医学的初级阶段。

科学实验思潮的掀起，大大地推动了生物医学的发展。生物医学在生理学、病理学、微生物学等领域相继取得了惊人的成就，使临床医学和预防医学的重大难题得到解决，由此推动整个医学的发展，外科学疼痛、感染和失血三大难题的攻破就是生物医学成就的典范。此前，外科医生对控制疼痛、感染、失血虽然积累了一些经验，但效果并不理想，如截肢手术死亡率高达 40%～50%。在药理学、病原微生物学、生理学等发展的基础上，难题逐渐被解决：1846 年发现病人吸入乙醚失去痛觉；1847 年创用氯仿施行麻醉；1882 年用可卡因作局部麻醉；1867 年英国医生李斯特在巴斯德关于有机物腐败是由微生物引起的启示下，作出了伤口腐烂和分解也是由微生物引起的推论，采用石炭酸溶液冲洗手术器械，用石炭酸溶液浸湿纱布覆盖创口，使截肢手术死亡率由 46% 下降至 15%，奠定了抗菌术的基本原则;1872年出现了止血带、止血钳;1877年德国医生柏格曼(Bergmann)采用蒸汽灭菌,建立了无菌术;1900年奥地利病理学家兰德坦纳(Landsteiner)发现了红细胞的血型系统,解决了输血造成死亡问题。这些成就增加了手术的安全性,减轻了病人的痛苦,使外科治疗技术得到了迅速发展。

在疾病预防领域,显微镜的发明并运用于寻找病原,微生物学实验证明细菌和病毒致病机制和由此发展起来的疫苗接种和化学治疗法,形成了宿主、环境和病原体相互作用的生态平衡概念,由此开始了第一次卫生革命。医学实验发现了不少致病性微生物,如结核杆菌、霍乱杆菌、立克次体、疟原虫、梅毒螺旋体等;由于免疫学和治疗的进步,通过预防接种、灭菌杀虫措施和抗菌药物学等,使急性、慢性传染病死亡率很快下降。全世界已消灭天花,在我国已基本控制了几种烈性传染病(鼠疫、霍乱等),部分传染病(疟疾、乙型脑炎、麻疹和血吸虫病等)的发病率大大降低,有些发达国家传染病死亡人数仅占总死亡人数的1‰以下。各国平均寿命,近50年来,已由30～40岁,增加到60～70岁,这都是与生物医学的进步分不开的。

由于生物医学的进步,产生的代表性理论有二元论和还原论。"二元论"认为研究人的身体和人的精神应有合理分工。医学应将注意力放在如何通过精密的技术测量细胞生物化学的变化,来解释病人的症状与体征,并干预这些变化来恢复病人的健康,不再从整体上去注意病人的心理社会状况。"还原论"进一步把人体分解为不同的器官、细胞、分子,认为复杂的生命现象必须用物理的、化学的方法来研究和解释功能改变的因果关系。疾病被当做一种静止的因果结局,而不是一个动态的变化过程。在此理论指导下,生物科学的发展进入了一个崭新的历史时期,生物学、解剖学、组织学、生理学、细菌学、生物化学、病理学、免疫学、遗传学等生物科学体系形成,以及现代分子生物学诞生。人们对生命现象及机体变化,以及健康与疾病的认识,完全从生物医学观点出发,并且运用生物医学的成就,防治威胁人类生命与健康的传染病,乐观地认为最终能解释所有的健康与疾病问题。

表2-2　19世纪下半叶细菌学研究的重大发现

发现者	发现年代	发现项目
李斯德	1852	传染(无菌外科)
巴斯德	1857～1862	酵母菌
	1877	鸡霍乱疫苗
	1881	炭疽疫苗
	1884	狂犬疫苗
科赫	1882	结核杆菌
	1883	霍乱弧菌
吕弗琉	1882	猪丹毒
	1883	白喉杆菌

(续表2-2)

发现者	发现年代	发现项目
伊培	1880	伤寒杆菌
范耳爱生	1854	丹毒链球菌
奈琴	1897	淋菌
魏书	1892	气性坏疽
欧培曼	1873	回归热螺旋体
布鲁	1887	布氏杆菌
志贺	1897	痢疾杆菌
北里	1894	鼠疫杆菌
鲍德	1900	百日咳杆菌

总之,生物医学模式(biomedical model)是建立在生物科学基础上,反映病因、宿主与自然环境之间的变化规律的医学观和方法论,认为每种疾病都必然并且可以在器官、细胞或分子上找到可以测量的形态学或化学改变,都可以确定出生物的或理化的特定原因,都应该能够找到治疗的手段。但是随着疾病谱和死因谱的转变,危害人类健康主要原因已是心血管疾病、恶性肿瘤、意外伤亡、呼吸系统疾病,这些慢性非传染疾病的致病因素已不再是单纯的生物病因,还有许多社会环境因素、个人行为、生活方式因素等。生物医学模式已无法完全解释和有效解决这些疾病的发生与发展,即使是生物因素为主要因素的传染性疾病(如性病、艾滋病和结核病)的流行与防治,也受到社会心理行为诸因素的制约,有许多疾病的生物因素要通过社会与心理因素而起作用。疾病的表现形式,已由单因单果向多因多果形式发展。与此相应,医学模式已逐步由生物医学模式过渡到生物-心理-社会医学模式(bio-psycho-social medical model)。

第三节 医学模式演变的规律

一、一般规律

医学模式的每一次转变都不是一个简单的替代过程,而是一次超越。任何科学的前进,总是在前人成果基础上起步的。生物-心理-社会医学模式是随着社会和经济及科学技术的发展,在生物医学模式的基础上形成的一种适应现代人类保健技术的新的医学模式。这个医学模式指导人们更全面更客观地认识和解决现代社会的医疗和保健问题,指导医学科学的发展。

由生物医学模式转变为生物-心理-社会医学模式的过程,是有着复杂的历史背景和社会背景的。人们对此也有一个认识过程。可以认为是人类获取的健康与疾病斗争的经验总结。

医学模式不是一成不变的僵死的教条,而是随着医学科学的发展与人类健康需求的不断变化而转移着。这种转移的最终极目标是运用医学模式思想指导,能最佳与最完善地满足人类对健康的追求。因此人类对健康需求不断提高,也迫使医学模式不断发展、变化与完善。

医学模式是人类获取健康与疾病作斗争的经验总结,在其发展过程中经历着曲折与反复,正如哲学的发展一样,也不是一帆风顺的。在人类一切活动中,正确与错误、片面与全面、缺陷与完善、低级与高级,都经历了历史无情的检验。实践是检验真理的惟一标准,医学模式也在人类医学实践中不断地充实、深化与完善。

目前正面临着由生物医学模式向生物-心理-社会医学模式的转变。这次转变将触动医学科学与卫生事业发展中许多领域内长期固守的生物医学观念,形成一次观念上的革命。生物医学模式固然有其存在的历史原因,对医学的发展也起到了巨大的推动作用。然而,由于生物医学模式只强调生物因素,忽视了人的社会心理属性,具有明显的片面性和局限性,已无法满足现代医学发展的要求。医学模式是动态变化的,每当社会发展到一个新阶段,医学模式也必须随之相应地改变。医学模式的转变,实质上就是医学观念和思维方式的变更,使之能够适合医学的时代特征。现代医学要求必须从生物、心理、社会三维角度认识健康与疾病问题,全方位、多层次把握医学发展方向,用现代医学观指导医学实践,解决现代社会面临的各种医学问题。

二、社会的进步和发展与医学模式的转变

生物-心理-社会医学模式的形成,使医学从象牙塔里走出来面对社会,使医学由传统的纯自然科学回归到自然科学与社会科学相结合交叉的应用性科学。医学与社会经济发展的双向性,决定了它作为社会可持续发展的组成部分,显现出作用的两重性。而医学所有的社会功能,又反过来表达了诸多医学的目的。

无论如何,医学模式的演变是客观存在的历史潮流,人们应当从现代观念、现代死亡方式和现代健康需求去把握医学的时代特征,把握医学发展的方向。只有这样,才能不断地摆正个体医学与群体医学间、生物医学与社会医学间、微观医学与宏观医学间、临床医学与预防医学间、防治医学与增进健康医学间、医学进步与社会发展间多种关系,进而解决现代社会面临的各类复杂的医学问题。

三、现代医学模式转变的作用

(一)医学与可持续发展的关系

随着科学技术的进步和商品经济的发展,包括医药科学技术和医疗卫生服务在内,人类在创造巨大财富和舒适生活的同时,越来越担心资源与环境的因素会限制社会的继续发展,昨天和今天的发展会降低我们这代和未来几代人的生存质量。这就是20世纪末全球关注的可持续发展问题。可持续发展(sustainable development)是指在满足当代人需要的同时,不损害人类后代满足其自身需要的能力。即可持续发展战略要解决资源的代际平等、人际平等。

基于可持续发展的思想和理论,医学的发展有赖于社会的持续发展,社会的持续发展对医学有着促进作用:社会可持续发展改善人类生存的环境和条件,有利于疾病谱的改变;社会可持续发展使医学科学技术有持续发展的经济基础;社会可持续发展最终改善人类的生存环境和生活质量。同时社会可持续发展的水平与速度也制约医学的发展,医学发展的经济需求不应超过社会经济发展的水平,应该考虑社会和个人的承受能力。根据公正和公平的原则,人不分种族、性别、等级、贫富,都有获得医疗的权利,当世界上还有许多人无法享受医疗资源时,医学必须满足全体人民的基本需要。因此,医疗模式应从治疗型转向预防保健型,从以疾病为主导转变到以健康为主导,从单个患者转向家庭和社区,使医疗防治目标转变为生理健康、心理健康与环境协调发展。医学除了研究人类疾病的发生、发展及其防治规律,更需要用生物-心理-社会医学模式来研究人类生命活动和外界环境的相互关系。医学发展应成为社会可持续发展的重要和积极组成部分。

(二)生物-心理-社会医学模式的医学目的

日新月异的医学技术,造成了日益膨胀的医学和医疗保健费用。很多技术,都是倾向于增加费用,通过提供以前没有的治疗方法,创造新形式的康复和延长生命的方法,使医学沿着以昂贵的治疗方法治疗少数人的疾病的方向前进。许多由技术发展带来的健康状态改善都是边缘性的,费用也是昂贵的,甚至很多诊断技术超越了治疗的可能性。由于医学传统地接受了治疗为主、治愈为目的的生物医学模式,昂贵地去谋求医疗的进步,这成为过去50年来医学的标志,也使得许多国家按照可持续发展原则,已经走到了医学可供性的边缘。

医学应该是社会供得起的和经济上可支撑的医学。医学应该努力使其目的适应经济现实,并使医学在可能的范围内交给公众。凡是供得起的医学,从长期来看就是可持续的。

医学应该是公正和公平的医学。医学应对所有人都是供得起的,而不仅是对那些能按市场价格支付的人。医学不应该继续研制那些只有富人用得起的药物和技术,也不应在不可避免的疾病的发生或死亡的边缘上挣扎。

医学应该是尊重人的选择和尊严。医学应尊重人的自由和尊严,应该对医学技能和知识的使用作出负责任的选择,应该由公众和病家作出治疗、生活态度和行为、终止维持生命的治疗的选择,以及稀缺资源的分配。

因此,医学的目的或者叫生物-心理-社会医学模式的医学优先战略是确立预防疾病和促进健康、解除疼痛和疾苦、治疗疾病和对不治之症的照料、预防早死和提倡安详地死亡等4项目的。

第四节 现代医学模式

一、生物-心理-社会医学模式的产生背景

(一)疾病谱转变

生物医学模式使传染病取得防治技术的突破,使一些烈性传染病得到控制,全球疾病和死因结构发生了显著改变。影响人群健康的主要疾病,在我国和发达国家已相类似,由传染病转化为慢性非传染病,恶性肿瘤、心脑血管病占据了疾病谱和死因谱主要位置(表

2-3)。这一转变驱使人们把视角由单纯考虑引起疾病的生物因素转向综合的生物、心理、社会因素。在传染病占据疾病谱和死亡谱主要位置时,人们专注于探讨特异性生物因素和有针对性的治疗方法,忽视社会经济因素的作用。疾病谱和死因谱的转变,把心理和社会因素的作用展现在人们面前,心脏病、脑血管病和恶性肿瘤等疾病的病因复杂,和人的性格、生活方式、情志因素乃至经济生活条件都有联系,必须从生物、心理、社会因素综合地研究和解决问题。

表 2-3 我国城市前五位死因谱的变化趋势

	1957 年 死亡率 构成比 ($1/10^5$)(%)		1963 年 死亡率 构成比 ($1/10^5$)(%)		1975 年 死亡率 构成比 ($1/10^5$)(%)		1985 年 死亡率 构成比 ($1/10^5$)(%)		1997 年 死亡率 构成比 ($1/10^5$)(%)	
1. 呼吸系统疾病	120.3	16.9	呼吸系统疾病 64.6	12.0	脑血管疾病 127.1	21.6	心血管疾病 131.04	23.39	恶性肿瘤 135.39	22.71
2. 传染病	111.2	15.4	传染病 57.5	10.7	恶性肿瘤 111.5	18.8	脑血管疾病 117.52	20.98	脑血管疾病 134.88	22.63
3. 消化系统疾病	52.1	7.3	恶性肿瘤 46.1	8.6	呼吸系统疾病 100.8	18.6	恶性肿瘤 113.86	20.32	呼吸系统疾病 99.99	16.77
4. 心血管疾病	47.2	6.6	脑血管疾病 36.9	6.9	心血管疾病 69.2	11.7	呼吸系统疾病 50.85	9.08	心脏病 84.00	14.09
5. 脑血管疾病	39.0	5.5	心血管疾病 36.1	6.7	传染病 34.3	5.8	消化系统疾病 23.34	4.17	损伤、中毒 36.84	6.18

当然,生物因素的作用不容忽视。最新的研究估计,15%的癌症新病例能通过预防相关传染病而被控制。当前发展中国家的疾病谱说明,占世界人口一半的这些国家,婴儿死亡率仍达 10% 左右,每天约有 4 万儿童死于传染病和营养不良。

联合国儿童基金会提出,发展中国家的传染病防治工作要同时实现技术和社会两重突破。传染病防治即使从生物学角度考虑,也需要通过改善人们自身的各种条件,才能有效地同生物病原作斗争。

(二)健康需求提高

随着生产的发展和生活水平的提高,人们的健康需求也日益多样化,他们已不满足于疾病的防治,而是积极地要求提高健康质量和生活质量,祛病延年,保持心理平衡,活得更有意义和价值,要求有利于身心健康的人际关系和社会心理氛围。这就要求扩大卫生服务的范围,由治疗服务扩大到预防服务,由生理服务扩大到心理服务,由院内服务扩大到院外服务,从技术服务扩大到社会服务。这种需求强烈地要求实现医学模式的转变,要求医疗卫生工作必须面对多样化的健康需求,要求卫生服务全面满足人们的这些健康要求。这种需求还会随着社会发展进一步扩展,成为促使医学模式转变的一大力量。

(三)医学社会化

医学是社会性的事业,承担着社会保健职能。但长期以来,它局限于个体疾病的治疗,即使预防,也主要是一种个体行为,限制了其他社会系统的参与,也限制了卫生服务的范围。随着城市化的发展,生产和生活消费行为的进一步社会化,公共卫生和社会保健的作用日益突出,人类与疾病的斗争日益突破个人活动的局限,成为整个社会关注的问题。许多健康问题局限在个人范围内已无法解决,必须采取社会化措施才能找到出路。整个社会系统都承担着保健职能,只有把卫生保健事业纳入整个社会范围内,通过医学的社会化,才能较好地得到解决。目前,人们越来越感到人类具有许多共同的健康利益,卫生工作全球化一体化的趋势正是这种共同健康利益作用的必然结果。人人享有健康,健康是基本人权已成为全球共识;生态环境保护问题,全球化一些高发病、严重传染病的共同防护,更使医学社会化的趋势不断增强。这种趋势必然要求突破生物医学模式的局限,形成全人类参与的社会健康工程,实现健康改善与社会进步的双向促进。

(四)医学学科的内部融合与外部交叉发展

卡尔·L·怀特(Kerr L. White)的《弥合裂痕——流行病学、医学和公共卫生》深刻地反映了临床医学与公共卫生分久必合的趋向,使预防和临床工作人员联系在一起,从不同角度有组织地进行活动,促使他们之间进行知识交流,彼此把对方带入与本专业有关但又不很熟悉的领域,打破惯性思维和保守倾向,换个新的视角观察问题,从整体角度考虑问题,进入更深层次的思考。这种不同知识结构的相互交流,使人们从经验思维、实验分析思维进入综合思维方式,形成立体化、网络化、多层次、多视角的立体思维方式,自然引起对生物、心理、社会因素综合作用的思考。

医学认识手段的现代化,使对疾病的认识在一定程度上摆脱了过分依赖个体经验,加强了分工协作,趋向于社会化,不同专业共同参与对疾病的考察,以及他们之间实现认识上的互补,为多学科参与医学实践提供了可能,为心理学家和社会学家参与医学认识与实践提供了可能。

现代医学中分子生物学、免疫学、遗传学的发展,揭示了宏观活动整体性的基础。特别是信息观点的引入,发现在人体内、人体与环境之间广泛存在着信息传递及交流,心理应激现象与激素分泌之间的联系,以心理活动为中介引起的社会因素与人体活动之间的联系,都促进了用生物、心理、社会因素综合考虑思路的发展。

所有这些医学学科内部的融合和外部的交叉,都把现代自然科学和社会科学的理论和技术带入医学领域,使人们观察健康与疾病问题的视角向社会和心理领域延伸和拓展。

二、生物-心理-社会医学模式的内容

社会的进步,在改变了疾病谱的同时,也改变了人们的健康需求。医学变得越来越社会化,与自然科学和社会科学有着密切的联系和融合交叉。现代医学模式正是在这种变化和交流中逐渐形成,并逐渐被人们所认识。

(一)布鲁姆的环境健康医学模式

1974年布鲁姆(Blum)提出了环境健康医学模式。他认为环境因素,特别是社会环境因素,对人们健康、精神和体质发育有重要影响,提出了包括环境、遗传、行为与生活方式及医疗卫生服务4个因素的环境健康医学模式。环境因素包括社会和自然的环境因素,是影响健康的最重要的因素。

(二)拉隆达和德威尔的综合健康医学模式

在布鲁姆环境模式的基础上,为了更加广泛地说明疾病发生的原因,拉隆达(Lalonde)和德威尔(Dever)对环境健康医学模式加以修正和补充后,提出了卫生服务和政策分析相结合的综合健康医学模式,系统地论述了疾病流行病和社会学相关的医学模式,用来指导卫生事业发展,作为制定卫生政策的依据。

三、影响人群健康的主要因素

按照现代医学模式指导思想,影响人类健康的因素包括以下几点:

1. 环境因素。人群的健康和疾病总是与环境因素密切相关。有害因素可以引起疾病从而影响健康。水、空气、食物等被污染,生产环境中的职业性危害,噪声及不安全的公路设计等均构成对人们健康的威胁。虽然人们对外界环境进行了改造,但新的危险因素不断产生。传统工业中,成千上万种的化学合成物质在生产中的危险因素成为对健康的严重威胁。

社会环境包括经济收入、居住条件、营养状况及文化程度等均对健康有着重要的作用。贫困者所面临的健康危险要超过富裕者;文化程度低的人所受危险因素的侵害要超过文化程度高的人。社会带来的工作紧张及生活压力、人际关系中的矛盾等,均能危害健康。

2. 生活方式及行为因素。吸烟、酗酒、滥用药物、缺乏体育锻炼、不合理饮食习惯等不良生活方式以及不良性行为等,均对健康带来直接和间接的影响。在美国人群前10位死亡原因中,有7种死亡原因与生活方式和行为危险因素有关。改变生活方式和行为,如不吸烟、少饮酒、参加体育活动、注意合理营养、保持乐观情绪等,可明显降低心血管病发病率和死亡率。

3. 生物遗传因素。有些疾病如血友病、镰状细胞贫血症、蚕豆病、精神性痴呆等直接与遗传因素有关。有些精神障碍性疾病、糖尿病和部分肿瘤、心血管疾病则是遗传因素与环境因素、生活方式和行为综合作用的结果。

4. 医疗卫生服务因素。医疗卫生服务的目的是防治疾病、增进健康、降低发病率与死亡率、延长寿命,服务的好坏直接影响人群的健康水平。医疗卫生机构布局是否合理,群众就医是否及时、方便,医疗技术水平的高低以及卫生服务质量的好坏,包括院内感染和药物滥用的控制,都会影响人群的健康和疾病的转归。因此,充分发挥医疗卫生系统在保护人群健康上的作用,是不可忽视的。

根据这一模式对全球的主要死因进行归类,世界卫生组织1991年调查显示,60%死亡是由于行为生活方式、17%为环境因素、15%为生物因素、8%为卫生服务。可见,与社会紧密相关的行为生活方式确已成为引起死亡的主要危险,成为新医学模式的客观佐证。

四、生物-心理-社会医学模式

在经历一系列的探讨和实践之后,1977年美国纽约州Rochester大学精神病学和内科学教授恩格尔(Engel)提出:生物医学模式应该逐步转变成为生物-心理-社会医学模式,生物-心理-社会医学模式又称恩格尔模式。生物-心理-社会医学模式基于系统论的原则,包括疾病、病人和环境,环境包括自然环境和社会环境。在这个系统框架中,可以把健康或疾病理解为从原子、分子、细胞、组织、组织系统到人,以及由人、家庭、社区、人类构成概念化相联系的自然系统。在这个系统中不再是二元论和还原论的线性因果模型,而是互为因果、协同制约的模型。健康反映为系统内、系统间高水平的协调。恢复健康不是健康的以前状态,而是代表一种与病前不同的系统新的协调。图2-1病例和图2-2病例,分别反映亚原子层次的失调和社会层次的失调在生物-心理-社会医学模式上的系统表现。

社会、国家	→	分配福利政策
↑文化		价值挑战、医治病人和资源的其他用途
↑社区		资源转移用来医治病人
↑家庭		情绪受创
↑人		不能进行复杂、协调的身心活动
↑系统		神经系统功能损害
↑器官		发育受阻
↑组织		显示形态变化
↑细胞		缺少分化指令
↑细胞器		染色体基因突变
↑分子		DNA模板变化
↑亚原子		配子受辐射

图2-1 辐射诱发配子突变的身心发育迟缓症

↓社会、国家	→	停止飞机制造的决策
↓文化	→	价值挑战,忠于政府和就业需要
↓社区	→	失去收入
↓家庭	→	经济上、情绪上的紧张
↓人	→	重新自我估价、再就业学习和新生活方式
↓系统	→	环境输入节奏破坏
↓器官	→	神经器官压抑
↓组织	→	器质性症状、体征,如失眠、疼痛、忧虑
↓细胞	→	神经细胞染色体改变
↓细胞器	→	染色体形态变化

图2-2 工程师失业引起的身心症

生物-心理-社会医学模式表明,每个层次系统既是由低层次系统构成的,本身又是更高层次的组成部分。各层次间存在着相互作用,包括向上因果作用和向下因果作用,任何层次的变化都会影响整个系统,并受到系统的作用。这种广义生物圈的系统需要用生物-心理-社会医学模式解释。

五、生物-心理-社会医学模式的健康观

健康观是建立在一定医学模式基础上的,随着医学模式的更新而改变的,研究健康与疾病的联系,是对健康和疾病的本质性认识。

传染病的发生和传播是生物体之间发生的变化,是宿主、致病因素和环境三者之间的平衡遭到破坏。人患了传染病,便失去了健康,而当传染病治愈,人又重新获得了健康。这种以传染病的发生、变化和转归为依据的疾病观是单因单果的健康疾病表现形式。"没有病"就是健康被称为消极的健康观,即生物医学模式的健康观。

在疾病谱和死因谱发生变化后,许多非传染性疾病和慢性病以及某些退行性疾病逐渐增加,主要有心脑血管疾病、恶性肿瘤等。要防治这些疾病不像防治传染病那么单一,而是要防治导致疾病发生的多种因素。这种多因单果(multiple cause/single effect)、多因多果(multiple cause/multiple effects)疾病形式,因果关系更加复杂。要消灭这类疾病,获得健康就不能单纯依赖治疗,而要更多或主要地依靠社会预防,降低和排除各种健康危险因素,以达到个体的身心平衡,并与环境协调一致,这样才能获得健康。世界卫生组织提出:"健康是指一种身体、心理和社会的完美状态,而不仅仅是没有疾病或虚弱。"根据这个积极健康观,健康可被理解为生物学、心理学和社会学三维组合的概念。从生物角度看人的健康,主要是检查器官功能和各项指标是否正常;从心理、精神角度观察人的健康,主要是看有无自我控制能力、能否正确对待外界影响、是否处于内心平衡的状态;从社会学角度衡量人的健康,主要涉及个体的社会适应性、良好的工作和生活习惯、人际关系和应付各种突发事件的能力。同样,对疾病的概念也作出了修正。恩格尔给疾病下了一个定义:"疾病可看做是整个生物体或其他系统在生长、发育、功能及调整中的失败或失调。"这一定义的局限性明显存在。疾病(disease)、病患(illness)及患病(sickness)是有区别的。疾病是一种病理状态(生物尺度),病患是病人说明病理状态的方式(感觉尺度),患病是病人对病理状态感觉的反应(行动尺度)。对一个人来说,在疾病过程中感觉是一个重要方面,而行动尺度对病人的反应及采取行动同样重要。实际上,不同观点的健康与疾病的定义是有差别的,表2-4列举了不同学派从不同角度提出的健康与疾病的定义。

表2-4 健康与疾病的定义

观点	健康	疾病
生理或生物观点	身体的良好状态	指一个医学概念,它表明身体的某一部分、过程、系统在功能和(或)结构上的反常
流行病学观	宿主对环境中的致病因素具有抵抗的状态	宿主对环境中的致病因素易感而形成的状态
生态学观点	人和生态间协调关系的产物	人和生态间关系不适应和不协调的结果
社会学观点	人在一个群体中认为身体和(或)行为是正常的	个体认为偏离了正常的身体和(或)行为状态
消费者观点	一种商品、一种投资,在某种程度上能够买到	通过购买保健服务可以治疗、控制及治愈的一种不正常情况
统计学观点	测量结果在正常值范围内	测量结果在正常值范围外

有关健康与疾病概念始终是医学模式的核心表现和争论焦点,除健康与疾病相对论观点外,近年来还衍生了亚健康、亚临床疾病等概念。

1. 健康与疾病相对的概念。所有生物体都会有病,都要经历生长、老化、死亡的过程。因此,可以把健康与疾病看做一个连续的统一体或分度尺。良好的健康在一端,死亡在另一端,每个人都在疾病-健康连续统一体的两端之间的某一地方占有一个位置,而且随着时间的推移在变化着。

2. 亚健康状态。这是近年来国际医学界提出的新概念,是指人的机体虽然无明显的疾病,但呈现出活力降低、适应力不同程度减退的一种生理状态,是由机体各系统的生理功能和代谢过程低下所导致,是介于健康与疾病之间的一种生理功能降低的状态,亦称"第三状态"或"灰色状态"。认定亚健康状态的范畴相当广泛,躯体上、心理上的不适应感觉,在相当长时期难以确诊是哪种病症,均可包括在其中。从预防医学、临床医学,尤其是精神及心理医学的临床实际工作中发现,处于这种状态的人群数量是相当多的。衰老、疲劳综合征、神经衰弱、更年期综合征,均属于"亚健康"状态范畴。

"亚健康"状态产生的主要原因是人体脏器功能下降,患者仅感到身体或精神上的不适,如疲乏无力、精神不安、头痛、胸闷、失眠、饮食欠佳等,但各种仪器和化验检查都没有什么阳性结果。"亚健康"状态极有可能发展成为疾病。医学界告示人们"亚健康"状态的存在,但是对其深入的研究是一个跨世纪的医学课题。

3. 亚临床疾病。这是健康观的另一概念,又称"无症状疾病"。认为疾病是改变了条件的生命现象过程。疾病过程中不仅有机体受损害、发生紊乱的病理表现,而且还有防御、适应、代偿生理性反应,这类病理性反应和生理性反应在疾病过程中不可避免地结合在一起,是很难人为进行分割的进程和结局。"亚临床疾病"与"亚健康状态"的区别在于前者没有临床症状、体征,但存在生理性代偿或病理性改变的临床检测依据。如"无症状性缺血性心脏病"可以无临床症状,但有心电图改变等诊断依据。

Chapter 2 Medical Model

Section 1 Medical Model Concept

Model is a symbolic logic concept in the beginning, expressing form logical theories with a series of formula within system. The philosophy course introduced and extended the concept of the model, used for analysis or to clarify the relation of the thing and essence, and made use of the realm of humanities social science and the natural science, becoming the core of the methodologies and Weltanschauung. Establishing the model is a kind of scientific investigative method. People establish the model to analyze and express the relation and essence, which leads people to observe, consider and solve problems. For this reason model can be comprehended a thought or mode for solving and understanding problems.

Medical model has been created based on the notion that medical practice is a total cognition of the medicine that human in the innumerable experiences fight with the various diseases and become acquainted with the life processes. This kind of highly generalized, abstract idealistic concept and thought way expressed the total construction characteristic of the medicine, and was a basic standpoint to guide medical practice. The medical model belongs to the nature's dialectics realm. It is the natural view and methodology that regards medicine as the object observed by people, analyzes and handles human health and disease problems with methods and standpoints of the dialectics and the materialism, is a scientific view about the phenomena of health and disease. The core of the medical model is medical view, which studies the medical property, function, structure and developing law.

Medical science studies and medical treatment practice are proceeding under the guidance between definite medical view and epistemology, such as from the single biological angle, or from biology, psychology and sociology all-directions to understand and observe the human health; from single biological angle or from multidimensional biology, psychology and sociology to handle and study the human diseases' prevention, treatment and health promotion. The difference among idea, cognition and method attributes to influences of the different medical models, and is also a virtual reflection of different medical science views. Since medical model embodies medical view, it also embodies methodology. The medical theories are produced tallying up of the medical practice but the medical practice is achieved under the guidance of particular medical thought to produce the medical behavior. Therefore, the medical view not only affects the medical thought and behavior, but also relates to the result of the medical behavior. Medical model has important influence on the human health protection, disease prevention and treatment and its result.

In 1977, Engel, the professor of psychiatry and internal medicine in Rochester University in New York State, pointed out "It is inevitable that the direction of medical development would turn from biomedical model into bio-psycho-social medical model gradually." This standpoint was introduced into China for the first time in National Medical Dialectic Conference in 1981, and our country medicine hygiene field began to pay attention to it.

Anyway, the evolvement of medical model is historical tidal current of objective existence. In the development process of medicine, people once created ancient Greece medicine, the representative of which was Hippocrates and a series of complete theories system of which Chinese medicine's *Internal Scripture* representative and holistic medical model was founded on the Yin-Yang and Five Elements theories. Along with the medicine progress, and the medical socialization course and the health demand advanced and changed, and the medical model changed several times. Reviewing the change process of the medical model will help people to comprehend better which the contemporary medical theories and practice are confronted with a change, namely biomedical model that uses the single biological angle to observe and handle medical problems, is changing to the modern medical model that uses the diverse bio-psycho-social angles to observe and handle the medical problems synthetically. Recognizing the concept that medical model changes will help to solve the relation of individual medicine and community medicine, biomedicine and social medicine, clinical medicine and preventive medicine, microscopic medicine and macroscopic medicine, prevention and treatment of disease and enhancement health, medical progress and social development.

Section 2　Historical Main Medical Model

1. Spiritualism medical model

Primitive medicine, which cannot be called science strictly speaking, had been attached to primitive religion, attributed to our ancestor, because people could not explain physiological phenomena, such as disease, death, dream, etc. Influencing the dream prospects, producing a kind of idea, thoughts and feelings were not a human oneself activities, but an activity of soul, which was independent of the body. Dream was a reflection of soul activity. Death was said to be a soul leaving body, body would die but soul was immortal. The reason, which resulted disease, could not be seen and could not touch, was thought to be the devils and ghosts, or parting person's soul breaking in. Ancestors thought God and spirits bestowed the human's life and health, and their punishment and condemnation were diseases and disasters. This is spiritualism medical model. Therefore, people mainly depended on begging God and spirits and praying for their bless and forgiveness to protect health and treat diseases. They also resort to some natural effective plants and minerals for medical treatment, although most of them were emetic and cathartic methods. Their dominant idea was to banish the spirits and ghosts who caused plague. Its responsibility and culture of spiritualism medical model achieved unification under social condition of the age.

2. Nature philosophical medical model

Religion was a result, which submitted to natural forces, and mystified it. Medicine was a process, which conquered natural forces, and cleared it. Along with the enhancement of productivity, mankind outshined others from the nature with subjective and objective integrated mass, finally producing the ego consciousness, becoming an independent one which could recognize object.

Prosperous philosophy thought in ancient Greece was accorded with the medical recognition for the essence of person and the disease origin. At that time, the philosophers usually were also doctors. Western medicine originator Hippocrates was influenced deeply by Alcmaeom and Empedocles, who were both famous natural philosophers and doctors in ancient Greece. Hippocrates put forward the theory in *About the Nature of Man* that the chemical element was like the water, fire, soil and spirit, which was thought to be the fountain of everything, corresponded to the mucus, blood, black bile and yellow bile of bodies. Person's health, disease and character were said to be the mixture of those body fluids and the result of that mixture determined the proportion of variation. Therefore, a doctor's job was only to maintain natural essentiality of man's body. Gradually, medical body fluid school was formed and it was developed to medical solid school. Those theories elementarily established that the recognition of human body was either body fluid or body configuration. These thought and theories of natural philosophy took their way out of spiritualism medicine, initiating the foundation of medical science.

Table 2-1 the comparison of Hippocrates' four kinds of body fluids

body fluid	source	characteristics	season	disease	treatment	idiosyncracy
mucus	brain	cold	winter	coryza/pneumonia, headache, pleuritis, stroke, painful urine	hotbath, hot gruel, diuretic, emetic	sticky liquid quality

(Table 2-1)

body fluid	source	characteristics	season	disease	treatment	idiosyncracy
blood	heart	summer-heat	spring	angina, arthritis, dysentery, lepra	bleeding, febrifuge, emetic	sanguineous quality
black bile	spleen, stomach	dryness	autumn	Edema, hepatitis, sciatica, macula, typhoid/malaria, canker	emetic, hot bath	hypochondriac quality
yellow bile	liver	dampness	summer	cholera, mouth ulcer, jaundice, tummy bug	bleeding, febrifuge, clyster, liquid food, anodyne	bile quality

Chinese medicine has been considered to be a medicine constructed based on epistemology and methodology of Confucianism and Tao. "Changes" was the mother of the medical principles. "Changes" contains three basic principles: simple Changes, easy Changes and no Changes. *The Internal Medicine Principles* and succeeding Chinese medicine theories had inherited and developed the Yin-Yang theories, established the pathological theories of Yin-Yang and Five Elements and the pathogenic theories of exogenous(wind, cold, summer-heat, dampness, dryness, fire) and endogenous(happiness, anger, sorrow, worries, sadness, fear, shock).

Whether ancient Greece medicine, or Chinese medicine theory, naive, dialectic, holistic contacts are observed and concerned in which health and disease are connected with the natural environment of mankind's living and social environment, and they are called nature philosophical medical model.

3. Biomedical model

European Renaissance has pushed natural science into technological advancement, bringing the high tide of the Industrial Revolution and the rise of experimental science, since the 15th century. Bacon, who was famous, experiment methods, "used experimental methods to research nature". Mechanics and physics obtained prominent advancement on the influence of experimental idea. Representative works of mechanistic ideology include Descartes's *Animal Is Machine*, Lamterry's *Human Is Machine*. They regarded person as machine, which starts up itself. Disease occurs when there is breakdown and when the body is out of order. Therefore, they needed to be repaired and perfected. This is mechanistic medical model. Medicine obtained definite progress on the influence of this model, such as the machine standpoint affecting the physiology to urge Harvey to discover blood circulation. The discovery of cell founded cell pathology. It put forward the idea that "all diseases have relation to cell", "the source of all kinds of diseases is cell's abnormal activities". Mechanism regarded life activities as machine movement, therefore protected health the same way as protecting machine. Mechanistic model can be the stage of entry-level into the medical science mode. The machine theory explains that the life activity is a machine to exercise, protecting the health is to protect the machine, and the machine theory can be regarded as the primary phase of modern biomedicine.

The thoughts of scientific experiment pushed the development of biomedicine tremendously. Biomedicine obtained the astonishing achievement one after another in physiology, pathology, and microbiology realms, resolving the grave puzzles of clinical medicine and preventive medicine and pushing the development of whole medicine. Three puzzles in surgery, namely, ache, infection and blood loss, had been conquered, which were paradigm of biomedical achievements. Before, although surgeon accumulated some experience to control ache, infection and blood loss, effect was not good, for instance, the death rate of osteotomy was up to $40\%-50\%$. The puzzle was resolved gradually on the basis of development of pharmacology, pathogens microbiology, physiology and so on. Researchers discovered that patient inhaling ether would lose the sense of pain in 1846, and used cocaine to make local anesthesia in 1882. In 1867, English doctor Lister created the theory which said that wound's decay and decomposition was caused by microorganism. Through this enlightenment that Pasteur gave theory about microorganisms causing the decay of organism, he adopted phenol to rinse the surgical operation apparatus, and to wet gauze to clean and cover wound. This theory decreased the death rate of osteotomy from 46% to 15%, establishing the basic principle of the asepticism; hemostatic bandage and hemostat appeared in 1872. Bergmann, a German doctor, adopted steam to sterilize, establishing asepsis in 1877; Landsteiner, an Austrian pathologist discovered the blood typing system of the red cell, resolving the problem which was caused by blood transfusion in 1900. These achievements increased the safety of the surgical operation and alleviated pain and sufferings of the patient, making the surgery treatment technique quickly advanced.

The invention of microscope and its use for finding pathogens, microbiological experiments proved the nosogenetic mechanism of bacterium and viruses, and vaccination and chemical therapy was developed on the basis of it, all of those forming the concept that the nature balances the interaction between host, environment and pathogen, for the first time starting hygienic revolution. Medical experiments discovered a lot of nosogenetic microorganism, such as tubercle bacillus, vibrio cholerae, rickettsia, malarial parasites, syphilis, spirochete, etc. Because of the advancement of immunotherapy, the death rate from acute and chronic infectious disease fell down very quickly by adopting vaccination, the disinfectants and insecticide measures and antibiotics. Smallpox have been exterminated in the world, a few violent infectious diseases (plague, cholera, etc.) have been controlled basically and the incidence of some of infectious diseases has fallen down consumedly (malaria, Type-B encephalitis, measles and schistosomiasis, etc.) in China, and the death from infectious diseases accounts for less than 1% of total death in some developed countries. The life expectancy of all countries has increased from 30 – 40 years old to 60 – 70 years old in 50 years, which tied up with the achievement of biomedicine.

Because of the advance of biomedicine, it founded the representative theories: dualism and restoration theory. Dualism thinks that there should be reasonable division of work for researching body and spirit. Medicine should put the attention to how to measure cell's biochemical changes by the precise technique, to explain the symptom and sign of the patient's, and to interfere changes to recover the patient's health. Medicine no longer gives its attention to the patient's psychological and social status. "Restoration theory" further disintegrates human body to different organs, cells, and numerators, thinking that complicated biological phenomenon must use physical and chemical methods to research and explain the causality of functional changes. Diseases were regarded as a kind of cause and effect with stationary outcome, not a dynamic variation process. By the guidance of that theory, the development of bioscience entered into the brand-new history period, forming the bio-scientific system: biology, anatomy, histology, physiology, bacteriology, biochemistry, pathology, immunology, genetics, etc. and producing the modern molecular biology. People used biomedicine standpoint completely to recognize biological phenomena, the changes of body, health and diseases, and to prevent and treat the infectious disease, which threatens human's life and health. People think optimistically that we can explain all problems of health and disease finally.

Table 2-2 The important discoveries of the bacteriology research in the second half of the 19th century

Discoverer	Years	Item
Lister	1852	infection(asepsis surgery)
Pasteur	1857 – 1862	microzyme
	1877	chicken cholera vaccine
	1881	anthrax vaccine
	1884	hydrophobia vaccine
Kohn	1882	tubercle bacillus
	1883	cholera vibrio
Klebs	1882	swine erysipelas
	1883	diphtheria bacillus
Eberth	1880	typhoid bacillus

(Table 2-2)

Discoverer	Years	Item
Fallesen	1854	erysipelas streptococcus
Neisser	1897	gonococcus
Weishu	1892	emphysematous gangrene
Oberman	1873	relapsing fever leptospira
Bruce	1887	Brucella bacillus
Shiga	1897	dysentery bacillus
Beilicaisanlang	1894	pestilence bacillus
Border	1900	chincough bacillus

In conclusion, biomedical model was established on the foundation of bioscience. It is the medical idea and methodology, which reflects the changes among pathogens, and natural environment. The model holds it is certain that in any of disease we can find measurable morphological and chemical changes on organ, cell or molecule and make sure of the biological, physical and chemical special causes; and therapeutic means can be found. But the changing disease chart and death chart showed that the primary reasons of endangering human health were cardiovascular disease, malignancy, accidental death and breathing system disease. The nosogenetic factors that caused chronic non-contagious diseases were not only due to single biological pathogens but also due to lots of social environment factors, individual behaviors and lifestyle factors, etc. Biomedical model could not explain and resolve the origination and development of the diseases completely. Even though the prevalence and prevention and therapy of contagious diseases (such as sexually transmitted disease, AIDS and tuberculosis) whose primary nosogenetic factor is biological factors are restricted with social, psychological and behavioral factors. Lots of diseases occur as a result of social and psychological factors' interaction. Disease expressional form is developed from single-cause and single-result to multi-causes and multi-results. Accordingly, medical model is transiting from biomedical model to bio-psycho-social medical model.

Section 3 The Evolution Law of Medical Model

1. General law

The transformation of medical model at every time is rather a surpassing than a process of simple substitution. Any of the scientific advancements is always accomplished through taking the first step on the basis of predecessors' achievements. The pattern of biological-psychological-social medicine is a new medical mode formed on the basis of the pattern of biological medicine along with the development in society, economy and science and technology, adapted to modern human health-care technology, i. e., the pattern of biological-psychological-social medicine. This medical mode will guide people to understand more comprehensively and more objectively the medical and health-care problems of modern society, and guide the medical science to develop.

The transformation process from the biomedicine mode to the pattern of biological-psychological-social medicine has the complicated historical and social backgrounds. It has also taken a long period for people to understand this transformation process. It can be regarded as the summary of experiences obtained by the human concerns on the health and the struggle against disease.

The medical mode is not an immutable or ossified dogma, but is continuously changed and transferred along with the development of medical science and the demands of human health. The ultimate target of this transference is to utilize the ideological guidance of medical mode to satisfy best and most perfectly the human pursuit of healthiness. Therefore, along with the mankind's continuously increasing demands for health, the medical mode has been forced to achieve constant development, change and perfection.

Medical mode is the summary of human experiences through the obtaining of health and the struggling against disease, and has been undergoing various twists and turns through its course of development, just like the development of philosophy, which is not of an unhindered advance. In every activity of the human being, those aspects have been examined mercilessly by the history, such as correctness vs. incorrectness, onesidedness vs. all-sidedness, imperfection vs. perfection and low grade vs. high grade. Practice is the sole criterion for testing the truth, and the medical mode is being continuously replenished, deepened and perfected in the course of medical practices of mankind.

Nowadays, we are faced with the transformation from the pattern of biomedicine to the pattern of biological-psychological-social medicine. This transformation will impact the concept of biomedicine inherent in various fields during the development of medical science and health-care undertakings, resulting in a revolution in concept.

No doubt that there was a historical reason for the existence of the mode of biomedicine and that the biomedicine played a great role in propelling the medical development. However, the mode of biomedicine emphasized only the biological factor and neglected the social and psychological attributes of human, thus presenting its one-sidedness and limitations and becoming unable to satisfy the demands of modern medical development. The mode of medicine is dynamically varying, and changes must take place in the medical mode once the social development steps into a new stage. The transformation of medical mode is virtually a variation in medical concept and mode of thinking, which adapts itself to the epochal characteristic of medical science. Modern medicine raises the requirement that we must base ourselves on the three-dimensional point of view, i.e. the biological, psychological and social angles, to understand the issue of health and disease, hold omni-faceted and multilevel grasp of the orientation of medical development, and apply the concept of modern medicine to guiding the medical practices so as to solve various medical problems faced with in modern society.

2. The advancement and development of society and the transformation of medical model

The formation of the pattern of biological-psychological-social medicine has resulted in the medicine marching from the ivory tower to the society, thus making the medicine, which was ever traditionally a purely natural science, revert to the reality. It is an applied science upon the combination and crossing of natural science and social science. The bi-direction between medicine and social and economic development decides the duality that the medicine is an integrant of the sustainable development of the society and is manifesting its role. Furthermore, all social functions of the medicine express various medical purposes in turn.

Anyhow, the evolution of medical mode is a historical trend of objective existence. People should grasp the epochal characteristic of medicine and the orientation of medical development from the angles of modern concept, modern way of death and modern health demand. Only by doing so can we correctly identify various relations between individual medicine and group medicine, biomedicine and social medicine, micro-medicine and macro-medicine, clinical medicine and preventive medicine, preventive and curative health-enhancing medicine as well as medical advancement and social development, and then solve various complicated medical problems faced with in modern society.

3. Role of the transformation of modern medical model

(1) Relationship between medicine and sustainable development

Along with the advancement in science and technology and the development of commodity economy, including the science and technology of medicine and pharmaceutics as well as the medical and health-care service, it has been noticed that while creating tremendous wealth and comfortable living, people are increasingly worrying about whether the factors of resources and environment will restrict the continuous development of our mankind society and whether the development of yesterday and today will reduce the living quality of our generation and the several future generations. This is the strategy of sustainable development drawing the serious attention of the whole world at the end of the 20th century. Sustainable development refers to the capability of satisfying the demands of the moderns without doing any harm to the future generations in satisfying their own demands in the meantime. The strategy of sustainable development needs to solve the problem of inter-generation and inter-personal equity in the aspect of resources.

On the basis of the ideology and theory of sustainable development, the medical development depends on the sustainable development of society, and the sustainable development of society plays an accelerating role in the medicine. The sustainable development of society improves the environment and conditions of mankind subsistence, thus being beneficial to the modification of disease spectrum. The sustainable development of the society provides the medical science and technology with the economic foundation for sustainable development. The sustainable development of society finally improves the subsistence environment and living quality of mankind. In the meantime, the level and the speed of social sustainable development exercises restraints on the medical development, and the economic demands of medical development should not exceed the level of social and economic development, and should take into consideration of bearing responsibility of the society and individuals. According to the principles of fairness and justice, all the people, regardless of race, sex, rank, richness or poverty, should have the rights to obtain medical service. When lots of people in the world are still unable to obtain the medical resources, the medicine must satisfy the basic demands of the whole people. Therefore, the medical model should transfer from the curative type to the preventive and health-care type, from the disease-oriented type to the health-oriented type, from the single patient to the family and community, so that the aim of medical prevention and cure will transfer to the coordinative development of physiological health, psychological health and environment. In addition to researching the laws of occurrence, development as well as prevention and cure of mankind diseases, the medicine should utilize the pattern of biological-psychological-social medicine to research the interrelation between mankind life activities and external environments. The medical development should become an important and positive integrant of social sustainable development.

(2) Medical purpose of the pattern of biological-psychological-social medical model

The rapidly changing medical technology has brought about increased expenses for medical and health services. Many technologies are always tending to the increase of expenses. By offering the curative methods not existing previously and creating the new methods for recuperation and life prolonging, the medicine has been making progress toward the direction of curing the diseases for the few through the expensive curative methods. Many of the improvements in health conditions caused by the technological development is marginal, and their efficiency is based upon costs, and many diagnostic technologies even go beyond the possibility of cure. Since the medicine had accepted traditionally the biomedicine pattern that gave priority to treatment and aimed at cure, and had always been pursuing the medical progress on the basis of expenses, this has become the medical symbol for the past 50 years. This has also brought many countries to reach the edge of medical availability according to the principle of sustainable development.

Medicine should be the one that can be afforded by the society and can be supported by the economy. The medicine should strive for adapting its aim to the economic reality, and can be handed over to the public to the possible extent. Any of the affordable medicine should be sustainable from a long-term point of view.

Medicine should be the one of fairness and justice. Medicine should be the one affordable to all the people rather than to those who can afford to pay the costs according to market prices. Medicine should not continue to research and develop those pharmaceuticals and technology affordable only to the wealthy people, and should not struggle against the occurrence of inevitable diseases or on the edge of death.

Medicine should be the one paying respect to the people's choice and dignity. Medicine should give respect to people's freedom and dignity and make the responsible choice in the application of medical skills and knowledge. The public and patients concerning the treatment, the living attitude and activity, and the termination of life-prolonging treatment, as well as the distribution of scare resources should make the choice.

Therefore, the medical aim, or the preferential medical strategy of the biological-psychological-social medical mode, lies in four aspects, that is, the determination of preventing the disease and accelerating the health; the release from pains and sufferings; the treatment of disease and the taking care of fatal sickness; the prevention of youthful death and the advocating of peaceful death.

Section 4　Modern Medical Models

1. Background of bio-psycho-social medical model

(1) Conversion of disease notation

Biomedicine model made the infectious diseases obtain the breakthrough of prevention technique and some violent infectious diseases have been controlled. The constitution of disease and cause of death have taken an obvious alteration. It seems that the main diseases influencing human health in our country and developed countries are the same. They all converted from the infectious diseases to chronic non-infectious diseases. For instance, malignant tumor and cardio-cerebral vessel disease occupied the major of position in disease notation and death notation. (Table 2-3) This change caused people to change their view in regarding the diseases that were caused by biological factors and that were also comprehensively caused by bio-psycho-social factors. When the infectious diseases held the main position in disease notation and death notation, people paid attention to studying specific biological factors and to aiming directly at therapy. They neglected the action of socioeconomic factors. With the change of disease notation and death notation, it showed the role of psychosocial factors to people and the etiological factor of cardiac disease, cerebral vessels, and malignant tumor have related with people's character, lifestyle, and even economy and living condition. So, we should synthetically study and solve problems with the bio-psycho-social factors.

Certainly, the role of biological factor cannot be neglected. The latest research estimated that 15% of new cases of cancer can be controlled by preventing some related infectious diseases. The current disease notation of developing countries showed that these countries occupy 50% of the world population, infant mortality still amounts to about 100‰ and every day nearly 40,000 children die in the infectious disease and malnutrition.

Table 2-3 the variety tendency of top five causes of death in China's towns

1957 Mortality Constituent ratio (1/100,000) (%)	1963 Mortality Constituent ratio (1/100,000) (%)	1975 Mortality Constituent ratio (1/100,000) (%)	1985 Mortality Constituent ratio (1/100,000) (%)	1997 Mortality Constituent ratio (1/100,000) (%)
1. Disease of respiratory system 120.3 16.9	Disease of respiratory system 64.6 12.0	Cerebrovasular disease 127.1 21.6	Cardiovascular disease 131.04 23.39	Malignant tumor 135.39 22.71
2. Infectious disease 111.2 15.4	Infectious disease 57.5 10.7	Malignant tumor 111.5 18.8	Cerebrovasular disease 117.52 20.98	Cerebrovasular disease 134.88 22.63
3. Disease of digestive system 52.1 7.3	Malignant tumor 46.1 8.6	Disease of respiratory system 100.8 18.6	Malignant tumor 113.86 20.32	Disease of respiratory system 99.99 16.77
4. Cardiovascular disease 47.2 6.6	Cerebrovasular disease 36.9 6.9	Cardiovascular disease 69.2 11.7	Disease of respiratory system 50.85 9.08	Cardiopathy 84.00 14.09
5. Cerebrovasular disease 39.0 5.5	Cardiovascular disease 36.1 6.7	Infectious disease 34.3 5.8	Disease of digestive system 23.34 4.17	Injury Intoxication 36.84 6.18

The United Nations Children Foundations held that the infectious diseases prevention in developing countries should realize the breakthrough of technique and society at the same time. Considering the infectious diseases prevention from biological angle, we should improve all kinds of condition. Then we can make the effective struggle with biopathogen.

(2) Health requirement rise

With the development of production and improvement of living standard, the health requirement diversifies increasingly. They are already not enough to prevent disease but actively require improving the quality of health and life, getting rid of disease and prolonging their life span, keeping the balance of psychology. They want their life more valuable and require the relationship with social psychology atmosphere that benefits mental health. These require us to expand the scope of health service. We should change from therapy service to prevention service, from physical service to psychical service, from hospital inside to outside, and from technical service to social service. This strongly requests to realize the change of medical model, the hygiene service should face the diverse health requirements of people, and the health services should completely satisfy these health requirements. With the development of society, this kind of requirement will be expanded further and become a strong power to cause medicine model conversion.

(3) Medical socialization

Medical career is a sociality career and assumes the function of social health. But in a long time, it is confined to individual disease treatment. Even though it has prevention, it is mainly an individual behavior, confined with other social system to participate in it and limiting the scope of health service. With the development of urbanization, manufacture and living consumption action are further socialized, and the effect of public health and social health stands out increasingly. The conflict between people and disease increasingly brought through the scope of individual activity and became the problems of focus in the whole society. Many health problems confine to the scope of individual that we cannot solve. So we can find pathway by taking socialization measure. The whole social system assumes the function of health care functional authority. So we must bring health care delivery into the whole range of society by medicine socialization, then these problems can be solved. At present, people are more and more sensible to having a lot of common health benefits. The tendency of whole globe in hygiene work is exactly the inevitable outcome of the function of this kind of common health benefits. It is basic human rights that everyone has the health and health has become the world's common ground. The problem of ecosystem environmental protection and common protection of some serious infectious diseases make the tendency of medicine socialization continuously enhanced. This tendency should break through the limitations of biomedicine model and form the social health engineering that everyone takes part in. Then it can realize the dual acceleration that improvement of health makes social progress.

(4) The internal integrate and exterior development in the medical science

Kerr L. White's *Abridge the Gap — Epidemiology, Medical Science and Public Health* deeply reflects the trend that the clinical medicine and public health will unite. This made the prevention and the clinical worker be contacted together. They take activity from different angles and make them exchange their knowledge. They take the other party into the domains that have relation with their specialty.

We should break the inertial thought and the trend of conservation, change a new visual angle to see the problem, think the problem from the whole angle and enter into the deep stratification thinking. This kind of different knowledge structure exchange makes people think the problem from the experience and experiment analysis into synthesis thinking method then form stereo, network, multi-stratification, and to multi-view angle stereoscopic thinking method. This tends to initiate synthesis-thinking function of bio-psycho-social factors.

With the modernization of medical science method, we know some diseases get away to a certain degree depending on the individual experience, and due to enhanced cooperation based on division of labor and inclination to socialization. Different specialty takes part in studying the diseases and realizes the complementation of knowledge. This provides the possibility that many scientists or psychologists and sociologists take part in medical science practice.

The development of the molecular biology, immunology, and genetics in modern medical science shows the background of macroscopic activity. Especially the information standpoint discovers that between the human body and environment there is extensive information delivering and exchanging. The correlation between psychological stress phenomenon and hormone secretion and psycho-activity cause social factor and human activity promotes the development of synthesized thinking in terms of bio-psycho-social factors.

All these factors integrate internally and external development takes its shape, through which natural science and social science theory and technique accumulates into medical science realm. They expand the visual angle of people observing health and disease problems in the social and mental realm.

2. The contents of bio-psycho-social medical model

With the advance of society, disease notation alternation at the same time also changed the requirement of health. Medicine became more and more social and came in close contact with natural science and social science. The modern medical model formed in this kind of alternation and gradually became known to people.

(1) Blum's environmental health medical model

In 1974, Blum brought up the environmental health medical model. He thought the environmental factors, especially social environmental factor, have an important influence on the growth of health, mind and physical quality. He brought up the environment health medical model that included environment, heredity, behavior, life style and medicine health service factors. The environment factors have social and natural environmental factor that is an important factor influencing human health.

(2) Lalonde's and Dever's synthesized health medical model

In order to extensively explain the cause of disease, on the basis of Blum environment model, Lalonde and Dever revised and completed the environmental health medicine model. They brought up the synthesis health medicine model by health service and policy analysis. It systematically discussed the disease epidemic and sociology related medical model. It was used to guide the development of health career and became the basis of the hygiene policy.

3. The main influence factor of the disease and health

According to modern medicine's model guiding principle, the factors affecting the human health are as follows:

(1) Environmental factor

The human health and disease always have correlation with environmental factors. Harmful factor can cause the disease that influences the health of people. The contamination of water, air, food, etc., the occupation hazards produced in environment, the noise and unsafe highway design, etc. all constitute to threaten human health. Although people have reformed outside world, the new risk factors will continuously form. In older industries, tens of thousands of chemically synthesized material productions have become the serious threats to human health.

The social environments include the income, living condition, and nutritional status, and culture degree. It will have an important role to human health. The poor faces the risk of health that exceeds the wealth they can spend on their health. The work tension, life pressure and the contradiction in social interaction can hazard people's health.

(2) Lifestyle and behavior factor

Smoking, alcoholism, drug abuse, lack of physical exercise, irrational eating habit, bad lifestyle and bad sexual behavior can directly and indirectly influence human's health. Among the top 10 causes of death in USA, 7 causes of death have correlation with lifestyle and behavior factors. When we change the lifestyle and behavior, say quiting smoking, temperance, taking part in physical exercise, reasonable nourishment, keeping optimistic emotion, we can obviously decrease the incidence rate and mortality from cardiac disease.

(3) Organism genetic factor

Some diseases such as hemophilia, sickle cell anemia, favism, psyche dementia, etc. directly correlate with genetic factor. Psychonosema disease, diabetes mellitus, and some tumor cardiac diseases are the comprehensive effect of genetic factor, environmental factor, life style and behavior.

(4) Medical health service factor

The aim of medical health service is prevention of disease, keeping salubrity, reducing incidence rate and mortality, elongating life span. The health service level will directly influence human health. Whether the medical health institution distribution is reasonable, receiving medical treatment is prompt and convenient, and medicine technical level and health service quality is good or not will affect the variety of health and disease. So the role of medicine health system cannot be neglected.

According to this model, we classify the main cause of death in the globe. In 1994, the research of WHO shows that 60% of death was due to behavior or lifestyle, 17% attributed to environmental factor, 15% because of biological factor and 8% health service. It is clear that the behavior or lifestyle has become the main risk to cause death and it is objective evidence of new medical model.

4. Bio-psycho-social medical model

After a long period of studying and practicing, in 1977 New York State Rochester University psychiatry and internal medicine professor Engel brought up that biomedical model should gradually turn into bio-psycho-social medical model. So bio-psycho-social is called Engel Model. The bio-psycho-social model is based on the principle of system theory. They include disease, patient and environment. The environment also includes nature environment and social circumstances. In this system frame we can take health or disease to think from the atom, molecule, cell, tissue, tissue system to person, and the conceptualized nature system in contact with person, family, community, mankind. In this system, there is no more dualism and recovery theory of linear cause and effect model, synergy restriction model. The health is the high level coordination between inside and outside system. The recruitment in health represents coordination in a new different system. Figure 2-1 and 2-2 cases reflect the maladjustment of the sub-atom level and the social level in bio-psycho-social medical model system performance.

society, nation	→	distribution welfare policy
↑ culture	→	value challenge, treatment patient and the other purposes of resources
↑ community	→	the resources transfer to use to cure the patient
↑ family	→	the emotion due to sufferings
↑ person	→	people cannot proceed to sophisticate and coordination activity in mind and body

↑ system	→	nervous system function be damaged
↑ organ	→	the growth be hindered
↑ tissue	→	show the morphologic change
↑ cell	→	lack of differentiation instruction
↑ organelle	→	chromosome gene mutation
↑ molecule	→	DNA template change
↑ sub-atom	→	gamete be radiated

Figure 2-1   The mind and body hypoevolution by radiation evoke gamete mutation

↓ society, national	→	decision to stop making the airplane
↓ culture	→	the value challenges, loyal government and the need of employment
↓ community	→	lose the income
↓ family	→	the tension in economic and emotions
↓ person	→	establishments of new values, reemployment study and new life style
↓ system	→	the environment input rhythm be damaged
↓ organ	→	the nerve organ be suppressed
↓ tissue	→	symptoms, physical sign such as insomnia, ache, apprehension
↓ cell	→	nerve cell chromosome changes
↓ organelle	→	chromosome morphologic change

Figure 2-2   Body and mind disease caused by the unemployment in enginear

The bio-psycho-social medical model shows that each layer system is constituted by lower level system and it is also a part constituting higher level of structure. Each level has some interactions that include upward and downward role of cause and effect. Any level of structure transformation would affect the whole system. The bio-psycho-social medical model would explain this kind of wider sense of a term as biosphere.

5. The health view of bio-psycho-social medical model

The health view is based on the foundation of certain medical model, and changes with the renewal of the medical model. It researches the contact of health and disease, and is the essential cognition of health and disease.

The change among organism and the disturbance of balance among host, pathogenic factor and environment lead to the happening and spread of communicable disease. People lose health after they have communicable disease, but regain it when communicable disease is cured. This kind of disease view, which is based on the happening, change and result of disease, is the expression form of single cause single effect disease. "Having no disease" is a negative health view, which belongs to biomedical model.

After disease pattern and cause of death pattern have changed, many uncommunicable disease, chronic disease and some regressive diseases increased gradually. Most of them are heart disease, cerebrovascular disease and malignant tumor. To prevent and cure these diseases is not the same as communicable disease. We should prevent and cure various factors, which lead to disease. These disease forms of multiple cause-single effect and multiple cause-multiple effect have complicated cause and effect relationship. To get rid of these diseases, we should more or mainly depend on social prevention, decrease and exclude various health risk factors to reach balance of individual body and mental, at the same time keep coordinate with environment. And we can't purely rely on treatment. World Health Organization has posed that "Health is a perfect state of body, psychology and society, but does not just mean having no disease or weakness." According to this active health view, health can be comprehended as a concept, which is composed by biology, psychology and sociology. From the angle of organism, health is judged by whether the function and each index of organs are normal or not; from the angle of mental and spirit, individual health is judged by whether he has the ability of controlling himself or not, whether he can treat outside influence correctly or not, and whether he is in a state of heart equilibrium or not; and from sociology angle, health mainly refers to individual social adaptability, good habit of living and work, human relationship and the ability of coping various sudden affairs. At the same time, the concept of disease is revised, too. According to Engel, "Disease refers to the failure or maladjustment of the whole living creature or other system in the process of growing, developing, function and adjustment." Limitation of this definition is apparent. Disease, illness and sickness are different. Disease is a pathological state (organism scale). Illness is the way patient illustrates pathological state (feeling scale). But sickness is a reaction when patient faces pathologic state (action scale). For each person, the feeling of the disease is an important aspect, but response and action of patient are also important. In fact, definitions of health and disease from different angles are distinguishable. Table 2-4 enumerates definitions of health and disease from different schools of thought and different angles.

Table 2-4　definitions of health and disease

Standpoint	Health	Disease
Physiology or biology	Good condition of body	Refer to a medical concept, it indicates functional and/or structural abnormality of a part, process, system of body
Epidemiology	The condition that host can resist pathogenic factors in environment	The condition that host is apt to be infected by pathogenic factors in environment

(Table 2-4)

Standpoint	Health	Disease
Ecology	The product of harmonic relationship between human being and ecosystem	The result of relationship between human being and ecosystem which isn't fit and harmonic
Sociology	A person in a community be considered that his body and behavior are normal	Individual deviates from normal state of body and /or behavior
Consumer	A kind of merchandise investment, which can be bought in a way	A kind of abnormal situation, which can be treated, controlled and cured by purchasing health service
Statistics	Measure result within the scope of normal value	Measure result beyond the scope of normal value

Concepts of health and disease are the core performance of medical model and the focal point of dispute from beginning to end. Besides relativity standpoint about health and disease, it has derived concepts such as subhealth, subclinical disease, in recent years.

①Relative concept about health and disease. All the organism will be ill, and will experience the process of growing, ageing and death. So health and disease can be regarded as a continuous unity or yardstick. Good health exists on one end, while death on the other end. Each person has a position at a place between the two ends, and the position will change with the pass of time.

②The situation of subhealth. It is a new concept raised by international medical field in recent years. It means that organism has no obvious disease, but presents a physiological condition of decreasing vitality and different reductions of adaptability. It is led by the lowering of physiology function and metabolic process of each system. It is a situation of decreased physiology function and between health and disease. So it is also called "the third state" or "grey state". The category to recognize this state is very extensive. The unfit feeling of body or mental, which can't be diagnosed exactly in a long time, can be both summarized in it. From clinical works of preventive medicine, clinical medicine, particularly spirit and mental medicine, it is found that the number of people who are in this kind of condition is huge. Senility, fatigue syndrome, neurasthenia and menopause syndrome all belong to the category of subhealth state.

The condition of subhealth is mainly caused by the degradation of the function of human body's organs. Patients only feel unwell of body or mental, such as mental uneasy, headache, tightly closed breast, insomnia, diet below the mark, etc. But they have no positive results after various apparatus and chemical checks. The condition of subhealth will probably develop into several diseases. Medicine barely notices people with the existence of subhealth. It needs a deep research in the medical field, which is beyond century.

③Subclinical disease. It is another concept of healthy standpoint. It's also called "no symptom disease". It believes that disease is a process of biological phenomena whose condition has been changed. In the progress of disease, there is not only organic damage, but also adaptability, compensative physiological reaction. These pathologic reactions and physiological response combine together inevitably in the process of disease, and are a kind of progress and result, which is very difficult to divide artificially. The difference between "subclinical disease" and "the state of subhealth" lies in that the former has no clinical symptom physical sign, but has clinical examination basis of physiological compensation and pathologic reaction. For example, some of "non-symptomatic ischemic heart diseases" have no clinical symptom, but they have diagnostic basis such as electrocardiogram changes.

第三章 社会因素与健康

社会因素对健康的影响非常广泛,在疾病的发生、转归和防治过程中起着非常重要的作用。社会因素是指社会的各项构成要素,包括环境、人口和文明程度(政治、经济、文化等)。随着社会经济发展、科学技术进步、居民生活及文化水平提高,人们对健康和疾病的认识在不断深化和发展。世界卫生组织宪章中对健康所下的定义是指身体、心理和社会适应能力的健全状态,而不仅仅是指没有疾病或身体虚弱。世界卫生组织又提出了衡量人体健康10个方面的具体标志:①精力充沛,能从容应付日常生活和工作。②处事乐观,态度积极,乐于承担责任。③善于休息,睡眠良好。④应变能力强,能适应各种环境的变化。⑤对一般感冒和传染病有一定抵抗力。⑥体重适当,体形匀称。⑦眼睛明亮,反应敏锐。⑧牙齿清洁、无缺损、无疼痛。⑨头发光泽、无头屑。⑩肌肉、皮肤富有弹性,走路轻松。不论从个体还是群体分析研究社会因素与健康和疾病之间的关系,都是社会医学最基本的研究内容。

第一节 社会制度与健康

社会制度是指在一定的历史条件下形成的,人们社会关系和行为的相对稳定的规范体系。一般来讲把社会制度分为两类:一类是本原的社会制度,另一类是派生的社会制度。本原的社会制度包括经济制度和家庭制度。派生的社会制度包括政治制度、法律制度、教育制度、宗教制度。社会制度会影响健康,主要途径有以下几个方面。

一、自由、民主的程度会影响健康

在专制社会中,人们言论和行为的自由受到极大程度的限制,即使学术争论也无法正常进行。人们不得不依附于统治阶级,个性受到压抑和摧残,影响了人们的身心健康。

二、医疗卫生保健制度影响健康

卫生保健制度,是指一个国家筹集、分配和使用医疗卫生保健资源,为个人和集体提供防病治病等医疗卫生保健服务的一种综合性措施和制度。卫生保健制度是社会制度的组成部分,一个国家实行哪种卫生保健制度,这种卫生保健制度是什么性质,采取什么具体形式,在很大程度上是由政治制度、经济制度等决定。医疗费用负担的形式主要有三类:一是公费医疗,医疗费用主要由国家支付;二是集资医疗,其主要形式为医疗保险,保险费用的来源又分为个体、集体和国家;三是自费医疗,费用主要由个体支付。我国目前医疗费用的负担形式正处于变革的过程中。享受不同程度医药费减免者在所利用的医疗卫生机构级别及其利用量方面存在明显不同,公费劳保者利用较高级别医疗卫生机构服务的比例、就诊率、住院率、住院天数以及医药费用均明显高于自费医疗者,而且公费劳保者能够获得定期的免费健康检查或疾病普查的机会,有助于及时发现潜在的不良健康问题。

三、社会制度影响人的行为

社会制度是一套规范体系,它把人们的社会活动纳入一定的轨道,以维持社会秩序,保证人类生活的正常进行,这是群体生活的需要。社会制度通过规定行为模式,以提倡或禁止某一行为的方式,把社会所需要的行为模式树立起来,使社会中的个人或群体知道应该怎样做,或不应该怎样做,使人们的社会行为有规可循。社会制度还可以通过理想行为模式的提倡使人们的行为受榜样的影响。社会制度通过调节个人行为而影响健康状况的作用是显而易见的。例如,一夫一妻制既保证人们享受性乐趣的权利,也赋予当事人对家庭和社会必须承担的义务。婚外性生活是感染性病、艾滋病的重要途径。婚外性生活因为直接伤害了自己的配偶,同时也可能对其他家庭成员生产不良影响,因而当事人常采用欺骗、说谎等不诚实手段。一方面受到良心的谴责,产生心灵深处的负罪感,另一方面因为有损自己的人格而丧失自尊,以至于精神涣散、意志消沉。而对性病和怀孕的担心又会形成很大的心理压力。在非婚性关系破裂时,还常引发一系列的感情纠葛和人际冲突,甚至自杀、他杀。我国明确规定严禁赌博。赌博的负面作用不可低估,不少人因赌博而走上犯罪道路,对个人心身健康和社会的危害非常严重。赌博对人体健康损害很大。赌博者高度紧张状态和严重消极情绪交替出现的心理活动,不分昼夜的沉溺于赌博之中的行为使体力和精力大量消耗。时间长了就会产生相应的内脏器官疾病,如高血压、冠心病等。对烟草生产的控制,对食品生产、加工和销售的管理,对吸毒、卖淫嫖娼等行为的禁止,都对维持人群健康产生重要作用。与此同时,社会制度通过教育来培养人们的良好的卫生习惯,宣传疾病预防和治疗的知识等促进人群健康。

第二节　社会经济与健康

经济是人类赖以生存和保持健康的基本条件。一定的经济条件是满足人们的基本需要,包括衣、食、住、行以及卫生保健服务和教育的物质基础,同时涉及生产体制、职业和社会阶层结构、福利与社会保障及其相互联系的社会心理状况。经济发展与人群健康是一种辩证统一的关系。一方面,经济的发展能为大众的健康水平提供物质基础,另一方面,人的健康对生产力的发展和经济的繁荣起着决定性的作用。在一般情况下,人均国民生产总值高的国家,科学技术水平高,劳动条件、营养状况较好,物质文化生活丰富,医疗保健和公共设施完善,有利于改善人群健康状况,提高人群健康水平。

一、经济发展水平与健康

统计资料表明,一个国家、一个地区的经济发展水平与居民健康之间具有非常密切的关系,这可以从时间跨度和地区跨度两个方面进行分析。从时间跨度看,第二次世界大战之后,随着世界各国经济的迅速发展,生物医学技术不断进步,人类平均期望寿命在短短的50年间有了很大的提高,全世界人口的平均寿命从1950年的48岁提高到2000年的67岁。中国人口的平均寿命从1950年的38岁提高到2000年的71岁。新中国成立后,随着社会经济发展,医疗卫生事业进步和人民生活水平的提高,中国人口死亡率明显下降,成为世界上死亡率下降速度最快的国家之一。1949年中国人口死亡率高达20‰,1990年已下降到6.28‰。与此同时,疾病谱和死亡原因谱也发生了重大的改变,在发达国家,慢性非传染性疾病如心血管疾病、脑血管病、恶性肿瘤已取代急性传染性疾病成为主要的死亡原因,在发展中国家,也已经或正在发生这样的转变。从地区跨度看,与发达国家比较,发展中国家的健康状况则要差得多。社会经济因素不仅可以直接影响居民健康状况,而且可以通过卫生服务间接地对居民的健康产生影响,不同的社会经济发展水平是造成不同国家居民健康水平差异的一个重要原因。据1985年我国农村卫生服务抽样调查结果,贫困居民组人年均就诊2.3次,温饱组为2.6次,宽裕组为3.2次,小康组为2.6次。人均年收入在200元以下者的年均住院天数为0.44天,200~299元者为0.34天,300~399元者为0.37天,400~499元者为0.78天,500元及以上者为0.52天。可见随着社会经济及文化的发展、生活水平的提高,人们对卫生服务的需要量和利用量会明显增加,并提出新的需求。

二、经济地位与健康

社会经济地位是影响一个人健康状况和期望寿命的最具有决定性的因素。社会经济地位包括收入水平、职业地位或声望和受教育水平。每个指标都可以从一个侧面反映一个人在社会结构中的地位。在健康和疾病状况的研究中,收入水平反映一个人的消费能力、住院条件、营养状况和医疗保健状况;职业可以反映一个人的社会地位、责任感、体力活动情况和与工作相关的健康风险的情况;受教育程度代表一个人获取积极的社会、心理和经济资源的能力。良好健康状况的最重要的决定性因素应该是受教育程度。受教育程度高的人总体上更了解健康生活方式的优点和预防保健的重要性,当他们出现健康问题时,他们能够更好地获得医疗服务。总之,良好的教育能促使人活得更健康,也能提高一个人解决问题的能力。例如,芬兰社会学家伊尔罗·拉荷马和塔帕尼·瓦尔科南在芬兰、丹麦、瑞典、英格兰和威尔士、挪威和匈牙利进行的有关健康状况的研究发现,在一个国家中,受教育程度最低的人群的死亡率最高。另外,一项在美国进行的重要研究发现,受教育程度高的人群与受教育程度低的人群相比,前者对于自己的生活和健康状况具有更大的调控力。受教育程度高的人通常较少吸烟,更多地参加体育锻炼,经常找医生进行体检,而且饮酒比较适量。

三、经济发展影响健康的途径

经济发展影响健康的主要途径有:①提供人们生活所必需的营养条件。评价居民营养状况包括居民摄入热量及食物的营养结构。前者是衡量人群摄入的食物能否能维持基本生命功能;后者则是分析摄入食物中各种营养比例的合理性。从世界范围来看,不同国家居民日平均摄入热量与健康状况关系密切。居民食物摄入量与平均期望寿命呈正相关。摄入的营养合理,就可防止疾病,促进健康。人均蛋白质、脂肪、碳水化合物三大营养素摄入的适合比例为 3:4:13。其中蛋白质以动物蛋白及植物蛋白各占 50% 为宜。这种标准既能保证机体对各种营养素的需要,又有利于预防常见的慢性病,如心血管疾病等。目前,发达国家居民膳食中,动物蛋白及脂肪的含量偏高;而发展中国家及不发达国家居民膳食中蛋白质及脂肪比例偏低。②保证了基本医疗保健费用的投入。③为人们的工作和生活提供较好的环境。

四、经济发展带来的新的健康问题

经济发展促进了人类健康水平的提高,同时也给人类带来了新的健康问题,主要表现在以下几个方面:①环境被污染和破坏。由于工农业生产和人群集居等活动对自然环境施加影响而造成的物理、化学以及部分生物因素,必然作用于人体,直接或间接影响人类健康。②生活方式的改变。交通运输发达,以车代步,走路减少;食品细化,使某些营养素丧失,消化功能减弱。出现诸如电视病、空调综合征、化妆品皮炎等新型疾病。③人口流动。经济发展必然伴随流动人口的增加,走亲访友、旅游、经商等活动增加。随着人口流动增加以及由此而导致的传染病发病率的增加,如"红眼病"、肝炎、传染性皮肤病等,给城市居民健康带来威胁。④心理问题。随着生产力水平的提高,知识经济时代的到来,社会竞争更加激烈,紧张、刺激及工作压力,使人们产生了不良的心理问题。

第三节 社会文化与健康

世界卫生组织在第六次报告中指出:"一旦人们的生活水平超过起码的需求,有条件决定生活资料的使用方式,文化因素对健康的作用就越来越重要了。"文化是人类社会特有的现象,美国文化人类家和社会学教授克来得·克鲁克洪说:"文化是无处不在的",它影响着人们的思维和行为,影响着健康。据世界卫生组织疾病监测中心统计,结核病、流感、肝炎、糖尿病、脑血管疾病、冠心病等常见病和多发病的死亡率与文化素养有着千丝万缕的联系。文化程度越高,患这些疾病的死亡率越低。挪威对冠心病的研究结果是最好的佐证,其研究发现,受教育时间短者,患冠心病的危险性比受教育时间长者高 2.3 倍。父母文化程度的高低也会对孩子产生影响。据有关资料报告,文盲妇女的婴儿死亡率是受过 10 年以上教育妇女的 2.5 倍。在美国,受过 16 年以上教育的母亲,生育低体重儿的比例要比受教育 9 年以下的母亲低 50% 左右。文化的内容非常广泛,明确文化的概念、类型、特点,才能认识文化因素由于健康之间的关系以及文化诸现象对健康的影响。

一、文化的概念、特性与功能

文化,英文是culture,广义的文化是指社会物质财富和精神财富的总和。狭义的文化即观念形态的文化,包括思想意识、道德规范、宗教信仰、哲学、艺术、习俗等所构成的领域。社会医学主要从狭义的文化概念出发,研究文化对健康的影响。

文化具有以下特点:①文化的超生理性和超个人性。所谓文化的超生理性,指任何文化都是人们后天习得和创造的,文化不能通过生理遗传。所谓文化的超个人性,指个人只有在与他人的互动中才需要文化、接受文化、影响文化。②文化的复合性。任何文化现象都不是孤立存在的,而是由多种文化要素复合在一起的。③文化的象征性。即文化现象具有广泛的意义,文化的意义要超出文化现象所直接表现的那个狭小的范围。④文化的传递性。即文化一经产生就要被他人模仿、效法、利用。⑤文化的变迁与文化堕距。文化不是静止不动的,而是时刻处于变化之中。

文化在社会上发挥重大的作用:①文化是社会或民族分野的标志。在不同的国家、民族或群体之间,文化所表现的区别要比人类的皮肤颜色或任何其他生理现象所表现的区别深刻得多。②文化有了系统的行为规范。有了文化,人类便有了行为标准。文化使人们相互间的行为功能协调和相互配合。③文化使社会团结有了重要的基础。有了社会要素还不等于一个社会,社会要素之所以能构成社会是靠了文化的联系作用。④文化塑造了社会的人。人由生物人转变为社会的人,最主要的就是一步步接受了文化。

二、文化诸现象与健康

文化因素对健康的影响常持续于生命的整个过程,甚至几代人或更长时间。哲学、教育、道德、风俗习惯、宗教信仰等文化现象对健康的影响不是仅限于个人,而是整个人群,它的广泛程度要大于生物、自然因素。

(一)哲学与健康

阴阳学说是中国古代的哲学思想。阴阳对立统一交互作用,是宇宙运动变化的源泉,是万物发生和变化的根源。阴阳学说是中医学整体观念的理论基础。中医学认为人体的健康和疾病,是在自然界大环境中进行的。阴阳对立统一的协调平衡,使自然界的人体处于相对稳定的状态,是人类生存和健康的必需条件。阴阳失去平衡,自然界就要发生自然灾害,人体就要生病。人无论是饮食起居、精神调摄、自我锻炼、药物作用都离不开协调平衡阴阳的宗旨,人的衰老,或为阴虚,或为阳虚,或阴阳俱虚。阴虚则阳亢,阳盛则阴虚,阴盛则阳病,阳盛则阴病。故防治衰老,贵在调和阴阳达到平衡。在中国哲学"天人合一"思想的影响下,中医主张把天文、地理、人事作为一个整体看待。人既是自然的人,又是社会的人。因此,影响健康和疾病的因素,既有生物因素,又有社会和心理的因素。

(二)教育与健康

教育水平是反映一个国家和民族文化水平及素质的重要指标。教育有助于感知疾病,改变不良的传统习惯,参与社会卫生和提高卫生服务的利用,使人们对生活中的危险因素具有更好的辨别能力。飞速发展的社会,要求生活在社会中的人不断调整自己的生活方式,造就新的生活技能,这样才能成为健康地生活于现代社会中的社会人。有人对不同受教育水平的国家进行比较,发现教育水平与健康水平呈现一定的正相关趋势。我国某地区的调查表明,在30~50岁年龄组的人群中教育程度与死亡率的关系是:大学文化程度组为0.36%,小学文化程度组为1.03%,文盲与半文盲组高达11.4%,是大学文化程度组的31倍之多。此外,受教育水平不但与自身的健康有着密切的关系,且对下一代健康也有明显的影响。据对106个国家的统计,母亲受教育水平与婴儿及儿童的死亡率有着很大的影响,受过教育的母亲,则其婴儿和儿童的死亡率低,其主要原因可能是:受教育的妇女容易放弃传统的观念,接受科学的儿童保健知识;易准确表达自己的思想,与医护人员沟通。

(三)音乐与健康

美国音乐治疗之父Gaston指出:"音乐是人类的感觉,这不仅仅因为人类创造了它,还因为人类创造了与它的关系。音乐是一个人类必不可少和有效的功能,它在几千年中影响着人类的行为和自身条件。"

不同的音乐可以使人的生理产生不同的反应,如心率和脉搏的速度、血压、肌肉电位和运动反应、皮肤电位反应、内分泌和体内生化物质(肾上腺素、去甲肾上腺素、内啡肽、免疫球蛋白)以及脑电波等等。音乐的节奏可以明显地影响人的行为节奏和生理节奏,例如呼吸速度、运动速度节奏、心率。不同的音乐可以引起不同的情绪反应。2000年8月16日,第三军医大学新桥医院成功地完成国内首例、国际第三例胸腹连体婴儿分离术。在整整8小时的手术中,电影《泰坦尼克》的主题曲一直在手术室回荡,事后就有医生说:"当优美的音乐响起时,我感到轻松自如。"同时音乐也是一种独特的交流形式,它是非语言的。Gaston指出:"音乐的力量和价值正在于它的非语言的内涵。"音乐的这一交流特点对于临床治疗来说是关键的重要因素,特别是当语言的努力归于失败时,音乐可以帮助建立起良好的医患关系,而这一关系正是治疗成功的基本动力。另外,由于音乐是一种存在于时间里和由物理结构形成的一种现实存在。这一现实存在是可以被听到、感到、测量到、用图表和符号表示出来的,因此音乐可以成为一个有效的媒介来帮助那些从现实和社会中退缩出来的病人重新回到现实世界中,建立起与外部现实世界的联系。

(四)风俗习惯与健康

风俗是指代代相延后而形成的风尚及习惯。风俗习惯是与人群健康联系最为密切的文化范畴,这是因为它与人的日常生活联系最为紧密,涉及人的衣、食、住、行等各个环节,良好的风俗习惯有益健康,不良的风俗习惯将直接危及和影响人群的健康。"非典"出现以后人们开始反思某些不良习惯,如西方人的分餐进食方式就比围坐一桌共享菜肴卫生得多,共食虽在一定程度上能密切感情、交流思想,但很容易传播某些疾病,弊大于利。又如随地吐痰,痰会传播许多疾病,危害甚大。痰是肺泡、支气管和气管的分泌物。某些细菌、病毒等病原微生物,在痰中能生存很长时间,成为传染病的源头之一。仅以肺结核为例,有学者报告,在一口痰里竟有5 000多万个结核杆菌;在患者一天所吐的痰中,结核杆菌可高达30多亿个。江苏省某医院曾调查过一个可容纳3 000多人的会场,在两个多小时的大会之后,发现痰迹800多处,从中取出91份痰液检查,就查到4份带有结核菌。结核菌在痰中的生存能力很强,在阴暗角落里可生存6~8个月,在6℃~10℃环境中可存活数月至数年,在阳光直射下也能活一天左右。痰干燥之后,被风刮起,可形成4~5 μm

的尘埃在空中漂浮,这种尘埃飞沫若被健康人吸入,就会感染肺结核。

(五)道德与健康

道德是调整人与人之间以及个人与社会之间的行为规范的总和,是一种依靠社会舆论、个人信仰、习惯和教育来起作用的精神力量。优秀的道德对人类健康和生存起着保护作用。中国健康教育研究所朱琪先生在《性与健康》中写道:泰国于1984年,中国于1985年,相继发现第一例境外传入的艾滋病患者,经过10余年的流行后,到1996年,泰国公布有85万艾滋病病毒感染者,而中国至1996年6月仅检测出5 157例感染者。所以泰国的流行速度是中国的200倍。在预防和控制艾滋病措施的力度上,泰国则明显比中国强。以经费投入为例,1996年泰国用于防治艾滋病的经费为8 230万美元,而中国为2 000多万人民币。按人口计算,泰国是中国的640倍。为什么泰国投入多而收效小,中国投入少而收效大呢?朱琪认为这就是传统道德的作用。他说,传统性道德是预防和控制艾滋病的巨大卫生资源和最有效的预防措施。

(六)宗教与健康

宗教是统治人们的自然力量和社会力量在人们头脑中的虚幻的、颠倒的反映,是由超自然实体即神灵的信仰和崇拜来支配人们命运的一种社会意识形态。宗教对健康的影响有积极的一面,也有消极的一面。宗教有心理调节功能,即通过特定的宗教信念把人们原来心态上的不平衡调节到相对平衡的心理状态,并由此使人们在精神上行为上和生理上达到有益的适度状态。不少西方学者把这种心理的调节功能称为信仰治疗,对健康有利。宗教的某些规定对健康也有积极作用,如犹太教对男性婴儿都要举行割礼,即包皮环切仪式,因此,犹太人几乎没有阴茎癌。但教徒的盲目信仰对健康也会带来危害。例如世界上曾发生过六次古典霍乱大流行,每次都源于印度。主要原因就是印度教教徒视恒河为"圣河",认为生前能饮其水,死后能用水浴身,便能除去一切罪孽。因此恒河水终年污染严重。时至今日,印度仍是霍乱威胁世界的疫源地。

第四节 社会心理、行为与健康

随着社会政治、经济、文化等的发展,社会心理对人类健康的影响越来越引起人们的重视。儒家创始人孔子曾提出一个著名的命题"仁者寿",这是中国古代最早的具有理论形态的养生学命题。在孔子看来,心平气和,才能延年益寿。这里,既讲了人的修养,又讲了人的健康,并把人的修养水平、精神状态作为健康的首要因素。养心的具体要求很多,其中较重要的一条是掌握"中庸"原则,以保持平衡的心态。人人都有喜怒哀乐的情感,无论这些情感是潜藏在心里,还是表现出来,都应使其适当适度,这就叫"中"、"和",凡是能以"中和"规范自己的人,就不会喜怒无常、哀乐失控,从而创造出一种使人与人、人与物相互统一的和谐气氛。这种和谐气氛下的心态平衡,对健康是极其有益的。马克思也说过:"一种美好的心情,比十服良药更能解除生理上的疲惫和痛楚。"好心情有助于防病防癌,好心情来源于人对客观事物的理解,好的情绪状态使大脑及下丘脑等神经系统通过激素、神经肽、神经递质等信息分子,作用于内分泌、旁分泌、神经分泌、自分泌等,影响免疫细胞,使其增强免疫功能,这对防病防癌非常有利。

社会心理因素是心身疾病发病的主要因素,是人们心理紧张对躯体作用的结果。如社会动乱、战争、自然灾害、瘟疫流行等,造成社会成员的精神紧张,从而引起心身疾病。社会医学把这种社会刺激因素叫做社会心理致病因素。由于社会心理因素的作用而引起的心身疾病,现已有十几种,最常见的心身疾病有冠心病、高血压、支气管哮喘、溃疡病、恶性肿瘤等。另外,社会心理因素也是导致精神病发作和自杀的重要原因。目前我国每年有近200万人自杀未遂,至少有25万人自杀死亡,自杀现已成为我国第五大死亡原因。这种给亲友带来难以愈合的心理创伤,同时带给社会巨大影响的死亡方式,由不受重视变成了不容忽视的重大公共卫生问题。随着世界卫生组织确定的2003年9月10日为首次世界预防自杀日,表明我国针对各类心理危机及预防自杀问题的心理干预也进入了新阶段。

人的行为是具有认识、思维能力的人对环境刺激所做出的能动反应。广义的行为分为内在行为和外显行为。内在行为即人的心理活动过程。外显行为是可以被人观察到的行为,如言谈举止。一般所谈的行为主要是指外显行为。要不断地认识、评价促进健康的行为和危害健康的行为,提倡健康行为,避免危害健康的行为。

(一)促进健康的行为

促进健康的行为是指个人或群体表现出的在客观上促进或有利于健康的一组行为群。对日常生活中的各种促进健康行为,有一定的判断标准,其主要依据为以下五大基本特征。①有利性。行为表现有益于自己、他人和全社会,如不抽烟、不酗酒。②规律性。行为表现有恒常的规律,如定餐。③和谐性。个体的行为表现有自己鲜明的个性(如选择运动项目),又能根据整体环境随时调整自身行为。④一致性。行为本身具有外显性,但它与内心的心理情绪是一致的。⑤适宜性。行为强度有理性控制,无明显的冲动表现。

从个体健康行为的角度,普遍认为以下几种行为有利于健康。①合理膳食。所谓合理膳食就是指膳食要符合个体生长发育和生理状态等特点,含有人体所需要的各种营养成分,且含量适当,全面满足身体的需要,能维持正常的生理功能,促进生长发育和健康。此外合理营养还要求食物易于消化,不含对机体有害的物质。②适度运动。运动有利于锻炼和增强人体各系统、各器官的功能;能增加肺活量,改善呼吸系统的功能;能促进肌肉发育,推迟骨关节、肌肉的老年性变化;能提高思维和反应能力,使神经系统处于良好状态;能改善消化系统机能,减轻体重,控制肥胖。运动要适度,过度运动容易产生不良后果。在奥林匹克运动的故乡——古希腊山上的岩石上,雕刻了这样的几句话:"你想变得健康吗?你就跑步吧!你想变得聪明吗?你就跑步吗!你想变得美丽吗?你就跑步吧!"③善于休息。精神焦虑和极度疲劳是催人早衰的重要因素。消除疲劳的方法主要有起居有序、适当放慢生活节奏、善于休息、主动变化行为方式等。

(二)危害健康的行为

危害健康的行为有三个特点:一是长期稳定的行为,如偶尔某天高盐饮食或抽一支烟不一定对健康造成危害。二是后天生活的习惯,是自愿的。三是有明显的健康危害。主要有以下几种。①不良生活习惯。表现在不良饮食习惯、缺乏运动等方面。②不良嗜好行为。表现在吸烟、酗酒等方面。世界卫生组织曾提出这样口号:"要吸烟还是要健康,任君选择。"这种选择当然是自由的,不过考虑到自身、家人和周围的人的健康和幸福,还是应戒烟。吸烟可引起癌症、心脑血管疾病、慢性支气管炎和肺气肿等多种疾病,同时还威胁周围不吸烟者的身体健康。因此,吸烟被世界卫生组织称为严重威胁人类健康的20世纪的瘟神。③成瘾行为。即不是由于医疗需要,个体出现强烈、被迫地连续或周期性地求得使用某种有害物质的行为,如吸毒。(4)不良性行为。

案例

在音乐中获得新生
——一个对抑郁症的音乐治疗案例报告

A女士,34岁,已婚,大学毕业,现为外企职员。她身材消瘦,愁云笼罩着一张苍白的脸,美丽的眼睛却暗淡无光。她在述说情况时面部始终没有表情,但我仍然可以从她的眼睛深处看到一种深深的悲哀。她告诉我,她从上初中时就开始了抑郁状态,情绪总是很低落,尽管学习成绩很好,但仍然充满了自卑,觉得自己不如别人,她7岁时曾自杀未遂。现在常有自杀的念头,但没有胆量实施,所以很羡慕那些已经自杀的人,觉得他们很勇敢。

根据她的情况,我诊断为抑郁症。根据弗洛伊德的精神分析理论,抑郁症的问题起源应在幼年时期,因此我又询问了关于母亲的情况。她说,母亲在自己出生不久就患了精神分裂症,在她仅7岁时就去世了。现在,母亲是什么样子都不记得了,跟母亲的那一段生活也不记得了。我决定把对童年经历的探索作为治疗的重点。我的治疗方法是先在缓慢放松的音乐背景下对A女士进行催眠,在她进入催眠状态后开始播放特别编排的音乐。这些音乐都是从世界经典作品中节选出来,然后又组合在一起的。在播放音乐的同时,引导她产生对童年生活场景的回忆。治疗每周一次。最后一次是第19次治疗,我引导她在优美的音乐中来到一片湖水旁,看看水中自己的倒影,因为这样可以反映出她对自己的认识和接受程度。

"我看到了草地上一片湖水,有点犹豫,想过去看看。(流泪)看到了自己在湖水里,白白的,挺文静的样子,为什么别人会不喜欢自己?他们为什么从小就告诉我,说我这么丑,这么坏?我觉得不管别人怎么说,我都要爱护自己。我下了决心,任何人说什么也阻止不了我。我要自己对得起自己。……我向草地上走去,心里挺宁静的,但是有点害怕。(我问:怕什么?)可能是怕别人。他们不许我爱自己,他们都告诉我自己是不重要的,他们总是用各种方法摧残我……我下定决心,不接受别人对我的侵犯,我要对自己好一点,为自己做些事情(流泪)……"

一个月后,A女士高兴地在电话中告诉我:"昨天早上我一出门,看到天空那么晴朗,阳光那么温暖,听到小鸟在歌唱,我心中突然冒出了一句话:'生活这么美好。'自己真的好感动,因为我从小到大从没有这种感觉。"从一个觉得自己"罪孽深重",活在世上"恬不知耻"的人成为接受自己、热爱生活的人,这是一个多么令人高兴的变化。我深深地为她祝福。

Chapter 3   Social Factors and Health

Social factors have a wide impact on health and play a crucial role in the course of disease like occurrence, outcome, prevention and treatment. Social factors are elements of all kinds of social components, which include environment, population and level of civilization (politics, economics and culture, etc.). With the development of social economy, the advancement of science and technology and the improvement of living and cultural level, people gradually deepen and develop the cognition of health and disease. The World Health Organization (WHO), in its constitutions, defines health as follows: health is a state of completely physical, mental and social well-being and not merely an absence of disease or infirmity. WHO also refers to detailed sign of 10 aspects which are used to assess personal health: (1) when a person has good energy and can respond to the varied experiences of life and work with flexibility; (2) when a person faces problems optimistically, has positive attitude and has courage to take on responsibility; (3) he is able to coordinate his life and to get good rest and high quality sleep; (4) he is well-adjusted and is able to adapt all kinds of environment; (5) he has some immunity to common cold and infectious disease; (6) weight is within the range of "normality" for the individual age and sex. Body structure is well; (7) he has good eyesight and brisk reaction; (8) he has clean teeth without absence and ache; (9) he has lustrous hair without scurf; (10) he has stretch skin and muscle and can easily coordinate bodily movements. It is always the basic content of social medicine to analyze and whether studying the relationship between social factors and health is based on individual or population.

Section 1   Social System and Health

Social system is a regular system formed under certain historical condition, in which the social relationships and actions of people are relatively stable. Generally speaking, social system is commonly divided into two types: one is the original social system, the other is the derived from social system. Original social system includes economy system and family system. Derived one includes politics system, law system, education system and religion system. Social system is able to affect health. There are three main approaches.

1. Degree of liberty and democracy can affect health

In despotic society, people's freedom of saying and behavior was extremely restricted. Even academic dispute was not able to carry out normally. People had to depend on the ruling class. Their personal traits were oppressed and wrecked. These had severely affected people's physical and mental health.

2. Health care system is affected and in turn affects health

Health care system is a synthetic measure and system, which is about how a country collects, allocates and utilizes the health resource, how to provide health service to individual or group as well. Health care system is a part of the social system. The type, quality and concrete form of the health care system are determined by political and economic system to a large extent. There are three ways to pay medicine cost. One is socialized medicine, and the cost for health service is paid by the government. The second one is collective medicine. Medical insurance is its main form. Insurance premium is gained from individual, collectivity and country. The third one is self-pay medicine, and patients pay for health service by themselves. At present, forms of socialized medicine are in the process of reform in our country. For people who enjoy different degrees of reimbursement for health service, the level of health institution and the quantity of health service they utilize are obviously different. For people who enjoy socialized medicine, the proportion, visit rate, hospitalization rate, hospitalization days and fee-for-service in higher medical health facilities are obviously higher than those for people who pay for health service by themselves. These people who enjoy socialized medicine is obviously higher than those who pay money for themselves in the proportion of utilizing high-level health institutions, rate of getting diagnosis, hospitalization rate, hospitalization days and cost for health service. Moreover, people who access socialized medicine are able to have opportunity to regularly get free health examination, which is contributed to discover underlying health problems.

3. Social system affects personal behaviors

Social system is a normative system in which people's social activities are brought into certain orbit to keep social order and guarantee normal life of human, which is necessary for group life. Social system, through regulating certain behavior model, advocating or banning certain behavior, sets up the needed one in society. By doing so, people obtain certain criteria in social behavior to follow so that individual or colony in society knows what should or mustn't be done. Through advocating ideal behavior mode, people's behavior is affected by model. It is obvious that social system affects health through adjusting personal action. For example, monogamy is marriage between one man and one woman. This system not only makes people enjoy right of erotic joy, but also requests the parties are responsible for family and society. Sexual life without marriage is the main approach through which people infect the STDs and AIDS. Sexual life without marriage not only directly damages one's own spouse, but also possibly brings some bad affection to family members. So the party often plays tricks or tells lies. On one hand the party feels guilty in deep heart for suffering self-reproach. On the other hand, the party loses self-esteem for decreasing own selfhood so that he becomes mull grubs and feebleminded. They worry about STDs and pregnancy, which bring huge mental pressure to them. When sexual relationship without marriage breaks, it often brings about a series of feelings problems and conflict, even causing tragedy of suicide or murder. There is unambiguous rule to ban gambling in China. We are not able to underestimate the effect of gambling. Gambling can extremely damage personal mental and physical health and society, even a great many people are willing to commit a crime for gambling. The gamblers experience the alternative psychological activities of high pressure and extreme disappointment, and indulge gambling all day and all night consuming a great deal of physical force and energy. If gamester does like this for a long time, it will bring relevant splanchnic organic disease such as high blood pressure, heart disease, etc. It has important effect on keeping public health to control tobacco production and manage the production, process and distribution of food and ban freak-out and the social evil, etc. Meanwhile social system is able to promote public health through education system to form healthy behavior and propagandize knowledge of disease prevention and treatment.

Section 2 Social Economy and Health

The economy is essential for human beings to survive and keep healthy. Certain economic conditions are necessary to meet the basic needs of humans. Basic needs include clothes, food, shelter, travel, health service and education, and also involve production systems, careers, social stratification, public welfare services, social security and related socio-psychological status. Economic development and population health are dialectically unified in a certain sense. On the one hand economic growth and development can provide the material conditions for people to improve their health standards, and on the other hand good health is a crucial factor for the development of productivity and economic prosperity. Generally speaking countries with a high GDP per capita and having advanced technology, good working conditions, sufficient nutrition, rich and colorful material-culture life, and perfect medical health care and public facilities, substantially contribute to improving population health and raising the standards of people's health.

1. Economic development and health

Worldwide statistics show that the level of economy of a country or a region has close relationships with the health of the local citizens. This finding can be found by an analysis of the relationships in different periods and in different regions. After World

War II, with the rapid economic growth of each country throughout the world and continuing progress of the bio-medical technology, human life expectancy improved significantly over the last fifty years. The life expectancy of the population worldwide rose from 48 in 1948 to 67 in 2000. In China the average life expectancy rose from 38 in 1950 to 71 in 2000. After 1949, with the development of the social economy, medical health care made great progress and the life expectancy rose, resulting in the mortality rate of the Chinese people to manifestly decrease and China became one among those countries with a rapid decline in the mortality rate. In 1949 the Chinese mortality rate was 20‰ but by 1990 it had greatly declined to 6.28‰. Meanwhile the disease spectrum and the death cause spectrum seriously changed. For example, in developed countries, the chronic and incommunicable diseases, such as A, B, C, instead of acute infectious diseases, became the main causes of death, and this has also occurred in developing countries. In comparison with developed countries the health situation in developing countries is far behind. The different economic level is the important factor, which causes this difference of health level in different countries or citizens. According to a sample survey of the countryside health service in 1985 poor citizens consult a doctor 2.3 times per capita, the subsistence citizen 2.6 times, the rich citizen 3.2 times and the well-off citizen 2.6 times. People with an annul income of less than 200 Yuan hospitalize for 0.44 day, those with an annul income of 200 – 299 yuan for 0.34 day, people with an annul income of 300 – 399 yuan for 0.37 day, people with an annul income of 400 – 499 yuan for 0.78 day and people with an annul income of more than 500 yuan for 0.52 day. Obviously with the development of social economy and culture, and improved living standards, people will substantially increase the need and utilization of health services, and in addition increase the demand for these services.

2. Economic status and health

Economic status is the most crucial factor that influences health and life expectancy. Economic status includes income, career status or reputation, and education background. Each indicator can show where a person's social status fits in the social class. In research on the health situation and disease, income reflects the capability of a person for consumption, for hospitalization conditions and for nutrition. Medical health care and career can reflect social status, sense of responsibility. Labor and health risk related to work and education background shows an ability to accept positive social, psychological and economic resources. Education background is a key factor in the importance of good health. Generally speaking the more education people receive the more they realize the benefits of a healthy life-style and the importance of preventive health care, and the better they can receive health services when required. To sum up, a good education background can contribute to a healthier lifestyle and increase the ability to resolve problems. For example, sociologists in Finland, A and B, carried out research on the health situations in Finland, Denmark, Sweden, England, Norway and Hungary and found that the mortality rate of people who received the lowest education is the highest in each country. In addition important research in the US shows that the group with a higher education can better control their own life and health care compared with people with a lower education. Well-educated people generally smoke less, drink moderately, take physical exercise and often see a doctor to take a physical examination.

3. How economic development can influence health

(1) The economy provides essential conditions for nutrition. An evaluation of citizen's nutrition involves energy and the component of nutrients. The former is used to weigh whether the foods taken by the population can meet the needs of basic life activities, and the latter is used to analyze whether the proportion of the nutrients of their foods is reasonable. Throughout the world the average energy taken by people per day is closely related and the amount of food taken by people and the average life expectancy are positively correlated. If people take reasonable nutrients they can prevent disease and promote health. The proper proportion of protein, fat and carbohydrate per capita is 3 : 4 : 13. Among these the quantity of animal protein should equal the quantity of vegetable protein, that is, each share 50%. This standard not only meets the needs of the body's nutrients but also is helpful to preventing the common chronic disease. At present in developed countries the content of animal protein and fat of the citizen's food is a little too high, but in developing countries and underdeveloped countries, the content of protein and fat is a bit too low.

(2) Economic development guarantees that basic medical health care is funded.

(3) Economic development provides people with a good working and living environment.

4. The major health problems caused by the economy

Economic growth and development like anything else has two sides. It promotes health but on the other hand raises the following new health problems:

(1) Environmental pollution and destruction. Because the activities of agriculture and of the population living together affect the environment in a negative way, they result in the physical, chemical and biological factors affecting people, directly or indirectly influencing the health of people.

(2) Changing lifestyles. Because of convenient transportation, people will often use their cars instead of walking. Food quality becomes better and better but many nutrients are lost thus leading to a weaker digestive function. And the new diseases appear, such as disease related with watching TV and syndrome caused by air conditioner, etc.

(3) Migration. Economic development of course is accompanied by increasing num-

bers of migrants, and the activities of meeting relatives and friends, travel and business. In turn, the incidence of infectious diseases rise, such as "red eye", hepatitis, infection skin diseases, etc. , which threaten people's health.

(4) Psychological problems. With a rise in productivity and the advent of the knowledge economic era, social competition becomes more intense which together with stress and working pressures causes many adverse psychological problems.

Section 3 Social Culture and Health

The World Health Organization points out in the sixth report: "Once people's living conditions exceed at least the necessary requirement, and they have conditions to determine how to use living materials, then culture factors become more and more important to health. " Culture is the human beings' special social phenomenon. Professor Keledo Kelukeho, a cultural humanist and sociologist in the United States of America, says, "Culture is everywhere, it affects people's thoughts, activities and their health. " According to statistics of WHO disease inspection center, tuberculosis, flu, hepatitis, cerebrovascular disease, coronary heart disease and other familiar disease's death rate have a strong connection with culture. The higher the degree of culture, the lower the death rate. Research results on CHD completed in Norway give significant evidence to show that people, whose formal education is shorter, have a 2.3 times higher risk to get CHD than those people with a longer time of formal education. Parents' degree of education also has a strong influence on their children. According to related reports, the infants of illiterate women have a 2.5 times higher death rate than those of women who have at least 10 years of formal education. In the United States mothers who have over 16 years of formal education have 50% lesser risk to bear low-weight infants than those mothers who have less than 9 years formal education. The content of culture is very extensive, and to know the concept, type and characteristics of culture can lead to a better understanding of the effects, which cultural factors have on health.

1. Cultural concepts, characteristics and functions

The meaning of culture in the broad sense points to the totality of both social material wealth and spiritual wealth. In the narrow sense the concept of culture consists of thought and consciousness, morals and norms, religion and faith, philosophy, art, and custom. The culture that social medical science is mainly set out from concern the narrow sense studies the influence that culture has on health.

Culture has the following characteristics: (1) the cultures beyond physiology and personal. The so-called culture beyond physiology character is that all cultures are exercised and created by people day by day; the culture can't exceed the physiology heredity.

The so-called culture's beyond-personal character exists only when people are interacting with others, when they need culture, accept culture, and influence culture. (2) Complexity of culture: Any culture phenomenon is not isolated and is reunited by many factors of various cultures together. (3) Symbolist of culture: The culture phenomenon has the extensive meaning; culture meaning must be beyond the narrow and small scope. (4) Delivering of culture: It points out that once culture is produced, it will be copied, followed, and used. (5) Changing of culture and culture lag: The culture is not static and changing every means.

Culture plays a significant role in society. (1) The culture is the mark of the society or race boundary. Among the different nations, races or communities, the differentiation for culture is deeper than that of skin color or any other of physiology phenomenon. (2) Culture contains the system on behavior norm. When there is culture, mankind then have the behavior standard. Culture makes people's behavior function moderately and match each other. (3) Culture is an important base of society to unite together. Social factor not being equal to society, the reason why social factor becomes a society is that society depends upon contact function of culture. (4) The culture molded the society. People become social ones from biological human mostly because they accept culture step by step.

2. Cultural phenomenon and health

The culture factor's influence on health often keeps on in the whole process of life, even several generations or longer time. Philosophy, education, morals, customs and habits, religion and faith, etc. influence health, which is not only limited to individuals, but the whole human being. Its extensive degree is larger than living creature and natural factors.

(1) Philosophy and health

The Yin-Yang theory is a philosophy of ancient China. Yin-Yang is the headspring of move and changes in cosmos and is source of creation and change. The Yin-Yang theory is the base of the whole concept of Chinese traditional medicine. It teaches people to think that human body's health or disease occurs in a big environment of nature. The coordinative balance on the opposition and unification in Yin-Yang makes the body in the relatively stable condition, and is the necessary condition for existence and health of mankind. Once Yin-Yang loses equilibrium, calamity will take place and people will get disease. Regardless of food and living, spirit modulation, exercise, medicine effects all cannot get away from the aim of the equilibrium of Yin-Yang. The person has decrepit because of weak Yin or weak Yang or both. The weak Yin means excessive Yang, and excessive Yang means weak Yin; excessive Yin makes people get Yang disease and excessive Yang makes people get Yin disease. Hence, prevention and treatment of decrepitude lie in adjusting Yin-Yang to attain equilibrium. Under the Chinese philosophy, nature and man are united as one thought's influence. The Chinese medicine supports considering astronomy, geography and person as a united one. Person is not only natural, but also a social one. Therefore, the factors influencing health and disease are not only within the biological factor, but also social factor and mental factor.

(2) Education and health

The education level reflects a nation with an important index of the level and character of race culture. The education is beneficial toes to know the disease, and to change bad traditional habit, participates in social sanitation and increases its efficiency, and makes people have the better discriminating ability to dangerous factor within life. A quickly developing society requests that who develop in the society continuously adjust their own life style, educate them new living techniques, and only they become healthily living-in-social people within modern society. Someone has made comparison of different education levels within different nations and discovered that education level and health level are relative. According to the inquisition of the certain area, the relation between education and death rate of 30 – 50 years-old group is: University culture degree set the death rate is 0.36%, grade school culture degree set is 1.03%, illiteracy and half illiteracy's set is high up to 11.4%, and is 31 times of university culture degree set. In addition, level of education not only has close relation with oneself, but also influences the next generation health. According to statistic of 106 nations, the influence of mothers' education upon infant and child's death rate is very great. Educated mothers' infant death rate is low. Its main reason may be that educated women are easy to abandon traditional idea, and accept scientific child-health-care knowledge, easily express their own thought, and communicate with medical personals.

(3) Music and health

Gaston, who is American music-treating father, points out: "The music is a kind of human feeling, and this is not only because mankind creates it, but also because mankind develops the relation with it." Music has an essential and official function for mankind, and it is music that influences people's behavior and oneself during several thousand years.

Different music can produce the different physiology reaction, such as the heart rate and pulse speed, blood pressure, muscle potential and sport response, the skin electric potential response, the endocrine and bio-chemicals (adrenaline, AN, adrenaline, immunity globulin) and brain wave, etc. The music's rhythm can clearly affect the person's behavior rhythm along with the physiological rhythm, for example, breathing rate, sport rhythm, and heart rate. The different music can cause very different motion reactions. On August 16, 2000, the New Bridge Hospital of the Third Military Medical University successfully completed the local head, chest and belly Siamese twin separation, which was the third of its kind in the world. During 8 hours' operation, the theme song of movie *Titanic* was played in the operating room. After the event, a doctor said: "When beautiful song is played, I feel relaxed. " Music is also a special communication; it's right and wrong at the same time. The Gaston points out: "the music's power consists in its non-phonetic connotation. " The characteristics of music plays a key role in the clinical treatment especially when the effort of language fails, the music is in aid of establishing good doctor-patient relation, and this relation is exactly the basic motive to treat successively. Moreover, the music exists with time and physical construction. This reality exists and can be heard, felt, measured, and represented with sign and chart, and for this reason music can become a valid medium to help those patients who draw back from reality and society to come back to real world and establish the contacts with reality of the external world.

(4) Customs and habits and health

The customs are formed from the vogue and habits continuing from generations to generations. They contact most with the population health, and this is because they contact with the person's daily life closely, dealing with clothing, food, shelter and travel and various coaches. Good habits are beneficial to health and bad ones will directly do harm to crowds' health. When SARS emerged, people began to think over some bad habits. For example, western meal taking is better, compared with round sitting at the table and sharing the food. Although eating together on a certain degree can add affection, exchange thoughts, it can easily spread some diseases. Fraud is bigger than benefits. Again spitting everywhere can spread many diseases, and the danger is terrible. The phlegm is the secretion of lung bulb, bronchus, and tube. Original microorganism of disease, some germs, virus, etc. , can exist in the phlegm for long hours, become one of the infectious disease's headstream. There is one scholar report regarding tuberculosis as the example, unexpectedly are there over 500 million tubercle rod bacteria in phlegm; In phlegm of a day, tubercle rod bacteria is high to amount to more than 3 billions. Conference holding more than 3,000 by some hospital of Jiangsu Province once was investigated and after two-hour meeting, they discovered phlegm vestige more than 800, and from 91 phlegm liquids drawn out, four were tubercle bacterium positive.

Tubercle bacterium is in the phlegm and breath, can exist in the dark corner for 6 – 8 months, at 6 – 10 ℃ environment can survive a few months to a few years, and can live about a day under the straight sunlight. But after phlegm is dry, it is carried by wind and forms the dust of 4 – 5 microns floating in the sky. If the healthy persons inhale this kind of dust, they can be infected with tuberculosis.

(5) Morals and health

The morals is the total of behavior norm on both person to person and person to society, is a kind of spirit power depending on the social public opinion, faith and education to work. The excellent morals of Chinese play a protecting role to human health and existence. Chinese health education school graduate, Mr. Qi writes *Sex and Health*: Thailand in 1984, China in 1985, discovered the first offshore-introduced AIDS example. After 10 years' prevalence, until 1996, the Thailand announced reach 85 out of 10,000 AIDS virus infection cases, but China in June 1996 only examined out 5,157 example infection cases. Therefore Thailand's spread rate is 200 times of China. On the prevention and control degree of the AIDS measure, Thailand is obviously stronger than China. Taking budget as example, in 1996 Thailand used the budget of 82.3 million dollars to prevent and treat AIDS, but China used only 200 million RMB. The per capita of Thailand is 640 times of China. Why is the output of Thailand is small despite of huge input and China's output comparatively large despite the little efforts? It is morale and tradition that functions. Zhu Qi thinks so. He says that tradition and morale is the most effective measure and big hygienic resources of controlling and preventing the AIDS.

(6) Religion and health

The religion is a shade and upside down reflection in people's brains by ruling people's nature power and social power, and is a social consciousness controlling people's fate by supernatural entity, namely the spirit's faith and social power. The religion influence towards health has both positive and negative aspects. Religion can regulate mental state. It is that through certain religion faith, religion modulates people from unbalance on the mindset to opposite equilibrium of mental state appearance, also this makes people attain the beneficial moderation appearance both in spirit and physiology. Many western scholars call this kind of function faith treatment. Some provisions of religion have some positive effects on health, such as the Judaism that holds the circumcision to male infant, namely the outer skin wreath slice the rites. Therefore, Jew almost have no penis cancer. But the belief of the blind followers of religion can bring harm to health. For example, in the world there were once 6 times big popular of classic cholera, and each time it came from India. The main reason is that Hinduism followers see the Ganges as the "saint river" so that if they can drink its water while living, and use the water to wash the body after death, they can abandon the whole sins. Thus it makes the Ganges water spread disease.

Section 4 Social Psychology, Behavior and Health

With the development of social politics, economy, culture, more and more people are concentrated on social and mental influences on mankind health. Confucius once brought up a famous theme "the long life of kind people", which is the most ancient

Chinese topics in the theory about the appearance regimen. To Confucius, calm can promise longevity. Here, we not only explain the person's accomplishment, but also speak of the person's health, and consider the person's accomplishment level, mental state as the first factor of health. Preservation of one's health requires a lot, among what is the most important is the "the doctrine of the mean" principle that holds balance. Everyone has happiness, anger, sorrow, joy, emotion. Whether these emotions are potential in mind or expressed out, we should make it appropriate, and this is called the "inside","with". Everyone who can control oneself with norm of "moderate", can't have unpredictable mood such as the sorrow and enjoyment, lose control, thus create a harmonious atmosphere in person to person, and person to thing. This kind of equilibrium under the diapason atmosphere is very beneficial to health. Marx also says, "A fine mood, comparable with ten good medicines, can relieve the physical exhaustions and pain more." The good mood is beneficial to defending the disease and cancer, originates from comprehension to objective thing and person, and the good motion appearance makes nervous system (the brain and the hypothalamus, etc.) through information numerator (the hormone, neuropeptides, neurotransmitter, etc.) work on the endocrine, secrete beside, the nerve endocrine, influences cell immunity, and enhances the function to build up immunity, by which it is very beneficial to defend the disease and cancer.

The social psychology factor is a main factor leading to the mental disorders and physical diseases. It results in that the strain mentality controls the body, such as social convulsions, wars, natural disasters, and plagues, which can lead to the change in intensity of the spirit of people in society. Social psychological factor is the stimulus for disease. Because of the function of the social mental state factor leading to the disease of brain and body, now there are more kinds of diseases, such as the coronary heart diseases, hypertension, bronchial asthma, the disease of abscess, and cancer. The social mental state is an important factor to cause the mental illness and suicide. At present about two million people attempt suicide in our country, at least 25 myriad people died, suicide now being the fifth cause of death. The death could bring to friends and relatives mental hurt which is too great to heal up, and bring the society great effect, so it becomes an important sanitation problem in public if neglected. Since the World Health Organization decided the first preventing suicide day on September 10th, 2003, our country has come into the new stage in preventing the various psychological states and suicide.

People's behavior means that everybody with the capability of cognition and thought can make motile response. The wider sense of behavior is divided into intrinsic behavior and extrinsic. The intrinsic behavior is activities of human being in body and mind, extrinsic behavior is the one that can be observed by people, such as conversation and deportment. The behavior that we often mention is the extrinsic one. We should continue to realize and evaluate the sanitary behavior, advocate healthy behavior, and avoid harmful behavior.

1. Behavior improving your health

The behavior improving your health refers to a kind of action showed by individual or group to promote or be in good health objectively. As to the various behaviors improving your health in the daily life, there are some certain standards which are characterized in the following five points: (1) Beneficial: These actions are good for oneself, other people and the whole society, for example, abstinence from smoking and drinking. (2) Regularity: These actions show fixed regularity, for example, your meals of fixed quantity. (3) Harmony: These actions show your own bright characters, for example, choosing sports games, and changing your own action according to the circumstances. (4) Communality: Actions sometimes can become visible but it is sometimes the same with your feeling inside. (5) Adaptability: The strength of actions has reasonable control without apparent impulse.

The personal action improves the health, and it is common that through the following actions health can be good. (1) Reasonable food: It refers to food that fits the character of one's growing and physiology and includes various nutrition composition which is proper, satisfies your need, keeps physiological function, improves growing and health. Besides, it also asks for the food that is easy to digest without toxin. (2) Proper treatment: Sports is good to treating and strengthening the function of every systems, and organs, the lung capacity, improving the growing of muscle, postponing aging of the muscle, bone and joint, improving the ability of thinking and response, letting the nervous systems in a good condition. It can also improve the digestive system, loose weight, control fat, but treatment must be proper. Overdoing can easily cause bad result. In the home of Olympics on the stones of the old Indian mountains, some words are caved, saying, "Do you want to become healthy? If so go running. Do you want to become wise? If so go running. Do you want to become beautiful? If so go running." (3) Being good at rest: Anxiety and overtiredness are two important factors of becoming old. The method to relax is regular sleeping and getting up early habits, slowing down the pace of life, being good at rest, changing the way of actions, etc.

2. Behavior endangering the health

The behavior endangering health has three characters: (1) long-time and steady behavior, occasionally having a high-salt dinner or smoking cigarette. (2) The acquired habit is of one's free will. (3) The obvious health bane primarily has several kinds: ① Bad life habit. Performance is in lack of sports and proper eating habits. ②Bad habit and behavior. Performance is the smoking, and drinking excess. The World Health Organization once brought forward the slogan "want to smoke cigarette or want health, term the gentleman choice." This kind of choice certainly is free. However in consideration of yourself, family and the health, happiness of surrounding person, you should quit smoking. Smoking cigarette can cause cancer, heart and brain blood vessel disease, chronic bronchitis, emphysema, and more diseases. At the same time, it can threaten the health of other people who do not smoke. Therefore, WHO refers to smoking as the serious threat to the 20th century's public health. ③Addiction behavior. It is without medical treatment demand, individual emerging as the strong, periodic begging the usage harmful material, such as the freak-out. ④Bad sexual behavior.

Case Example

A Case Reported — Using Music as Treatment for Blues Syndrome

Lady A, 34 years old, married, and graduating from university is now working for an oversea enterprise. Her figure is emaciated with a pale face covered with anxiousness and beautiful eyes with no interest. When she talks her face has no expression and there is a profound sadness from her eyes. She told me she had been depressed during junior school and her actions were always very slow. Although her study scores were very good she was still filled with shame, feeling unequal to other people. When she was seven years old she attempted to commit suicide. Now she often entertains thoughts of committing suicide but has no courage to put it into practice and envies people who do suicide, feeling they are very brave.

According to her circumstances, I diagnosed Blues Syndrome. As the psychoanalytical theories from Sigmmnd Freud, Blues Syndrome should originate from childhood period; therefore I inquired about the circumstances concerning her mother. She said her mother had schizophrenia soon after she was born and died when she was only seven years old; she no longer recalled her mother's appearance nor the period of her life when she lived with her mother. I decided to place treatment emphasis on exploring her childhood experiences. My treatment method is firstly to use a slow-moving and loose music background to hypnotize the lady and after she enters the hypnotic state I broadcast specially arranged and ordered music. All of this music is selected from classical works of the world and combined together. This guides her to recollect childhood scenes. The treatment is given once a week. In the most recent treatment session, the 19th treatment, I guided her with beautiful and serene music to arrive at a lake and to see her own reflection in the water, because this could reflect her recognition herself and a degree of acceptance. I came in sight of the water in the lake and was a little hesitant, wanting to go over and have a look.

Seeing myself reflected in the lake water, white, gentle and quiet, why would other people not like me? Why would they tell me I am ugly and bad in my childhood? I feel that regardless of what other people say I should take good care of myself. I make a firm decision and others will not hinder me. I want myself right place... I go to the lawn, with mind quiet, but a little afraid. (I ask :What am I afraid of? Why care other people?) They forbid me to love myself, they all tell me I am of no account, and they always trample upon me. I made a firm decision with every means, and did not accept other people's interference. I must do something for myself (tearing)...

A month later the lady rang me happily and told me on the telephone: "Yesterday morning when I went out, seeing the sky so clear, and the sunlight so warm, hearing the birds singing, one thought suddenly burst into my mind. 'life is so fine', and I was so moved because since a little child I never had this kind of feeling before."

It is such an exciting change that she shifted from a person who felt "her sin deep and heavy" and had a sense of "shame while living in this world", to one who accepted and loved herself.

第四章 社会卫生状况

第一节 社会卫生状况评价

了解社会卫生状况,犹如了解社会政治、经济形势一样,是十分重要的。只有看清我们当前面临的主要社会卫生问题,才能作出正确的社会卫生"诊断",开出解决问题的社会卫生"大处方"。

一、社会卫生状况及其评价

(一)社会卫生状况的含义

社会卫生状况是指人群的健康状况,以及影响人群健康的相关社会环境的状况。生物-心理-社会医学模式指出,人群健康状况不仅要受到生物遗传因素的影响,而且要受到自然和社会环境、心理因素、生活方式以及卫生服务等因素的影响。从根本上说,影响健康的因素是社会因素。因此,社会卫生状况的评价主要包括两大方面:人群健康状况评价、与人群健康有关的社会环境因素评价。

(二)社会卫生状况评价的意义

社会医学的基本任务,是对人群的健康状况作出判断,找出影响人群健康的因素,特别是社会因素,从而制定社会卫生策略,促进人群的健康。只有充分地认识人群健康状况和社会因素对人群健康的影响,才能找出主要的社会卫生问题、发现重点保护的人群及重点防治的对象;有助于科学地制定改善社会卫生的措施,动员有限的卫生资源,最大限度地促进人群的健康。

(三)社会卫生状况评价的程序

社会卫生状况评价,基本上可以分为4个步骤。

1. 确定社会卫生状况评价的项目及内容。例如,对于人群健康状况的评价,应依据"生物—心理—社会"三维健康的概念全面地进行评价,而不是单纯评价躯体健康。对于健康影响因素,应当侧重社会环境的状况,包括社会经济水平、文化水平、生活方式和卫生服务等。

2. 确定适宜的评价指标。指标应当具备有效、可靠、灵敏和特异4个特征。"有效"指的是指标能够真实地反映所研究的内容,"可靠"指的是测量的可重复性好,"灵敏"指的是随着健康状况的微小变化,指标发生改变、反映该变化的程度高,而"特异"则说明指标有针对性。

3. 开展资料搜集工作。根据所选定的指标,制定搜集有关资料的计划,开展资料搜集工作。搜集的方法有文献法和调查法。

4. 分析指标,归纳结果。把来自调查和文献的资料加以整理,统计分析,形成指标;把指标归类,形成结果。通过对结果的综合分析,评价社会卫生状况,得出评价的结论。

二、社会卫生状况评价资料来源

(一)文献资料

1. 生命统计资料。生命统计资料是一种重要的和基本的资料来源,包括出生、死亡等。我国可以从户籍登记机构(公安局)中获得相应地区的人口出生、死亡统计资料,在设立死因监测点与疾病监测点的地区内的医院保健科负责对居民死因的调查核实。

2. 人口普查资料。人口普查资料是社会、经济和人口统计情报的重要来源。如居民的性别、年龄别人口数、死亡率、出生率、人口自然增长率和平均期望寿命等指标都可以从人口普查资料中获得。人口普查常规为每10年进行一次,在此期间每年有1次5%或10%的抽样调查,以适应数据更新的要求。

3. 卫生服务常规登记。有关人群健康状况的指标,如疾病别的发病率、患病率和死亡率,儿童生长发育指标和卫生服务提供指标等,可以通过查阅卫生服务常规登记资料获得。

4. 疾病登记。疾病登记常常可以提供某个系统或某种疾病的发病、死亡、治疗和其他信息。例如,一些专科医院对某些具有特殊意义的疾病如肿瘤、高血压病、地方病或传染病以及罕见疾病的发病和死亡情况制订专门的表格进行登记。

5. 卫生相关部门的资料。这是卫生部门以外与健康相关的其他部门的资料,或者是非卫生专业人员协助搜集的资料。如自然环境情况,可以来自气象、环保等部门;社会经济情况,可以来自统计局、工农业生产部门以及计划、民政、教育等部门。

(二)调查和监测资料

1. 调查资料。有些资料无法从常规登记资料中获得,需要组织专题现场调查。例如,对居民亚健康状况的了解,就要通过症状功能评价来分析;对居民生活质量的评估,也要通过专门的家庭询问调查来完成。常用的现场调查方法有三种:家庭调查、机构调查和典型调查。

2. 监测资料。一些传染病和慢性非传染性疾病,如结核、高血压、肿瘤等疾病的控制是一个社会或者一个社区防治工作的重点,要获得这些疾病的发病和患病的资料,就必须建立疾病监测点,及时获得有关这些疾病的发生、流行情况,制定有效的措施防治疾病的发生和发展。计算机技术的发展和网络的应用,将会使疾病监测系统更加完善。

此外,联合国、世界卫生组织等国际组织和我国卫生部等国家机构已有很多现成的文献资料可以供我们使用。表4-1列出了一些相关文献资料的名称和网址。

表 4-1 世界和中国卫生状况的部分文献资料来源

资料名称	出版机构	网址
The World Health Report	世界卫生组织	www.who.int
The State of the World's Children	联合国儿童基金会	www.unicef.org
Demographic Yearbook	联合国	www.un.org
中国统计年鉴	国家统计局	www.stats.gov.cn
中国卫生年鉴	卫生部	www.moh.gov.cn
中国人口年鉴	中国社会科学院人口研究所	www.cass.net.cn
中国环境年鉴	国家环境保护总局	www.zhb.gov.cn

三、社会卫生状况评价指标

指标(indicator)是对某一事物或现象的标记或反映,是衡量变化的变数,亦是实现既定目标的进度的标志。

社会卫生状况指标由两部分组成,一是人群健康状况指标,二是一些影响人群健康状况且已指标化了的社会因素指标。可归纳为下列六类。

(一)卫生政策指标

近几年来,这一类指标的重要性越来越被各级政府和研究人员所认识,成为分析社会卫生状况不可缺少的指标。例如:

1. 各级政府及其领导对人民健康的政治承诺,例如有关政策、法律、法规、条例等。
2. 资源分配,例如卫生经费占国民生产总值的百分比。
3. 卫生资源分配的公平、合理程度,例如各地区人均卫生经费,各地区每千人口拥有的医院床位数、医师数和其他卫生人员数等。

(二)与卫生有关的社会、经济指标

这一类指标反映社会经济、人口、文化、居住条件及食品供应等状况。例如:

1. 经济指标,例如人均国民生产总值(GNP per capita)、人均国内生产总值(GDP per capita)、劳动人口就业率等。
2. 社会指标,例如人口负担系数、妇女识字率、学龄儿童入学率、人均居住面积、人均热量的供应等。

(三)卫生保健服务指标

这一类指标比较多,例如:

1. 初级卫生保健普及面指标,主要有农村行政村的初级卫生保健普及率、城镇社区的初级卫生保健普及率等。
2. 安全饮用水普及率。安全饮用水系指感观性状良好,无毒无害,流行病学安全,煮沸后可以饮用的水。
3. 医疗卫生服务需要量,主要有两周每千人患病人数、患病次数及患病日数、因病卧床日数、休工日数和休学日数等指标。

(四)卫生资源指标

这类指标包括每千人口拥有医师、护士和其他卫生人员的数量,每千农村人口拥有乡村医生、卫生员、经培训的接生员的数量,每千人口拥有病床数,以及各类医疗卫生保健机构具有2000元以上的设备件数等。

(五)卫生行为指标

常用指标有每千人口中吸烟人数、每千人口中饮酒人数、每万人口吸毒人数、每万人口患性病人数等。

(六)人群健康状况指标

1. 单一指标(传统指标):对于人群的生、老、病、死通常使用出生率、死亡率、死因别死亡率、婴儿死亡率及孕产妇死亡率等指标进行评价。

2. 复合指标(新指标):复含指标是指由两个或以上的指标组成的指标(指数)。由于单一指标只能单纯地测量一部分社会卫生状况,如平均期望寿命的观察点是死亡,它只反映死亡作为健康最坏的极端状态给人的寿命带来的影响,只反映生存的时间数量,不反映生存的健康质量。这是传统寿命表方法的最大不足。所以,已有很多新发展的寿命表评价方法,考虑了早死、残疾、疾病状况对健康的影响,对传统的疾病和死亡指标加以改进,以弥补传统寿命表的不足。例如:

(1) 减寿人年数(potential years of life lost,PYLL):减寿人年数是指某一人群一定时期内(通常为一年)在目标生存年龄(通常为70岁或出生期望寿命)以内死亡所造成的寿命减少的总人年数。该指标基于这样一种观点:同是死亡,但死亡年龄不同所反映的社会卫生问题也不同。低年龄死亡是"不合理"的死亡,在用死亡状况来反映健康水平时,应给"早死"以较大的权重,以提高危害低年龄组健康和致命疾病在所有疾病中的重要性,突出过早死亡的危害。减寿人年数的计算公式为:

$$减寿人年数(PYLL) = \sum a_i \times d_i$$

其中:$a_i = L - x_i$,L是目标生存年龄(可根据不同地区的平均期望寿命来确定,或直接用70岁);x_i是i年龄组的平均年龄,例如1~4岁组的$x=(1+4)/2=2.5$;d_i是目标生存年龄内各年龄组死亡人数。

减寿人年数就是全体死者因早死而损失的人年数。标准化减寿人年数可以用于国际比较。减寿人年数是衡量居民健康状况的重要指标,而且可以根据各死因损失寿命年数的大小顺位来判断导致"早死"的原因。

(2) 伤残调整生命年(disability adjusted life year,DALY):伤残调整生命年是衡量健康生命损失情况的单位,用年数表示,是疾病死亡损失健康生命年与疾病伤残(残疾)损失健康生命年相结合的指标,是生命数量和生活质量以时间为单位的综合性指标。目前,全球疾病负担均以DALY为单位进行测算。

伤残调整生命年所考虑的死亡是"早死",即减寿人年数。这里的"早死"定义为低于发达国家模型寿命表的理想潜在寿命,日本是全球平均预期寿命最高的国家,其平均期望寿命女性为82.5岁,男性为80岁。实际死亡年龄与发达国家模型寿命表的理想潜在寿命的差额表示一例死亡所带来的寿命年损失。伤残调整生命年还考虑了以下两个条件:①年龄权数,即生命年的年龄相对值,指各年龄组的人健康地存活一年的价值。年龄权数从出生时的 0 开始,随着年龄增加急剧上升,在 25 岁时达到最高峰,然后随年龄增加而下降。②年龄贴现率,即生命年的时间相对值,指现有伤病对健康的毁损过程长达数年或数十年,因而需要决定如何为相对于现在的未来健康定值。

伤残调整生命年所考虑的残疾与无残疾期望寿命的原理相同,代表着因病伤而在未来将失去的健康寿命。但是其内容得到了进一步的扩展,残疾的程度用权重表示,对残疾严重程度确定的等级权数由代表健康的 0 至代表死亡的 1。预期残疾年数(直到康复或死亡)乘以一个度量残疾与死亡相比的严重性权数,分为 7 等残疾。例如,第四等级残疾,包括膝下截肢和耳聋,其严重性系数为 0.24～0.36。

"早死"所导致的健康生命年损失为 YLLs(years of life lost),残疾所导致的健康生命年损失为 YLDs(years lived with disability)。把两者结合起来,就形成 DALY。

$$DALY = YLLs + YLDs$$

DALY 主要有以下方面的用途:①找出某地区严重危害健康的疾病和主要的卫生问题,即对不同地区、不同对象(性别、年龄、职业等)、不同疾病进行 DALY 分析,可以确定高发地区、重点人群及主要疾病;②通过干预前后 DALY 指标的比对,可评价某项措施是否得力;③比较几种干预措施的 DALY 效果,选择最佳的方案来控制重点疾病,以达到使用有限的资源,而取得最大成效之目的;④进行全球疾病负担(global burden of disease, GBD)分析。

(3) 健康期望寿命(healthy life expectancy, HALE):这是由世界卫生组织开发的一个最新的衡量健康的指标,在《2000 年世界卫生报告》中被称为伤残调整期望寿命(disability adjusted life expectancy, DALE),可以理解为"完全健康(full health)期望寿命",是扣除了死亡和伤残影响之后的平均期望寿命。因为其计算结果是期望寿命,所以比DALY 更容易理解,它采用无残疾期望寿命的 Sullivan 方法,即用一般寿命表,结合抽样调查的方法,获得人群健康状况(如完全健康、轻微残疾、中度残疾、重度残疾、极重度残疾)的流行率,就可以计算该指标。需要注意的是,健康状况流行率部分地来自自我评价的健康,当用于国家间或地区间比较的时候应当进行校正。

HALE 是评价人群健康状况的正向指标,它扣除了死亡、残疾和疾病对于健康的影响,衡量的是完全健康的期望寿命。HALE 的开发,使得在充分考虑失能的基础上进行人群间的比较成为可能。该指标还用于评价卫生体系的运行效果,并在《2000 年世界卫生报告》中得到应用。

第二节 全球社会卫生状况

20 世纪的后半叶,人类在健康状况改善方面取得了巨大成就。从 1995 年至 1997 年,全球人口平均期望寿命从 48 岁提高到 66 岁,婴儿死亡率从 148‰ 降低到 57‰,5 岁以下儿童死亡率从 210‰ 降低到 75‰,孕产妇死亡率从 $620/10^5$ 降低到 $230/10^5$。

一、人群健康状况

世界卫生组织在《2000 年世界卫生报告》中,根据各成员国的复合健康指标——伤残调整期望寿命(DALE)(或称健康期望寿命,HALE)衡量各个国家国民的健康水平,并按照该指标的高低,把 191 个成员国排序。从表 4-2 中可以看出,DALE 基本上能够代表各个国家实际的健康水平,它所表现出来的国家间健康水平差距,与其他常用的健康指标(如婴儿死亡率、孕产妇死亡率、平均期望寿命)所表现出来的差距是一致的,发达国家的健康水平要远远高出发展中国家。

表 4-2　世界卫生组织部分人口大国* 1999 年健康指标

国家	总人口数(百万)	婴儿死亡率(‰)	孕产妇死亡率($1/10^5$)	平均期望寿命(岁)	残疾调整期望寿命(岁)	WHO 排序(2000 年)
日　本	126.5	4	8	81	74.5	1
美　国	273.1	7	8	77	70.0	24
中　国	1 259.1	33	56	71	62.3	81
俄罗斯	145.6	21	50	66	61.3	91
巴　西	165.4	36	160	67	59.1	111
印　度	977.5	69	410	63	53.2	134
尼日利亚	109.0	112	-	48	38.3	163

资料来源:《2001 年中国统计年鉴》,《2002 年世界卫生报告》;* 人口在 1 亿以上。

二、社会因素对健康的影响

在过去的 50 年间,因全球社会经济的快速发展,人类贫困状况的改善幅度比过去 500 年还大,全球人口增长了 1 倍,人均国内生产总值增长了 2.5 倍。世界各地区的成人识字率从 1970 年的不足 50% 提高到 1995 年的 77%,尤其是发展中国家,已经提高到 70%,截至 2000 年底,全球人均国民收入已经达到 5170 美元。

表 4-3 表示世界卫生组织部分人口大国的国民收入和卫生资源状况。人均国民收入水平较高的国家,卫生投入相对较多,健康水平较高。

表 4-3　世界卫生组织部分人口大国的经济和卫生资源状况

国家	人均国民收入(美元) 2000 年	世界银行排名(位) 2000 年	每千人口医师(人) 1990~1998 年	每千人口医院病床(张) 1993 年	人均医疗卫生费用(美元) 1990~1998 年	卫生经费占 GDP(%) 1990~1998 年
日　本	35 600	5	1.8	16.2	2 379	7.1
美　国	34 100	7	2.6	4.0	4 080	13.9
中　国	840	141	1.3	2.4	33①	4.8②
俄罗斯	1 660	114	4.6	12.1	130	5.7
巴　西	3 580	82	1.3	3.1	359	7.3
印　度	450	159	0.4	0.8	18	5.2
尼日利亚	260	186	0.2	1.7	9	0.7

注:①世界银行估计数;②卫生总费用占 GDP 的百分比。
资料来源:世界银行《2000 年世界发展指标》,《2002 年世界发展指标》。

三、21世纪面临的主要健康问题

(一)健康状况存在着普遍的不公平性

首先,在国家之间存在着健康不公平。从平均期望寿命看,1997年全球平均期望寿命为66岁,但发达国家为74岁,发展中国家为67岁,最不发达国家为53岁;从婴儿死亡率看,发达国家为13‰,发展中国家83‰,最不发达的国家为144‰;从传染病死亡所占比例来看,穷国占60%,富国仅占8%～10%;从死亡年龄分布来看,穷国有一半以上的死亡发生在15岁之前,而在富国仅占4%。其次,在国家内部也存在着健康状况的不公平。不论是穷国还是富国,不同阶层人群的健康状况有着明显的差别,如英国的研究表明,社会经济地位较低者的死亡率与较高者的死亡率之间存在着差异,而且这种差异存在梯度关系。在不发达和发展中国家,这种差异主要取决于卫生保健服务提供的公平程度;而在发达国家,则主要取决于社会经济地位的公平程度。

(二)疾病谱和死因谱发生重要改变

人类的主要死亡原因已经由过去的传染病、寄生虫病和营养缺乏性疾病逐渐转为心脑血管疾病、恶性肿瘤和意外伤害。用DALY计算的疾病负担分析,从1990年至1999年,传染病、寄生虫病和营养缺乏性疾病死亡从占全部DALY损失的45.8%下降至42.8%;而慢性非传染性疾病从42.2%增加到43.2%,意外伤害从12.0%增加到13.2%。在发达国家,心脑血管疾病死亡所占比重已经有所下降,但是仍然占近一半;在发展中国家,虽然传染性疾病仍然是最主要的健康威胁,但心脑血管疾病和恶性肿瘤的危害也正在逐步加大。表4-4显示了全球主要死因构成的变化。

表4-4 全球主要死因构成变化(%)

死亡原因	发达国家			发展中国家		
	1985	1990	1997	1985	1990	1997
传染病与寄生虫病	5	4	1	45	44	43
循环系统疾病	51	48	46	16	17	24
恶性肿瘤	21	21	21	6	7	9
呼吸系统疾病	4	3	8	6	7	5
围产儿及孕产妇疾病	1	1	1	10	9	10
其他疾病	18	23	23	17	16	9
合计	100	100	100	100	100	100

(三)健康问题的复杂性

在很多地区,降低传染性疾病危害,对付传染病、寄生虫病和营养缺乏性疾病的任务仍然艰巨。同时,曾经一度被控制的结核病、疟疾等传染病,由于耐药菌的出现又开始肆虐;新的传染性疾病如艾滋病,正在全球呈明显的蔓延之势。与人类社会经济、人口城市化和老龄化、行为和生活方式有关的非传染性疾病又成为很多发达国家和发展中国的主要死因。旧的健康问题尚未解决,新的健康挑战已经出现。所以健康问题将成为继人口、环境之后,关系可持续发展的又一个全球命题。

第三节　中国社会卫生状况

一、人群健康状况

（一）健康水平显著提高

建国 50 多年来，中国取得了超越经济发展水平的卫生成就，健康水平显著提高。从 1949 年至 1999 年，平均期望寿命由 35 岁提高到 72 岁，婴儿死亡率由 200‰ 下降至 33‰。我国居民的总体健康水平已经远远超过同等经济水平的发展中国家，一些主要健康指标接近发达国家的水平。

（二）人群健康状况存在明显的地区差异

由于各地社会经济发展和自然历史条件的制约，人群健康状况存在明显的地区差异。根据死亡谱的构成，大体可以分成三类地区：

第一类为发达型，主要是大城市和沿海发达地区，接近发达国家。以心脑血管疾病、恶性肿瘤和意外伤害为主要死因。

第二类为发展型，主要是中小城市和大部分农村地区，主要死因处于从传染性疾病向心脑血管疾病和恶性肿瘤的转型期。

第三类为欠发达型，主要是一些经济欠发达农村、边远地区、山区和少数民族聚居区。传染病、寄生虫病和营养不良性疾病仍然有相当高的死亡率。

2000 年我国部分市、县居民前十位死亡原因，见表 4-5。

表 4-5　2000 年我国部分市、县居民前十位死亡原因

顺位	部分城市居民			部分县居民		
	死亡原因	死亡专率 $(1/10^5)$	占死亡总人数的（%）	死亡原因	死亡专率 $(1/10^5)$	占死亡总人数的（%）
1	恶性肿瘤	146.61	24.38	呼吸系病	142.16	23.11
2	脑血管病	127.96	21.28	恶性肿瘤	112.57	18.40
3	心脏病	106.65	17.74	脑血管病	115.20	18.40
4	呼吸系病	79.92	13.29	心脏病	73.43	12.37
5	损伤和中毒	35.57	5.91	损伤和中毒	64.89	11.03
6	消化系病	18.38	3.06	消化系病	23.89	3.98
7	内分泌、营养、代谢及免疫疾病	17.99	2.99	泌尿、生殖系病	9.27	1.51
8	泌尿、生殖系病	9.01	1.50	肺结核	7.39	1.19
9	精神病	6.70	1.11	新生儿病	697.05	1.14
10	神经病	5.53	0.92	内分泌、营养、代谢及免疫疾病	6.84	1.11
	十种死因合计		92.18	十种死因合计		91.46

资料来源：《中国卫生年鉴》(2001 年)。

(三)面临传染病和慢性非传染性疾病的双重挑战

近年来,旧传染病如鼠疫、霍乱呈局部活跃之势,而新的传染病如传染性非典型肺炎(SARS)给人民健康带来新的威胁,也使防治工作面临窘境;一些曾经得到较好控制或者相对稳定的疾病,如性病、结核病、血吸虫病等又有死灰复燃迹象;由于卖淫、嫖娼、吸毒人群的出现,我国面临着艾滋病大面积流行的潜在威胁;病毒性肝炎等疾病发病人数众多,危害已相当严重;与环境、营养等因素密切相关的疾病,如地氟病、地甲病、大骨节病等仍未得到有效控制。同时慢性非传染病已成为居民常见病、多发病,精神疾病患病率持续增加;各种由职业危害所致的急、慢性职业病居高不下。传染病与非传染病双重夹击已成为威胁中国人群健康的主要问题。

(四)城乡居民卫生需求发生新变化

1998年国家卫生服务调查结果与1993年比较,城乡居民两周患病率增加6.9%,显示居民卫生服务需要量增加;一些慢性非传染性疾病患病率有较大程度上升,成为居民常见病、多发病,如糖尿病、高血压病在城市分别上升53%和32%,而农村升幅更高,分别达到128%和36%;疾病危害程度增加,全国居民患病总天数增加24.5亿天,劳动力人口平均每人每年休工天数增加1.8天,因病伤失能总人数达8 500万,需要社会和他人帮助的残障总人数达1 600万。卫生已越来越凸现出对社会经济的影响力。

(五)意外伤害的发生呈上升趋势

目前,我国交通事故的发生呈上升趋势,已经成为各种事故中的第一位原因。在2002年各种事故中,交通事故死亡人数占78.5%,死亡10.9万人,万车死亡13.71人,大大高于发达国家及某些发展中国家。此外要关注"溶剂中毒"。近年来,多种多样的溶剂在我国建筑业、制鞋业、箱包制造业、玩具制造业等行业广泛使用,但缺少防护措施;由于超标接触苯、正己烷、甲醛、四氯化碳等溶剂而引起的中毒时有发生。曾有报道,广东省涉外企业中,溶剂中毒者占职业中毒总人数的64.4%,94.6%的严重中毒是溶剂所致。

二、影响健康的社会因素

(一)社会经济状况

从1978年至2000年,我国人均GDP由379元增加到7 084元;城市人均居住面积由3.6 m² 增加到10.3 m²,农村由8.1 m² 增加到24.8 m²;学龄儿童入学率由1952年的49.2%上升至2000年的99.1%。

(二)人口状况

人口城市化、老龄化的速度加快。从1978的至2000年,城镇总人口已经由1.7亿增加到4.5亿,城市化水平由17.9%提高到36.2%,预计在未来的20年内,中国城市化水平将达到60%。中国人口老龄化的速度之快,是中国人口生育率在短时期内迅速下降的结果。1990年,60岁及以上人口占总人口的8.6%,2000年达到10%,预计2020年将达到15.6%。老年人口绝对数目增加,将对整个社会经济和卫生体系带来沉重的压力。

(三)卫生服务状况

建国50多年来,我国的卫生机构、卫生人力数量增加很快。目前每千人拥有病床2.4张、医师1.3人,人均医疗卫生费用33美元。卫生总费用占GDP的4.8%,卫生事业费占国家财政支出的 2.1%。但这些指标与发达国家还有很大的差距,如发达国家每千人口医师数为 2.87 人。从卫生总费用的筹资结构看,1990~1995 年,全国卫生总费用中,政府预算卫生支出所占比重从 25% 下降至 17%;居民个人支出从 27% 上升到 50%。而同期发达国家卫生总费用占 GDP 的比例从 9% 上升到 12%,政府预算卫生支出所占比重普遍较高,如英国为 80%。

(四)行为与生活方式

1991 年的抽样调查显示,中国 15 岁及以上人口的平均吸烟率为 30.5%,而男性为 61.0%,女性为 7.0%。中国男性人口占全世界总人口的 10%,却消费了全世界香烟的 30%;1990 年,中国有 80 万人死于吸烟。1989 年的一项估算结果显示,我国与吸烟有关增加医疗卫生开支约为 69 亿元。如果不采取措施的话,预计 30 年后,我国每年将有 200 万人死于吸烟。另有抽样调查显示,我国城市居民酒精依赖患病率达到 3.7%,一些少数民族地区慢性酒精依赖的患病率明显高于其他地区。目前我国的嗜酒者达到 1.16 亿,每年酒精中毒者达 10 多万,死亡近万人。

近年来,我国艾滋病传播呈快速增长的趋势。据估计,从 1985 年发现首例艾滋病病毒感染者到 2002 年底,我国艾滋病病毒感染者累计已达 104 万,其中病人数累计达 20 万以上。根据世界卫生组织统计:截至 2001 年底,包括中国在内的西太平洋地区艾滋病病毒感染者总数为 120 万,其中我国居该地区第 1 位、亚洲第 4 位和世界第 17 位。其他性传播疾病如梅毒的患病率也以每年几十倍的速度递增。

三、21 世纪我国面临的主要卫生问题

1. 传染病防治工作不能放松,慢性非传染病防治任重道远。
2. 实现"人人享有卫生保健",必须尽快解决我国广大农民的基本卫生服务,这项任务尚十分艰巨。
3. 城镇化进程加快,对卫生机构应对现代公共卫生问题的能力带来挑战。
4. 社会主义市场经济体制的建立与完善,对公共卫生监督职能提出了更高要求。
5. 人口老龄化逐渐成为我国社会发展的突出问题,迫切要求对现行卫生服务体系和服务模式进行调整。
6. 意外伤害形势严峻,交通事故、中毒、火灾及矿井事故时有发生,必须进一步加强社会预防措施。
7. 我国进入全面建设小康社会的新阶段,社会要求卫生部门提供多层次、多样化的卫生服务,以满足社会各阶层人群的需求。
8. 由于"知识爆炸"、生活节奏加快、社会竞争激烈,精神卫生问题应引起广泛的重视。

Chapter 4　Social Health Condition

Section 1　Evaluation of Social Health Condition

Understanding the social health condition, just as understanding social, political and economical situation, is very important. Only when major social health problems we confront are clearly seen, can a right "social health diagnosis" then be made and a "big prescription of social health" for solving problems be prescribed.

1. Social health condition and its evaluation

(1) The connotation of the social health condition

Social health condition is about the crowd health condition and some related social environments, which affect the crowd health. Bio-psycho-social medical model points out that the crowd health condition is influenced not only by biological, inheritable factors, but also by nature and social environment, mental state, life style and health service factors, etc. Basically speaking, it is social factors that affect health.

Therefore, the evaluation of the social condition includes two major aspects, evaluation of the crowd health condition and evaluation of the social environment factors which concern crowd health.

(2) The significance of the social health condition evaluation

The basic mission of the social medical science is doing the judgment to the crowd health condition, finding out the factors that affect the crowd health, especially social factors in order to make out social health strategy and promote the crowd health. Only knowing the crowd health condition and the influences of the social factors on health adequately, we can find out the major social health problems and discover major crowd who need protection and major object who need prevention and cure, which is beneficial to scientifically making out and improving social health measures, mobilizing limited health resources and promoting crowd health to the maximum.

(3) The procedure of the social health condition evaluation

The social health condition evaluation can be divided into 4 steps:

①Defining items and contents of the social health condition evaluation. For example, to evaluate the crowd health condition should be according to "bio-psycho-social" three dimensional health concept, not be confined only in body health. As to factors which affect the health, we should lay emphasis on the social environment, including the social economic level, cultural level, life style and health service, etc.

②Defining index for evaluation. The index should have validity, reliability sensitivity, specificity. Validity means that index can really reflect what is studied; Reliability means measures have good re-measured results; Sensitivity means along with slight changes of the health condition, the index changes and the index can correctly reflect the changes to a great extent; Specificity means the index has a special object to aim at.

③Doing data-collecting work. According to index selected, a plan should be made for data-collection and doing data-collecting work. The source of the data includes looking through documents and investigation.

④Analysing the index and inducing the results. Sorting out the data from documents and investigation and analyzing the data with statistics so as to form the indexes — categorizing the indexes and forming the results. Through comprehensive analysis on results, we can evaluate the social health condition and get a conclusion of evaluation.

2. The data source of the social health condition evaluation

(1) Document data

①Life statistics. Life statistics is a kind of important and basic data source, including birth, death, etc. In our country, we can acquire population statistics about birth and death from the household register organization (police department) in the region we choose. The region, which has established the monitors of death causes and disease and the health care section in hospital, is in charge of investigating and verifying death cause of residents.

②Census data. The census data is an important source for information of society, economy and population statistics. For example, sex, population with different age, death rate, birth rate, natural population-growing rate and life expectancy can be acquired from the census data. As usual, the census is made once every 10 years. In this period, 5% or 10% sampling is made once a year for data-renewing.

③The conventional health service register. Index concerns the crowd health condition, such as incidence rate with different diseases, prevalence rate with different diseases, death rate with different diseases, child growth index and health service index, etc. All these can be acquired by checking the conventional registered data of health service.

④The disease registers. The disease register can usually provide incidence, death, treatment and other information of some system or some disease. For instance, some special hospital can make out special table for registration according to the incidence and death of some disease with special meaning, such as tumor, hypertension, endemic disease, infectious disease as well as rare disease.

⑤The data from the section related with health. These are data not from health section, but from other section related with health or from collection by non-professional health people. For example, the natural environment circumstance can come from the meteorological, environmental protection section, etc. ; Social economic circumstance can come from statistic bureau, industry and agriculture productive departments, plan, domestic affairs and educational section, etc.

(2) Investigation and monitoring of data

①Investigation of data. Some data can't be acquired from conventional register and can be acquired through investigating special subject on the spot. For instance, understanding the secondary disease in resident condition must be done by evaluation of symptom function. Evaluation of the life quality of the resident must also be done by special family inquiry. The three conventional investigation methods are family investigation, the organization investigation and typical model investigation.

②Monitoring data. The control of some infectious diseases and chronic, non-infectious diseases, such as tuberculosis, high blood pressure, tumor, etc. , is a key point of prevention and cure work of a society or a community. To acquire incidence and prevalence data of these diseases we must establish the disease monitors so as to acquire something about their occurrence and prevalence in time, work out effective measures to prevent disease from occurrence and development. With technical development of computer and the application of the network, our disease monitor system will be more and more perfect.

In addition, the United Nations, the World Health Organization and our Health Department, etc. have a lot of ready-made documents to meet our demand.

Table 4-1 listing the names of documents concerned and their Web addresses.

Table 4-1 source of part documents about health condition of World and China

Data name	Publishing house	Web addresses
The World Health Report	WHO	www. who. int
The State of the World's Children	UNICEF	www. unicef. org
Demographic Yearbook	UN	www. un. org
Year Report of China Statistics	National Statistic Bureau	www. stats. gov. cn
Year Report of China Health	Health Department	www. moh. gov. cn
Year Report of China Population	Population Graduate School of China College of Social Science	www. cass. net. cn
Year Report of China Environment	Total Bureau of National Environment Protection	www. zhb. gov. cn

3. The index of social health condition evaluation

Index is marking or reflecting something or phenomenon, a variable which measures change and a sign of degree of progress to realize decided target.

Social health condition index is divided into two parts: one is indexes of crowd health, the other is some social factor indexes which affect the crowd health condition. All above can be divided into six types:

(1) Health policy index

Recent years, the importance of index of this type is understood by more and more governments and researchers at all levels. The index has become the indispensable index in analysing social health condition.

①Political commitment of governments and leaders at all levels to people's health, such as relevant documents, law, regulation and some other measures.

②Resource allotment. For example, the health budget accounting for percentage of GNP.

③The equal, reasonable degree of the health resource allotment. For example, health budget per person in different areas, bed numbers, doctors and other health people of hospital per thousand people in different areas.

(2) Social, economic index related with health

The index of this type reflects the social economy, population, culture, living condition and food supply, etc.

①Economic index. Such as GDP per capita, GNP per capita, person employment rate of labour force, etc.

②Social index. Such as the population burden coefficient, rate of women knowing words, rate of children at school age entering school, living housing area per person, calories per person, etc.

(3) The index of health care service

This type of index is used more.

①Index of primary health care — universal rate of primary health care of the village, universal rate of primary health care of town community, etc.

②Universal rate of safe drinking water. The safe drinking water means to feel well, not poisonous or harmful. Its boiling water can be drunk.

③Demand of medical treatment and health service includes prevalence rate, prevalence times, prevalence days per thousand people in two weeks, days in bed for ill, days of non working for ill and days of non studying for ill, etc.

(4) Health resource index. Including numbers of doctors, nurse and other health members per thousand people, numbers of doctors, health members, trained assistant for childbirth per thousand people in village, numbers of hospital bed per thousand peo-

ple and numbers of equipments above 2000 Chinese dollars the various organizations of medical treatment and health care.

(5) Health behavior index refers to numbers of smoker per thousand people, numbers of drink men per thousand people, numbers of drug addiction per ten-thousand people, numbers of sexual disease per ten-thousand people, etc.

(6) Crowd health condition index

①Single index sign(traditional index) is used to evaluate birth, aging, ill and death with indexes as follows: birth rate, mortality rate, mortality rate with different causes, infant mortality rate, maternal mortality rate, etc.

②Compound index (new index). A compound index is constituted by two indexes or more. Single index only evaluates some parts of social health condition. For example, observation point of life expectancy is death, which is a big shortcoming of the traditional life table. It only reflects the influence by death as the worst extreme health state, only reflects quantity of survival time, does not reflect survival quality. So, there has been many new developed methods of life table which can reflect the health condition influenced by early death, disablity, disease and improve the traditional index of disease and death so as to overcome the shortcoming of the traditional life table.

A. Potential years of life lost (PYLL). PYLL means in some crowd and period (usually a year), within target survival age (usually for 70 years old or birth life expectancy), the total years of life lost resulted from death. The index bases itself on that standpoint: the death results are the same, but different death age reflects different social health problems. The death at low age is unreasonable, while the death condition reflects health level. We should give death at low age a heavier weight to increase importance of harmfulness to health in low age group and mortal diseases in all diseases, and give prominence to the harm of early death. The calculation formula of PYLL is:

$$PYLL = \sum a_i \times d_i$$

Among them, $a_i = L - x_i$, the L is a target survival age (changing according to the life expectancy of different areas or using 70 years old directly). The x_i is an average age of i age group, for example, in 1-4 years old age group, $x=(1+4)/2=2.5$; The d_i represents the death numbers of different age groups within a target survival age.

PYLL is years of life lost of all dead people at low age. Standard PYLL can be used for the international comparison. PYLL is an important index to measure resident health condition and can judge the causes resulting in early death according to order of life lost years of different dead causes.

B. Disability adjusted life year (DALY). DALY, expressed by years, is a unit to measure healthy life lost. It is an index of "years of life lost (YLL)" combined with "years of lived with disability(YLD)" and a comprehensive index of life quantity and life quality in form of time unit. At present, the global burden of disease is calculated with DALY.

The death DALY considers is "early death", namely, years of life lost (PYLL). The early death here is defined as lower than ideal potential life years of life table of developed countries' model. Japan is a country which has highest life expectancy in the world. Its life expectancy is as follows: female is 82.5 years old; male is 80 years old. The difference between the actual death age and ideal potential life years of life table of developed countries' model expresses as years of life lost resulted from one case of death.

DALY also considers the following two terms:

a. Age weight, namely relative age value of life years, which means the value of healthy living for one year in different age groups. The number of age weight starts from 0 of birth and increases steeply with aging, and at 25 years old, it goes up to the highest, then goes down with aging.

b. Age discount rate, namely relative time value of life years, which means the process of current disability and disease derogating health is long up to several years or decades. Therefore, how to measure the value for future health needs to be decided.

The disability DALY considers has the same principle as life expectancy without disability does. It represents the healthy life which would be lost in future because of disability and sickness. But its contents have been further enlarged. The degree of disability can be expressed by weight. The grade weight are: 0 represents health; 1 represents death. The years of disability expectancy (until recovery or death) multiply seriousness weight which measures the ratio of disability to death form seven grades of disability. For example, the fourth grade disability includes knee limbed and deaf, and its seriousness coefficient is 0.24 – 0.36.

Early death results in YLLs (years of life lost); disability results in YLDs (years lived with disability). Putting the both together forms DALY.

$$DALY = YLLs + YLDs$$

The DALY mainly has some uses as follows:

a. Finding out the diseases which are seriously harmful to health and main health problems in some areas, namely to analyse different areas, different objects (sex, age, occupation, etc.), different diseases with method of DALY so as to make sure the areas of high incidence rate, major crowd and major diseases.

b. Through self-comparing of DALY before and after interference, we can evaluate whether some measure is effective or not.

c. Comparing the effects of DALY interfered by several measures can choose the best project to control the major disease in order to get the best effective result by using limited resources.

d. Analysing global burden of disease, GBD.

C. Healthy life expectancy, HALE. This is a brand-new index to measure health developed by World Health Organization. *World Health Report in 2000*, it is called "disability adjusted life expectancy, DALE" and can be understood to be "full health life expectancy" which is an average life expectancy after throwing away the influences from disability and death. Because its calculation result is life expectancy, it is more easily understood than DALY. It uses the Sullivan method without disability, namely ordinary life table together with the method of sampling to acquire epidemic rate of the crowd health condition (such as full health, slight degree disability, middle degree disability, heavy degree disability and the very heavy degree disability), then index HALE can be calculated. What need to be noticed is that epidemic rate of health condition partly comes from health self-evaluation, and when used for comparing among countries or areas, it should be corrected.

The HALE is a positive index which evaluates the crowd health condition. It throws away the influence to health from death, disability and disease. What it measures is life expectancy of full health. HALE's development makes it possible to compare each other in crowds on the basis of fully considering efficiency-losing. The index is also used to evaluate the effects of health system running and has been applied *World Health Report in 2000*.

Section 2 The Global Social Health Status

In the late 20th century, human being made great achievements on improving the health status. From 1995 to 1997, the average life expectancy in the world increased from 48 years old to 66. The mortality of infant reduced from 148‰ to 57‰ and the children under 5, reduced from 210‰ to 75‰. The pregnant & maternal mortality decreased from 620 people per 100,000 to 230 per 100,000.

1. The population's health status

World Health Report in 2000, WHO estimated people's health level of every country according to the compound health indicator — disability adjusted life expectancy (DALE) or healthy life expectancy. It also sorted the 191 member countries in terms of this health indicator. From table 4-2, which showed the health indicators of some big population countries of WHO in 1999, it was seen that DALE basically represented every country's real health level. The difference of health level in different countries represented by DALE was the same with the difference represented by another commonly used health indicators, such as infant mortality, pregnant & maternal mortality and average life expectancy.

Table 4-2 Health indicators of some big population countries* of WHO in 1999

Country	Total number (million)	Infant mortality (‰)	Pregnant & maternal mortality (1/100,000)	Average life expectancy (year)	Disability adjusted life expectancy (year)	Sort by WHO (the year 2000)
Japan	126.5	4	8	81	74.5	1
America	273.1	7	8	77	70.0	24
China	1,259.1	33	56	71	62.3	81
Russia	145.6	21	50	66	61.3	91
Brazil	165.4	36	160	67	59.1	111
India	977.5	69	410	63	53.2	134
Nigeria	109.0	112	-	48	38.3	163

Material source: *Chinese Statistics Annual in 2000*, *WHO Report in 2002*.

* Country which has a population over 100 million.

2. The influence on health caused by social factors

In the past 50 years, because of the quick development of global society and economy, the degree of improving poverty status of humans was higher than the total of the past 500 years. The global population doubled and the gross domestic product per capita (GDP per capita) grew two and a half times. The literacy rate of adults in the world increased from less 50% in 1970 to 77% in 1995, especially in developing countries, rose to 70%. Up to end of 2000, the global average national income had achieved US $5,170. Table 4-3 shows the national income and health resource status in some of the WHO's big population countries. The higher of the average national income of a country, the bigger of the health investment, and the higher of the health level.

Table 4-3 The economy and health resource status in some WHO's big population countries

Country	Average national income (US $)	Sort by World Bank (position)	Doctors per 1,000 people (people)	Hospital beds per 1,000 people (bed)	Average medical & health cost (US $)	Proportion of health cost to GDP (%)
	Year 2000	Year 2000	Year's 1990 – 1998	Year 1993	Year's 1990 – 1998	Year's 1990 – 1998
Japan	35,600	5	1.8	16.2	2,379	7.1
America	34,100	7	2.6	4.0	4,080	13.9
China	840	141	1.3	2.4	33	4.8

(Table 4-3)

Country	Average national income (US $)	Sort by World Bank (position)	Doctors per 1,000 people (people)	Hospital beds per 1,000 people (bed)	Average medical & health cost (US $)	Proportion of health cost to GDP (%)
	Year 2000	Year 2000	Year's 1990－1998	Year 1993	Year's 1990－1998	Year's 1990－1998
Russia	1,660	114	4.6	12.1	130	5.7
Brazil	3,580	82	1.3	3.1	359	7.3
India	450	159	0.4	0.8	18	5.2
Nigeria	260	186	0.2	1.7	9	0.7

Note: ①estimated number from World Bank; ②the proportion of total health cost to GDP.
Material source: From the World Bank *The World Develop Indicators in 2000*, *The World Develop Indicators in 2002*.

3. The primary health problems in the 21st century

(1) Health status is unjust universally: Firstly, unjustness existed health between different countries. The average life expectancy in the world in 1997 was 66 years old. But it was 74 years old in developed countries, 67 in developing countries, and 53 in the less developed countries. The infant mortality was 13‰ in developed countries, 83‰ in developing countries and 144‰ in less developed countries. The proportion of death of infectious diseases was 60% in poor countries, however, only 8%－10% in rich countries. Seeing from the age distribution of death, poor countries had more than half of their people died before 15 years old. However in rich countries, this phenomenon happened only 4%. Secondly, health unjustness exited within one country. Whatever poor countries or rich countries, there was obviously different health status between people at different social classes. For example, British researcher showed the death rates was different between the people with lower socioeconomic status and those with higher socioeconomic status. And this difference existed in gradient relationship. In undeveloped and developing countries, this difference was mainly decided by the equity provided by the health care service. In developed countries, however, it was mainly decided by the equity of socioeconomic status.

(2) The pattern of disease and the pattern of cause of death have changed greatly: Human's main causes of death gradually transferred from the infectious disease, verminosis and nutritional deficiency disorder in the past to cardiovascular disease, malignant tumor and unintentional injuries. Using the disability adjusted life year (DALY) to calculate the burden of disease, it was found that from 1990 to 1999, the proportion of

death of infectious disease, verminosis and nutritional deficiency disorder to the total DALY loss decreased from 45.38% to 42.8%; the proportion of death of chronic non-infectious disease to the total DALY loss increased from 42.2% to 43.2%; the proportion of death of unintentional injuries increased from 12.0% to 13.2%. In developed countries, though the proportion of death of cardiovascular disease had reduced, it still accounted for 50%. In developing countries, though infectious disease was still the most important health problem, the harm of cardiovascular disease and malignant tumor was gradually increasing. Table 4-4 shows the changes of global main causes of death.

Table 4-4 Changes of the composition of main causes of death in the world (%)

Causes of death	Developed countries			Developing countries		
	1985	1990	1997	1985	1990	1997
Infectious and parasitic disease	5	4	1	45	44	43
Disease of circulatory system	51	48	46	16	17	24
Malignant tumor	21	21	21	6	7	9
Disease of respiratory system	4	3	8	6	7	5
Disease of perinatal baby and pregnant & parturient woman	1	1	1	10	9	10
Other disease	18	23	23	17	16	9
Total	100	100	100	100	100	100

(3) The complexity of health problem: In many areas, it is still a hard task to deal with the infectious disease, verminosis and nutritional deficiency disorder and reduce their harms. At the same time, some infectious diseases such as tuberculosis, malaria which have once been controlled are coming back again because of the appearance of drug resistant bacteria. New infectious disease, such as the AIDS, is spreading fast in the world. Some non-infectious diseases, which are related with society, economy, urbanizaion, aging, behavior and life style, become the main causes of death in many developed and developing countries. The former health problems are unsolved, yet the new ones are coming. So health problems will arouse another global attention after the population and environmental problems.

Section 3   The Social Health Status in China

1. People's health status

(1) The health level enhanced greatly: since the establishment of People's Republic of China(PRC), China has made great health achievements which have surpassed the economic development and its health level enhanced significantly. From 1949 to 1999, the average life expectancy rose from 35 years to 72 years; the infant mortality decreased from 200‰ to 33‰. The total health level of Chinese people has far exceeded the level of developing countries that have the same economy. And some main health indicators have approached the developed countries' level.

(2) People's health status exhibits obvious regional difference: According to the death notation, it is divided into three regions:

The first is the developed form: It is mostly distributed in big cities and prosperous areas along coast, which is close to the developed countries. Its main causes of death are cardiovascular disease, malignant tumor and unintentional injuries.

The second is the developing form: It is mostly distributed in middle or small cities and most rural areas. It is on the period that the main causes of death is changing from infectious disease to cardiovascular & cerebrovascular disease and malignant tumor.

The third is the less developed form: It is distributed in some poor villages, remote areas, mountain areas and habitat of minority ethnic group. The death rates of infectious disease, verminosis and nutritional deficiency disorder are still high. Table 4-5 shows the top 10 causes of death of people in some Chinese cities and counties in 2000.

Table 4-5   The top 10 causes of death in some Chinese cities and counties in 2000

No.	Dwellers in some cities			Dwellers in some counties		
	Causes of death	Special death rate (per 100,000 people)	Proportion of death to the total death number (%)	Causes of death	Special death rate (per 100,000 people)	Proportion of death to the total death number (%)
1	Malignant tumor	146.61	24.38	Disease of respiratory system	142.16	23.11
2	Disease of cerebral vessels	127.96	21.28	Malignant tumor	112.57	18.40
3	Cardiac disease	106.65	17.74	Disease of cerebral vessels	115.20	18.40

(Table 4-5)

No.	Dwellers in some cities			Dwellers in some counties		
	Causes of death	Special death rate (per 100,000 people)	Proportion of death to the total death number (%)	Causes of death	Special death rate (per 100,000 people)	Proportion of death to the total death number (%)
4	Disease of respiratory system	79.92	13.29	Cardiac disease	73.43	12.37
5	Injury and toxication	35.57	5.91	Injury and toxication	64.89	11.03
6	Disease of digestion system	18.38	3.06	Disease of digestion system	23.89	3.98
7	Endocrinopathy and nutritional, metabolizable and immune system disease	17.99	2.99	Disease of reproduction system	9.27	1.51
8	Disease of reproduction and urinary system	9.01	1.50	Pulmonary tuberculosis	7.39	1.19
9	Mental disease	6.70	1.11	Disease of neonate	7.05	1.14
10	Neuropathy	5.53	0.92	Endocrinopathy and nutritional, metabolizable and immune system disease	6.84	1.11
	Total of ten causes of death		92.18	Total of ten causes of death		91.46

Material source: *Health Annual of China in 2001*.

(3) Facing the double challenges of infectious disease and chronic non-infectious disease: In recent years, the former infectious diseases, such as plague, cholera, become active in some local places. At the same time, the new infectious disease, such as Serious Acute Respiratory Symptom (SARS), makes new threat to people's health and makes awkward situation to the work of prevention and cure. Some diseases that have once been controlled well or steadily, such as venereal disease, tuberculosis, schistosomiasis, are rekindled. Due to the appearance of prostitution, going whoring and drug

use, China is facing the latent risk that the AIDS will be spread widely. There are numerous people who developed viral hepatitis and other diseases which have very serious harm. Some diseases which have close relationship with environment and nutrition, such as endemic fluorosis, endemic thyromegaly and Kaschin-Beck disease, have not been controlled effectively. At the same time, chronic non-infectious diseases have become popular and common among people. The prevalence rate of mental disease increases constantly. Various acute and chronic occupational diseases caused by the occupational hazard are still very high. The double threats coming from both infectious disease and non-infectious disease become the most important health problem in China.

(4) Health demand of inhabitants in cities and villages changes: The national health service survey in 1998 indicates the prevalence rate of disease in two weeks increased 6.9% compared with that in 1993, which shows the health demand of inhabitants are increasing. The prevalence rate of some chronic non-infectious diseases ascends greatly and these diseases become more popular and common among inhabitants. For example, the prevalence rates of diabetes and hypertension in cities have ascended to 53% and 32% respectively. And the rates in villages are much higher, which have reached 128% and 36% respectively. The risk degree of disease expands. The national people's total days of being sick increase to 2.45 billion days. The average rest days of a worker per year increase 1.8 days. The total number of disabled people caused by disease and injury is 85 million. The total population of physical disabilities who need society and other people's help is 16 million. Health has showed more and more influence on the social economy.

(5) The unintentional injuries become ascending: Now the traffic accidents are ascending in China, which has become the first cause of all the other accidents. In 2002, the death number of traffic accidents was 109,000, which held 78.5% of the total death number of all kinds of accidents. The mortality was 13.71 people per 10,000 cars. It was much higher than that in developed countries and some developing countries. In addition, solvent intoxication makes much attention. Recently various kinds of solvents are widely used in construction, shoemaking, box & bag manufacturing industries. But they are lack of defending measurements. Intoxication often happens because of over-contact with the benzene, formaldehyde and CCl_4, etc. It was once reported that in some foreign capital enterprises of Guangdong Province, the number of people caused by solvent intoxication accounts for 64.4% among all of the occupational intoxication. There were 94.6% of serious intoxications that were caused by solvent.

2. The social factors that affect health

(1) The status of social economy: From 1978 to 2000, GDP per capita in China rose from 379 RMB to 7,084 RMB. The average living area in city increased from 3.6 to

10.3 square meters, and 8.1 to 24.8 square meters in countryside. The enrollment rate of children who reached the school age ascended from 49.2% in 1952 to 99.1% in 2000.

(2) Population status: Population's urbanization and aging are speeding. From 1978 to 2000, the total population of cities and towns increased from 17 million to 45 million. The urbanization level rose from 17.9% to 36.2%. It is anticipated that within the coming 20 years, the urbanization level will arrive 60%. The cause of aged population speeding in China was the result of rapid decreasing of bear rate in China in short times. In 1990, people who were 60 years old or over 60 occupied 8.6% of the total, while in 2000 they occupied 10%. It is anticipated that in 2020 they will attain 15.6%. The absolute number increased in aged people will bring heavy pressure to the whole social economy and health system.

(3) Health service status: After the building up of PRC, the number of health institution and health officer augment fast. Now there are 2.4 hospital beds and 1.3 doctors per 1,000 people. The average medical cost of a person is US＄33. The whole health cost accounts for 4.8% of GDP. The health service cost accounts for 2.1% of the nation financial expenses. But these indicators are still less than those of developed countries. For example, there are 2.87 doctors per 100 people in developed countries. The financing formation of total health cost showed that from 1990 to 1995, the proportion of government budget of health expenses to the whole nation health expenses reduced from 25% to 17%. The inhabitant's individual expenses increased from 27% to 50%. However, the proportion of total health cost to the GDP in developed countries at the same period ascended from 9% to 12%. The proportion of government budget of health expenses in these countries is generally high. Take the British as an example, its proportion was 80%.

(4) Behavior and life style: The sampling survey in 1991 indicates the average smoking rate of Chinese people at or over 15 years old was 30.5%, and 61.0% in males, 7.0% in females. The population of Chinese male occupied 10% of the male in the world. However, they had consumed 30% of cigarettes in the world. In 1990, there were 800,000 Chinese people died of smoking. An estimation in 1989 showed that the increased health cost related with smoking in China was 6.9 billion RMB. It is predicted that in 30 years there will be 200,000 people in China who die of smoking if no actions are taken. Another sampling survey showed the prevalence rate of alcohol dependence of city people in China was 3.7%. The prevalence rate of chronic alcohol dependence in some areas where minority ethnic group live was much higher than that in other places. Now in China, the addicted alcohol users are 116 million and there are more than 10,000 people who have got alcohol intoxication. About 10,000 people die of it.

In recent years, the spread of AIDS in China was quick. From 1985 when the first HIV-infected person was found to the end of 2002, it was estimated that there were 1.

04 million people who were infected by HIV in China, and more than 200,000 AIDS patients among them. It was reported by WHO, till the end of 2001 the total number of HIV-infected persons were 1.2 million in west Pacific Ocean Area where included China. And China was on the first place in this area, the 4th place in Asia and the 17th in the world. The prevalence rate of other sexually transmitted disease (STD) such as syphilis increased decade times per year.

3. The primary health problems faced in China in the 21st century

(1) The prevention and cure to the infectious disease can't be loosened. And the road of prevention and cure to the chronic non-infectious disease is heavy while the way is long.

(2) Realize the goal that everyone receives health care. It must be resolved that most farmers in China receive the elementary health services, which is a hard task.

(3) Urbanization speeds, which brings challenge to the health institutions on how to cope with the modern public health problems.

(4) The establishment and perfection of socialistic market economy system bring higher requirements to the function of public health supervision.

(5) The aging problem becomes prominent gradually as the society develops in China. It is urgent to adjust the current health service system and service mode.

(6) The situation of unintentional injuries is serious. Traffic accident, intoxication, fire disaster and mine accident often happens. So the social preventive measurements should be strengthened more.

(7) China has entered into the new stage of constructing the rich and comfortable society. It is required that health institution should provide multiplayer and various services to meet the demand of people at different social classes.

(8) Because of the knowledge exploding, life rhythm speeding and intense social competition, the mental health problem should be given comprehensive attention.

第二篇　社会病理现象

Part 2　Social Pathologic Phenomena

第五章 疾病流行中的社会医学问题

人具有两种属性:生物属性和社会属性。疾病发生与流行不仅受生物学因素、自然因素和生态因素的影响,而且与社会因素息息相关。社会因素对疾病的影响广泛而深刻,一是因为各种疾病的流行无不与人类活动的足迹紧密相连,二是在任何一种疾病的发生、转归和防治过程中,社会因素常常起着极其重要的作用。因此,无论从个体,还是从群体角度去分析疾病流行中的社会问题,都是社会医学要研究的重要内容。

第一节 传染病流行中的社会因素

一、概述

传染病是指在宿主之间直接通过媒介互相传播,具有传染性、暴发性和流行性等特点的疾病。传染病的发生和流行必须具有传染源、传播途径和易感人群三个环节,并受社会和自然两大因素的影响。随着时代的变迁,传染病的传播与社会文化因素的关系更加密切。传染病的特点在于它的致病因子是活的病原微生物,在生物长期进化过程中适应了定居于人或者其他宿主的一定组织和器官。传染病就是病原体和宿主两种生物在一定环境中相互作用的结果;传染病的发生是千万年来病原体与人类机体长期进化和适应的结果,两者是矛盾的统一体,是彼此消长、相互斗争、不断适应的过程。机体对病原体产生免疫力、抵抗力的过程,也是病原体发生相应的变化对抗人体的免疫力的过程。

因此,我们必须重视社会因素对传染病的发生发展的重要影响,从社会根源上探究其发病原理。传染病同其他事物一样有其发生、发展和消亡的客观规律。既有内因,又有外因。内因是变化的根据,外因是变化的条件。造成传染病重新抬头的影响因素既有生物因素,又有社会环境因素。生物因素是指微生物的进化与变异,是内因。社会环境因素包括自然因素与社会因素,是外因。在人类改造自然、改变生态环境时,社会因素往往作用于自然因素。社会因素既是促使传染病传播蔓延的重要因素,又是有效防治及消灭传染病的关键所在。近年来,越来越多的学者认识到社会因素在传染病产生和流行过程中所起的决定性作用。很多生物因素是在社会因素影响下出现的,终极根源还是社会因素的影响。即使是病原微生物本身(内因)的改变,如致病性的增加和对抗生素抵抗力的增强,也是社会因素所影响的。因此用社会医学的方法去认识传染病的病因,对于制定传染病的综合防治措施、促进人类健康具有重要的意义。

二、社会因素影响传染病流行的表现形式

社会因素包括生产、生活条件、医疗卫生状况、经济、文化、生活方式、人口和社会制度等。社会因素通过作用于传染病的三个环节而影响其流行过程。社会因素对传染病的流行过程既有正向作用亦有负向作用。

(一)社会经济对传染病的影响

社会经济既是人类社会发展的主体形式,又是人类赖以生存和保持健康的基本条件,同时它是一把双刃剑,对传染病防治起着双向的作用。

一方面,社会经济的发展将大大提高其他社会要素的水平,直接为公共卫生事业提供物质保障;由于公共卫生具有效益外在性和福利性的特征,因此政府应该在这方面的物质投入上承担相应的责任,增强居民战胜传染病的能力。传染病流行的控制依赖于对传染病流行的三个环节的干预。其中,对易感人群接种有效疫苗是控制传染病流行的关键措施,而研制新型疫苗需要大量人力和物力,没有科技和经济作后盾是办不到的,实践已证明社会经济和科技的发展对预防传染病最直接有效的结果是产生用于防治传染病的新疫苗;而切断传播途径、消除传染源有赖于社会经济的发展,发展公共卫生基础设施也依赖于政府物质的投入。现代社会经济的进步和发展,使得人类的生活质量和健康水平有了很大的提高,也将大大增强人类抗病能力。但是,如果忽视对公共卫生事业的投入,使预防医学处于"讲起来重要,办起来次要"的状态,新老传染病就会联手卷土重来,使卫生工作的重心再次向第一次卫生革命倾斜。艾滋病流行和非典型肺炎在中国的暴发就是深刻的教训。

另一方面,经济发展促进了人类健康水平的提高的同时,也对人类防治传染病和人类的健康问题提出了新的挑战,主要表现在以下几个方面:

(1) 环境污染和破坏。现代工业对人类的生活、生产环境造成了严重的污染和破坏,由此产生的公共卫生问题及潜在的危害广泛存在。

(2) 生活方式的改变。随着社会经济的发展,行为模式的改变和不良生活方式也成为传染病发生的重要因素。对于一些发达国家居民来说,健康问题已不再来自营养不良、劳动条件恶劣和卫生设施落后,而主要来自不良的生活方式,如吸毒、性乱导致的艾滋病的流行。例如2003年SARS在我国的暴发流行,首先发生在广东省,据初步估计,就与食用野生动物有一定的关系,因为现已发现多种动物身上携带有SARS病毒。

(3) 大量合成化学物质进入人类生活。为改善人类生活条件不断使用一些新的化学物质,使人类在吃、穿、住、行方面无时无刻不与化学物质接触,这些化学物质无疑将会对人类的健康产生负面影响,降低了他们抵抗传染病的能力。

(4) 社会流动人口增加。经济的发展必然伴随着流动人口的增加,也将给传染病防治增加了难度。

(二)科学技术对传染病防治的影响

科学技术总是与传染病相伴而生、此消彼长,科学技术对传染病的控制一直发挥着关键性的作用。科学上的每一次发现,都是人类从必然王国迈向自由王国的一步。尤其是20世纪初以来,在短短100年里完成了医学史上95%以上的发明和发现,使导致人口大量死亡的传染病得到了有效控制。现代科学飞速发展使得人类在跟传染病较量过程中的力量对比发生了根本变化。人类对传染病从病原到发病,再到人体如何抵抗它,有更深入、更进一步的了解。一方面,科学技术的进步发展带来了高新医药生物技术领域的革命,一批控制重大传染病的基因治疗包括基因工程药物、基因工程疫苗相继问世将大大缩短人类与传染病斗争的历程。从艾滋病到SARS,我们可以看出现代医学、现代科学技术飞速发展所带来的深刻变化。人类从发现艾滋病到不断深入研究再到不断发现有效的治疗方法,经过了10年时间。此次与SARS的斗争,从2003年2月份SARS在广东流行到4月16日,仅两个月的时间,中外科学家就成功地找到了病原,这就为研制特效药物指明了方向。正如胡锦涛主席所说的:"战胜非典,我们主要依靠的是科学技术。"

另一方面,营养学和卫生学的进展使人类找到了改善营养、增强体质的有效途径,科技进步改善了人的健康状况,减少了人的机体遭受疾病侵害的广度与频度,延长了人的个体生命存在和持续的时间。科学还间接地通过促进社会经济的发展,全面改善人类的生活状态,增长人类的福利,从而增强了人体抵抗传染病的能力和促进了社会的繁荣稳定。

(三)人口因素与传染病

人口不仅是社会存在和发展的要素,而且与人类的健康息息相关。世界卫生组织指出:"健康、人口和发展是相互不可分割的,发展的成功,取决于资源的平衡。迅速增长的人口正在威胁着这种平衡。"人口的过快增长对人类传染病预防工作提出了空前的挑战。这主要表现在以下几个方面:

1. 加重社会负担,影响卫生资源投入。世界很多地区由于人口的增长速度超过了经济增长速度,致使大批居民营养不良,社会卫生状况恶化,大量失业人口存在和生活条件下降,也对居民的身心健康造成了严重的损害。这样必然导致社会财富主要用于维持温饱,而减少对公共卫生、教育和医疗保健的投入,最终使得预防传染病的防线出现漏洞。

2. 加重环境破坏,造成新旧传染病的肆虐。由于人类不仅需要维持生活的物质条件,而且需要生活和生产空间,导致人类对自然界的干预和破坏达到空前规模。人类社会工业化过程造成的污染,改变了生态平衡,使得很多生物死亡,对生态系统中生物链产生很大影响。全球气候变化和旱涝灾害都是传染病发生的重要因素。药物滥用、血液制品的污染和捕食野生动物也造成了传染病的发生。最近30年,人类发现了30多种以前不知道的传染病。尽管有了现代医疗手段,传染病不再像以前那样会引起大量的死亡,但是新的传染病产生的速度比以前更快了,这是现代社会的发展对生态的破坏所造成的。

3. 人口流动和经济全球化,加剧了传染病的传播。人口流动和经济全球化是现代社会普遍存在的现象。随着工业化的进展,世界人口聚集居住的都市化现象也越来越普遍,且速度有增无减。联合国人口统计局最近的统计表明:城市人口已占全球人口的一半,而且这一比例还在不断增加。人口集中化和爆炸性增长最大的危险就是传染病的大流行,城市的密集人口是传染病大流行的温床,人口的高度密集容易导致传染病通过空气传播、饮水传播和直接接触传播。人口增长速度过快而经济发展滞后则使预防措施不到位和公共设施难以满足人群的需要；伴随着人口的剧增，世界各大城市饱受生活垃圾的侵扰，"垃圾围城"不仅成为城市卫生环境的第一"世界难题"，也成为滋养传染病的温床。经济全球化导致的人口大流动也使传染病在全球范围内四处传播。全世界每年约有 4.5 亿人从一个大洲到另一个大洲去旅游，其中至少包括 110 万 HIV 感染者。正如美国哥伦比亚大学新兴传染病专家赫斯蒂芬·莫尔斯所说："SARS 表明我们未来可能遇到什么。使病原体传染大量人口并扩散到全球各地的条件近年来不断发展，而且还会继续发展。"

4. 卫生服务与传染病防治。卫生服务是卫生部门为一定目的合理使用卫生资源向居民提供服务的过程，在这里主要是指向居民提供传染病防治所需服务的过程。与传染病防治紧密相关的卫生服务有传染病防治服务需要量、相关的卫生资源配置情况、利用情况、评价体系以及服务体制。由于长期以来受急功近利思想的影响，使与传染病的防治有关的卫生服务处于从属地位，大大地淡化了"预防为主"的指导思想，使传染病的防治工作出现了漏洞。我们应该从 2003 年非典型肺炎的暴发中吸取教训。

5. 其他社会因素对传染病影响。生活方式、风俗习惯、宗教信仰、文化素养等其他因素也可影响传染病流行过程。例如，我国有些地区居民喜欢吃生的或半生的水产品而引起肺吸虫病、华支睾吸虫病、绦虫病、甲型肝炎等病发生；新疆察布查尔锡伯族自治县流行的察布查尔病（肉毒杆菌引起的肉毒中毒），是由当地锡伯族人生吃面酱的半成品"米送糊糊"所致；缺少饭前便后洗手卫生习惯者易发肠道传染病；在早期推行全球消灭天花计划及近期实施消灭脊髓灰质炎的计划过程中，某些国家个别地区的宗教势力有干扰免疫接种计划的推行事例发生，因而对当地的灭病计划也有一定的影响。

因此，面对传染病对人类健康生存的挑战，需要全球采取共同行动，不仅从卫生防疫上，更要从社会系统工程这一大思路上寻找答案。

第二节　传染病控制的社会医学策略

从艾滋病到"非典"，都在提示和指向医学模式的多元化趋向，新的传染病和死灰复燃的传染病将会更加危险和凶残。21 世纪，我们将面临着以预防控制传染病为重点的第一次卫生革命和以预防控制慢性非传染病为重点的第二次卫生革命的双重挑战，形势十分严峻，任务极为繁重。因此，应该制定正确的传染病控制策略。

一、一定要有与传染病长期斗争的思想准备

从历史上看，人类跟传染病的较量是个漫长过程。人类与微生物以及其他生物，都是在自然界中共存的，因此它们之间是相生相克、互相制约的关系。传染病长期存在也符合辩证法。

世界卫生组织 1980 年 5 月 28 日郑重宣布：全球已经消灭了天花！于是一些专家提出世界医学模式正在发生变化，即由生物医学模式转变为社会——心理医学模式，也就是说以前人类疾病主要是生物因素引起的传染病，而后主要是社会和心理等因素引发的慢性病。这一理念曾一度得到了世界卫生组织的认同。然而，5 年之后，首先在美国发现一

种新传染病——艾滋病。正是这种迄今人类还无法对付的传染病,不仅使专业人员也使普通大众意识到,传染病永远不会绝迹,传染病并未退出历史舞台;而非典型肺炎的出现则说明,新传染病并非仅仅一种,很可能成双成对或大量出现,故此两种或多元医学模式将在今后并存。人类社会和自然界是一个多元的综合体,传染病种类亦呈多元状态,人类与传染病的斗争将是艰苦而又漫长的。

二、传染病的防治必须坚持现代大卫生观

大卫生观体现了社会医学的系统观,大卫生观强调各级政府要充分认识到公共卫生工作对维护社会发展和稳定的重要作用,并承担起相应的责任。具体到传染病防治,就是要突出预防工作的系统性、整体性、协调性和社会性。但是迄今为止,我们对传染病的研究仍主要停留在生物学方面,而对社会、心理、行为、环境等因素与传染病发生、发展的相互作用研究较少。近年来,传染病在世界范围内有愈演愈烈之势。这表明,在遏制传染病传播上抗生素已显得越来越"力不从心",而社会因素在现代传染病的流行与控制中越发显得突出。所以人们在进行传染病控制时,不仅要考虑生物因素,更要重视环境、社会、心理和行政手段等方面对疾病的影响。通过对传染病的社会因素分析,我们可看出,生物因素所占的比例在逐步变小,而社会政治、经济因素、个人行为、生活方式所占的比重越来越大。我们必须确立以全体社会人员为服务对象,以优化生态环境、改善社会环境为目标的社会大卫生观,唤起各行各业的社会大众担负起预防传染病滋生与传播的责任。建国50多年的历史证明,社会大卫生观是我国传染病防治工作取得辉煌成绩的根本,这一观念一旦淡化,就会造成传染病防治网的破损和工作滑坡,对人民健康和正常的社会经济秩序造成不良后果。我们应看到,它不仅仅是人类面临的医学问题,而且是一个严峻的社会问题。大卫生观突出强调发展经济、改善人民物质生活条件,对防治传染病的重要意义,但也重视对群众加强科学文化教育和精神文明教育,提高人口素质,加强公共卫生建设,使其改变不良生活习惯,增强自我保健意识,降低与社会环境密切相关的传染病的发病率及死亡率。同时还强调加强生态环境保护、控制人口增长、促进社会的可持续发展对控制传染病的现实意义。

三、加强控制传染病的各个方面的技术合作,形成预防传染病的合力

本着"分工明确、加强合作、优化配置"的原则统筹安排传染病的预防工作。首先,应该加强传染病的基础和应用研究。在控制传染病的基础研究中应当把微生物的变异作为重点,尤其是微生物基因组工程。病原体的最后确诊依赖于实验技术的应用,用核酸扩增技术和先进的抗原抗体血清学检验方法有助于这一问题的解决。传染病学是随着分子生物学、免疫学和流行病学的发展而发展的。传染病的应用研究应将实验研究和流行病学研究相结合,以完善和优化防治措施。同时,控制传染病必须重视有关预防、治疗、诊断新方法的开发研究。

其次,应该加强传染病的全球合作和监控工作。经济的全球化进程加快,使传染病的传播模式也出现了新局面。传染病的传播是无国界的,仅仅在某一国家和地区消灭或控制传染病是不现实的,消灭传染病是全球的共同责任,消灭传染病必须依靠全球的通力合作,实现信息与技术的交流和共享。为此建立一个全球性的传染病监测体系势在必行。在中国,还要相应健全各省市传染病流行监测组织;加强控制传染病创新技术的培训与推广;重视流行病学人才的培养,并采取相应的激励措施;要使生物信息学首先用于预防医学,实现全国性传染病监测网的联网。

再次,发挥政府职能优势。要注重早期预防和早期控制,公共卫生基础建设、环境保护、城市规划和国境检疫必须着眼于未来,处理好经济发展与人类利益的关系,并特别应当注意机构、体系的完善和人才培养、储备,建立规范的科学研究程序,充分利用先进的科学技术平台,发展先进的传染病防治技术,并加快科技应用步伐,把传染病的预防和控制当做一个影响健康社会和经济发展的重要因素来看待,并在政策制定过程中加以体现。同时大力加强传染病防治工作法制化建设。乔治敦大学法律及公共卫生中心的负责人 Lawrence O. Gostin 表示:"公共卫生法制的改革已经迫在眉睫。对监控、防疫、治疗、隔离、检疫等都应有一套明确的规定,使卫生机构能在法律的框架下有充分的决定权去应对突发卫生危机。"

总之,传染病不再仅仅是一个纯医学问题,而已成为一个社会问题,对世界所产生的后果难以估量。展现在我们面前的传染病形势是严峻的,预防和控制传染病的工作任重而道远。

第三节 慢性病流行中的社会因素

随着我国社会经济的发展以及人民生活水平的提高和卫生事业的进步,疾病谱已发生了变化。在传染病逐步得到控制的情况下,慢性病正严重影响着人民的生命和生活质量,已成为严重的公共卫生问题。慢性病主要包括:①心脑血管疾病;②恶性肿瘤;③代谢性疾病;④精神异常和精神病;⑤遗传性疾病;⑥慢性职业病;⑦慢性气管炎和肺气肿。据世界卫生组织估算,1999年,上述疾病造成的死亡大约占全球死亡总人数的60%,占全球疾病负担的43%,到2020年时,这类死亡预计占死亡总人数的73%,占疾病负担的60%。因此,加强慢性病的防治管理已成为疾病控制的重要任务。

一、社会因素对慢性病作用的规律

慢性病是社会经济发展的主要产物,即"现代文明病"(the diseases of modernization),它的发病机制和发病原理带有明显的社会原因。社会因素影响慢性病主要是通过心理感受这个中心环节发生作用的。社会因素被人的感知器官系统纳入,经过中枢神经系统的调节和控制,形成心理折射,产生心理反应及行为、社会适应和躯体机能的变化,从而改变了人的健康状况。社会因素对慢性病的影响具有如下规律和特点。

1. 泛影响性。泛影响性是指作用的发散性,是指一种社会因素可导致全身多个器官及系统发生功能变化。

2. 恒常性与积累性。社会因素广泛存在于人们的现实生活中,对人类慢性病产生具有稠密和持久的作用,即作用的恒常性;而社会因素长期作用于人体可形成应答累加及功能损害累加或健康效应累加。

3. 交互作用。社会因素作用于人体健康导致慢性病发作常常是以交互作用的方式产生效应，这主要是由其因果的多元性所决定的。

二、社会因素对慢性病作用的表现形式

慢性病是多种致病因素综合作用的结果。由于人类具有整体性和社会性的特点，人体处于内环境与外环境各种因素相互联系、相互作用的生态关系之中，我们对社会因素与慢性病的关系思考也应该坚持全方位化和多层次化。

(一)社会经济对慢性病的作用

社会经济的发展，提高了人们受教育层次，优化了人们的职业结构，增加了人们可支配的收入，促进了人类整体健康水平的提高，同时也给人类带来了新的健康问题，加重了慢性病的发展。主要表现在以下几个方面：

1. 环境被污染和破坏。现代工业给人类生活和生产环境造成了严重的污染和破坏，使人类的吃、穿、住、行和工作等环节都无时无刻不与化学物质接触，由此产生的健康问题及潜在的危害广泛存在。环境与慢性病的发作的关系是复杂的，环境中的化学、生物、物理因素以及其他因素相互交织，可产生对人体间断的或持续反复的侵袭。环境化学物对人体损害可以分为特异性损害和非特异性损害两种，前者包括急慢性中毒和特殊毒性反应，后者多表现为某些慢性病、多发病的发病率增加，慢性病病情加重，人体抵抗力和劳动能力明显下降等。

2. 生活方式的改变。随着社会经济的发展，人类的健康主要受不良生活方式的威胁。不良的生活方式已成为慢性病最重要的致病因素。早在 1993 年 WHO 的专家们就指出："大约 20 年以后，发展中国家和发达国家的死亡方式将大致相同，生活方式疾病将成为世界头号杀手。"生活方式疾病是由不良习惯造成的，而且一种不良习惯对健康有着多种危害。比如，吸烟和不适当的膳食结构，不仅会导致患心脏病、中风、高血压，而且会增加结肠癌、胃癌的发生率。尽管生活方式疾病还被认为主要属于西方发达国家的疾病，但目前从绝对人数来看，此类疾病的死亡率发展中国家比发达国家更高。在发达国家里，每年约有 820 万人死于心脏病、中风、癌症等生活方式疾病，而第三世界中每年此类疾病的死亡人数大约为 1 170 万。死于生活方式疾病的人数现在占发展中国家总死亡人数的 45% 左右。到 2015 年，预计将上升到 60%。而发达国家预计将达到 75%。

3. 心理因素与慢性病。心理因素包括社会心理、个性心理以及对应激、生活事件的情绪反应。随着生产力水平的提高以及知识经济时代到来，社会竞争更加激烈，导致工作、生活节奏的加快，紧张、刺激及工作压力给身心健康带来了不良影响。大量研究表明，许多有害的社会心理因素可能是躯体疾病和精神疾患的致病因素。相反，良好的社会心理因素对疾病的预防治疗和康复起着重要作用。个性心理主要包括能力、气质和性格三个方面，能力主要是指人的智力和技能，而气质和性格则与慢性病的发病有着直接的联系。例如，20 世纪 50 年代 Friedman 和 Rosenmen 等提出 A 型性格模型以来，它与冠心病的关系已有了多门学科的研究，被认为是与高胆固醇血症、吸烟及高血压并列的冠心病危险因子之一。人们对不同生活事件会用不同的情绪反应，愉快积极的情绪可对人体的生理机能起到良好的作用，可以发挥人的潜力，有利于人的健康；而消极情绪可能使人的心理失去平衡,严重的会导致神经系统功能紊乱、机体病变。

(二)人口因素对慢性病的影响

人口因素对慢性病的影响也不可忽视,尤其是人口老龄化问题,因为慢性病患者主要人群是中、老年人。我国慢性病问题之所以如此突出,人口老龄化是一大原因。随着人们生活水平的改善,人均寿命已从20世纪40年代末的35岁增加到1998年的71岁;60岁以上人口从1991年的9.35%增至1998年的10.52%。老龄人口增多了,再加上城市化进程的加快,生活节奏也明显加快,城市拥挤症、综合征等精神卫生疾病也使得人们(特别是老年人)感到不适应。慢性病低龄化的趋势也不容忽视,虽然现在的慢性病主要患病人群仍是中、老年人,但年轻人比例呈上升趋势。美国是慢性病防治做得较好的国家,慢性病总体比例在下降,但其年轻人的比例却呈上升趋势。足见慢性病的低龄化是一个全球性的问题。在现代大城市中有许多青少年喜食高糖、高脂食品和快餐(欧美国家称之为垃圾食品)导致肥胖,肥胖会使心脑血管疾病、心脏病、高血压、糖尿病等主要慢性病的发病率大大增高;还有一些青少年有吸烟、喝酒等不良习惯;随着科技的发展,电子产品增多,许多孩子整天呆在家里上网聊天或玩游戏,活动量不够,再加上应试教育的不良影响,在学校就只有一周一次的体育课,身体的运动和锻炼很不够。这就为其以后慢性病的发作留下了隐患。

(三)社会关系与慢性病

人是社会人,人是生活在有一定社会关系结合而成的社会群体,包括家庭、邻里、朋友和工作团体之中的。这些基本社会群体构成了社会网络。人在社会网络中的相互关系是否协调,是否能得到相互支持,不仅是影响健康的因素,而且是健康的基本内容。因为社会关系的好坏直接影响人的心理健康和情绪反应,而慢性病与人的心理和社会因素有着重要的联系。社会关系包括两个方面——社会支持和家庭关系。社会支持(social support)是指一个人从社会网络中获得的情感、物质和生活上的帮助。支持是一个人的基本的社会需要,获得社会支持不是被动的,而是一个互动的过程。影响社会支持的因素主要有人际关系、社会网络和社会凝聚力。家庭是以婚姻和血缘关系为纽带组成的基本社会单位,家庭结构、功能和关系是否完好对于家庭成员的身心健康有着重要的影响。如果长期处于关系紧张家庭环境中,不良的刺激会对人的健康产生稠密和持久的影响,即作用的恒常性和积累性,从而引起人的神经-内分泌-免疫系统调节的紊乱,最终引起人躯体机能的变化和慢性病的发作。

(四)其他社会因素与慢性病

其他社会因素包括卫生服务、文化教育等因素。卫生服务不仅仅是治病救人,而且要维护和促进人群的健康。在现代社会,卫生服务被列入社会保障的范畴,卫生事业是社会发展的重要方面。卫生服务对慢性病防治的基本功能包括保健功能和社会功能,保健功能是通过预防保健、治疗、康复及健康教育等措施,降低人群的慢性病的发病率和死亡率,维护人群健康,提高生命质量;社会功能是通过对慢性病患者进行医疗服务,使其恢复健康,提高生活质量和社会生产力,维护社会的稳定和发展。由于不同国家卫生资源和卫生服务配置以及人群健康状况不尽相同,WHO提出要本着社会公平的精神和国际合作的原则在全世界,特别是在发展中国家实施初级卫生保健,尽量减少各类疾病的发生。文化的特征决定了它对健康影响的广泛性和恒常性,文学艺术、教育、道德规范、风俗习惯、宗教信仰等文化诸现象对健康的影响不仅仅局限于个人,而是整个人群,其广泛程度远远大于生物、自然因素;另一方面,文化作为精神产物,影响人的思想意识、观念,这种影响作用一旦发生,绝非短期内能消失。因此,文化因素对健康的影响常持续于生命的整个过程,甚至几代人或更长时间。文化的各个方面直接影响着人们的生活环境、劳动条件、生活方式和心理状态,对人的生理健康和心理健康产生广泛的影响,进而对人们控制慢性病起到积极的作用。

第四节 慢性病控制的社会医学策略

慢性病通常为终身性疾病,病痛和伤残不仅影响人的劳动能力和生活质量,而且治疗费用高昂,给家庭、社会和国家带来了沉重的负担。因此,在慢性病的防治过程中仍要坚持预防为主的方针,而选择适当的、切实可行的预防策略和措施,对于慢性非传染性疾病的控制具有举足轻重的作用。具体说来,预防策略的选择要从以下几个方面入手。

一、慢性病的三级预防策略

慢性病的疾病自然史(natural history of disease)可以粗略地分为发病前期、发病期和发病后期三个阶段。在发病前期,虽未发病,但已存在潜在的危险因子,如血清胆固醇高是冠心病(CHD)的危险因子,吸烟是肺癌的危险因子,肥胖是糖尿病的危险因子。发病前期也可有某种病理生理的改变,如血管粥样硬化等。在发病期,一般都有轻重不一的临床表现。在发病后期,其结局可能是痊愈或死亡,也可能会留下后遗症甚至残疾等。在疾病自然史的每一个阶段,都可以采取措施防止疾病的发生或恶化。因而预防工作可以根据疾病自然史相应地分为三级:第一级预防为病因预防;第二级预防为"三早"预防,即早发现、早诊断、早治疗;第三级预防为对症治疗、防止伤残和加强康复工作。

第一级预防也叫初级预防(primary prevention),主要是针对致病因子(或危险因素)采取措施,也是预防慢性病的发生和消灭疾病的根本措施,其中包括自我保健和健康教育。自我保健即在发病前期就进行干预,以增强人的健康状况,促进健康。健康教育是以教育手段促使人们主动采取有利于健康的行为,从而消除危险因素,预防疾病,促进健康。第一级预防还包括保护和改善环境,旨在保证人们生产和生活区的空气、水、土壤不受工业"三废"——废气、废水、废渣和生活"三废"——粪便、污水、垃圾,以及农药、化肥等的污染。

第二级预防(secondary prevention)又称"三早"预防,它是发病期所进行的防止或减缓疾病发展的主要措施。为了保证"三早"的落实,可采用普查、筛检、定期健康检查、高危人群重点项目检查以及设立专科门诊等措施。

第三级预防(tertiary prevention)主要为对症治疗,防止病情恶化,减少疾病的不良作用,防止复发转移,预防并发症和伤残;对已丧失劳动力或残废者,通过康复治疗,促进其身心方面早日康复,使其恢复劳动力,病而不残或残而不废,保存其创造精神价值和社会劳动价值的能力。

二、慢性病预防的社会策略

1. 加强领导，坚持改革，加强慢性病防治的组织建设。慢性病防治是一项巨大的社会系统工程，没有行政领导的观念更新和高度重视，没有坚强有力的组织机构，没有整个社会的积极参与，单靠卫生部门少数医务人员孤军奋战，控制慢性病只能是美好的空想。

2. 以综合卫生观念进行慢性病防治。综合卫生是WHO针对生活方式疾病的规划，即共同防治由不健康生活方式的共同原因引起的疾病。这样可以更为经济有效。这是WHO于1990年在赫尔辛基发起的，其思想基础是：同一病因（即某种不健康的生活方式）造成的疾病不应分别处理，而应一起处理。WHO估计，实施综合规划，提倡健康的生活方式，至少可以使死亡率降低一半，即每年可拯救数百万人的生命。

3. 加强慢性病病因的流行病学调查。寻找危险因素及保护因素，阐明确切病因和疾病形成模式，以明确预防什么和如何预防。

4. 改变和避免不良的生活方式和行为，建立良好的健康的生活方式和行为，从而达到预防慢性病、增进健康的目的。不良的生活方式和行为主要包括吸烟、饮酒、不合理的膳食、钠摄入过多、钾摄入过低、精神紧张、长期坐位的生活方式、体力活动少等等。其中最为重要的是吸烟和不合理的膳食。天津市控制慢性病提出了"不吸烟，少吃盐，合理膳食，适当锻炼"的倡议后取得了良好的效果。

5. 以健康教育为主导措施，以降低危险因素为目标。这是国内外公认的一条低投入、高效益的战略决策。健康教育是通过传播媒介来提高人们的健康知识水平和自我保健能力，激励人们采取有益于健康的行为和生活方式，避免危险因素，进而达到增进健康的目标。健康教育既重视健康知识的传播，又强调行为的改变。健康教育已成为各国实现人人享有卫生保健这个战略目标的一个重要支柱，也是当前许多国家正在设法摆脱日益增长的巨额医药费财政开支的一条有效出路。北美、澳大利亚和北欧等许多国家正在积极推进这种新的健康促进模式，在预防和控制高血压、CHD以及与生活方式密切相关的恶性肿瘤等方面，都取得了令人鼓舞的成绩。

6. 从娃娃抓起，强调对人的一生的连续不断的健康管理。学校教育是在最理想的场所，进行健康教育效益最高、时机最佳。医学技术已证明，CHD、脑卒中和恶性肿瘤等疾病的某种病理变化和危险因素始于生命早期。我国某城市调查发现：3～6岁儿童33%血脂过高（主要是高胆固醇），儿童偏食率很高，以喜食肉食、拒食蔬菜类而导致的肥胖儿童的检出率在大城市有不断上升趋势，吸烟率近年亦有增高趋势。1978年澳大利亚阿德雷德市（Adclaide）在学校开始了一项10岁儿童改变生活方式的规划，首先从加强体力活动入手。该规划使儿童体力活动能力有所改善，同时有社会心理方面的好处，而学生学业成绩并未下降。的确值得我国借鉴。

7. 依靠城乡三级医疗预防保健网。在我国，医疗预防保健网已遍布城乡，城乡三级医疗预防保健网在防治疾病、保障人民健康上发挥了巨大作用。在慢性病防治中，无论是第一级预防、第二级预防还是第三级预防都必须紧紧依靠三级网，发挥其在健康教育、基线调查、干预措施的实施、信息管理、治疗、康复等多方面的作用。

8. 社区预防和高危人群预防策略。社区预防是指对全体居民的预防；高危人群预防是对危险性高的人员、家庭和集体作为特殊重点的预防。因为现代公共卫生规划，特别是防治与和生活方式有关的疾病，必须得到社会的理解与支持，通过融合到当前社会和卫生服务结构中去而受益。社区干预的策略主要在于减少社区人群普遍存在的危险因素。从流行病学观点看，社区模式的优势在于它在减少患病率方面要比强化的高危人群干预更为有效。从行为学和社会学观点看，社区模式的优势在减少植根于人们生存环境中的危险因素。因此，人群要形成永久性的健康生活方式，必须在社区范围内改变其不健康的生活方式。

案例

艾滋病引发的官司

欣欣妈妈分娩欣欣时医院给她输了 400 毫升血。出院后没有多长时间她就口腔溃疡、发烧、腹泻，且久治不愈，病情不断恶化。最后经检验，确认她患有艾滋病。后来连自己得了什么病都不知道就离开了人世。灾难接踵而至，当时只有两岁的欣欣经检验证实也因母乳喂养被感染艾滋病。为了清白，为了两条人命，为了今后的生存，欣欣爸爸决定讨回公道，他不相信妻子的一条命、孩子的未来、一个家庭的幸福就这样被简简单单地打发了，他决定运用法律维护全家人的权益。他找了许多律师，大家虽然同情但考虑到案件难度大，再加上艾滋病的恐惧和欣欣爸爸拿不出律师费等原因，没有人肯代理。欣欣和爸爸慕名来到北京大学法律系妇女法律研究与服务中心，中心决定给他们提供法律援助。在他们的帮助下，欣欣和父亲向法院提起了民事赔偿诉讼，并提出缓交诉讼费的请求。

终于开庭了，欣欣和爸爸能挺直腰板和医院对簿公堂了。庭审从早晨 8 点一直持续到下午 7 点，双方辩论激烈。一审法院判决被告——医院给付 36 万元赔偿费。欣欣父亲激动得流下了眼泪，他知道，等到这一天是那么多认识的和不认识的人共同伸出援助之手的结果。

思考 1. 艾滋病流行的社会因素有哪些？

思考 2. 通过本案例，对控制艾滋病你还有那些启发？

厦门：随地吐痰一律罚款 50 元

从 4 月 6 日开始，为严防"非典"病毒通过痰液传播，厦门市市容环境卫生监察大队将加强执法力度，对公共场所随地吐痰的不文明行为加大罚款额度，对在公共场所随地吐痰者，一律罚款 50 元，并将责令其将痰迹清除干净。昨天，有关部门共出动 100 名执法人员上街，对随地吐痰者进行处罚。市容监察执法人员称，对于随地吐痰等不文明行为，在已出台的《厦门市城市市容和环境卫生管理办法》中有规定，对随地吐痰者可处 10～50 元的罚款。为此有关部门通过加大执法力度，提高处罚额度，以加强震慑作用。

思考 1. 与"非典"流行有关的生活方式有哪些？

思考 2. 除了通过罚款帮助人们树立正确的卫生习惯外，还有哪些有效的方式？

Chapter 5   Social Medicine Problems of Disease Prevalence

Mankinds have two kinds of properties, biology and society. Disease occurrence and spreading not only are affected by biology factors, nature factors and ecological factors, but also are related social factors. Social factors exert extensive and deep influence on diseases. One cause is that every kind of disease prevalence is related with the human activity closely, the other is that social factors play an important role in any disease's occurrence, changing and prevention. Therefore, no matter from the angle of individuals or population to analyze social problems of disease prevalence, all these are important roles that social medicine needs to study.

Section 1   Social Factors of Infectious Diseases Prevalence

1. Summary

Contagion is a kind of transmitted disease by media, with the property of infectivity outbreak and epidemic. The necessary links of contagions are sources of infection, route of transmission and susceptible herd, simultaneously affected by social and natural factors. With changing of times, the transmission of infectious diseases has been simultaneously affected by social and cultural factors. And the characteristic of infectious diseases is that their pathopoiesia is live pathogenic microorganisms, which have adapted some tissues and organs of mankind or animals during the long-term evolutions. Therefore, the infectious diseases are the results produced by the struggles between pathogens and hosts under certain circumstances. Also, the happenings of them come from evolution and adapt between pathogens and mankind in thousands of years, which are entities of contradictions with the course of mutual growth and decline, struggle with each other and continuous adaptation. When the organisms have immune resistances against pathogens, pathogens react against our body.

So we should pay attention to the social factors' strong effect to infectious diseases. What's more, we should carry out social diagnosis and prescriptious from social roots. And infectious diseases have the same objective rules during the course of occurrence, development and extinct as other matters, which have internal causes and external causes. And the former is basis, the latter is condition. There are both biologic and social factors leading to infectious diseases' prevalence. Biologic factors refer to the evolution of pathogen. Social factors include natural factors, namely internal causes, which play an important role on natural factors, when people rebuild nature and change environment. So social factors are important causes that result in the infectious diseases' transmiting rapidly, as well as the key point to prevent and exterminate infectious diseases. More and more scholars have realized the vital role that social factors play, during the course of infectious diseases' occurrence and prevalence. Many biologic factors occur under the influence of social factors, but ultimately as the result of them. Even though there are some changes of pathogen, such as the increasing of pathogen and resistance to drugs, eventually resulting from social factors. So it is of great significance for making the comprehensively preventive measures and promoting the health of people if we use the methods of social medicine to study pathogen of infectious diseases.

2. The embodying forms of social factors affecting infectious diseases' prevalence

Social factors should include productions, living conditions, status of health, economy, culture, life style, population and social systems. Social factors affect infectious diseases' prevalence by their three links. So social factors have both positive and negative effects on them.

(1) Economy effect on infectious diseases

Economy is both the main body of society and basic living conditions and maintaining health. Meanwhile it is also a double-edged sword, exerting both-way effect on disease control. Because the development of economy can promote the standard of other social factors greatly, the public health cares are provided with material security. And governments should take responsibility for these investments to enhance their inhabitants' resistances against diseases, which is grounded on externality of health benefit and property of welfare. Disease control depends on the intervention of the three links, and among them the key is effective vaccine. But technology and economy are necessities, because improving advanced vaccines need large amount of manpower and material resources. All these measures, including cut-off route of transmission, eliminating source of infection and improving infrastructures of public health, depend on the devotions of governments. The life quality, health level and resistance against disease of people have been improved a lot, thanks to progress of modern society. But if the devotions are neglected, accordingly preventive medicine will be set in a state of "importance of being discussed, sub-importance of being practiced." So the prevalence of AIDS and SARS in our world provide us profound lessons.

On the other hand, when economy promotes people's health levels, it also produces new challenges on preventing infectious diseases and health issues, mainly including following aspects.

①Environmental pollution and deterioration. Modern industries bring about serious pollution to lives and product surroundings. Therefore, the public health issues and potential hazards are pervasive.

②Changing of life style. With improvement of economy, changing of behavior style and harmful life style has become an important factor attributing to infectious diseases. For some developed countries, the health issues mainly come from harmful life styles. For instance, drug taking, epidemic AIDS resulting from sexual disorder, instead malnutrition, bad working condition and hygienic facilities. For example, in 2003, the outbreak of SARS in Guangdong, China, partially related to eating wild animals by preliminarily predicting. Because SARS virus is found in some wild animals.

③Lots of synthesized chemical materials assessing our lives. In order to improve our lives, newly produced chemical materials have been used, which make people contact with them constantly. Undoubtfully these matters will produce negative effect on our health and reduce our resistance against diseases.

④Increasing of floating population. Increasing of floating population is inevitablely accompanied with development of economy, which can produce difficulty for preventing infectious diseases.

(2) Influence of preventing infectious diseases by science and technology

Science and technology have always played a vital role in disease control, which has a close relation with infectious diseases. Each finding in science makes human stride from confined kingdom to free kingdom greatly. Especially since the 20th century, people have fulfilled 95% inventious and findings of medicine history, which control deadly infectious diseases effectively. And the ratio between human beings and infectious diseases has changed ultimately. Human beings have far-reaching knowledge about pathogen, outbreak and treatment of the diseases.

The development of science and technology is revolutionary for the high-tech medicines and biology fields. As a result, a batch of gene treatments for controlling fatal infectious diseases comes out, including gene protecting medications and vaccines, which greatly shortens the struggling course between man and infectious diseases. So from AIDS to SARS, we can feel the profound changes that modern medicine and technology bring to. As we can also see, it took ten years to accomplish the course from finding first AIDS patient and now still studying in depth to getting effective treatment. But as for SARS, scientists only spent two months on finding out the pathogen successfully, which provided correct direction for improving specific medicine. Just as Chairman Hu Jintao appreciated "Overcoming SARS mainly depends on science and technology".

On the other hand, the developments of nutriology and hygiene help people find effective ways to improve nutrition and build up constitution. Science and technology contribute greatly to people, including improving the status of people' health, decreasing the extent and frequency of organisms' suffering from diseases, prolonging individual life span, promoting development of economy indirectly, improving people's life status roundly, increasing human welfare, which all consequently improve the ability of resisting infectious diseases and promote prosperity and stabilization of society.

(3) Population and infectious diseases

Population is not only a key element of society existence and development, but related closely to human health. WHO pointed out that "health, population and development are indivisible. But the rapidly increasing population is threatening the balance of resources, which decide success of development". Unprecedented challenges are put forward for prevention of infectious diseases, because of over-many population. There are aspects as follows:

①Aggravating society burden and affecting health resource input.

In many places of world, increasing speed of population exceeds that of economy, which results in malnutrition for many inhabitants, deterioration of public health, unemployment, decline of living conditions and serious hazard for inhabitants' health. All these above will ultimately lead social wealth to maintain basic dressing and food, but decrease the input to public health education and health care. So there are inevitable leaks in line of defence against infectious diseases.

②Aggravating environment disruption, resulting in all kinds of infectious disease unbridled.

Because of needing material conditions to maintain lives and spaces for living and manufacture, man unprecedentedly intervene and destroy the nature. Pollution resulting from industrialization, have changed balance of nature, leading some creatures extinct, which exerted significant influence on ecological links. So climate changing, drought and flood are all the key factors resulting in infectious diseases. And drug abuse, blood pollution and eating wild animals are also prime culprit. More than 30 kinds of unknown infectious diseases have been found in recent 30 years, although modern treatment can prevent infectious diseases as much mortality as before, speed of the new propagations are much more faster. All these attribute to ecological destroys.

③Floating population and globalization aggravating their transmission.

Population floating and globalization are very common nowadays. With increasing of industrialization, congregating urbanization has been more and more popular, what's more, its speed is steadily increasing. It was showed by PSB of UN that population of urban area have accounted for half of the whole world, and its proportion is increasing. The most dangerous thing is pandemic infectious diseases, resulted from congregation and explosive increasing of population. The dense urban population is the hotbed of the pandemic, because the highly dense population readily result in infectious diseases spreading by air, water and contact. Overmuch population and laggard economy can't ensure the timely preventing measures and public facilities meeting population. With the great increasing of population, the whole world metropolises are suffering from life garbage, so garbage encircling is not only the first worldwide problem of city sanitation, also the hotbed of fostering infectious disease. Movement of population makes them spread throughout the world. For instance, every year there are about 4.5 hundred million people traveling trans-continently, among of whom are at least 1.1 million people with HIV. Just as newly rising expert on infectious disease, H. Molth in Colombia University, USA said "SARS manifested what we would get in future. The conditions that make pathogen infect people even throughout the world are increasing continualy, What's more, they do go further."

④Health care and preventing

Health care is the process that health department offers health services for habitants for some specific purpose, here mainly referring to preventing infectious diseases. What relates closely to the preventing should include demanding quantity, allocation of health resource utility, assessing system and servicing organism. Because of being affected by quick success and instant benefit, the health care related to the preventing is disposed in secondary situation. The guideline of "giving priority to preventing" is desalinated and flaws appears in defence line of preventing. So we should get enough lessons from the outbreak of SARS in 2003.

⑤Other social factors of infectious diseases

Life style, customer, religion and culture, all can exert influence on prevalence of infectious diseases. For instance, in China, some of inhabitants like eating raw or uncooked aquatic food, which result in paragonimiasis, distoma japonicum, cestodiasis and hepatitis A. There was a kind of strange disease, namely Chabuchaer, which was resulted from eating raw sauce by Xinjiang local people. People who have no sanitary habit can readily be infected intestinal diseases. And even some religious forces intervened the enforcement of vaccination in some countries, when early program of exterminating smallpox and infantile paralysis was carried out. So cial factors eventually exerted negative influence on eliminating diseases.

Therefore, when faced with the challenge to the health of people, preventing infectious diseases need the co-operations of whole world. We should seek the answer not only from preventing systems but from the socially systematic project.

Section 2 Social Medical Strategies on Preventing Infectious Diseases

The outbreaks of AIDS and SARS all indicated and suggested that medical model have the trend of multi-element, Moreover, old and new infectious diseases are becoming more hazardous and fierce. In the 21st century, we are facing double challenges, including the medical revolution and the medical revolution. The former aims to control infectious diseases, and the latter to chronic diseases. So the situation is very serious and the task is very heavy. Accordingly, we must make valid controlling strategies.

1. Ensure the ideal of long-term struggle with infectious diseases

According to history, the struggles between human and infectious diseases are natural and endless. Because man and other micro-organisms have co-existed in nature, they have shown mutually controlling relationship, which also coincides with dialectics. On May 28, 1980, WHO solemnly stated that smallpox had been eradicated. So some experts draw this conclusion that the world medical model have transferred from biology medicine to society-psychology medicine. Namely the former mainly results from biological factors, and the latter from chronic diseases related to social and psychological factors. Even this idea has been recognized by WHO organizations for a long time. But after 5 years, a new infectious disease — AIDS was found in US which hasn't been coped with effectively. And it makes both professional staffs and normal people realize that the infectious diseases will never vanish from historical arenas. And SARS shows that new infectious diseases are not single but twin even mass. So the double or multi-element medicine model will exist for a long time. Essentially, society and nature are entity of multi-element, and the species of infectious diseases are diverse. So the struggles between man and infectious are arduous and endless.

2. Maintain the methodology of "modern health" in preventing infectious diseases

The methodology of "Modern Health" embodies the systematic method of social medicine, which emphasizes that all levels of governments should fully realize the importance of public health to maintain the development and stability of society, accordingly take responsibilities. As for preventing, we should highlight the system, integrity, harmony and social character. But so far, studying about infectious diseases mainly focuses on the biological factors, less on the interaction between infectious diseases and society, mental behavior, environment. In recent years, the situation of infectious disease has been deteriorating world-wide, which shows that antibiotics have increasingly lost their advantages, but social factors are standing out. So when infectious are controlled, biological factors, as well as environmental, social, mental ones, should be concerned. On the analysis of social factors, we can find the proportion of biology is shortening, but the others are arising. So "Modern Health" should be established, aiming to service the whole people, optimize environment, improve social settings, and evoking all levels of public to take the responsibilities of preventing infectious diseases. More than 50 years of history since liberation shows that Modern Health is the foundation of great achievements, but if once neglected, the nets of preventing will be damaged and bad effects on people's health and social orders are also produced. So it is not only a medical issue, but a severely social one. Modern health IS emphasizes the importance of developing economy and improving people's living conditions as well as educating public for scientific, technical and spiritual civilization, in order to improve the population qualities, strengthen public health, abandon harmful life styles, enhance self-protection, reduce the incidence rate and mortality rate of infectious diseases related to social environment. Meanwhile, we should stress that environmental conservation, population control and sustainable development have realistic significance for controlling infectious diseases.

3. Strengthening all levels of technical co-operations and forming joint forces to prevent infectious diseases

Abiding by the principles of clear division of work, strengthening co-operation, optimizing allocations, preventing infectious diseases should be planned as a whole. Firstly, fundamental and applying researches should be strengthened, especially microbial variability and genome projects. Because confirming pathogen eventually depends on testing technologies, nucleate extended technology and antigen antibody serology can be helpful. Epedemiology improves with molecular biology and immunology, so laboratory researches combined with Epedemiology aim to improve and optimize the preventing measures for applying researches of infectious diseases.

Global co-operation and supervision should also be enhanced. New situations appear in transmitting models of infectious diseases with globalization. Because there is no boundary for the transmissions, it is not realistic to eradicate or control them within some countries, so it is our common duties, which depend on global joint efforts and achievements to share with information and technologies. So it is imperative to establish a global surveillance systems, which accordingly each province and city should follow. At the same time, innovative technology for disease control should be trained and popularized, training epedemiology stuff should be taken into account with according stimulant measures, biological informatics should be firstly applied to preventing medicine, so as to connect the nationwide surveillance nets.

Take advantage of government functions. Early prevention and control, public health infrastructure, environmental protect, town planning and quarantine should have far sights to future. We should also handle well the relations between economies and human interests, especially improvement of institute and system, as well as professional training and reservations. Infectious diseases preventing should be regarded as an important factor affecting society and economy, meanwhile embodied in policy making, so regulatory and scientific procedure should be built. Scientific and technological platform should be made use of. Advanced technology should be developed and applied. All these should be legalized. Dr. Lawrenceo, Gosin, head of Law Public Health Center in Gorgetwon University, said "Reform of public health legislations is extremely urgent. There should be a series of definite regulations, including surveillance, prevention, treatment, isolation and quarantine. So the health institutions have full power to handle outburst crisis of public health."

In brief, infection is not merely a pure medical issue, but also a social one, which produces unestimated results to the world, so the situation is serious, the preventing shoulders heavy responsibilities.

Section 3 Social Factors in Chronic Diseases' Prevalence

With the development of economy, living level and health care, great changes have taken place in disease spectrum. Under the circumstance of increasing control, chronic diseases have replaced infectious ones to imperil people's lives and qualities. Chronic diseases mainly include such aspects as angiocardiopathy cancer, metabolic disease, mental disease, hereditary disease, chronic occupational disease, chronic tracheitis and emphysema. It is estimated by WHO that in 1999, these mortalities accounted for 60% of global total death, 43% of global disease burden, and that by 2020, the former will be more than 3%, and the latter will be 60%. Therefore, strengthening chronic diseases' prevention and management has become an important task of disease control.

1. How social factors work on the chronic diseases

Chronic diseases are also called the diseases of modern civilization, of which the mechanism and principle of their initiation mainly results from the development of social economy. Social factors work to influence chronic diseases through the principal step called psychoeonsciousness. Social factors are firstly in-taken by the sense-organ system of person. Then through regulation and control of the CNS, the psycho-reflection is formed, which results in alteration of psycho-reaction, adaptation to society and function of the body, thus changing the condition of people's health. The principle and characteristic of how the social factors influence on chronic diseases is mentioned below:

(1) Pan-affection refers to the dispersion of the influence and social factors upon chronic diseases. In other words, pan-affection of social factors means one social factor can result in functional disorders of more than one organs or systems of our body.

(2) Cumulativeness and constancy universally dwell in social lives of all people, which may densely and lastingly work on people's chronic diseases, to form response accumulation, function-injuring accumulation and health effect-accumulation.

(3) Reciprocal action exerts on human health to promote the occurrence of chronic diseases usually by the pattern of interaction between the factors and the diseases mainly due to the pluralistic relationship of the causes and their outcomes.

2. The pattern of how social factors act on chronic diseases

Chronic diseases result from the generally intercourse of multiple disease-causing agents. We should think about the relationship of social factors and diseases in a way of comprehensiveness and multi-strata concerns, because human beings have the character of comprehensiveness and sociality and also because people are positioned in an ecologically related web, in which various internal and external factors are interrelated and interacting.

(1) The influence of social economy upon chronic diseases

Side by the development of social economy that has enhanced people's education level has optimized the structure of their occupations, improved their income, and promoted the health level as a whole. It also brings people some new health problems that aggravates chronic diseases as follows:

①The destruction and pollution of environment

Modern industry has brought tremendous destruction and fearful pollution to the environment in which people work and live. People have to contact with great variety of chemical substances along with their eating, clothing, housing, traveling and working and hence provoke many health-related problems and some potential harm. The relationship between environment and chronic diseases is complex. The chemical, biological and physical factors of the environment can interweave together to exert intermittent or continuous incursion on human bodies. The harms of environmental chemicals to human body can be categorized into two different groups, namely specific and nonspecific. The former includes chronic toxication and special toxicity response, while the latter consists of raising the incidence of some chronic or other diseases, the acceleration of some chronic diseases and the degeneration of the resistance and work force of the body.

②The alteration of life style

With the development of social economy, the health of human being hinges mainly on the treat of hazardous life styles. Unhealthy mode of life has become the principal cause of chronic disease. Early in the year 1993, experts of WHO predicated that the mode of death in developing countries will be proximately equal to that of the developed countries after 20 years, that diseases caused by the mode of life will become the primary killer of the world. Diseases caused by the mode of life are wrought by some mal-habits and one mal-habit will lead up to several damages to human health. For example, smoking and disordered structure of diet can not only cause heart diseases, stroke vascular hypertension, but also increase the incidence of cancers. Although diseases caused by the mode of life are thought to be boasted by the developed countries, the death of such diseases are higher in developing countries than developed countries at present. If the absolute number of death is taken into account, in developed countries about million of people die of heart diseases, stroke, cancer, and so on, each year, while in the third world countries, the number of death of such diseases is about 11 - 70 million each year. In developing countries the proportion of death caused by life-mode-related diseases among the total death is about 45%. By the year 2015, the proportion will soar up to 60% and 75% in developing countries and developed countries respectively.

③Mental factors and diseases

Mental factors comprise of social mind, individual mind, and the response to life events. Along with the improvement of the level of productive force and the advent of information economy, social competition is more and more impetuous and makes the work and life rhythm much faster, which can bring people stress and stimulation and thus bring bad influence upon body and mental health. A plenty of study has revealed that many harmful social-mental factors are the causes of body or mental disorders. On the contrary, good social-mentality can take excellent affect on the protection or recovery from illness. Individual mind is composed of ability, temperament and disposition. Ability refers to one's intelligence and skill wherein temperament and disposition concern the occur of chronic diseases. For instance, Friedman and Rosenmen in the last century set forth the mode of type-A disposition which invoked science to study to find that A-typed disposition is regarded as one of the risk factors of coronary heart disease paralleled with the factors such as hyper-cholesterol, smoking and hypertension. People usually yield different responses to different affairs in their daily life and while positive and pleased feelings bring about favorable effect on physical mechanisms of people, negative and depressed mood result in the loss of mental equilibrium. Positive feelings can help to extend one's potential power and keep good health on while depressed feelings will plunge the nerve system into chaos and increasingly forge ailments.

(2) Population factors and chronic diseases

The influence of population factors upon chronic diseases should not be neglected, especially the aging problem, because chronic diseases often attack middle-aged and old people. As the level of life has been increasingly advanced, life expectancy had increased from 35 years old in later 1940s to 71 years old in 1998. The proportion of over-sixty year old among the total number was 9.35% and 10.52% in the year 1991 and 1998 respectively. Plus the acceleration of life rhythm, various other syndromes often make the aged discomfort and ill. On the other hand, the victim of chronic diseases has changed from old to young and the number of younger patient is soaring. The VSA is the country that copes very well with the problem of chronic diseases prevention and the general percent of chronic diseases is decreasing, but the percentage in young people of this country shows a rising tendency. This is in document that chronic diseases are a global issue. More and more youth are pleased to intake high-carbohydrate and high-fat diet as well as fast food in some American countries. It is referred to as trash food, which leads up to the more up of the incidence of obesity. And obesity is the main factor of heart disease, diabetes and so on. There are some adolescent with habits of smoking and alcohol abuse. With the development of science and technology, various conducts are mushrooming, which give a chance to children to stay all day at home lodging the apartment or playing games. In addition, the ill-influence of education for the sake of examination makes schools give only one physical exercise curriculum each week. All these issues result in lack of enough movement and exercise, which is the inducement of chronic diseases

(3) Social relation and chronic diseases

Individuals are living in social groups of all forms, such as family, friends, workmates, which on the whole form the social web. Whether or not the relationship between person and person in the web is supportive, it is important not only to determine one's health but also to be the basic control of health. Social relation comprises social support and family relation. Social support means that one can cure from social web emotional or substantial help, which is a basic demand for a person. Obtaining the social support is an interactive process. We regard interpersonal relation, social web and social coherence as factors which influence social support. Family relation is the basic social unit formed by marital relations. The perfection of family structure, of family function and of family relation is important to the mental and body health of the family members. If the family environment is always strained, it can produce dense and lasting response which further induces the upset of nerve-incretion-immunity system and which eventually induces the alteration of physical function as well as the occurrence of chronic diseases.

(4) Other social factors and chronic diseases

These factors include health service, education and so on. The errand of health service is health promotion. In a modernized society, health service is affiliated to the field of social security and health business to the aspect of the development of society. The function of health service for chronic diseases is health care and social function. Health care can decrease the incidence and death rate of chronic diseases by way of health protection, therapy recovery and health education to maintain population health and promote the quality of life. The social function of health service manages to recover the patients from chronic diseases to advance the quality of life and the power of production and thus keep the development and stability. In view of the difference of health resource, allocation of health serve and the status of population health among different countries, they urge the primary health care in all over the world especially in the developing countries in a spirit of social fair and based on the role of global collection to minimize the occurrence of various diseases. It is the character of certain that determines its influence upon human health has the property of constancy. The influence of literature, art, education ethics custom and religion upon health takes effect in not only individuals but also the whole population. The cultural factors are more effective than biological and natural factors in the formation of chronic diseases. On the other hand, culture can constantly be in charge of people's mind and concept in that the time when culture factors take their effect is all life or even several generations long. The aspects of one culture directly affect the environment of life and work, the mode of life as well as the mind. In brief, cultural factors can exert comprehensive influence on the mental health and physical health and they are positive in the controlling of chronic diseases.

Chronic disease is a common all-life disease. Ailment and disability not only affect people's ability of labor and quality of life, but also cause the expensive lost, which leads a heavy burden to the country and society. So we should take preventive policy in the first place during the chronic disease-prevention. But it's important for chronic in non-infectious disease-prevention to select to adjustable policy, namely, we should begin from the following routes, when we select preventive strategy.

Section 4 Social Medical Strategies in Prevention of Chronic Disease

1. Three-grade prevention of disease

Chronic disease can be classified into the primary stage, mid-term and third-phase of pathogenesis. In the primary stage it haunts pathogenesis but all kinds of risk factors have already existed. For example, the high cholesterol in blood is the risk factor of CHD. Smoking is the risk factor of lung cancer. Fat is the factor of DM. The primary stage includes some changes of pathological physiology, such as change of blood vessel. During the mid-term, there is high, heavy clinical embody. In the another phase, he can be fully recovered from an illness death or even have disability. In every stage of natural history of disease, the policy can be taken to prevent the beginning or aggression of disease. So the work of prevention can be classified into three grades according the natural history of disease. The primary prevention is first prevention. The secondary prevention is three early prevention, early discovery, early diagnosis, early treatment. The third stage prevention is providing patients medicine and remedy to prevent disability and improving the recovery. The first prevention is also called primary prevention which mainly takes policy to the risk factor and is the basic policy in order to prevent the beginning of chronic disease. It includes self health care and health education. Self health care takes prevention in the primary stage to enhance healthy situation. Health education can lead man to take healthy behavior by education which can eliminate the risk factor, prevent disease and enhance health. The first prevention also includes protecting and improving the environment which aims to keep air, weather, soil, people life and production that are from three wastes in industry (waste waterf, waste gas, residue) and in life (stool waste water, garbage and pollution caused by insecticide and tank).

2. The social strategies of preventing chronic diseases

(1) We reinforce leading, insist on reform and enhance organizational construction of chronic disease. Chronic prevention is a systematic social project, if there isn't regenerating idea and strong organization and all chronic disease prevention is only a good imagination by a few medical staff.

(2) Chronic disease prevention by the policy of comprehension health

Comprehensive health is norm to the disease of life style by WHO, that is to say, we should prevent diseases caused by unhealthy life style which is more useful and economical. This was launched by WHO in 1990, its basic idea being diseases caused by common factor should be controlled at a time. By the estimation of WHO the death rate can at least reduce 50% by implementing comprehensive norm. Enhancing healthy life style can save millions of people's life.

(3) Eahance epidemiology investigation of cause of chronic look for risk factor and protective factor and clarify definite factor in order to think how to prevent.

(4) We should change and avoid unhealthy life style and behavior, find ones that aim to prevent chronic disease and enhance health unhealthy life style that mainly includes smoking, alcohol, unreasonable food, much intake of sodium and little intake of potassium, nervous mind, prolonged sitting life style and little exercise. The most important is smoking and unreasonable food. CDC in Tinjin launch no smoking little reasonable food and exercise, which makes good effect

(5) Health education as a main policy, to reduce of risk factor as a main aim

It is acknowledged by all the world for low cost and high effect policy. Health education improves man's health knowledge and self-health by media, encourages people to take healthy behavior and life style, avoids risk factor and aims to gain health. Health education not only treasures the propagation of health knowledge but also underlines the change of behavior. Health education has become a mainstream that all people enjoy health care and is a way that many countries get rid of heavy medical cost. Many countries are passively taking the new healthy mode. They made encouraging progress in preventing and controlling high pressure, CHD and malignant cancer caused by life style.

(6) From child, health manage should be underlined during all one's life

School is the most ideal place to educate, where the effect of health education is the most high and the effect is the best. It has been proved by medical technology that some pathological changes and risk factor of CHD stroke and malignant cancer appear during the early stage of life. Investigations shows 33% in 3 to 6-year-old children have high blood fat. Fat children prefer food preference (mainly meat) and refuse vegetable and fruit. Smoking rate has a trend of rising among them. In 1978, the school in Australia takes a norm of changing life style in teens, which can change children's exercise has goodness social psychology but the scores of student don't fall. It's worth studying.

(7) By three-grade net in health care for medicine in city

In our country, prevention and health care in medicine have spread in city, which has an effect on preventing diseases and protecting health. During chronic disease prevention, however, primary prevention, second prevention and tertiary prevention all depend on three-grade net tightly, which has an effect on health education line, investigation of policy, information management, treatment and recovery.

(8) The policy of community prevention and the prevention of high risk people

The community prevention is all residents' cause. The prevention of high risk person is a specially important prevention which aims at high risk person, family and group. Because the norm of modern public health and life style which has something with diseases must get social comprehension and support, only if so can people benefit from the organization of social and health service. The aim of community prevention is to reduce of risk factor. From the point of epidemiology, the mode of community prevention in reducing sickness rate is more effective than high risk person prevention. From the point of behavior and sociology, the mode of community prevention aims to reduce the risk factor in environment. So if the men want to develop lifetime healthy life style they only need change unhealthy life style in community.

Case Example

Case by AIDS

Xinxin's mother was transfused in 400cc blood. When she delivered not long after she discharged from the hospital she had ulcer fever and diarrhoea and couldn't recover after a long treat. At last she was diagnosed AIDS. But when she died she even didn't know which disease she died of. At that time, Xinxin was only two years old and she was also diagnosed AIDS by breast feeding. For the truth, the two lives and the living, Xinxin's father decided to suit. He didn't believe that his wife's life, his child' future and his family were simply damaged, so he decided to protect the family's interest with law. He looked for many lawyers. But no one wanted to accept the case, because they thought the case very difficult and was afraid of

AIDS. They also thought that Xinxin's father couldn't afford the pay. They came to the center of Research of Women's Law and Service, Department of law in Beijing University. The center decided to offer legal service. With its help, they asked for pay in the court and asked for paying for the cost of suit lately.

Finally, the court began to handle the case. Xinxin and her father could sue a charge against the hospital. The case beguned 8:00 am, ended at 7:00 pm. The two sides discussed fiercely. At last, the court asked the defendants — the hospital — to give 360 thousand yuan RMB. Xinxin's father was moved to weep. He knew it was the outcome of many known and unknown men's help.

Questions to answer:

1. What social factor is the prevalence of AIDS?
2. What is your inspiration in controlling the AIDS by the case?

Forfeit 50 Yuan RMB on Those Who Spit Anywhere

To control the prevalence of SARS, which can be transmitted in air by spit, from April sixth supervising group in environment health in Xiamen would enact the enforcement fine on anybody who spit anywhere, anyone who spit anywhere would be fined 50 yuan RMB and be asked to clean the floor. Yesterday there were one hundred persons who went out and fined anyone who spit anywhere. They said,"Crude behavior, for example, spitting anywhere, will be fined." It was from *The Idea of Management Environment Health in Xiamen*. Some departments agreed the enforcement and improved the amount of fines, so it could enhance deterring ability.

Questions to answer:

1. Which factor is the prevalence of SARS having something with?
2. Is there any useful way to help people found good habits, except for by fine?

第六章 社会病

第一节 社会病概述

一、社会病的概念

社会病是指社会因素起主导作用,并与个人的行为生活方式密切相关的疾病或社会病理现象。社会因素主要包括社会制度、经济、教育、法律、社会风俗、道德、行为生活方式以及卫生保健等。

人类健康不仅受到生物因素、环境因素的影响,更重要的是受到社会因素的影响。当前,医学模式已由生物医学模式转变为生物-心理-社会医学模式,生物因素、环境因素已不再是影响健康的主要原因,而与社会密切相关的行为生活方式则成为人类死亡的主要危险因素。据 WHO 的调查,全球所有死因中的 60% 是不良行为生活方式。由社会因素起主导作用的一些健康问题已成为当前危及人类生命和健康的主要威胁。这些问题主要有意外伤亡(自杀、车祸)、酗酒、吸毒、性传播疾病、青少年妊娠等。研究社会病就是运用社会医学研究方法,研究社会因素致病机制,找出社会因素与社会病之间的关系,为预防社会病提供有效的依据。针对某种社会因素,采取相应的社会防治措施,保护和促进居民的健康水平。

二、社会病的特点

(一)广泛性

社会病是一个广泛存在的问题,几个病例不能形成所谓社会病。例如,一个地区如果只有为数不多的几个人吸毒,充其量只能作为个人的不良行为生活方式,而不能称其为社会病。但是如果有几十万甚至上百万的人吸毒,那就是一种社会病。

(二)时代性

任何一种社会病的产生都与时代的发展密切相关。例如,自杀和车祸是在近代才被看做一种社会病,吸毒是随着毒品的产生并扩散才成为一种社会病,而网络成瘾更是近几年刚刚出现的问题。

(三)复杂性

这里的复杂性包括三点:一是社会病自身的复杂性。如自杀现象至今仍是一个谜。二是社会病病因的复杂性。社会病是多种因素综合作用的结果,其致病机理也极为复杂。三是社会病防治的复杂性,如对成瘾问题的控制,其反复性较大,需要认真研究对策。

(四)危害性

社会病不仅影响个人的心身健康,更重要的是对家庭和社会都具有严重的危害性。如自杀、吸毒、性传播疾病等,既危害个人健康,影响生活质量,又会破坏社会稳定,妨碍经济发展。

(五)社会性

社会性有三方面含义:一是社会因素如经济、教育、道德、行为生活方式等起主导作用;二是引发一定的社会问题,对社会产生危害后果;三是社会病的防治是一项社会系统工程,单靠卫生部门很难取得良好的效果,需要政府和其他部门齐抓共管。

三、社会病的致病因素

(一)经济因素

经济的快速发展在一定程度上提高了人类健康水平,但同时也带来了一系列问题。经济的发展使城市化速度加快,生活节奏加快,社会竞争激烈,工作压力增大,人际关系复杂。这些很容易造成人们精神紧张、焦虑,从而影响身心健康。

(二)人口因素

人口的快速增长加重了社会负担,还可能造成失业人数增多,使社会不稳定因素增加,人们的就业压力增大,从而引发一些心理疾病。地区间、国家间的人口流动则使一些传染病如艾滋病等的传播速度加快。

(三)家庭因素

良好的家庭关系可使人保持身心健康,有利于青少年的健康成长。家庭关系破裂、过分溺爱孩子、虐待弱势群体等,则会对家庭成员产生不良的心理影响。几乎所有的社会病都与家庭环境有密切关系。

(四)文化因素

文化习俗、思想意识、教育水平等对社会病的产生均有一定影响。病态的思想观念必定引发病态的社会行为,如自杀、吸毒、性乱等行为与人们的人生观、道德观密切相关。受教育水平不同的人健康观也不同,提高教育程度有助于消除人们的不良生活行为,提高健康水平。

(五)心理因素

心理问题可引发社会病。如抑郁症患者是自杀的高危人群,性情急躁的A型性格人容易发生车祸。心理健康的人在遇到挫折时会迎难而上,解决问题,而心理素质差的人往往会选择自杀、吸毒等方式来逃避现实。

四、社会病防治原则及措施

社会病的防治应采取包括社会、家庭和个人在内的综合性措施。

(一)社会医学措施

1. 在全社会开展健康教育,普及卫生保健知识,教育人们改变不良卫生习惯,建立健康的生活方式。

2. 改善社会条件,加强社会预防。对高危人群进行筛检,及时发现,及早治疗。建立健全社会性防治组织,如心理咨询机构等。加大社会支持力度。

3. 健全卫生法律法规。对一些不良行为除进行健康教育外,还应通过法律手段来禁止。如吸毒、嫖娼等必须通过立法来严禁。

(二)家庭医学措施

1. 维护和谐的家庭关系。家庭关系和谐,有利于家庭成员的生理、心理健康发展,减少心理疾病发生的危险,防止社会病的发生。

2. 维持正常的家庭功能。家庭是孩子的第一课堂,家长必须加强对孩子的教育和培养,使孩子具有良好的心理素质和行为品质,防止其形成不良行为方式。

3. 关注高危家庭。高危家庭主要包括不和睦、酗酒、吸毒家庭,单亲家庭,有长期慢性病或精神疾病患者的家庭,功能失调或濒于崩溃的家庭等。这些家庭中的成员往往容易引发社会病,应给予高度重视。

(三)行为医学措施

1. 建立健康的行为生活方式。做到不吸烟,少饮酒,合理营养和平衡膳食,规律生活,遵守交通规则,锻炼身体,定期健康检查,养成清洁卫生的习惯。

2. 增强心理健康,保持良好的情绪反应。现代生活的激烈竞争给人们的心理带来一定压力,保持健康的心理和愉快的情绪,可对人体的生理机能起良好的作用,有利于人的健康。

3. 保持积极的应对方式。积极应对是指人对紧张刺激可能出现结果的一种积极反应。保持积极的应对方式,可使人们在面对挫折或困难时不至于过分紧张或焦虑,以一种平静的心态来看待问题,可减少心理疾患的发生。

第二节 自杀

自杀是指由于社会心理冲突而产生的一种蓄意终止自己的生命,有目的、有计划的自我毁灭性行为。WHO报告全球每年约有100万人死于自杀,中国2002年底进行的一次大规模调查显示,我国平均自杀率为 $23/10^5$,全国自杀死亡人数占全部死亡人数的3.6%。在1995~1999年全国人口最重要的死因中,自杀居第5位。而在15~34岁人群的死因中,自杀更是第一原因。1999年中国/世界卫生组织精神卫生高层研讨会明确提出,预防自杀是中国目前迫切需要解决的三大精神卫生问题之一。自杀已经成为我国公共卫生领域中一个亟待解决的问题。

一、自杀的流行病学分布

(一)地区分布

一般来说,发达国家自杀率高于发展中国家,欧洲高于美洲和大洋洲,非洲最低。我国已成为自杀的高发国家,而且我国的自杀率表现出一种独有的特征:农村的自杀率是城市的 3 倍,全国 90% 的自杀发生在农村。有专家指出,这可能与我国农村居民文化水平相对较低以及普遍使用农药有关。

(二)时间分布

法国社会学家杜尔凯姆认为,自杀的高发期为夏季,其次为春、秋季,冬季自杀率最低。他认为这主要是由于夏季社会活动比其他季节更加紧张的缘故。我国农村则主要在秋季高发,这与秋季开始喷洒农药,容易获得自杀材料有关。在每个季节,绝大多数的自杀发生在白天。在每个周中,自杀率在每周开始(星期一)时较高,而在接近周末(星期六)时开始降低。这可能与白天及每周开始时社会活动开始变得紧张、人们心理负担加重等有关。

(三)人群分布

1. 年龄。自杀一般有随年龄增长而增高的趋势,老年人的自杀率高于青年人。但不同国家之间也有差异。我国自杀年龄分布在城乡大为不同,农村自杀有两个年龄高峰,即青年组和老年组。城市则没有中青年高峰期,男女均表现为老龄后自杀增多。

2. 性别。中国和加拿大两国科学家研究的最新结果表明,世界范围内男性的自杀率是女性的 3.6 倍,而在我国女性自杀率比男性高 25%,其中农村妇女又比城市高 3~4 倍,这是中国特有的现象。原因可能是农村妇女的文化层次较低,又缺乏完善的社会支持网络,使她们在遇到问题后首先想到的是自杀。

3. 文化状况。国外报道文化程度高者一般自杀率也较高,我国则为文化程度低者自杀较多。我国成年人自杀者中多为文盲,青少年自杀者多为初、高中文化,原因可能是这部分人缺乏沟通和社会支持,青少年可能还存在其他因素,如学习压力、家庭问题(父母不和、分居、离婚)等。

二、自杀的社会病因

(一)遗传因素

国外关于自杀的遗传学研究已有 50 多年,但至今尚无确切的定论。目前对自杀的遗传研究有三种见解:①自杀的遗传是通过抑郁症或其他精神疾病而体现的。②自杀的遗传是独立于抑郁症和其他精神疾病之外而传递的。③自杀是"冲动"这一心理特质的遗传发挥作用的。

(二)精神疾病

由精神疾病所致的自杀为全部自杀的 30%~50%。我国 2002 年的调查显示,63% 的自杀者患有不同程度的精神障碍。在各种精神疾病中,抑郁症的危险性最大,其自杀率为一般人口的 50~80 倍,其次分别为精神分裂症、神经症和人格障碍、酒精中毒等。

(三)生活事件

据调查,我国人群中最为常见的自杀原因包括 5 个方面:家庭矛盾、恋爱受挫、人际关系紧张、失业和考试失利。家庭矛盾最主要的是夫妻矛盾和婆媳矛盾,因家庭矛盾而自杀者以女性居多;恋爱受挫自杀者在男性和女性中都比较常见;人际矛盾也很容易将人推向绝路,如阮玲玉因"人言可畏"而自杀;失业主要对男性青年自杀影响较大;考试失利则是许多学生自杀的原因,几乎每年高考发榜后都有学生自杀。

(四)心理传染

受心理传染而自杀者多数为青少年,他们缺乏社会经验,没有形成成熟的人格,判断能力较差,容易产生"目标性求同作用",以至于模仿现实生活或文艺作品中的相似人物,走向自杀死亡。比较典型的模仿自杀事件是在1774年歌德《少年维特之烦恼》问世后,许多青少年模仿维特自毙,形成一股青少年自杀风潮,精神分析学家Pbillps将此称为"维特效应"。

(五)社会环境

战争期间自杀率一般较低,因为战争会使社会归属意识增强,攻击性倾向完全外向化,因而自杀减少。战争结束,从紧张状态到松弛,内部倾轧增加,自杀率开始上升。社会政治动乱和经济萧条时期自杀一般较多,如第二次世界大战后一段时期柏林经常处于政治不安定局面,自杀率随之上升。

(六)政治目的

政治性自杀往往有着很明确的政治意图,每个自杀者背后都代表着一个利益集团,他的牺牲能够为这个集团带来更大的利益。许多恐怖主义行为都与政治自杀有很大的关系。如恐怖分子制造的"9·11事件"、巴勒斯坦人体炸弹就是明显的政治性自杀。

三、自杀的社会防范措施

(一)维持社会稳定

保证社会政治和经济的稳定,防止动荡不安的局面,减少因迷茫而产生的自杀。保持经济快速发展,减少贫困、失业等自杀的危险因素。

(二)做好社会性预防工作

主要是在全社会开展健康教育,改善人们的精神健康。尤其要加强青少年学生的心理卫生工作,增强他们的心理素质,提高他们的社会适应能力和应对挫折的能力,帮助他们树立正确的人生观和价值观。此外,应严格控制和管理自杀工具,如枪支、农药、老鼠药等。

(三)及时进行心理干预

实践证明,当一个人产生自杀意念时,如果能及时进行心理干预,给予精神支持,可以有效地防止自杀。因此,可在城市中设立自杀干预中心和心理咨询机构,免费对社会上烦恼绝望者给予心理咨询和心理疏导,指导当事人克服危机。目前,美、英、日及欧洲不少国家均在大城市设立了生命电话服务机构,其宗旨就是对濒临自杀者进行干预,防止其自杀。我国2002年成立了第一个专门自杀干预的机构——北京心理危机研究与干预中心,说明我国对自杀问题开始重视。

(四)高危人群筛选

采用心理测试量表,将有自杀意念、情绪障碍(焦虑、抑郁等)、心理障碍等的高危人群筛检出来,及时发现,以防范自杀。如采用Eysenck人格度量表和Bech-H无望量表可将有自杀倾向或意念的高危人群找出来,采用自评抑郁量表(SDS)和自评焦虑量表(SAS)可以将自杀率发生较高的抑郁症和焦虑症患者检查出来。

(五)防止自杀的复发

研究表明,自杀未遂再次发生自杀行为者占10%~15%,因此,防止自杀未遂者再次自杀有重要意义。对自杀未遂者要加强监护,除对其及时进行医疗急救外,还要进行心理及情感治疗,协助进行适当感情宣泄,恢复心态平衡,消除危险因素,以防止自杀行为的复发。

第三节 车祸

车祸是指车辆在街道、公路上行驶过程中发生碰撞、碾压、翻覆、落水、失火或驶出路外造成人畜伤亡、车物损坏的事故。车祸也是一种社会病,它是生理、心理和社会等多种因素综合作用的结果,其中心理和社会因素对车祸的发生起决定作用,车祸的控制也必须采取以社会性措施为主的综合治理方法。

目前,全世界每年约有70万人死于车祸,约300万人在车祸中受伤。我国2002年共发生车祸77万多起,因车祸而引起的死亡人数近11万、受伤人数为56万,造成的直接经济损失超过33亿元。而且车祸主要危及低年龄组及青壮年人群,对社会劳动力的影响特别大,由此带来的间接经济损失也不可忽视。随着现代交通运输业的迅速发展,车祸的发生率也在继续增长,有专家指出,车祸在我国已成为危害公共安全的首要因素。

一、车祸的流行特征

(一)时间分布

不同国家地区由于地理、气候条件不同,车祸的时间分布也不同。北欧国家在冬、秋季的车祸较多,可能与冬天冰雪盖道、车轮易打滑及秋天旅游人多、交通拥挤有关。我国高温季节(6~8月份)车祸发生较多,可能是由于气候炎热,驾驶员易疲劳、注意力不易集中。美国、香港等地的调查还发现,车祸以周末为最多,可能是因为周末人们活动较频繁,导致交通拥挤。

(二)地区分布

据统计,多数发达国家的车祸发生地点主要集中于郊区,城区内车祸相对较少。这可能是因为郊区的交通不如城市发达,交通管理也较城市薄弱。我国车祸发生地段多在城市与郊区交界处和公路干线。国内研究发现公路等级越高,交通事故死亡人数越多,原因是路况越好车速越快,从而导致驾驶员的视野窄、应激反应不良,而且相应的安全设备没有跟上。

(三)人群分布

我国近几年统计表明,3年以下驾龄司机制造的交通事故占事故总量的47.38%,直接导致的死亡占41.28%;导致的伤亡占47.06%,造成的经济损失占44.85%。而且重大车祸肇事者,主要集中在持有2~3年驾照的司机身上。

车祸主要危害儿童、青少年和老年人,对儿童、青少年的危害尤为严重。在日本,车祸在儿童、青少年的主要死因中占首位。我国成都市调查还发现,农民发生车祸的比重较大,占1/3左右。

二、车祸的社会病因

(一)交通状况

目前,发展中国家人口、车辆增长很快,但道路却增加较慢,导致人、车、路发展比例不平衡。此外,有关部门对道路管理重视不够,交通管理人员和交通管理设施缺乏,交通管理较为落后,这是车祸快速增长的重要原因。

(二)驾驶员的不良行为

酗酒是引起车祸的一个重要因素,在发达国家,酗酒是导致车祸的首要原因。酒精能影响司机的操作能力,使司机接受和感知信息的能力下降,视野变窄,认识和判断能力下降,自我控制和综合定向能力下降,反应时间延长,操作的准确性下降。用药和吸毒也容易引起车祸,服用某些药品后产生的催眠等副作用以及吸毒后产生的幻觉等,均可导致车祸的发生。

(三)疲劳与瞌睡

新西兰有学者指出,疲劳对车祸的发生具有潜在的危险,其危害不亚于酒后驾车。英国的一项调查表明,29%的司机承认自己在驾车时有睡觉的经历,而10%的交通事故与疲劳有关。美国有人统计,在4.8万起无外界条件因素引起的车辆交通事故中,10%与疲乏有关。我国2001年发生的特大交通事故中,驾驶员疲劳驾驶是肇事的主要原因。

(四)驾驶员违章驾驶

违章驾驶主要包括不使用安全带(摩托车驾驶员不戴头盔)、超速行驶等。在美国,13%的车祸是司机未系安全带所致,在中国这个比例则更高。尤其在新建的高速公路上行驶,很多司机不系安全带,使车祸发生的危险性增加。

(五)驾驶员的生理、心理状况

一般认为,驾驶员的最佳驾驶年龄段为30~49岁。随着年龄的增长,驾驶员的体力、耐力、反应速度、视力等都会不同程度地下降,增加了发生车祸的危险。另据研究,车祸的发生与驾驶员的性格、情绪等因素有关。发生车祸的驾驶员性格多为不随和,人际关系不良,易冲动,情绪不稳定,紧张过度等。

(六)行人自身的原因

25岁以下青少年、50岁以上老年人、农村人口(城市民工)是车祸中伤亡的主要人群。其表面原因是青少年外出机会多,老年人听力下降、行动迟缓、反应较慢,农村人口对城市拥挤的交通状况不适应。但更深层次的原因则在于:这些人交通安全意识较为淡薄,不能适应复杂的交通环境。

三、车祸的社会防范措施

(一)加强交通立法

建立健全交通法律法规,规定司机必须系安全带(摩托车驾驶员必须戴头盔),规定领取驾驶执照的年龄限制;规定司机血中酒精浓度(BAC)的标准;严格规定司机每天开车的时间,严禁疲劳驾车;严厉查处吸毒司机;对违规的驾驶员要给以相应处罚。

(二)改善交通条件和汽车性能

改善交通状况,增设先进管理设施,培训管理人员。在公路标志、信号、监控等方面采取措施,建立有效的公路保护系统,加强对公路交通的管理。不断地研究、开发和采用先进的汽车主动、被动预防事故技术,如改进刹车系统、配置安全气囊和电子防撞系统等,提高车辆应付事故的能力。

(三)做好驾驶员的选拔工作

据调查,我国交通事故的原因构成中,人的因素占92.8%。因此,做好驾驶员的选拔工作对减少车祸的发生极为重要。驾驶员的选拔不仅要看其体格,还应重视心理素质,应对司机的性格、神经类型等进行测验,尽量做到生理素质、心理素质都过关。

(四)加强对高危人群的安全教育

我国儿童、青少年是车祸发生的高危人群,在学校进行驾驶和交通安全知识教育,让青少年掌握交通规则和交通安全知识,这对于防止车祸的发生是有效的。对司机应投入更多的时间和精力,进行职业技术培训,使他们认识到自己的行为直接影响别人的生命安全。

(五)改进医疗急救措施

有研究发现,在车祸死亡者中,有20%是可以通过及时抢救而免予死亡的。可见,建立急救中心,加强急救医疗系统,对车祸损伤进行及时处理是极为重要的,可减少车祸的致残率和死亡率。美国和欧洲许多国家都有较完善的急救系统,许多长途客车上备有担架和其他急救器材,车祸发生后伤员可尽快得到抢救。我国也应加强急救系统如医院急诊室、"120"急救等的建设。

第四节 性传播疾病

性传播疾病(STD)是一组主要由性接触或类似性行为接触为主要传播途径的传染病。1975年世界卫生组织常任理事会通过,确定用"性传播疾病"来代替既往习惯上所称的性病。以往的性病主要是梅毒、淋病、软下疳及性病淋巴肉芽肿,亦称经典性病。现在的性传播疾病种类逐渐增多,我国目前主要防治的性传播疾病有淋病、尖锐湿疣、非淋菌性尿道炎、梅毒、艾滋病、细菌性阴道炎、生殖器疱疹感染、软下疳、性病性淋巴肉芽肿、腹股沟肉芽肿、乙型肝炎等。

一、性传播疾病的流行概况

(一)患病情况

由于种种原因,STD的准确数据很难获得。WHO在20世纪90年代末估计,全球新增病例约为4亿个,其中淋病6 200万、梅毒1 200万、HIV感染3 000万、衣原体感染8 900万。截至2001年,我国8种法定报告的STD累计报告人数近550万,排在前四位的分别是淋病、非淋菌性尿道炎、尖锐湿疣、梅毒。近几年艾滋病的发展尤为严重。自1981年美国发现首例艾滋病人,AIDS已在全球广泛流行。据WHO估计,全球HIV感染者已达到6 000万。我国目前约有100万HIV感染者,如果不采取积极有效的措施,到2010年将达到1 000万。

（二）地区分布

世界不同地区STD发病率及病种差别很大，发展中国家由于诊疗技术有待改善，因此STD流行率较高。艾滋病发病最严重的是非洲，其次是亚太地区，东欧和中亚地区则是艾滋病增长最快的地区。城市化较快的地区STD发病较多，我国东南沿海开放城市人口流动较大，发病率上升较快。2000年8种STD报告最多的省份依次为江苏、浙江、广东、安徽和四川。艾滋病则仍然以云南等西南边境地区发病最为严重，目前已蔓延至全国大多数省份。

（三）人群分布

1. 年龄。我国STD病例多数为青壮年，其中，20～39岁组占总人数的92.4%。HIV感染者中，年龄在15～49岁者占93.9%。近几年，STD发病年龄段有从青年向儿童蔓延的趋势，儿童STD患者在逐渐增多。

2. 性别。大多数的STD发病率均是男性高于女性，1987～1989年我国监测的STD病例男女之比为2:1，至2000年降为1.4:1，这可能与女性主动就诊的人数增加、诊疗水平提高和女性实际发病数也在不断增加有关。艾滋病感染者中男女之比为4.6:1。

3. 职业。我国STD发病以工人最多，约占1/3，无业及待业青年占20%，个体工商业者占15%，服务行业及供销人员占10%。近年来，机关干部及公职人员患病人数增长最快，农民患病者也在增加。HIV感染者主要是农民、归国劳工、无业游民及个体从业者，长途司机感染者近几年增长快速。

二、性传播疾病的社会病因

（一）社会状况

随着经济的发展，对外交往的增多，西方"性开放"思想传入，对我国传统的伦理道德观念产生一定的冲击。国际旅游业的发展，国际商业交往的频繁，为STD的传播提供了条件。第三产业和个体经济迅速发展，大量服务业和个体工商业出现，形成一个经济上比较富裕但文化素质较低的社会阶层，这是STD的一个高危人群。

（二）人口流动

我国每年有0.8亿～1.2亿流动人口集中于密集地区，这些人多为性活跃人群。人口的高度集中和大量迁移、流动，为STD的传播提供了机会。

（三）嫖娼、卖淫

嫖娼、卖淫是STD流行的重要社会原因。泰国是色情业发达的国家，STD流行极为猖獗。我国暗娼和嫖客的STD检出率平均为39.9%。近年来不少夜总会、美容院、按摩院开始出现娼妓活动，应引起有关部门的重视。

（四）吸毒、贩毒

吸毒者中STD检出率为32.5%，女性患病率为43.25%。2002年我国报告艾滋病毒感染者中有63.9%是静脉注射毒品，吸毒已成为我国艾滋病传播的最主要途径。

（五）色情作品的泛滥

色情作品（文学、影视、音像制品、网络文化等）能够导致道德败坏，特别容易引起青少年的好奇心和仿效。因此，不可低估淫秽宣传作品在STD流行中的影响。

（六）自我保护意识差

许多人缺乏自我保护的基本卫生知识和防范意识，由于现代口服避孕药和宫内避孕方法的普遍应用而不使用避孕套，失去对STD感染因子的物理保护。

（七）性病医疗市场混乱

社会上许多无照行医者、个体游医，他们技术和卫生条件差，又不报告疫情。一些病人碍于颜面怕暴露身份，求助于这些非法行医者。结果性病长期不愈，这些病人又作为传染源而长期蔓延。

三、性传播疾病的社会防范措施

（一）加强健康教育，普及性教育知识

加强性健康教育和生殖健康教育，使广大居民对性传播疾病有充分的认识和了解，认识到STD对个人、家庭和社会的危害以及STD的预防措施，提高居民的自我保护意识。教育内容应包括性道德教育、性生理知识和健康性心理的自我培养、正确使用避孕套等避孕工具、洁身自好、认清性乱等异常性行为方式的危害等。青少年应是宣传教育的重点对象，青少年的性教育是全社会都应重视的问题。

（二）综合治理，进行全方位防范

STD的防治必须多个部门齐抓共管，综合治理。卫生、公安、司法、民政、宣传等部门应加强配合，取缔嫖娼卖淫活动，对艾滋病患者应实行强制治疗；加强流动人口的管理；对各种色情文化要坚决予以打击，视其情况没收或罚款；整顿医疗市场，禁止非法行医。

（三）加强立法，完善疫情报告制度

我国1991年颁布了《性病防治管理办法》，规定艾滋病、淋病、梅毒、尖锐湿疣、非淋菌性尿道炎、软下疳、生殖道疱疹、淋病性淋巴肉芽肿8种性病为必须报告的疾病。各地要严格执行这一规定，发现病例应及时上报，防止疾病的扩散。

（四）切断性接触以外的其他传播途径

除性接触外，STD的传播途径有血源感染、母婴传播、医源性传播、日常生活接触传播等。要严格保证血液制品的安全可靠，供血者须绝对健康；预防新生儿感染，已明确患有STD的孕妇最好能中止妊娠；注意做好浴池、旅店、理发店、游泳池的消毒卫生；医务人员应注意自身防护，严守操作规程，防止医院内感染的发生。

（五）做好STD的监测工作

加强对性传播疾病的监测，以及时掌握STD的流行动态，了解其传染的来源，调查各方面的影响因素，为制定预防措施提供依据。主要做好高危人群（如卖淫者、同性恋者、药瘾者及一些特殊服务行业人群等）的监测、重点疾病（如艾滋病、淋病、梅毒等）的监测。

第五节　成瘾性社会病

成瘾是指个体不可自制地反复渴求从事某种活动或滥用某种药物，虽然这样做会给自己或已经给自己带来不良后果，但仍然无法控制。成瘾主要包括物质成瘾和行为成瘾。

物质成瘾是通过具体物质作用于人体而引起的,又称物质依赖,如吸烟、酗酒、吸毒等;行为成瘾则是对某种行为产生强烈的依赖性,如赌博、盗窃成瘾、购物成瘾、网络成瘾等。

成瘾行为有三个主要特征:①已成为成瘾者生命活动中的必需部分,由此产生强烈的心理、生理、社会性依赖,并且不择手段地去获取致瘾源。所谓致瘾源,即引起成瘾的某种物质或行为。②成瘾行为一旦中止,将产生明显的戒断症状。而且一旦恢复成瘾行为,戒断症状将很快消失。③对个人、家庭和社会都产生危害后果。

不论是物质成瘾还是行为成瘾,其致病机制是相同的。一般都经历四个阶段:①诱导阶段,开始与某种成瘾物质或行为接触,并感到欣快;②形成阶段,行为不断重复,逐渐形成依赖;③巩固阶段,成瘾行为已经巩固,并成为生命中必需的一部分;④衰竭阶段,生理、心理都出现明显的损害。

目前,成瘾性社会病已成为社会关注的热点问题,也是社会医学研究的重要课题。本节主要介绍目前危害较为严重的吸毒和新出现的网络成瘾问题。

一、吸毒

吸毒是指麻醉品、止痛药、迷幻剂等非法毒品滥用现象。毒品一般可分为合法毒品和非法毒品两大类,通常所说的吸毒是指滥用非法毒品,如大麻、海洛因、可卡因、迷幻剂等。吸毒同自杀的根源是相仿的,都是个人想用忘掉或毁掉自身存在的办法来逃避痛苦和不幸,都是由于人们对物质或精神上的不满足或感到不幸福而引起的。

(一)吸毒的流行特征

据联合国禁毒署2002年公布的数字,目前世界上约有1.85亿人吸毒。我国1998年吸毒人数约为5万,而到2002年内地累计登记在册的吸毒人数已达到100万,加上估算的隐性吸毒人数,共计500万左右。其增长速度增长之快,令人震惊。

1. 人群分布。我国对6个吸毒严重的地区近10年的调查显示,男性吸毒人数高于女性;吸毒者文化程度较低,初中以下者占78.95%;流动性职业是吸毒最重要的危险因素,下岗、无业、个体户、司机等人群吸毒率比干部、教师、农民、工人等有固定职业的人群和学生高11倍。近几年吸毒人群趋于低龄化,来自国家禁毒委员会办公室的数字表明,我国最近几年青少年吸毒占吸毒总人数的比例始终为80%左右。

2. 地区分布。吸毒现象从边境向内地,从农村向城市蔓延。20世纪90年代初,我国的吸毒现象还仅限于云南边境地区的少数村寨,随着国际毒品贩子向我国境内的加紧渗透和国际吸毒通道的开辟,吸毒现象迅速蔓延,目前已祸及全国大部分省、市、自治区。

(二)吸毒的危害

吸毒不仅对个人,而且对家庭、整个社会都会产生严重的危害。

1. 吸毒严重损害身体健康。可卡因可引起失眠、体重减轻、鼻黏膜坏死等,长期使用可产生呼吸衰竭,最终导致死亡。海洛因对消化系统、呼吸系统、神经系统等都会产生明显伤害。迷幻剂LSD可使人心理损伤,产生超自然幻觉,促使人自杀。因长期吸毒引起的"戒断综合征"更使多数吸毒者无法忍受。

2. 吸毒常导致婚姻家庭破裂。长期吸毒成瘾之后,吸毒者会变得十分自私且不诚实,性格变得烦躁易怒,情感变得淡漠厌世,沉溺于对毒品的追求之中。他们淡漠了对配偶的关心体贴,淡漠了对家庭的责任和对子女的教育,而且根本不能顾及家庭捉襟见肘的经济困境,反而会变卖家庭财产来维持吸毒,很容易造成家庭的破裂。

3. 吸毒危害社会安定。国内外的毒贩为了保证他们的毒品的贩运,已屡屡使用武力。而吸毒者为了获得毒品,常常铤而走险,进行各种犯罪活动。据统计,大多数省(市、区)抢劫、盗窃等侵财性案件30%以上是吸毒人员所为,一些毒情严重地区甚至接近70%。此外,因吸毒而造成的艾滋病的传播已对全社会构成了极大威胁。

(三) 吸毒的社会病因

1. 好奇心是吸毒的最早冲动。许多吸毒者都是在一开始怀着好奇心而进行吸毒尝试的,尤其是青少年,他们具有强烈的好奇心和探索欲望,但又缺乏必要的科学知识和辨别是非的能力,当听说吸毒后"其乐无穷"时便想试一试。一项调查表明,在青少年吸毒者中,80%以上是在不知道毒品危害的情况下吸毒成瘾的。

2. 无知和追求享乐是吸毒的另一个原因。这在一些文化水平较低而暴富的人群中尤为突出。在沿海地区,有些大款视吸毒为时髦,为潮流,为一种身份。有的农民企业家竟然以海洛因招待客人。在南方一些贵族学校,不少学生把抽海洛因当做高档消费和富贵的象征。这些实际都是无知的表现。

3. 哥儿们义气是吸毒的一种心理力量。许多青少年一开始就是因为碍不过朋友的面子而陪着吸毒,认为对朋友应该讲义气,不能搞特殊,大家都吸自己也不能例外,从而一步步走上吸毒之路。正是由于这种原因,吸毒者一般都有自己的圈子,有自己的毒友。武汉抽样调查发现,单独吸毒者只占21.9%,而共同吸毒者占72.3%。

4. 不良的家庭环境是一个重要影响因素。除了家庭成员的吸毒行为直接成为青少年吸毒的原因外,一些家庭父母离异或者长期外出,孩子得不到正常的教育;一些经济条件好的家庭,父母过分溺爱孩子,无条件地满足孩子的物质要求,使孩子有充分的物质条件去寻求毒品的刺激等等,都可能是导致青少年吸毒的原因。

5. 生活中的失意感容易诱发吸毒。人们在生活中受到挫折、感到失意时,一般都会采取不同的方式宣泄。一些青少年由于父母离异、家庭缺少温暖、学习压力大等不顺心的问题,引起精神苦闷,便通过吸毒麻醉自己来逃避现实。

6. 毒贩子无孔不入。贩毒分子要扩大毒品市场,销售其毒品,不能通过广告推销,只能用诱骗的手段。最常用的方法是送烟,将毒品巧妙地用名牌香烟包装起来,让人在不知不觉中吸上瘾,最后不得不求助于送烟的人。许多青少年就是在学吸烟的日子里染上了吸毒。在云南边境还有人将毒品掺入口红或食物中,让人在舔唇或吃饭过程中不知不觉沾上毒品而成瘾。

(四) 吸毒的社会防范措施

1. 加强精神文明建设,提高国民素质。国学大师王国维先生早在《禁毒》一文中指出,禁毒之要点是提高国民素质。只有加强精神文明建设,提高国民整体素质,真正认识到毒品对个人、家庭和社会的危害,在全社会共同抵制毒品,才能真正赢得禁毒之战的胜利。

2. 加强对青少年的健康教育。青少年是吸毒的高危人群,也是危害最深重的人群,做好对青少年的健康教育对防范吸毒有重要意义。首先,要使青少年明白,毒品一旦沾染，便永远无法摆脱，切不可轻易尝试毒品，不能天真地去设想吸了再戒。其次，要对青少年加强吸毒危害性的健康教育。目前我国国家禁毒委和教育部已联合开展了"禁毒知识一堂课"活动，在全国大、中、小学校举办专门的禁毒教育课，使每一位公民在走向社会前都接受毒品预防教育。此外，还应加强对青少年的心理健康教育，提高他们应对生活挫折的能力。

3. 加强有关禁毒的立法工作。制定有关禁毒和打击走私贩毒的法令，对毒品原料如罂粟和大麻等种植，要坚决予以取缔，逮捕业主，焚毁果实。打击毒品走私集团和毒品犯。吸毒问题已不是哪一个国家、哪一个民族的问题，而是整个人类共同面对的问题，要加强国际间的合作，共同开展有效而持续的打击毒品斗争。

4. 对吸毒者应及时治疗。心理学家指出，吸毒实际是一种病。对吸毒者不应歧视，而应给予同情和关怀。除了戒毒所进行常规治疗外，社会、家庭都应加强对吸毒者的人文关怀，使他们摆脱滥用毒品的生活模式，恢复正常的生理和心理以及社会功能，重返社会，成为有用的社会成员。

5. 加强对吸毒成瘾和复吸心理机制的研究。所谓心理毒瘾，是一种心理状态，即人吸毒在生理毒瘾戒断后，仍然控制不住自己的吸毒欲望，并对重新吸毒有着难以控制的欲望。大多数吸毒者都认为，在戒毒后已经没有那些痛苦的生理反应，但仍然抑制不住想要再次吸毒的那种"想瘾"。防止复吸是戒毒成功的关键，但目前国内复吸率达95％以上。因此，研究吸毒者戒毒后复吸的心理毒瘾机制，对戒毒有重大意义。

二、网络成瘾

（一）概述

网络成瘾是指无节制地花费大量时间和精力在网上冲浪、聊天或进行网络游戏，并且这种对网络的过度使用影响生活质量，降低学习和工作效率，损害身体健康，导致各种行为异常、心理障碍、人格障碍和神经系统功能紊乱等消极后果。

1994年，纽约市的一名精神病医生声称自己发现了一种新的心理障碍疾病，并把它命名为"互联网成瘾症"（IAD）。IAD很快引起了精神病学家和临床心理学家的关注。在1997年多伦多和1998年旧金山两届美国心理学会年会上，研究者们专门讨论了IAD成为正式诊断的可能性。

虽然正式的IAD诊断标准尚未出台，但研究者们一般认为，要诊断一个人患有IAD，必须在过去12个月内表现出下列7种症状中的三种以上：①耐受性增强：病人要不断增加上网时间才能达到同样的满足程度，也就是网瘾越来越大；②戒断症状：如果有一段时间（从几小时到几天不等）不上网，病人就会变得明显的焦躁不安，不可抑制地想上网，时刻担心自己错过了什么，甚至做梦也是关于网络；③上网频率总是比事先计划的要高，上网时间总是比事先计划的要长；④企图缩短上网时间的努力，总是以失败告终；⑤大量时间花费在和互联网有关的活动上，比如安装新软件、整理和编码下载的大量文件等等；⑥上网使病人的社交、职业和家庭生活受到严重影响；⑦虽然能够意识到上网带来的严重问题，病人仍然继续花大量时间上网。

(二)网络成瘾的危害

1999年8月,在美国心理学协会年会上公布的一项调查显示,在全球2亿多网民中,大约有1 140万人是IAD患者,占6%左右。我国北京师范大学的一次调查表明,北京市约有14.8%(13.65万人)的未成年人患有网络成瘾症。据估计,我国至少有22.5万人不同程度地患有网络性心理障碍,患者年龄一般为15~45岁,男性患者占总发病人数的98.5%,女性仅占1.5%,其中年龄在20~30岁的单身男性为易感人群。

因特网成瘾病的患者,从某种意义上来说与染上吸毒、酗酒或赌博等恶习没有什么区别。心理学家研究发现,在对外界刺激没有控制能力这个特点上,网络成瘾与赌博是极为相似的。研究还发现,使用因特网会导致一个人在学习、社交、财政以及工作上出现混乱状态,这一点与我们熟知的赌博、饮食不规律和酗酒是极其类似的。

网络成瘾会给人的生理、心理带来一系列负面影响。生理方面的影响主要有:食欲减退,易疲劳,消化不良,大脑血流量减少。此外,长时间僵坐在电脑前会使个体缺乏适当的锻炼,容易引起腕关节综合征、背部扭伤和眼睛疲劳等不良身体反应。心理方面的影响主要有:兴趣产生偏离,对网络依依不舍,排斥其他事物,精力长时间过分集中于某个方面。而且一旦停止上网,则产生不安、焦躁、失眠、情绪低落、心情不佳、思维迟钝等类似戒断症状。

网络成瘾还会给家庭和社会带来一定的危害。许多网络成瘾者为享受网上乐趣而不惜支付巨额上网费用,宁可荒废学业或事业甚至抛弃家庭,也要与电脑为伴。目前美国因上网而离婚的人数已占离婚人数的1/3。网络瘾患者由于长期脱离现实生活,容易产生精神紊乱导致抑郁症,影响正常的学习、工作和生活,同时给社会增加了不安定因素。专家预测,在21世纪网络成瘾对社会的危害决不亚于今天的海洛因成瘾。因此,重视网络成瘾的研究,是当前社会医学的一项重要课题。

(三)网络成瘾的社会病因

1. 网络自身的诱惑。网络最大的特点就是它的虚拟性。在网络的虚拟环境中,人的内心准则和社会规范的制约性大大削弱或不复存在,人们的网上行为表现出一种解除抑制的特点,可以随心所欲地发表自己的言论,做出许多平常想做而不敢做的事情。网络游戏也是吸引人的一个重要因素。在网络游戏中,人们可以充分发挥自己的主观能动性,使心理得到满足。

2. 网吧管理不规范。有关网吧的政策法规不够完善,缺乏可操作性。不少网吧经营管理人员缺乏必要的专业技术、法律知识,网络安全意识淡薄,在实际经营中疏于管理。有关部门在日常监管中也存在权限交叉、职责不清的现象,给违法经营者以可乘之机。有的网吧无视《互联网上网服务营业场所管理条例》的规定,仍然对18岁以下未成年人开放,使一些青少年沉溺其中。

3. 家庭环境的影响。据北京市的调查,27%的家长对孩子玩游戏不管;19%的家长虽然知道孩子玩游戏,但不知道具体的游戏内容;而54%的中学生对家长隐瞒了自己玩游戏的真实情况。调查还显示,网络成瘾者与父母的文化程度和职业有关,父母亲为高中文化程度的成瘾者居多,工人家庭的学生成瘾者比例偏高,这与父母了解、指导孩子使用计算机上网的认识及能力有关。

4. 上网者自身的原因。青少年学生是上网的主力军,他们这一年龄段生理上、心理上都不够成熟,自我控制能力较弱,很容易迷恋于网络游戏之中。许多青少年甚至把网络世界当成逃避现实的地方,当他们遇到家庭不和睦或生活中不顺心的事件时,就会到网吧中去宣泄。有专家指出,网络成瘾与孤独、抑郁等人格因素有关,国内对大学生上网成瘾的调查显示,网瘾与"卡特尔十六种人格因素测验"中推理能力和支配性有关,显示大学生网瘾者智力水平相对较低。

(四)网络成瘾的社会防范措施

1. 加强对网吧的管理。2002 年我国颁布了《互联网上网服务营业场所管理条例》,明确规定了对网吧等场所的管理规则。各地工商、公安、文化等部门应加强合作,对网吧进行综合治理,控制网吧总量,完善网吧布局规划,坚决关闭无证无照的非法网吧,对违反《互联网上网服务营业场所管理条例》的网吧一定要严肃追究。同时应规范对进口游戏软件的管理,大力开发具有中国文化特色、内容健康、情节生动的电子游戏产品,以取代那些充满暴力、色情内容的游戏。

2. 加强宣传教育工作。要教育上网者以理智的态度控制上网时间和上网费用。对那些色情图片或信息,应保持洁身自好,切莫掉入色情陷阱。对青少年更应加强教育,学校应让学生了解电脑是传播信息的机器,网络只是进入虚拟世界的一种手段而已,学生应不断充实人的各种体验,在现实和虚拟之中取得均衡。青少年要以健全的心态进入网络,对网络游戏及各种网络信息应抱有正确的态度,强化防范意识,抵御网上的各种不良诱惑。

3. 鼓励上网者积极参加社会活动。上网者每天应保持正常而规律的生活,娱乐有度,不可过于迷恋网络。严格控制上网时间,每天应至少抽出 2～3 个小时与同事、家人进行现实交流;通常连续操作电脑 1 小时,就休息 5～10 分钟,逐步摆脱对网络的依赖;闲暇时,可以和大家一起运动、娱乐或外出旅游,时刻感受自然界的美好事物。

4. 加强家庭教育指导。家长要向孩子传授正确的网络知识和使用网络的方法,让孩子全面地认识网络。帮助孩子合理安排学习和上网时间,适当限制他们接触网络的次数。经常和孩子交流沟通,鼓励或者陪伴他们进行适当的体育活动。鼓励孩子多交现实中的朋友,给他提供交友的方便和支持。有条件的家庭,可让孩子在家中上网,并且和孩子一起在网络上获得一些娱乐、体育、市场等方面的信息。这样既可以增加双方的沟通,也使网络成为家庭娱乐和信息的来源。

案例

网络成瘾

武汉某学院大三的小华入学成绩在班上排前两位,大一下半年迷恋上网络游戏《帝国时代》,开始阶段经常通宵达旦上网,后来发展到一周甚至半月不回寝室,吃在网吧住在网吧,校方多次劝说不改。后来其父得知情况,来学校劝其改过,谈及贫寒的家境和跨出农门的不易,父子一阵唏嘘,小华当面保证以后决不再玩网络游戏。但其父前脚刚走,他后脚又进了网吧大门。最终导致多门功课成绩挂红灯,不得不自动退学。

在有一段时间里,小华也曾想收回心来好好学习,可是由于他在网络游戏中确实占有霸主的地位,只要一有什么大的网络游戏比赛,以前的网友总是千方百计找到他,因为他不出征,他们所组的战队就无法获胜。无奈,小华就得继续出征,而一发不可收拾。虽然在现实中小华已经找不到成功的感觉,但是在网络游戏中他绝对是"大哥大",受人追随和受人尊敬。就这样,小华最终走向了网络成瘾的深渊。

究竟是什么原因让他对网络如此迷恋?为揭开这个谜团,有记者专门与小华进行了一次对话,从中,我们似乎可以读懂一点什么。

记者:长时间上网对学习、对身体都有不良影响,每次你去上网的时候,没有想过这些吗?

小华:想过,当然想过,但是我没有办法控制自己。

记者:你现在是大学生,难道这点自制力都没有?

小华:这不是自制力的问题。大学和高中相比,空余时间太多了,而且也没有家长和老师的督促,感到很无聊,所以只有去上网,到网上去发泄自己。

记者:听说你上网大部分是玩网络游戏,难道你不觉得网络游戏与现实相差太远了吗?玩网络游戏不感到无聊吗?

小华:对于网络游戏,我只能说"乐在其中,不可言喻"。

记者:大学生马上就要步入社会了,应该面对现实啊!

小华:在现实中,有很多事情自己是无法改变的,而在网络中,那种经过努力,最终夺得第一的快感,在现实中是永远无法实现的。

思考1. 从记者与小华的对话中,我们可以发现引起小华对网络迷恋的原因有哪些?

思考2. 在对话中,小华提到了现实的无聊及网络的乐趣,针对这个问题,我们应如何实现现实与网络虚拟世界间的平衡?

Chapter 6 Sociopathy

Section 1 The Summary of Sociopathy

1. The concept of sociopathy

Sociopathy is a disease and social pathologic phenomenon, which is dominated by social factors and closely related to the behavior and life style of individual.

Social factors primarily include social systems, economy, education, the law, social customs, morality, behavior and life style and health care, etc.

Human health is influenced not only by bio-factors and environmental factors, but also mainly by social factors. Currently, medical model has already changed from bio-medical model, bio-factors to a bio-psycho-social medical model. Environmental factors are no longer main reasons that influence health, behaviors and life style closely related to society. However, they have become main dangerous factors in the cause of human death. According to WHO's survey, about sixty percent of the cause of death in the world results from bad behavior and life style. Some health problems dominated by social factors which include accidental casualty(suicide, traffic accidents), alcohol abuse, drug addiction, sexually transmitted diseases, adolescent pregnancy, etc., have become the main threat to endanger human life and health. A study of the sociopathy is to research the mechanism about how social factors lead to diseases, find out the relationship between social factors and sociopathy, provide an efficient basis for the prevention of sociopathy by using the research methods of social medicine, and adopt corresponding social preventive measures to protect and promote residents' health level aiming at a certain social factor.

2. The characteristics of sociopathy

(1) Universality

Sociopathy is an extensive phenomenon. Several cases cannot form the so-called sociopathy. For example, a small number of drug addicts in one region cannot be named sociopathy, but regarded as individual's bad behaviors and life style at most. However, millions of people taking drugs can be viewed as a sociopathy.

(2) Time characters

The appearance of each sociopathy has a close relationship to the development of times. For instance, suicide and traffic accidents are considered as sociopathy in modern times, drug taking is viewed as sociopathy with the spread of drugs, and Internet addiction is a yet more recent problem occurring in these years.

(3) Complexity

Complexity includes three meanings. First, the complexity of sociopathy itself, suicide, for example, is still an enigma. Second, the complexity of social causes, sociopathy is a result of synthesis of various factors, and its pathogenic mechanism is extremely complicated. Third, the complexity of prevention and treatment. For instance, the control of addiction problems need to be studied seriously because of its repetition.

(4) Harm characters

Sociopathy causes grave harm to families and society besides the influence on individual's physical and mental health. For example, suicide, drug taking, STDs, etc., not only hurt individual's health and quality of life, but also disrupt social stability and hamper economic development.

(5) Sociality

Sociality includes three implications. First, social factors, such as economy, education, morallity, life style, are the leading causes. Second, sociopathy can result in some social problems and lead to some harmful consequences. Third, the prevention of sociopathy is a socially systematic engineering. Merely the department of health cannot improve it. It needs synthetical work by government and other departments.

3. Factors that cause sociopathy

(1) Economic factors

The rapid economic development improves human health level to a certain extent, and at the same time, it brings a series of problems. The development of the economy expedites the trend of city evolution, quickens the life rhythm, intensifies the social competition, increases work pressure, and complicates relationship among people. All these issues easily make people nervous and anxious, and affect human physical and mental health.

(2) Population factors

Rapid increasing population weighs the burden of society, and may result in a rise of the number of unemployed, add to the unsteady social factors, and increase the pressure of job-hunters; therefore, it causes some psychological disorders. The population flowing among districts and nations speeds up the transmission of some infectious diseases such as AIDS.

(3) Family factors

Good family relationship can maintain physical and mental health and benefit the teenager's growth. The break-up of family relationship, spoiling excessively the child, maltreatment of feeble member, however, would produce a mentally ill influence on all family members. Almost all of sociopathy is closely related to the family environment.

(4) Cultural factors

Cultural customs, ideology, education levels and so forth have certain influence on sociopathy. A morbid attitude necessarily causes abnormal social behaviors, some of which such as suicide, drug addiction, and sexual abuse, are closely related to the philosophy and moral fiber of people. People with different education levels have different concepts of health. The improvement of education level is beneficial to eliminating people's ill life behaviors and improving health level.

(5) Psychological factors

Psychological problems can cause sociopathy. Melancholy people, for example, are susceptible to suicide. People with type A character who have a precipitate temper are vulnerable to traffic accident. People who have a good mental quality are able to face the difficulties and solve the problems when they meet frustration. Those who have a bad psychological quality, on the contrary, usually escape reality by suicide or drug addiction.

4. The principle and measures of prevention and cure for sociopathy

The integrated measures, including society, families and individuals aspects, should be taken for the prevention and cure of sociopathy.

(1) Social medical measures

①Health education should be carried out in the whole society to popularize sanitation knowledge and educate people to get rid of the bad habits of hygiene and to form healthy life style.

②Social conditions and social preventive measures must be improved. High-risk people should be screened to discover and cure as soon as possible. Social organizations of prevention and cure, such as the institutions of mental consultation, are supposed to be established and strengthened. Social sustaining degree ought to be enhanced.

③Strengthening the sanitation legislation. The legal means must be used to forbid some ill behaviors, besides health education. For example, drug addiction and going whoring must be forbidden by legislation.

(2) Family medical measures

①Preserving harmonious family relations. Harmonious family relations benefit the physical fitness and mental exuberance of the family members. It can also reduce the risk of mental disorder and prevent the occurrence of sociopathy.

②Maintaining normal family function. Family is the first class for children; parents must educate and cultivate children to form a good mental quality and characters, so as not to form the bad behavior pattern.

③Pay attention to the high-risk families. The high-risk families primarily include the families of inharmoniousness, intemperance or drug addiction, single parent families, the families with members who have long-term chronic diseases or mental diseases, families with some relation problems or on the verge of break-up. Members in such families are vulnerable to sociopathy. Therefore, attention must be paid to these families.

(3) Behavior medical measures

①Forming healthy behavior and life style. Be sure not to smoke. Drink little, eat reasonable nourishment, follow a good life style, observe the traffic regulations, carry on exercise, examine the body periodically, and develop healthy habit.

②Improving mental health and keeping positive emotional reaction. The intensive competition in modern living brings people certain mental pressure. So it can be helpful to human physical energy and health to keep healthy mentality and happy emotions.

③Keeping positively reactive way. Positive response refers to a positive reaction to consequences caused by tense stimulus. Keeping positively reactive way can help people remain calm when they face frustration or difficulties, and treat the problems with a quiet mood. So it can reduce the occurrence of mental illness.

Section 2　Suicide

Suicide refers to self-destruction behaviors with purpose and design that premeditatedly terminate life because of social and mental conflicts. The WHO reports that there are about one million people dying of suicide every year on the earth, and in China, a large-scale survey at the end of the year 2002 shows that the average suicide rate is 23 out of 100,000, and that the suicides account for 3.6% of the whole death toll. Suicide is the fifth cause of death among the most important death causes of the population in China from 1995 to 1999. And it even is the leading cause of death in the 15 – 35-year age group. The China/WHO advanced seminar about spiritual health in 1999 brought forward that the prevention of suicide is one of three most important problems of spiritual health that need to be solved urgently. Suicide has become a problem to be solved exigently in the field of public health in our country.

1. **The epidemiological distribution of suicide**

(1) District distribution

By and large, the suicide rate in developed countries is higher than that in developing countries. In Europe, it is higher than in America and in Oceania, and the lowest rate is in Africa. China has become the country with high suicide rate, and the suicide rate in our country shows a particular character: suicide rate in village is three times more than that in city, 90% of suicides in China happened in village. Some experts point out that it may be related to the relatively less education of village residents and the widespread use of pesticides in the village.

(2) Time distribution

French sociologist Emile Durkheim considered that the season with highest suicide rate is summer, and the next is spring and autumn, the lowest is winter. He thought it is primarily because the social activities in summer are much more intensive than in other seasons. The season with high suicide rate in village of China, however, is autumn. This phenomenon is related to the fact that suicidal materials are easily obtained because of crop-spraying in autumn. Most of the suicides happened in the daytime in all seasons. Suicide rate is relatively higher at the beginning of every week (Monday) and becomes lower near the weekend (Saturday) of every week. Because the social activities begin to become intensive in the daytime or at the beginning of week, therefore it weighs people's mental burdens.

(3) Population distribution

①Age. Suicide rate generally increases when people grow old. The suicide rate of the old is usually higher than that of the young. But there are differences among various countries. The distribution of age is distinct between village and city. There are two suicidal age peaks in the country, i.e., young group and old group. In the city, however, there's no young peak. Suicide rates of both men and women become high when they are aging.

②Sex. The latest outcome researched by scientists in China and Canada shows that male suicide rate is 3.6 times as much as female's in the world. However, female suicide rate is 0.25 times higher than male's in China, and women rate in village is 3 - 4 times as much as that of in city. This phenomenon is particularly true in China. The reason why women in the country select suicide as the first solution to problems may be because they have little education and lack perfect social support network.

③Cultural condition. Foreign report shows that highly cultured people usually have a high suicide rate, but the suicides in China are more the illiterate. The adult suicides are mostly analphabetic, and the adolescent suicides are mainly students of junior or high school in our country, which may be because the illiterate people are short of communication and social support. Meanwhile, the adolescent may have other factors, such as study pressure, family problems (parents with enmity, separation, divorce).

2. Social causes of suicide

(1) Heredity factor

There are more than fifty years of research about the suicidal genetics in foreign countries, but it has yet no clear conclusion till today. There are three opinions about suicidal genetics at present.

①Suicide is embodied by depression or other mental diseases. ②The heredity of suicide is independent of depression or other mental diseases. ③Suicidal genetics work through mental characters of impulse.

(2) Mental diseases

The suicides caused by mental diseases roughly account for 30%–50% of all. The survey in our country in 2002 shows that 63% of suicides have mental aberration in different degrees. Depression is the highest risk among all the mental diseases, and the suicide rate of depressive people is 50 – 80 times as much as the ordinary population. The next is respectively schizophrenia, neurosis and personality aberration, alcoholism, etc.

(3) Life affairs

The suicidal reasons usually include the following five factors among Chinese people according to survey, family conflicts, love frustration, strained interpersonal relations, unemployment and examination failure.

The conflicts between husband and wife and between mother-in-law and daughter-in-law are the prime collision, and the suicides due to family conflict are mostly women; the suicides resulted from love frustration are common in male and female; the interpersonal conflicts can make people suicide. Ruan Lingyu, for example, commits suicide because gossip is a fearing thing; unemployment affects mainly male youths; the defeat of examination is the suicidal reason of some students. Many students commit suicide after the result of college entrance examination almost every year.

(4) Mental infection

The suicides suffered from mental infection are mostly teenagers. They lack social experiences and mature personality, and their judgmental ability is comparatively low. So they tend to form "object-agreement function". They even imitate the similar person in reality or literature works and step to suicide. The typical imitating suicidal affair happened after the publication of the *The Sorrows of Young Werther* by Johann Wolfgang von Goethe in 1774. Many youngsters imitated Werther to suicide, and a suicidal agitation was formed. Psychoanalyst Pbillps called it "Werther effect".

(5) Social environments

The suicide rate usually decreases during period of warfare, because warfare can build up the consciousness of attachment and the trend of attack completely externalizes. So suicide rate descends. When warfare ends, the emotion becomes relaxed from strain and the interior conflicts increase, suicide rate begins to ascend. There are generally more suicides during the period of political disturbance and economic depression. The suicide rate in Berlin, for example, rose as a result of long-term political instability after World War Ⅱ.

(6) Political purposes

Political suicides usually have a definite political intention. Each suicide represents an interest group, and one's sacrifice can bring larger benefits for a certain group. Much terrorism has a great relation to political suicides. The "9 · 11" event made by terrorists and Palestinian body bomb, for example, are obvious examples of political suicide.

3. The social preventive measures to suicide

(1) Maintaining social stability

The society should guarantee the stability of social politics and economy, prevent the turbulent situation, and reduce the suicide caused by daze, keep rapid economic development, reduce the suicidal factors such as poverty and unemployment, etc.

(2) Carrying out good social preventive measures

Health education should primarily be carried out in society so as to improve people's mental health. Younger students' psychological health especially needs to be enforced in order to build up their mental quality and increase their ability to adapt to society and face frustrations, help them to set up right philosophy and values. In addition, the suicidal tools, such as guns, pesticides, rat-poisons, must be strictly controlled and managed.

(3) Timely mental interference

Practices prove that suicide can be prevented effectively if the mental interference and spirit support are given in time when one forms suicidal ideas. Therefore, suicidal interference centers and psychological consultation organizations should be established in city, giving people who are in trouble or in despair free mental consultation and appeasement, directing them to conquer crises. Many countries like USA, UK and Japan have established organizations of life telephone services in some big cities at present. Their aim is to interfer with the people on the verge of suicide and prevent suicide. Our country's first special institution of suicidal intervention, Beijing Mental Crises Research and Intervention Center, was established in 2002, which manifests that China begins to attach importance to suicide.

(4) Screening high risk people

People who have suicidal idea, emotional disorders(anxiety, depression), mental disorder, etc., can be screened by using the psychological measure scale in order to discover them and prevent suicide. People with suicidal inclination or idea, for example, could be found by Eysenck personality scale and Bech-H despair scale. The melancholic and the anxious who have a high suicide rate could be discovered by self-evaluation depression scale (SDS) and self-evaluation anxiety scale (SAS).

(5) Prevent re-suicide

It is very important to prevent would-be suicides from re-suicide, for 10%–15% of all would-be suicides can re-suicide according to a research. In order to prevent re-suicide, the custody must be enforced to would-be suicides. Besides timely emergency treatment, the mental and emotional cure should be taken so as to help them relieve their feeling, recover the psychological balance and eliminate dangerous factors.

Section 3 Traffic Accidents

Traffic accidents refer to accidents caused by collision, crush, overturn, drowning in water, fire or deviating the roadway in the course of vehicle's running in the street or road which often lead to the casualty of people or livestock and the loss of vehicle or other things. Traffic accidents are sociopathys, too. They are synthetical result caused by physiological, psychological and social factors, etc., among which the psychological and social factors are the decisive ones, and the synthetical measures, mainly including social measures, must be taken to prevent the traffic accidents.

At present, about 700,000 people die and about 3,000,000 people are hurt in traffic accidents in the world every year. There were approximately 770,000 traffic accidents in our country in 2002, which cause almost 110,000 deaths and some 560,000 injured. The direct economic losses caused by traffic accidents exceed 3,300 million yuan RMB. And the traffic accidents primarily endanger the young and middle-aged, which have an obvious influence on social labor force. So the resultant indirect economic loss should not be neglected. The traffic accidents rate is continualy increasing with the rapid development of modern traffic and carrying trade. Some experts said that the traffic accidents have become the leading factor that affects severely the public safety.

1. The prevalent character of traffic accidents

(1) Time distribution

Time distribution differs with different geography and climate in different countries. The nations in Northern Europe have more traffic accidents in winter and autumn, which possibly is because that the wheels tend to slide resulting from covering of snow on the ground in winter, and traffic becomes crowded with the increase of tourists in autumn. In China, traffic accidents usually occur more in the high temperature seasons from June to August, which may be because the weather is hot, drivers are inclined to be tired and find it difficult to concentrate. The survey of some countries and regions, like the United States, Hong Kong, etc., also discovered that the traffic accidents occur more at the weekends, which may be due to the crowded traffic because of frequent activities at the weekends.

(2) Area distribution

According to statistics, traffic accidents mainly occur on the outskirts in most developed countries, compared to less traffic accidents in city. This may be because the suburban traffic condition and traffic management is not well compared to that in the city. In China, traffic accidents occur largely in the area connecting city and suburb and the trunk-road. The domestic research discovers that the higher highway grade is, the more deaths there are, the better road is, the quicker drivers speed. This accordingly gives drivers a narrow visual field and bad response. At the same time the corresponding secure facilities are lacking.

(3) Population distribution

The drivers under 3-year driving experiences are involved in about 47.33% of more serious traffic accidents. The dead and the injured in the accidents caused by them respectively account for 41.28% and 47.06%, and the consequent economic losses account for 44.85%. Serious traffic accidents are mainly caused by the drivers with 2 - 3-year driving license. Traffic accidents primarily endanger children, teenagers, and old people, especially affect badly the children and teenagers. In Japan, traffic accidents are the leading cause of death among children and teenagers. The research in the city of Chengdu, China, discovered that peasants have a comparatively large proportion of the occurrence of traffic accidents — about one out of three.

2. Social causes of traffic accidents

(1) Traffic conditions

At the moment, highways develop slowly compared to the rapidly increasing population and motor vehicles in developing countries, which cause unbalance of population, vehicles and highways. In addition, the departments concerned attaching no importance to the road management, the lack of traffic administrators and facilities with transportation, the lag of traffic management are also the reasons of rapid increase in traffic accidents.

(2) The bad behaviors of drivers

Drinking is an important factor causing traffic accidents. It is the chief reason for traffic accidents in developed countries. Alcohol can affect drivers' ability to operate and decrease their ability to accept and perceive information, make the visual field narrow down, and reduce both the ability to recognize, judge and the capability of self-control and synthetically orientation, prolong the reactive time; reduce the operative accuracy. The use of medicine and drug abuse is also vulnerable to the traffic accidents. The side effect such as hypnosis brought on by taking some medicines and the hallucination produced by drug abuse may cause traffic accidents.

(3) Tiredness and nap

Some experts in New Zealand point out that tiredness has a latent danger for the traffic accidents, and that its hazard is no less than driving while intoxicated. A survey in England shows that 29% of drivers acknowledge their sleeping experiences when steering, and 10% of traffic accidents are related to fatigue, 10% of which have a relation to tiredness in 48,000 traffic accidents without outside conditional factors, according to the statistics in the United States. In China, driving with tiredness is the main reason of traffic accidents among the gravest traffic accidents in 2001.

(4) Motoring offense of drivers

Motoring offenses primarily include non-use of safety belt and helmet, speeding, etc. In the United States, 13% of drivers who cause traffic accidents do not wear safety belt, and the proportion is higher in China. Particularly when driving on the newly built freeway, a lot of drivers do not wear safety belt, therefore adding to the risk of traffic accidents.

(5) The state of drivers' physiology and psychology

Drivers' physical strength, stamina, reactive velocity, sight, etc. can decline to different extent while aging, which increases the risk of traffic accidents. Another research shows that the occurrence of traffic accidents has a relation to drivers' personality, motion, etc. Drivers who cause traffic accidents usually have the personality of not easy-going, bad interpersonal relation, easiness to impulse, unstable emotions, excessive strain, etc.

(6) The reason of the pedestrians

People mostly injured in traffic accidents are the young under 25, the old above 50, and the people in village or peasants working in city. The superficial reason is that the young have more opportunity for outing, the old have a poor hearing, tardy action and slow reaction, peasants don't adapt to the crowded traffic conditions in city. But the deeper reason is that these people are indifferent to traffic safety and are not able to adapt to the complicated traffic environments.

3. The social preventive measures of traffic accidents

(1) Strengthening traffic legislation

Measures should be taken to establish and strengthen traffic legislation and regulate drivers to wear safety belt and helmet, prescribe the drivers' age limit of drawing driver's license, set the standard of blood alcohol consistency (BAC), restrict rigidly drivers' driving time in each day and prohibit driving while they are tired, check and penalize the drivers addicted to drugs. The corresponding punishment should be given to the motoring offense drivers.

(2) Improving traffic conditions and motor function

We should improve traffic conditions, establish advanced managerial facilities, and train traffic control personnel. We should take some measures in road symbol, signal, supervision, etc., to establish effective road protection system, and strengthen the control of highway transportation. We should constantly study, develop and adopt advanced active or passive accidents-prevention technique, for example, improving brake system, installing the safe gasbag and electronic defense system, etc., therefore increasing the vehicles' ability to cope with the accidents.

(3) Selecting drivers carefully

Personal factor accounts for 92.8% among the components of the reasons of traffic accidents in our country, according to a research. Therefore, selecting drivers well is very important to reduce traffic accidents. When we select drivers, their psychological quality must be considered besides noticing physique, and drivers' characters, temperament type, etc., should be tested in order that their physiological and psychology quality can pass as far as possible.

(4) Enhance the safety education to high risk people

Children and teenagers are prone to be injured in traffic accidents; it is effective for the prevention of traffic accidents to educate the young to know traffic regulation and traffic safety knowledge by teaching them knowledge of driving and traffic safety. More time and energy should be spent on drivers for occupational technique training, making them realize that their behaviors directly influence others' lives.

(5) Improving measures of medical emergency

Some researches discover that 20% of the injured in the traffic accidents can avoid death by timely treatment. Therefore, it is extremely important to improve the first aid system and deal with timely injury in traffic accidents. It can reduce the rate of disability and death. The United States and many countries in Europe have comparatively perfect first aid system, many coaches have stretcher and other emergency equipments, and the injured can get salvage as early as possible after traffic accidents. Our country should reenforce the establishment of first aid such as the hospital emergency ward, "120" emergency treatment, etc.

Section 4　Sexually Transmitted Diseases

Sexually Transmitted Diseases (STDs) are a group of infectious diseases transmitted mainly by sexual contact and analogously sexual contact. The World Health Organization permanent council decides that the venereal diseases were replaced by Sexually Transmitted Diseases in 1975. Former venereal diseases, mainly including syphilis, gonorrhea, soft chancre and venereal lymphogranuloma, are also called classical venereal diseases. The kinds of Sexually Transmitted Diseases now are gradually increasing. The primarily preventive Sexually Transmitted Diseases in our country include gonorrhea, condyloma acuminatum, ungonococcus urethritis, syphilis, acquired immunodeficiency syndrome (AIDS), bacterial colpitis, genitals herpes infection, soft chancre, venereal lymphogranuloma, groin granuloma, hepatitis B, etc.

1. The epidemiological overview of STDs

(1) General situation of prevalence

It is difficult to acquire accurate data of STDs due to some reasons. WHO estimates at the end of the 1990's that the newly added cases are about 400 million, among which the gonorrhea is 62 million, syphilis is 12 million, HIV infection is 30 million, chlamydoaoan infection is 89 million. In China, the cumulative reported cases of eight legal reportorial STDs are nearly 5.5 million up to 2001, and the first four are respectively gonorrhea, ungonococcus urethritis, condyloma acuminatum, syphilis. The prevalence of AIDS is particularly severe in these years. AIDS has become widely prevailed in the world since the first AIDS case was discovered in the United States in 1981. WHO estimates that the total amount of HIV infection on the earth has reached 60 million. In China there are presently about 1 million people infected with HIV, and it will reach 10 million up to 2010 if active and effective measures are not taken.

(2) Area distribution

There are varied prevalence rate and kinds of STDs in different areas in the world; in developing countries there is a high prevalence rate of STDs because the technique of diagnosis and treatment needs to be improved. The gravest prevalence of AIDS occurs in Africa, the next is Asia and Pacific area, and the east Europe and middle Asia area have the most quick increasing rate. The area with rapid city evolution has a high STDs prevalence rate. The southeast littoral open cities in our country have a rather large population flow and a rather quickly increasing prevalence rate. Among provinces that reported the eight legal reportorial STDs cases in 2000, the first five ones are respectively Jiangsu, Zhejiang, Guangdong, Anhui and Sichuan. The gravest areas of AIDS occurrence are still in southwest border such as Yunnan, and it has spread to most provinces in the whole nation.

(3) Population distribution

①Age. The STDs cases in our country are mostly the young and middle-aged. The 20 - 39-year age group account for 92.4%. Among HIV infection cases, the 15 - 49-year age group account for 93.9%. In recent years, STDs prevalence has the tendency to spread to children, and the number of children who have STDs are increasing.

②Sex. Male prevalence rate is higher than female in most STDs, and the proportion of men to women was 2 : 1 among the STDs cases inspected in 1987 - 1989 in our country, and it declined to 1.4 : 1 in 2000, which was possibly because that the female who actively see the doctor are on the increase, the level of diagnosis and treatment improve and the female actual cases increased. The proportion of men to women among AIDS infected people is 4.6 : 1.

③Occupation. Workers who have the highest prevalence rate of STDs account for about one-third, the young people without job or waiting for a job account for 20%, the individual businessmen account for 15%, the people engaged in services or supply and marketing account for 10%. The cadre in department and the official personnel have a quickest infection rate in recent years, and the peasants infected are increasing, too.

The HIV infected are mainly peasants, homecoming laborers, hobos, and individual practitioners. The number of long-distance drivers infected increase quickly in these years.

2. Social causes of STDs

(1) Social conditions

Along with the economic development and the increase of external intercourse, the introduction of west concept of sex free to China has a certain impact on the traditional moral concept in our country. The development of international tourism and frequency of international commercial intercourse offers opportunities to the transmitting of STDs. The rapid development of the third industry and individual economy and the appearance of lots of service occupations and individual industry and commerce result in a social class with high economic salaries and little education. They are high risk population of STDs.

(2) Population's flow

There are 80 million – 120 million flowing people crowded in dense areas in China per year. These people are mostly in the sexually active phase. The high density and the massive move and flow bring opportunities for the spread of STDs.

(3) Going whoring and prostitution

Go whoring and prostitution are cardinal social causes of spread of STDs. The Thailand is a nation with developed erotic vocation and the prevalence of STDs is extremely rampant. The check rate of STDs among unlicensed prostitute and whore master in our country averages 39.9%. In recent years, whoring occurs in many nightclubs, beauty parlors and massage parlors, which should be regarded by some departments concerned.

(4) Drug taking and drug trading

The check rate of STDs among drug addicts is 32.5%, and the prevalent rate of STDs in the female dope-addict is 43.25%. 63.9% of HIV infected are drug addicts by mainline according to the report in China in 2002. Drug taking has became the main path of spread of AIDS.

(5) Pornographic deluge

Pornography, including the literature, film and TV, phonetape and videotape, network culture, etc., can corrupt morals, and specially tend to cause the teenagers' curiosity and imitation. Therefore, the influence of pornography on STDs should not be underrated.

(6) Lack of consciousness of self-protection

Many people lack basic sanitation knowledge and consciousness of self-protection. They do not use condoms because of the widespread use of the modern oral contraception and intrauterine contraception and, therefore, lose the physical protection against the STDs infection factors.

(7) Chaotic medical market of venereal disease

There are many practitioners without license and quacks in society. They have bad techniques and sanitary conditions, and they do not report epidemic situation. Some infected turn to these illegal practitioners for fear of loosing their face and exposure of identity. As a result, the infected are still with STDs chronically and continue to spread the STDs as the source of infection.

3. The social preventive measures of STDs

(1) Increasing health education and popularize sex knowledge education

The sex health education and procreation health education should be increased in order to fully acquaint most residents with knowledge of STDs, and to make them realize the harm of STDs to individual, families, society and know the preventive measures of STDs, therefore, increase the resident's self-protection consciousness. The contents of education should include sex morals education, self-cultivation of sex physiological knowledge and sexual healthy psychology, right usage of contraceptives such as condom, etc., preserving moral integrity, realizing the abnormally sexual behaviors such as sex abuse. The sex education for teenagers who should be major object of propaganda and education is a problem that ought to be regarded in whole society.

(2) Comprehensive management and overall prevention

The prevention of STDs needs to be administered by many departments. Ministry of Health, public security, justice, civil administration, propaganda should cooperate to ban whoring and prostitution, to compel the people with AIDS to accept treatment, to control strictly the mobile population, to suppress firmly the pornography, confiscate or forfeit them according their conditions, and to restructure the medical market and prohibit illegal practitioners from doctoring.

(3) Strengthening lawmaking and consummating system of epidemic situation report

Our country has enacted *The Regulation of Prevention and Cure of Venereal Diseases* in 1991 which prescribes that the diseases which must be reported are respectively AIDS, gonorrhea, syphilis, condyloma acuminatum, ungonococcus urethritis, soft chancre, genitals herpes infection, venereal lymphogranuloma. Each local authority ought to perform strictly this regulation and report to the leadership in time when finding cases so as to prevent them from spreading.

(4) Cutting off other routes of transmission besides sex contact

Besides sex contact, the routes of transmission of STDs contain blood infection, vertical transmission, iatrogenic infection, contact infection in daily life, etc. The blood produces' safety and credibility and the blood donors' health must be guaranteed; to prevente the infection of neonates, the pregnant women who was diagnosed as having STDs had better end the pregnancy; the piscine, hotels, beauty salons and swimming pools are supposed to do well the disinfectious work; doctors should pay attention to self-protection, and abide strictly by operation regulations to prevent the iatrogenic infection.

(5) Doing well the surveillance of STDs

Reinforcing the monitoring of STDs can master in time the prevalent trends of STDs, find out the source of infection and investigate all-sided influencing factors and offer basis for the establishment of preventive measures. The surveillance objects mainly include high-risk people (such as harlots, queers, drug addicts and some other people worked in special services industry, etc.) and emphatic diseases (such as AIDS, gonorrhea, syphilis, etc.).

Section 5 Addictive Sociopathy

The addiction refers to the overwhelming need to repeatedly engage in some activities or misuse of some drugs, though such drugs or behaviors will result or have resulted in various adverse consequences. The addiction primarily includes materials addiction and compulsive behaviors. The material addiction, also called materials dependence, is caused via the action of concrete materials on human body, such as smoking, drink, drug taking, etc. The behaviors addiction is a strong dependence on some behaviors, such as gambling, theft addiction, shopping addiction, network addiction, etc.

Addictive behaviors contain three main characteristics: (1) It has become a necessary part of life activities of addicts. Therefore, it causes strong dependence of psychology, physiology and society on addicts and urges them to acquire the source of addiction by all means, the source of addiction are some materials or behaviors that cause addiction. (2) The obvious withdrawal syndrome will occur when people stop addictive behaviors. And it will quickly disappear once they resume addictive behaviors. (3) It will bring severe consequences to individual, families and society.

The pathological mechanism is alike no matter material addiction or compulsive behaviors. It generally experiences four stages: (1) the stage of inducement, when the person begins to contact some addictive materials, and feels pleasure; (2) the stage of formation, when dependence gradually forms with the continued repetition of actions; (3) the stage of consolidation, when the addictive actions have been strengthened and become a necessary part in life; (4) the stage of decline, when the obvious damages occur in physiology and psychology.

Nowadays, the addiction sociopathy is a hotspot that people pay close attention to and an important topic of social medicine. This chapter mainly introduces drug taking that has a severe damage and network addiction that appears recently.

1. Drug taking

Drug taking refers to the phenomena of abuse of illegal drugs such as narcotic drugs, anodyne, hallucinogen, etc. The drugs generally include two kinds, namely legal drugs and illegal drugs. Drug taking that we usually call refers to the abuse of illegal drugs such as cannabis, heroin, cocaine, hallucinogen, etc. The root of the drug taking, like suicide, is that individual wants to escape agonies or misfortunes by force of forgetting or destroying himself, and it is caused by individual's material or spiritual dissatisfaction or unhappiness.

(1) The prevalent characters of drug taking

There are about 185 million dope-addicts in the world according to the figures announced by UN Drug Forbidden Office in 2002. In China, the inland registered drug addicts reached nearly 1 million in 2002, compared to about 50,000 in 1998, and the actual figures are possibly 5 million if estimated recessive drug addicts are included.

The quickly increasing speed is shocking.

①Population distribution. The research into six regions where drug taking is very severe in our country for nearly 10 years shows that male outnumbers the female; drug addicts have little education, 78.95% of whom don't attend junior high school. Mobile jobs are the most important risk factor of drug taking, and the drug taking rate of lay-offs, the unemployed, individual households, drivers, etc. is 11 times as high as the rate of fixed occupations such as cadres, teachers, peasants, workers, etc. The age of drug addicts has become younger in these years, and the data from national drug forbidden committee office show that the proportion of young drug addicts accounts for about 80% in recent years in our country.

②District distribution. The phenomena of drug taking have spread to inland from border and to villages from cities. At the beginning of the 1990's, the phenomena of drug taking are only confined to few villages in the border provinces such as Yunnan, but nowadays they spread quickly and have endangered most of provinces and municipalities of China with the international drug dealers' pervasion to inland and the open of channel of international drug taking

(2) The harm of drug taking

Drug taking is very harmful not only to individual, but also to families and society.

①Drug taking badly damages health. Cocaine can cause insomnia, loss of weight, membranae pituitosa necrosis, etc., and it can bring respiratory failure and result in death if used overtime. Heroin can produce obvious harm to digestive system, respiratory system, nervous system, etc. The hallucinogen LSD can hurt people's mentality, bring people supernatural hallucination, and urge them to commit suicide. The withdrawal syndromes caused by long-term drug taking especially make most drug addicts unendurable.

②Drug taking often results in the break of marriage and families. Drug addicts can become very selfish and dishonest after long-term drug addiction, their characters will go worried and irritable and their emotion will become indifferent and world-weary. They are completely addicted to the pursuit of drug. They lack the care for their mates and are apathetic to family duties and their children' education. Furthermore, they do not consider the economic crisis in their family at all. On the contrary, they will sell off family fortune to sustain drug taking, and all these are likely to result in the break of the family.

③Drug taking also breaks social peace. The domestic and international drug dealers have repeatedly used force in order to guarantee their drug traffic. And drug addicts often go various criminal activities neck or nothing to acquire drugs. Above 30% of law cases of property torts are caused by drug addicts in most provinces or municipalities, and in some regions where drug taking is very serious even reach 70%, according to statistics. In addition, the spread of AIDS resulting from drug taking has become a very grievous threat.

(3) The social causes of drug taking

①The curiosity is the first impulse of drug taking

Many drug addicts, especially the youth, beginning to take drugs out of curiosity, have strong curiosity and desire of quest and lack necessary scientific knowledge and the ability to distinguish right from wrong, want to try it when they heard that drug taking can make people greatly pleased. A survey expresses that above 80% of the teenagers are addicted to drugs because of having no idea of the harmful effect of drugs.

②Ignorance and the pursuit to enjoyment is another reason of drug taking

It's particularly highlighted in some upstarts with little education. In some littoral special districts, some moneybags view drug taking as a vogue, tide, and status. Some farmer entrepreneurs even treat guests to heroin. At some noble schools in the South of China, many students regard taking heroin as a symbol of advanced consumption and richness and honor. In fact, all these phenomena result from ignorance.

③Personal loyalty of pals is a mental power of drug taking

It is to keep friends' face that many teenagers start to take drugs accompanying friends. They consider that friends should have personal loyalty, and they should not be an exception, therefore, they walk on the way of drug taking step by step. It is for this reason that drug addicts usually have their circle and partners. Single drug addict only account for 21.9%, compared to 72.3% of co-drug addicts, according to the sampling survey in Wuhan.

④Bad family environments are important influential factors

Besides influenced directly by family members' drug taking, some teenagers, whose parents have divorced or stay out long, cannot get normal education; some children, who live in a rich family and are terribly spoilt by parents that satisfy material need unlimitedly, have full material qualification to seek for excitement of drugs. All these could be the reason why the teenagers take drugs.

⑤Chill in life tend to induce drug taking

When encountering frustration or chill in life, people generally take various ways to release it. Some teenagers, who have many unsatisfactory problems such as want of a warm family, suffering from parents' divorce and having great study pressure, etc., tend to become mental pang and want to escape reality by taking drugs.

⑥Drug dealers penetrate everywhere

Drug dealers cannot advertise for sale promotion but they can achieve their aims by the way of decoy to extend drug markets and sell drugs. The most used methods are giving cigarettes to drug dealers who pack the drugs skillfully. Therefore, the smokers become addicted unconsciously and have to turn to the persons who send cigarettes at last. It is during the time of learning smoking that many teenagers are addicted to drug. Some people in Yunnan border put drugs into lipsticks or foods, and cause people to be addicted to drugs by licking lip or eating.

(4) The social preventive measures of drug taking

①Strengthening spiritual civilization and increasing citizens' diathesis

Wang Guowei, the great master of national theory mentioned in the book of *Drug Forbidding* that the key of drug forbidding is an increase in citizens' diathesis. The war of drug forbidding cannot be won unless strengthening spiritual civilization, increasing citizens' integral diathesis, and making them recognize indeed the harm to individual, families and society, and resist drugs in the whole society.

②Strenthen teenagers' health education

It is very important for the youth, who are high risk and badly injured population of drug taking, to strengthen their health education to prevent drug taking. First, make them understand that they can't attempt rashly to take drugs and they shouldn't think childishly they can abstain from drugs after addicted, because drugs cannot be get rid of after addicted. Second, strengthen the health education of teenagers and warn them of drugs' harm. Nowadays the National Drug Forbidding Committee and Ministry of Education have taken the actions of "the knowledge of drug forbidding for one lesson", and carry out the special education lesson of drug forbidding in colleges, middle schools and elementary schools in our country, which make each citizen receive the preventive education of drugs before they step into society. In addition, the mental health education should be strengthened for teenagers so as to increase their ability to deal with frustration in lives.

③Strengthen the legislation concerning forbidden drugs

The laws about forbidden drugs and blow of drug trade are supposed to be enacted; the planting of drug materials such as poppy, cannabis, etc. must be banned firmly and the planters should be arrested. The fruits ought to be burned down. The group of drug smugglers and drug criminals must be beaten. Drug taking is not a problem of any single country and nation, but a problem the human race should face. Therefore, the effective and continuous measures to beat drugs should be taken by strengthening international cooperation.

④Timely treatment for drug addicts

Psychologists point out that drug taking is an illness in nature. The drug addicts should not be discriminated against, but be sympathized and cared for. Besides the normal treatment by the bureau of drug abuse control, society and families had better increase humane care to drug addicts to help them get rid of the life mode of drug abuse, and recover normal physiological, psychological and social function. Then they can return to society and become useful social members.

⑤Enhancing the research of mental mechanism of drug addiction and re-drug taking

The so-called mental drug addiction is such a mental state when drug addicts can not control their desire for drug taking, and have an overwhelming desire for drug re-taking, though they have abstained from physiological addiction. Most drug addicts admit that they are unable to control the "desiring addiction", namely can't help desiring drug re-taking, despite having no anguished physiological response after abstaining from drugs. Preventing drug re-taking is the key to abstain from drug taking, but the drug re-taking rate in our country is above 95%. Therefore, it is significant for abstinence from drugs to research drug addicts' mental addition mechanism of re-drug addiction after they abstain from drugs.

2. Internet addiction

(1) Summary

Internet addiction refers to spending much time and energies immoderately in surfing, chatting, or playing internet games on the network, and the excessive usage of network affects living quality, lowers the efficiency of study and work, impairs health, and results in some negative consequences such as abnormal behaviors, mental disorder, personality disorder, dysfunction of nervous system, etc.

In 1994, an alienist Iva Kimberger claimed that he had discovered a new mental disorder and named it "internet addiction disorder" (IAD). The IAD arouses the attention of psychiatrists and clinical psychologists very quickly. Researchers specially discussed the possibility that IAD becomes formal diagnosis on the two American psychology academy annual conventions in Toronto in 1997 and in San Francisco in 1998.

Although the formal IAD diagnosis was not fixed on, researchers generally considered that to be diagnosed as having IAD, a person must meet criteria as follows. ①Tolerance increasing: This refers to the need for increasing amounts of time on the Internet to achieve satisfaction, namely the network addiction becomes more serious. ②Withdrawal symptoms: The reduction of Internet use or cessation of Internet use (from several hours to several days) will cause psychomotor agitation and obsessive thinking about what is happening on the Internet and fantasies or dreams about the Internet. ③ The Internet is often accessed more often, and the time on Internet is longer than was intended. ④The attempt to reduce time on network always ends in failure. ⑤A significant amount of time is spent on activities related to Internet, e. g. , installing new software, sorting and coding large quantity of downloaded files, etc. ⑥The surfing on network influences badly on social, occupational, family lives. ⑦Much time is spent on Internet though the person can realize the serious problems of Internet.

(2) The harm of network addiction

A survey announced in American psychology association annual conventions in August, 1999 shows that about 11.4 million people are having IAD among the 200 million surfing people in the world, and that the proportion is about 6%. There are about 14.8% of minors (136.5 thousand) who are having IAD in Beijing according to the research by Beijing Normal University. There are at least 225 thousand people that are having Internet mental disorder in different degree in our country by estimation, who are generally 15 – 45 years old. The male account for 98.5% of the total IAD people, the female account only for 1.5%, and the single male at 20 – 30 years are more inclined to having IAD.

The Internet addicts, to some extent, are the same as being addicted to some bad habits such as drugs, alcohol or gambling, etc. The research by psychologists discovers that network addiction is extremely similar to gambling characteristics that cannot resist temptation. The research also finds that the use of Internet can lead one to confounding state on the learning, social intercourse, public finance and the work, which is greatly analogous to the well-known gambling, erratic diet and excessive drinking.

Network addiction can cause a series of negative influence on individual's physiology and psychology. The influence on physiology primarily includes anorexia, tiredness, dyspepsia, decreasing of cerebral blood flow. In addition, the lack of proper exercises because of staying before computer for long easily causes some bad physical response such as carpal syndrome, back sprain and eyestrain, etc. The influence on psychology primarily includes the deviation of interest, unwillingness to part from network, exclusion of other things, concentration to a certain aspect for long. And once they stop surfing Internet, the symptom, like withdrawal syndrome, such as unease, anxiety, insomnia, down-heartedness, bad emotion, tardy thought, will occur.

Network addition can bring certain harm to families and society. Many network addicts spend a huge amount of surfing charges enjoying the interest of network. They go with computer at the expense of desolation of school work, careers and even families. In the United States the number of divorced people because of network accounts for one-third of all divorced people at present. Network addicts who separate from reality for long are vulnerable to psychological disorders and melancholy, influencing normal learning, work and living, and adding the unstable factor to society at the same time. Experts forecast that in the 21st century the harm of network to society is no less than today's heroin addiction. Therefore, paying attention to the research of network addiction is currently a cardinal task of social medicine.

(3) The social causes of network addiction

①The allure of the network

The biggest character of the network is virtualization. In the virtual environments of network, the conditionality of people's inner standard and social norm can be reduced or eliminated and people's behaviors in network express a character of freeing from restraint. They can deliver their views, follow their inclinations and do many things that they want to do but dare not do at ordinary time. The network game is also a cardinal factor that attracts people. In the network game, people can exert fully subjective activities to satisfy their mentality.

②The management to network bars is not normative

The policy and statute about network bars are not perfect and lack maneuverability. Not a few network bar managerial personnel lack necessary professional technique and juristic knowledge, and they often neglect management in practice on account of lack of consciousness of network safety. There is an opportunity given to operators because the phenomena of crossing purview and unclear duties exist in departments concerned. Some network bars still open to minors under 18 year-old regardless of the rules of *The Management Statute for Business Place of Internet Surfing Services*, and many teenagers indulge themselves with Internet.

③The influence of family

According to a survey in Beijing, 27% of parents do not restrain their children from playing games; 19% of parents do not know about the concrete contents of games although they know their children play games; The survey also shows that network addiction has a relation to parents' education degree and occupations. The students whose parents have a senior high school education or whose parents are workers usually have a high addiction proportion, which is related to parents' knowledge and ability to know and guide children to surf.

④The reasons of people who surf the Internet

Teenage students are the main force surfing the Internet. They are not mature both in physiology and psychology, and they have poor control ability. So they tend to indulge in Internet games. Many teenagers, however, regard the Internet as the place of escapism, and they often go to network bar to release their emotion when encountering family fiction or some unsatisfactory things in life. Some experts point out that network addiction has a relation to personality such as solitude, depression, etc. The inland investigation of college students shows that network addiction is related to ability to reasoning and domination in "the trial of cartel sixteen personality factors". This shows the addicts of college students have a relatively lower intelligence level.

(4) The social preventive measures of network addiction

①Strengthening the management of network bars

The promulgation of *The Management Statute for Business Place of Internet Surfing Services* in 2002 ordains definitely the managerial rules to places such as network bars. The departments of business, public security, culture, etc. in each local authority should reinforce cooperation to govern network bars synthetically, to control the amounts of network bars, and to consummate the topological design. The illegal network bars without licenses must be closed and the network bars that disobey *The Management Statute for Business Place of Internet Surfing Services* must be searched question. At the same time, the imported game software must be managed normatively, and the Chinese game software with Chinese cultural characters, healthy contents and dramatic plot are supposed to be developed to replace the games full of violence and eroticisms.

②Strengthening the work of propaganda and education

People surfing Internet should be educated to control time and expenditure on network in sensible manner. They ought to preserve their moral integrity and avoid on the hook of eroticism to those erotic pictures or information. Teenagers are supposed to be given yet more education, they must know that computers are only machines of transmitting information and Internet is merely a means of entering virtual worlds, they should enrich various experiences to get the balance between reality and virtualization. The youth need a right mentality when surfing in network and have a correct attitude to various network games and information, so they can reinforce preventive consciousness to defend all kinds of bad allure.

③Encouraging people who surf in Internet to participate in social activities

People who surf the network should keep a normal and regular life, their entertainments should have a degree, so avoid indulging in Internet. The time spent on network must be controlled, at least 2 – 3 hours per day ought to be spared to communicate with colleagues and folks; in order to get rid of the dependence on network gradually, they should rest for 5 – 10 minutes after operating computers continuously for one hour; when being at leisure, they can take some exercises, amusement or outing travel with others to feel the good things in the whole of nature.

④Strengthening guide of home education

The parents had better teach children the right Internet knowledge and the method of using Internet, and make them know roundly the network. And they must help children to arrange reasonably the time of study and surfing on Internet, and restrict them properly the time of contacting Internet. In addition, parents should often communicate with children, encourage or accompany them to do proper exercises, encourage them to make friends in reality, give them the convenience and support for making friends. In some qualified families, children can surf on Internet at home, and parents can accompany them together to acquire some information such as entertainment, sports, markets, etc. In this way, the Internet can not only add bilateral communications but also become the source of family amusement and information.

Case Example

Network Addiction

Xiao Hua, whose study grades rank the first or second just entering college, is a junior in a college in Wuhan. He became infatuated with the Internet game *Imperial Age* in the latter half of the first year in college. At first, he often surfed on the network all night. Afterward, he did not go back to his dormitory for a week even half a month, but ate and slept in network bar. His father went to college to advise him to give up surfing after the invalidity of school's advice. When hearing of the poverty of their family and the difficulty of striding out of farmhouse, they all sighed, and Xiao Hua guaranteed in his father's presence that he would not play Internet games any longer. However, after his father left, he again entered network bar. At last, he was taken away from school because of his failure of many subjects.

Xiao Hua wanted to study wholeheartedly at one period, but his former network friends always turned to him when there was important competition of Internet games because their group couldn't win without him due to his overlord in Internet games. Thus, Xiao Hua had to continue to play games and became irremediable. He was the absolute hegemony in Internet games and was respected and followed by others, although he had no sense of success in reality. In this way, he walked toward the abyss of network at last.

What on earth made him so indulged in Internet? Some reporters take a special conversation with Xiao Hua in order to uncover the enigma. We may know something from the conversation.

Reporter: When you surf on network, do you take account of the harm to your study and health?

Xiao Hua: I considered it of course, but I couldn't control myself.

Reporter: You are a college student, haven't you the capability for controlling yourself?

Xiao Hua: It is not a problem of capability for controlling. There is much spare time and short of urging of parents and teachers in college compared to high school. I felt bored and had to surf on the network to release feelings.

Reporter: I heard that you often play games when you surf on Internet, don't you think that Internet games are very different from reality? And don't you feel the Internet games boring?

Xiao Hua: As to Internet games, what I want to say is merely "it is too pleased to say".

Reporter: As a college student, you will step into society soon, you had better face the reality.

Xiao Hua: Many things in reality are unmodifiable. In the network, however, the sweet feeling of taking first after endeavor could not be achieved in reality.

Question 1: What reasons can we find from the conversation between reporter and Xiao Hua that make Xiao Hua indulge in the network?

Question 2: Countering the problem of humdrum in reality and interest in network that Xiao Hua mentioned in the conversation, how do we keep the balance between reality and the virtual world?

第七章 特殊人群社会医学

特殊人群是指具有特殊的生理、心理特点,或处于一定的特殊环境中,自我保护能力较差,容易受到各种有害因素的作用,患病率较高的人群。主要包括妇女、儿童、老年人、残疾人等。这些群体近年来又被称为弱势群体。他们的健康问题有着广泛的社会根源,是社会医学必须加以关注的群体。

第一节 儿童和青少年社会医学

儿童一般是指 0~12 岁的人群,占总人口的 30% 左右。世界卫生组织对青少年的定义为:10~19 岁为少年期,20~24 岁为青年期,这一年龄段的人口占总人口的 25% 左右。儿童青少年人数众多,处于形体上、生理上和心理上不断发生变化的时期,是一生中生长发育最快的阶段,也是奠定身心健康的基础阶段。因此,是必须加以特殊关注的人群。

一、儿童和青少年的身心特点及健康问题

(一)儿童的身心特点及健康问题

根据不同年龄段儿童生长发育过程中所表现的特点,可将儿童分为婴儿期(出生~1 岁)、幼儿期(1~3 岁)、学龄前期(3~7 岁)、学龄期(7 岁及以上),各期儿童的身心发育特点及健康问题有所不同。

1. 婴儿期的特点及健康问题。由于婴儿期的生长发育比任何时期都快,因此,对能量和蛋白质的要求特别高,否则易发生营养不良和发育落后;进食多,以乳类为主,但消化和吸收功能发育不完善,易发生消化不良和营养紊乱;从母体得到的免疫力逐渐消失,而后天获得的免疫力很弱,易患感染性疾病。

2. 幼儿期的特点及健康问题。幼儿期处在刚断奶之后,如不注意饮食营养,则容易发生营养不良。此时,幼儿的神经精神发育迅速,表现在语言、动作明显发展,与成年人交往增加,往往表现出违拗性。由于幼儿已能控制大小便,活动范围逐渐加大,发生意外事故和接触感染的机会增多。

3. 学龄前期与学龄期的特点及健康问题。这两个时期儿童的生长较缓慢,速度平稳,6 岁以后乳牙松动脱落,恒牙长出。学

龄前期神经精神发育迅速,语言、动作发展逐渐成熟。免疫系统及消化系统功能逐渐成熟,传染病及消化道疾病减少,意外事故和免疫性疾病增多。进入学龄期的儿童的环境变化较大,与教师、同学的接触和正规的学习过程影响着儿童的身心发育。

(二)青少年的身心特点及健康问题

青少年是处于青春发育期的人群,青春期是从儿童到成年人所经历的一个转变时期。处于这一时期的青少年生理和心理都发生较大的改变,从生理特点来看:①身高、体重、胸围等发育加速;②各系统和内脏的发育加快,功能增强;③生殖系统发育成熟,第二性征出现。在心理特点方面,青春期是充满独立与依赖、自觉与幼稚等错综复杂的矛盾时期。10～14岁的青春早期,一方面保持着儿童的某些心理特征,表现为幼稚,另一方面已具有成年人的某些心理特征,思维活动逐渐完备,情感更为复杂和热烈,对异性开始萌发爱慕之情。15～19岁的青春晚期,是少年向成年人的过渡阶段,心理发育逐渐成熟。青少年时期常见的健康问题有近视、意外伤害、青春期心理卫生问题等,少女月经异常也较为多见。

二、影响儿童和青少年健康的社会因素

(一)经济因素

经济因素是影响儿童青少年健康的重要社会因素。经济发达的国家,儿童青少年的健康状况优于不发达的国家。据世界卫生组织《2000年人人健康全球策略》资料,发达国家的婴儿死亡率仅为19‰,而不发达国家为160‰。2001年我国统计资料显示,北京、天津、上海等大城市婴儿死亡率和5岁以下儿童死亡率均低于10‰,而云南、贵州、青海等经济发展较为落后的省区婴儿死亡率在30‰以上,5岁以下儿童死亡率为40‰左右。一项对58个发展中国家的抽样调查指出,在其他条件相同的情况下,人均收入下降10%,则婴幼儿死亡率上升2‰～3.5‰。

(二)家庭因素

家庭是以婚姻和血缘关系组成的社会基本单位。家庭是儿童青少年生长发育和受教育的重要环境。父母是儿童的第一任教师,儿童性格气质、卫生习惯、生活方式、饮食习惯等或多或少会受到父母的影响。家庭的经济状况会影响到儿童青少年的营养状况,从而影响健康,父母的文化程度,尤其是母亲的文化程度对儿童的健康影响也很大。美国的研究表明,母亲的文化程度对婴儿死亡率的影响大于家庭经济状况的影响。来自非洲13个国家1975～1985年的资料表明:妇女的识字率增加10%,儿童的死亡率则下降10%。在25个发展中国家的调查表明:在其他条件相同时,即使母亲仅有1～3年受教育的文化程度,也能使儿童死亡率下降约15%。

(三)行为因素

与儿童青少年健康有关的行为因素包括体育锻炼、生活作息方式,也包括吸烟、酗酒等有害健康的行为。营养是生长发育的物质基础,运动是生长发育的源泉。在营养得到保证的情况下,通过积极、合理的体育锻炼可以促进机体的生长发育、提高免疫功能、增强体质。青少年时期是长身体也是长知识的时期,如果不能够合理地安排生活作息方式,保证足够的睡眠和户外活动时间,学习负担的加重就有可能影响到他们的健康。青少年是求知欲最强的人群,具有极大的好奇心和模仿欲,如果不加以正确的引导,一些有害健康的行为,如吸烟、酗酒,甚至吸毒将对他们的健康产生极大的危害。

三、儿童青少年的社区保健措施

(一)对学龄前期的儿童开展儿童保健系统管理

学龄前期儿童的社区保健主要是以社区为基础开展儿童保健系统管理,其内容如下:

1. 建立儿童保健系统管理的保健卡(册)。婴儿出生后即建立系统保健卡(册),做到一人一卡(册),并交由承担系统保健的机构管理。

2. 开展新生儿访视。婴儿出生并返家后,由妇幼保健人员到产妇家中随访,作好记录,填写系统保健卡(册)。在新生儿期要求访视 3~4 次,至少应访视 2 次(初访、满月访),对体弱儿应酌情增加随访次数,并专案管理。访视中,除了解和观察一般情况外,要进行全身检查,指导合理喂养和护理。

3. 定期健康体检。儿童在 1 岁以内每季度 1 次,1~2 岁每半年 1 次,3~6 岁每年 1 次,体检时填写保健卡(册、表)。有条件的地方可适当增加体检次数和项目。体弱儿应专案管理。

4. 定期计划免疫。按照儿童计划免疫,定期进行预防接种,按规定必须接种的 4 种疫苗是卡介苗、脊髓灰质炎活疫苗、麻疹活疫苗、百白破三联制剂,以预防结核病、脊髓灰质炎、麻疹、百日咳、白喉、破伤风等 6 种疾病。

5. 生长发育监测。为了及早发现生长缓慢现象,适时采取干预措施,保证儿童健康成长,要使用小儿生长发育监测图来进行生长发育监测。连续地测量小儿体重,绘出体重曲线,即可动态观察婴幼儿生长发育趋势。要求 1 岁以内测体重 5 次,1~2 岁内测 3 次,2~3 岁内测 2 次。

6. 体弱儿的管理。对发现和筛选出的体弱儿要进行专案管理。体弱儿是指低体重儿(出生体重小于 2 500 克),早产儿、弱智儿、佝偻病活动期,Ⅱ度以上营养不良,中度以上缺铁性贫血,反复感染,以及患先天性心脏病、先天畸形、遗传代谢病等疾病的儿童。对体弱儿要采取针对性措施,定期访视,指导家长正确护理喂养,注意保暖,防止感染等。要督促患儿就医,建立专案病历,制订治疗方案,定期复诊治疗。待恢复正常情况和疾病治愈后,转入健康儿童系统管理。

7. 健康教育。要采取多种形式,利用各种媒介大力宣传优生、新生儿护理、科学喂养、营养、疾病防治、健康行为等儿童保健知识和儿童优教知识,提高广大群众的保健意识,养成良好的卫生习惯,适时利用医疗保健服务,促进儿童健康成长。

(二)对学龄期的儿童开展学校健康教育

学校健康教育是指以学校为单位,以学生为对象,以促进学生健康为目标开展的有组织、有计划的教育活动。其目的是引导学生树立健康意识,养成良好的卫生行为和生活方式,使学生身心得以健康发展。学校健康教育不仅在学校开展,而且需要家长和学校所属社区内所有成员的参与。学校健康教育的对象包括学龄前儿童、中小学学生以及大学生。其中学龄儿童处于成长发育阶段,行为的可塑性很大,教师的一言一行对学生具有较强的权威性,比较容易养成健康的习惯和形成健康的生活方式,因此具有更重要的意义。

开展学龄儿童健康教育有多种途径。可以采用儿童喜闻乐见的方式通过学校健康教育课程系统传授适宜的医学科学知识及保健知识,培养学生正确的判断和评价能力,树立正确的健康信念；可以对学生进行健康行为指导，帮助学生把学到的卫生知识运用到日常生活中；开展学校健康服务，如学生生长发育监测，健康检查，牙齿检查，视力、听力检查，免疫接种和传染病管理，常见病预防和身体缺陷的纠正，突发性疾病的紧急服务，意外事故的应急措施，心理咨询以及为伤残学生提供必要的服务等。此外，还要营造有利于学生身心健康的学校环境，包括良好的学校人际关系、合理的教学制度及符合卫生标准的学校物质环境。

(三)对青少年开展青春期保健及心理咨询

青春期是儿童向成年人过渡的关键时期，因此，生理和心理保健相当重要。此期的保健工作包括以下几个方面。

1. 合理营养指导。青春期是身体各器官、系统发育较为快速的时期之一，因此需要较多的蛋白质即热量，所需的热量比成年人多20%～50%，细胞、激素、抗体及促进体内化学变化的酶等物质的形成都需要蛋白质的参与，另外，性腺的发育、神经兴奋能力的加强也都离不开蛋白质。因此，食物应该保证有足够的热量并富含蛋白质。

2. 心理卫生及健康行为的指导。这个时期，青少年逐步进入社会独立生活，容易受环境因素影响，因此有人称此时期为"危险时期"，故应该加强心理卫生和健康行为的指导，包括环境适应指导、重视性教育、杜绝不良嗜好等。

3. 培养良好的个人卫生习惯。包括合理地安排作息时间，积极、合理的体育锻炼等。女性还应注意经期卫生。

第二节　妇女社会医学

妇女是指15岁以上的女性人口，约占总人口的1/2。她们分布在每个家庭。做好这部分人群的保健工作，关系到人口的大多数，关系到每个家庭的幸福。

妇女一生中要经历青春期、孕产期、产褥期、哺乳期和更年期等一些特殊的生理时期，在这些时期，妇女全身各系统，特别是内分泌系统的变化较大，容易发生感染性、损伤性疾病，对环境中的危害因素也比较敏感。并且，妇女的健康影响人口的发展，健康的母亲才能孕育出健康的子女。因此，应该重视妇女的健康及保健工作。

一、妇女的身心特点及健康问题

(一)孕产期的身心特点及健康问题

妇女在不同的生理时期有不同的特点及健康问题，尤其是在孕产期，生理和心理都发生较大的改变，可能出现一些特殊的健康问题。妊娠期间由于胎儿发育的需要，母体发生一系列适应性生理变化，生殖系统、乳腺、心血管系统、血液、呼吸系统、泌尿系统、消化系统、皮肤、内分泌系统等，包括新陈代谢都可能发生变化。由于孕妇肾上腺皮质激素分泌增加，易有情绪波动、烦躁不安、焦虑、悲伤等反应。尤其是孕早期内分泌改变，可能引起胃肠功能紊乱、妊娠呕吐，导致上述心理变化加重，心理活动平衡失调。在此期间，由于全身器官负担加重，易发生各种妊娠并发症，也可能使孕妇原有的一些疾病复发或加重。分娩时易发生的问题包括产道的损伤、产后大出血及产后感染等。在产褥期，产妇既要进行自身的恢复,又要担负起哺育和照看新生儿的重任,会由于较重的生理和心理负担而出现健康问题,尤其是不能尽快适应角色的转变,极容易出现心理障碍,如发生产后抑郁症。

(二)更年期的身心特点及健康问题

更年期是妇女从生育功能旺盛走向衰退的过渡时期,是一个逐步变化的过程,一般可以分为绝经前期、绝经期以及绝经后期。由于卵巢内分泌减退是逐渐发展的,并有个体差异,一般绝经前期始于45岁左右,持续2~4年,即进入绝经期,绝经后期持续6~8年,卵巢分泌日益减少,以至达最低水平。故更年期的全过程为8~12年。

更年期的各种生理及解剖上的变化均与卵巢的功能衰退有关。由于卵巢分泌的性激素特别是雌激素减少,引起机体一些器官的功能发生改变。生殖道、乳房、泌尿道、皮肤与毛发等相继发生变化,月经周期紊乱,经量减少,甚至绝经。同时,由于内分泌平衡失调,导致下丘脑及植物神经系统功能紊乱,可引起血管舒缩功能障碍等,出现更年期综合征,骨质重吸收增加可引起骨质疏松。由于下丘脑及植物神经系统功能紊乱,还可能产生不同程度的心理反应,如焦虑、悲观、个性及行为改变等,甚至出现更年期抑郁症。

二、影响妇女健康的社会因素

(一)经济因素

经济因素主要通过影响妇女能够享受到的卫生保健、教育、食物营养等进而影响妇女的健康。据统计全世界每年大约有50万名孕产妇死亡,平均每天死亡约1 400名,其中99%的孕产妇死亡发生在发展中国家与不发达国家,这些国家的孕产妇死亡率平均高达$800/10^5 \sim 1\,000/10^5$,而在发达国家平均仅为$30/10^5$,在欧洲及北美的发达国家更低。联合国儿童基金会报道,1991年加拿大的孕产妇死亡率为$5/10^5$,美国为$10/10^5$,爱尔兰为$2/10^5$。2001年我国统计资料显示,北京、天津、上海等大城市孕产妇死亡率不到$20/10^5$,而云南、贵州、甘肃、青海等经济发展较为落后的省区,孕产妇死亡率在$100/10^5$左右。

(二)文化因素

我国经历了漫长的封建社会,一些封建道德观念如"三从四德"、"男尊女卑"等仍然影响着一部分人的思想观念,尤其是边远贫困的农村地区,这些封建道德观念影响妇女接受教育、参加社会活动、享受社会保障的权利,影响到妇女的身心健康。目前,在我国农村,妇女往往要承担农活、家务劳动和养育孩子三大重任,劳动时间长、强度大,但得到的营养物质在家庭成员中为最少。据世界银行1980年世界发展报告介绍,种种事实表明,在多数发展中国家,妇女得到的伙食占其所需要的比例比男子低。城市妇女也肩负着工作和家务劳动双重负担。有调查表明,女性的家务劳动时间明显长于男性。上述种种状况的形成与人们的道德观念、风俗习惯等有密切的联系。因此,必须提高妇女的地位包括政治地位、法律地位与经济地位,做到妇女与男人在政治、受教育机会、就业机会、社会价值认同等方面的平等,确认妇女在社会中的作用和妇女生育的特殊价值,才能使妇女的健康得到保证。

(三)妇女受教育程度

从世界范围来看,妇女受教育程度低于男性,全世界文盲男女之比为1:2。我国多年来一直关注妇女的地位及教育,但从2000年的人口普查资料来看,妇女的文盲率为13.47%,而男性仅为4.86%。受教育程度低有可能影响妇女的保健意识和享受保健的能力,从而影响她们的健康。2001年全国统计资料显示,孕产妇的死亡原因主要是产后出血,约占总死亡的55%。产后出血引起的死亡可以通过做好孕产妇的产前检查工作及产后访视,提高住院分娩率来预防和控制。我国一些地区的研究表明:妇女的文化程度越高,接受产前检查率也越高。

(四)行为因素

影响妇女健康的行为因素包括吸烟、酗酒、求医行为、性行为及生育行为等。吸烟对健康的危害早已证实,吸烟除了是肺癌等疾病的危险因素外,孕妇吸烟会造成婴儿出生体重减轻、宫内胎儿发育迟缓、孕期缩短、自发流产率增高、妊娠和产时并发症增多、围产儿死亡增高等。据世界卫生组织报告,在许多国家,男子吸烟有减少的趋势,而妇女吸烟却有增多的趋势。

不良的性行为可能导致性传播疾病的发生,不但影响妇女的健康,还可能通过母婴传播影响儿童的健康。不良的性行为还有可能通过破坏家庭结构和功能影响妇女的身心健康。不良的生育行为也会影响妇女的健康。普遍认为,母亲生育时太年轻、生育时年龄太大、怀孕间隔太密、怀孕次数太多等4种情况增加了妇女死亡的危险。因此,通过有计划的生育可以促进妇女的健康。我国推行计划生育以来,妇女生育年龄提高,生育数减少,大大减轻了妇女怀孕哺乳的负担,也减少了与妊娠、生育有关疾病的发生。

三、妇女社区卫生保健措施

(一)关注影响妇女健康的社会问题

要提高妇女的健康水平,需要全社会参与,关注影响妇女健康的各种社会问题,并采取相应的社会卫生措施加以解决。包括进一步提高妇女的社会经济地位,尤其是在我国的农村地区,更应对此加以关注,使女童与男童具有同样的受教育机会;给与妇女更多的生殖健康保健服务,在城市应该将此任务与社区卫生服务工作结合起来,在农村应该通过进一步完善原有的三级妇幼保健网,落实妇女生殖健康保健服务。

(二)重视妇女的健康问题,提供相应的保健服务

针对妇女健康状况和存在的卫生问题,提供相应的保健服务。服务的内容在不同的社区可以有所不同,但主要内容应包括以下几个方面。

1. 健康教育和健康咨询。采用多种形式向社区居民宣传妇女保健工作的重要性,使社区居民尤其是妇女本人了解妇女在不同时期的健康问题,掌握基本的预防保健方法,并及时解答她们所关心的问题。

2. 生殖健康保健。既包括性健康教育,普及优生优育知识,进行孕前、孕期教育等;也包括在知情选择的情况下提供适宜的避孕药物和避孕工具,提供适宜的人工流产技术和绝育与输卵管复通术,开展节育手术质量管理,开展手术并发症的防治和并发症病人的管理等。

3. 定期的健康体检。妇女健康体检主要包括常规妇科检查、宫颈涂片检查、白带检查、乳房检查及一些特殊检查等。

(三)加强孕产妇保健系统管理

孕产妇保健系统管理运行的程序为:孕妇怀孕3个月前检查一次;3个月后每4周检

查一次;7个月后每2周检查一次;9个月后每周检查一次。凡经确诊为怀孕的孕妇应填写孕产妇系统管理保健手册,定期到所属医院或社区保健机构进行产前检查。妊娠到36周后持保健手册到医院住院分娩,出院后母婴一同转入社区保健机构进行产后第3天、第7天、第14天、第28天、第42天随访检查登记,发现问题及时处理。如发现孕妇有高危因素时,按高危妊娠专案管理。

第三节 老年社会医学

联合国1956年出版的《人口老化及其经济意义与社会意义》一书中提出以65岁作为老年人的起点。1982年7月联合国在维也纳召开的"老龄化问题世界大会"提出以60岁及60岁以上为老年人的标准后,包括我国在内的许多国家都采纳了这一标准。其中60~69岁者为低龄老人,70~79岁者为中龄老人,80岁及以上者为高龄老人。联合国规定:一个国家和地区,年满60岁及以上的老年人数占总人口数的10%以上,或年满65岁及以上的老年人数占总人口数的7%以上,即可称为老年型社会。

1990年全国第四次人口普查显示,我国60岁及以上的老年人口为9 739万,是世界上老年人口数量最多的国家,占总人口的比例已达8.59%。2000年第五次全国人口普查,60岁及以上的老年人口已达12 997万,占总人口的比例为10.45%,我国已经进入老龄化社会。老龄化问题研究及老年保健问题必须加以重视。

一、老年人的身心特点及健康问题

(一)人口老化是必然的规律

人的生长发育在20~25岁达到成熟期,此时各种生理功能达到最高储备、活力及潜力状态。随年龄增加,30岁左右各系统、器官的形态结构和生理功能逐渐出现退行性变化,60~65岁老化速度加快。老化是一种正常的生命过程,具有以下4个特点:①普遍性,老化或迟或早都要发生,没有一个人可以幸免。②内源性,如同诞生、发育、死亡一样,老化是人体固有的、非外界的力量所能变更的一种过程,是机体内在的遗传等生物因素决定的。③进行性,老化具有渐进而不可逆转的性质,一旦出现和产生,便不能复原。④危害性,老化直接导致生理功能的下降,影响人的身心健康,并最终走向死亡。

(二)老年人的身心特点

随着机体的衰老,老年人在体表外形、器官功能、机体调节控制能力等方面都有所改变。体表外形的改变主要表现为须发转白、脱落稀疏,皮肤出现皱纹,牙齿松动脱落,关节活动不灵等。器官生理功能的下降主要表现为视力、听力、嗅觉、味觉减退,肺活量、胃酸分泌量、心肺排血量下降,免疫功能也会降低。随着机体调节控制能力降低,老年人的动作和学习速度减慢、操作能力和反应速度降低。由于社会接触相对减少,心理上会产生失落感、孤独感、被遗弃感等。

(三)老年人的健康问题

由于生理机能衰退、免疫功能降低,老年人发生疾病的概率增加,表现为老年人的患病率高于其他人群。据1996年全国卫生服务调查资料,老年人的两周患病率(250‰)和慢性病患病率(540‰)以及住院率(61‰)均远高于其他年龄的人群。并且,老年人的疾病主要以慢性非传染性疾病为主,许多老年人处于长期带病生存的状态,同时患有多种疾病的老年人也较多。国内资料统计,住院老年病人中,同时患有两种以上重要疾病者占85%左右,有三四种疾病者占50%左右。因此老年人的保健服务需求较大,但由于各种社会经济方面的因素导致他们实际得到服务的比例较小,老年保健服务不足的问题比较突出。

二、影响老年人健康的社会因素

(一)经济收入

我国1987年的抽样调查表明,老年人经济收入增长速度低于在职职工工资的增长速度,两者的差距还在扩大。老年人再就业是补助经济不足的重要方式,但在社会高速发展和科学技术不断进步的今天,老年人再就业的难度加大,再就业率很低。随着经济收入的减少,城市老人的家庭经济地位也随之下降。农村老人的经济收入无固定保障,主要来源于自己劳动和子女接济,经济收入低的问题更为突出。低收入严重影响老年人的营养、生活条件和医疗保健等。1995年6月,北京市老年学会调查发现,北京市城区仍有44.4%的老年人就医困难,其中近40%与经济因素有关。

(二)婚姻和家庭

人到老年,从社会转向家庭。家庭对老年人具有物质支持、精神安慰和生活照顾三大功能,成为影响老年人健康的重要因素。完整的家庭结构、和睦的家庭气氛、尊老爱幼的优良传统有利于老年人的身心健康。反之,则会严重损害老年人的健康。目前,家庭变化的趋势是由大家庭向小家庭发展,核心家庭及独居家庭逐渐增多。2000年我国人口普查,核心家庭占45.92%,独居家庭占8.30%,两者合计占50%以上。小家庭的增加虽然降低了家庭矛盾的发生,但有可能影响到对老年人的赡养和及时照料,尤其是精神赡养。

(三)社会交往

脱离工作岗位以后,老年人与同事及同所从事工作有关人员的联系骤减以至于中断,与朋友的交往也因行动不便而逐渐减少,与邻居、亲戚交往开始增多。原先的与他人进行利益交换、工作交流和事业探讨的需求退至其次,代之以主要为了交流、沟通感情,排遣心中的抑郁、不快或分享彼此的愉悦的"互相慰藉"的目的。这种交流与沟通,多在同龄人之间进行,"共同"点多者,相互交往也多。相对而言,文化程度高者,参加社会活动的能力较强,有较多的社会交往,日常生活丰富、充实,精神较为愉快。值得注意的是,城市老人的社会活动,社会交往圈较大,社交活动已扩展到了亲缘关系之外的情感性联系和地缘关系之外的功利性联系。其中,老年男性的非亲缘、非地缘关系的交往均多于女性。

(四)社会支持

世界上许多国家在解决老龄问题时都制定了相应的政策和对策,建立了管理老年人的机构和为老年人服务的组织,增加了老年人需要的商品以及医疗卫生保健设施。我国于1996年制定了《中华人民共和国老年人权益保障法》,1999年成立了全国老龄工作委员会,为发展我国的老龄事业奠定了基础。由于我国老年社会保障体系不完善,老年福利设施不足,加上传统文化习俗的影响,95.3%的老年人在遇到困难时由子女或配偶照料,2.3%向亲友求助,很少有人向社会求助。因此,应该充分发挥社区及社会力量的作用,使老年人获得必要的社会支持,包括医疗保健照顾与其他福利,以提高老年人的生活质量。

三、老年人社区卫生保健措施

(一)建立和健全老年社区保健网

我国的老年保健组织行政机构有:①老龄委员会。从中央到省、市、县、乡各级都建立了老龄工作办事机构;②民政部门。从国家民政部到省市级民政厅局、县级民政局、乡镇民政干事,组成了负责管理老年人福利事业的机构;③卫生部门。从国家卫生部医政司的老年卫生康复处到省、市、县卫生厅、局的医政处、科以及乡镇卫生院负责老年保健的专职人员。目前全国范围内还没有形成老年医疗保健网,但有的城市已设有老年病医院或综合医院老年病科。为了老年社区保健工作的开展,在城市应该切实将老年保健工作纳入社区卫生服务的工作范畴,在农村可在三级医疗保健网的基础上,将老年医疗保健工作纳入服务范围。

(二)开展老年人系统管理

在建立健全老年人健康档案的基础上,通过掌握社区老年人和社区资源的基本情况,对老年人开展系统管理。其内容包括以下几个方面。

1. 对社区内的老年人登记建册,建立个人健康档案。

2. 定期进行健康检查及生命质量评价,根据检查及评价结果,对老年人实行分级管理和提供服务。

(1) 社区老年医疗保健三级监护。将社区内的老年人,根据其生活自理能力、年龄、患病情况,逐个进行分析,划分为三种类型,分别进行医疗保健监护。

(2) 社区老年医疗保健的三段服务。对患病的老年人,根据疾病发展的过程,在各个阶段提供不同的服务。对急性病与慢性病复发的患者提供医疗服务;对疾病的恢复期、慢性病的迁延期和各种残疾患者提供康复服务;对预后不良的危重患者和老年多器官衰竭患者提供临终关怀服务。

(3) 参照国外资源利用分类系统(RUG),更细地将老年人划分为多个不同的组别,分别提供不同类型的服务。

(三)提供社会服务

1982年联合国召开的世界老年人会议的结论指出:"对老年人的照料不能只局限于疾病,而应包括整个老年幸福生活。要考虑物质、精神、社会、环境等因素相互依存的关系。"故老年社区保健不应只局限于提供医疗卫生服务,还应包括其他的社会服务如老年人的照料、赡养、婚姻介绍、娱乐等。

(四)建立社区非正式支持组织

社区非正式组织是指社区内的一些对老年人具有帮助和支持作用的群众组织,其名称和具体形式可多种多样,如退休科技人员协会、老年人协会、孤老包产组、老年人体育协会、老年人读书会等。非正式支持组织通过组织老年人开展有益身心健康的文体活动、互助互济活动等在老年社区保健工作中发挥着巨大作用。我国是发展中国家,卫生资源不足,国家财力有限,更应注意发挥非正式支持组织在社区老年保健中的作用。社区基层管理机构是社区老年保健工作的中坚力量。

Chapter 7 Social Medicine of Special Population

Special population refers to those population who have special physical and mental features, or are in the special circumstance, weak in protecting themselves, easily affected by all of the harmful factors and have a high prevalence. It mainly includes women, children, the old and the disabled. In recent years, they are called weak population. Their health problems have rooted extensively in society and they are those population social medicine must pay more attention to.

Section 1 Social Medicine of Children and Adolescent

Children generally refer to the 0 – 12-year-old population, which account to about 30 percent of the total population. According to the adolescent's definition given by WHO, 10 – 19 years are called juvenile, 20 – 24 years are called youth, and the population of this age period account about 25 percent of the total population. Children and adolescent have a great population, and it is this period that they keep on changing in shape, physique and mind. It is this period that they develop in the highest velocity in their lives and it is also the foundational period in basing the physical and mental health. So they are the population demanding special attention.

1. Physical and mental features and health problems in children and adolescent

(1) Children's physical and mental features and health problems

According to the different features in the different growing ages of children, children are divided into periods, namely infant period (birth to 1 year), nursling period (1 – 3 years), pre-school-age period (3 – 7 years), school-year period (above 7 years), in which children have different physical and mental developing features and health problems.

①Features and health problems in the infant period

Since the growth in infant period is the fastest than others, children have a special high demand on energy and protein, or malnutrition and drooping-growth will easily occur; they have taken much food, mainly milk food, and because of the incomplete growth in digesting and absorbing system, mal-digestion and nutrition disorder may easily occur; the immune function got from their mother dies down gradually and newly acquired one is still very weak. So children can easily get infectious diseases.

②Features and health problems in nursing period

Nursing period is just after ablactating. If parents fail to pay attention to the nutrition of food, malnutrition may easily occur. Meanwhile, nursling's neural system develops rapidly, manifesting obvious development in language and act and disobey when affiliating with adults. Because nursling cannot control their bowels, their activity ranges in expanding gradually and chances of accident happening and infection increasing.

③Features and health problems in pre-school-age period and school-year period

In the two periods, children grow comparatively slowly with steady speed, and after 6 years their milk teeth begin to loose and fall off and their permanent teeth begin to grow out. In pre-school-age period their neural system develops rapidly and language and act development becomes mature gradually. With the gradual maturation of immune system and digesting system, infectious diseases and alimentary canal diseases are declining and accidents and immune diseases are increasing. Children's circumstance changes greatly when they enter school and the contact with teachers and classmates and the formal learning process have great effect on their physical and mental development.

(2) Adolescent's physical and mental features and health problems

Adolescent are the population in puberty, which is a transition period from children to adults. Great changes have taken place in physique and mind of adolescent in this period. Physical features are ①the development of height, weight and circumference and so on speeding up. ②the development of each system and viscera speeding up and their function being strengthened. ③the reproductive system has developed maturely and the secondary sex characteristic occurs. In mind, puberty is a period of full independence and reliance, self-knowledge and babyhood and so on. During the earlier period of puberty, from 10 to 14 years, adolescent maintain some child psychological characteristics, manifesting childhood, and on the other hand adolescent have some adult psychological characteristics, such as their mental activities gradually becoming complete, having complicated and strong emotions and initially having ardour feelings on their opposite sex. During the late puberty, from 15 to 19 years, adolescent, who are experiencing transitions period from adolescent to adult, become more and more matured mentally. The common health problems in adolescent period include near-eyesight, accident and puberty psychological health problems etc. and the girls' abnormal menses also common.

2. Social factors affecting children and adolescent's health

(1) Economic factors

Economic factor is an important social factor affecting children and adolescent's health. In developed countries, the health status is superior to that of the developing countries. According to the data from WHO the global strategy of all people's health in 2000, the infant mortality in developed countries is only 19‰, while that in developing countries is 160‰. In our country, the statistics data of 2001 shows that the infant mortality and children (under 5 years) mortality in big cities, such as Beijng, Tianjin and Shanghai, are all under 10‰, whereas in the comparatively backward provinces such as Yunnan, Guizhou and Qinghai, the infant mortality is above 30‰ and the children (under 5 years) mortality is about 40‰. A survey carried out in 58 developing countries shows that under the same other conditions, when the income drops by 10%, the infant mortality will raise 2%- 3.5%.

(2) Family factors

Family, composed by marriage and consanguinity, is the basic social unit. And it is also the important environment of children and adolescent's growth and education. Parents are the first teacher of children, affecting children's personality, health habit, life style and diet habit more or ness. Family economic status will influence children's nutrition status and then their health, mother's educational level also having great effect on children's health. And according to an American study, the latter has greater effect than the former on the infant mortality. The data of 13 African countries, 1975 to 1985, shows that when women's literacy rate increases 10%, children's mortality will drop 10% correspondingly. And a survey in 25 other developing countries shows that under the same other conditions, even if mother has 1 - 3 years school education, the children's mortality will drop about 15%.

(3) Behavior factors

Behavior factors related to children and adolescent's health include physical exercise, life style and some behaviors harmful to health, such as smoking and drinking. Nutrition is the material basis of growth and exercise is the source of it. Only ensured nutrition and active and rational physical exercise can promote organism's growth, immune function and constitution. And adolescent period is the period both of growing body and of enlarging knowledge. If adolescents fail to arrange a rational work and rest scheme to guarantee adequate time for sleep and outdoor activities, their health may be affected with the increasing learning burden. Adolescent, a population with a strong desire to learn and great curiosity and imitating tendency, should be correctly guided, or they will be affected greatly by some harmful behaviors, such as smoking, drinking and drug addiction.

3. Community health care measures to children and adolescent

(1) Carry out health care system management to pre-school-age children

The pre-school-age children community health care carries out the health care system management based on community, its content including the following:

①To establish children health care system management card and to establish system health care card as soon as an infant is born, each card for one infant and then hand it to the system health care institute to manage.

②Carry out interview to newly born infant when the baby returns home. Maternal and child care staff will visit the lying-in woman, take notes and fill in the system health care card. During the newly born infant period, visits 3 or 4 times are necessary, at least twice (initial one and first month one). But to the weak infants, visit times should be increased and special files should be established to manage. During the visit, we should know and observe the common situation. In addition we should examine baby from head to foot and guide mother to rational raise and care.

③Regular health examination once per quarter of child under 1 year, once per half a year of child 1 to 2 years, once per year of child 3 to 6 years, and fill in the health care card during examination. In some districts, the examination times and items can be increased if possible. We should establish special files to weak children.

④Regular planning immunization according to the child. Planning immunization is essential to carry out vaccination regularly. The four vaccines that must be inoculated according to the regulation are BCG vaccine, poliomyelitis vaccine, measles vaccine and DPT to prevent six kinds of diseases, namely tuberculosis, poliomyelitis, measles, whooping-cough, diphtheria and lockjaw.

⑤Growth supervising. Use infant growth supervising chart to supervise growth to detect growth delay as soon as possible and take some intervening measures in time to ensure children to grow healthily. Constantly measure children weight and draw weight curve to display infant's grow trend. This should be done 5 times for children under 1 year, 3 times for those under 1 to 2 years and twice for those under 2 to 3 years.

⑥Weak children's management. Set special files to the weak children. The weak children refer to children who are with low weight (the born weight under 2,500 gram), premature, with mental defect, in active period of rickets, with malnutrition (above II degree), in intermediate level iron-deficiency anemia, infected repeatedly as well as who are suffering from congenital heart disease, congenital malformation and congenital metabolizing disease. Take pertinence measures to them, such as regular visit, to direct parents to raise their children correctly, to pay attention to keeping them warm, to prevent infection and so on. Urge the sick children to be hospitalized, and set special case files and treatment scheme to carry out regular consultation. When they restore, shift them to healthy children system to manage.

⑦Health dissemination. Adopt multi-form and make use of all kinds of media to disseminate child-care information and child-education information to promote people's care idea, form good health habits, enjoy medical service in time and promote child to grow in health.

(2) Develop school health education to school-age children

School health education refers to the organizing and scheming educational activities, which are based on the school unit, make student objects and aim at students' health promotion. It aims to direct students to set health awareness and form good health habit and life style and then to promote them to develop healthily both in mind and physique. School health education does not only need to be carried out in school, but requires the participation of parents and all members of the community, to which the school belongs. The object includes pre-school-age children, primary and intermediate school students and college students. And it is significant that teacher's words and behavior have authority on the school-age children and help them easily form healthy habits and life style, as they are in the developing age, with great behavior plasticity. There are kinds of approach to carry out school-age children's health education. In school health education, we can adopt methods which children like to impart medical and health-care information, cultivate their ability to judge and evaluate correctly and set correct health awareness; also we may lead them to health behaviors and help them apply the heath information, which they have learned, to daily life, carry out school health service, such as height supervising, health examining, dental examination, eyesight and hearing examination, immunity inoculation and infection managing, preventing common disease and rectifying physical defect, emergent service to the outbreak diseases, emergent measures to accidents, psychological consultation and essential service for the disabled students. Besides, good school circumstance must be formed, which benefits students' physical and mental health, including good social relationship in school, rational teaching system and material circumstance.

(3) Carry out puberty health care and psychological consultation to adolescent

Puberty is a critical period for children to become adults. Therefore, both physical and psychological cares are vital. Health care tasks include:

①Rational nutrition direction. All organs and systems are developing rapidly in puberty. Therefore, much more protein is needed, which can produce energy (the energy adolescent needs is more than that adult needs by 20%-50%), participate the formation of cells, hormone, antibody and enzyme, which promote the chemical reaction in organism, and play an irreplaceable role in the gonad development and strengthening the nerve's exciting ability. Therefore, adequate energy and protein should be ensured and contained in food.

②Psychological health and healthy behaviors direction. In this period, adolescents are gradually involved in society to live independently and easily influenced by surroundings. Therefore, this period is called Dangerous Period, and psychological health and healthy behaviors direction must be reinforced, which includes circumstance adaptation direction, emphasis on sex education, good hobbies, etc.

③Cultivating good individual health habits. This includes rational work and rest scheme, active and rational physical exercise, girls' attention to menstrual health, etc.

Section 2 Social Medicine of Women

Women refer to female over 15 years old, which account for half in the total population and exist in every family. It will benefit most of the people to provide enough health care to this group, which also plays a quite important role to the health and welfare of each family.

During their lives, women will experience some special physical periods such as adolescence, pregnancy and delivery period, puerperium, lactation period and climacteric. In these periods women's various systems, especially the endocrine system, will change greatly and become easy to get infectious and traumatic diseases, and sensitive to the environmental risk factors. Furthermore, women's health is relevant to the development of population and only healthy mother can gestate healthy baby. Therefore, women's health problems and health care should be paid more attentions to.

1. **Women's physical and mental characteristics and health problems**

(1) Physical and mental characteristics and health problems in pregnancy and delivery period

Women have various characteristics and health problems in different physical periods. Especially in pregnancy and delivery period, great physical and mental changes take place and result in some special health problems. In gestation, a series of adaptive physical changes take place as a result of the demands for fetus development, such as changes in reproductive system, galactophore, cardiovascular system, blood system, respiration system, digestive system, endocrine system, and so on. Even metabolism is likely to change. Due to the increase of cortin in body, the pregnant are easy to be emotion waving, .dysphoria, anxiety and sadness. Especially in the early stage of pregnancy, the changes in endocrine system possibly lead to dysfunction in digestive system. The vomit will aggravate these mental changes and break the mental balance. During this period, all the organs bear a heavier burden than before and the pregnant are easy to get various complications, their primary diseases relapse or they are aggravated. The common problems while delivering include birth canal trauma, postpartum hemorrhage and postpartum infection, etc. In puerperium, mother takes on the important task to feed and take care of the newborn, at the same time to recover herself. So health problems tend to appear due to the heavy physical and mental burdens, especially when she can't adapt the role transition as soon as possible. It's much easier to get mental obstacle, such as postpartum depression.

(2) Physical and mental characteristics and health problems in climacteric

Climacteric is the interim in which women's bearing function changes from strong to weak. It's a stepwise changing process and can be generally divided into three phases, which are pre-climacteric, climacteric and post-climacteric. As the endocrine function of ovary becomes weak step by step and this process is different between individuals, pre-climacteric starts at 45 commonly and lasts for 2 – 4 years, then climacteric starts and post-climacteric lasts for 6 – 8 years. The secretion of ovary decreases day by day till to the lowest level and the whole climacteric will last for 8 – 12 years.

All the physical and anatomic changes in climacteric are relevant to the functional weakening of ovary. Some organs function changes as a result of the decreasing secretion of sex hormone, especially the decrease of estrogen. Birth canal, breast, urinary tract, skin and hair change one after another, menstrual disorder, then decrease of climacteric. At the same time, the endocrine dyscrasia leads to hypothalamus and vegetative nerve functional disorders, thus brings vasomotor disorders as well as climacteric syndrome. The increase of bone absorption can cause rarefaction of bone. Due to the hypothalamus and vegetative nerve functional disturbance, women will have mental responses in different degrees such as dysphoria, sadness, characteristic and behavior changes, even climacteric depression.

2. Social factors that influence women's health

(1) Economic factors

Economic factors influence women's health mainly through influencing the health care, education, food nutrition, etc. whom women can access to. Based on the statistics, about 500,000 pregnant and maternal women died every year and the average number is 1,400 women per day, among whom 99% are in developing and underdeveloped countries. The MMR in these countries is high at (800 – 1,000)/100,000 while only 30/100,000 averagely in developed countries, and even lower in those developed countries in Europe and North America. According to the UNICEF reports, in 1991, the MMR is 5/100,000 in Canada, 10/100,000 in USA, 2/100,000 in Ireland. In 2001, Chinese statistics data showed that the MMR was less than 20/100,000 in such big cities as Beijing, Tianjin and Shanghai. However in those underdeveloped provinces in term of economy such as Yunnan, Guizhou, Gansu and Qinghai, the MMR was about 100/10,000.

(2) Culture factors

China has undergone the lengthy feudal society. Some feudal morality concepts, such as treatment of females as inferior to males, etc., still affect some people. Especially in some remote and poor countries, these feudal morality concepts influence women's right to get education, join social activities, and access to the social guarantee, thus influence women's physical and mental health. In present rural areas in China, women sometimes bear three hard jobs, namely farm work, housework and feeding the children. The work takes a long time and with great intensity. However, they get least nutrition among all the family members. Based on the World Development Report from World Bank in 1980, in most developing countries the proportion of food women get was lower than that of man. Women living in city also bear two burdens, namely work and housework. According to a relative survey, women's housework time is obviously longer than men's. The formation of these situations is closely related to people's morality concepts and customs. Therefore women's status, including political status, job status and economic status, should be improved. Try to make women and men equal in getting political and educational opportunity, opportunity of obtaining employment and the acknowledgement of social value. Thus women's health situation can be guaranteed.

(3) Women's educational background

Women's educational backgrounds are poorer than men's, and the number of illiterate women is twice as large as that of illiterate men in the world. Recent years women's status and education have been paid much attention to in China. However, according to the national census data in 2000, woman illiteracy rate was 13.47%, while male illiteracy rate was only 4.86%. The poor educational background is likely to influence women's health care awareness and the ability to access health care, thus influence their health situation. That national statistic data showed in 2001 that in China the prior cause for maternal mortality was postpartum hemorrhage, which accounted for 55% of all the causes. Death caused by postpartum hemorrhage can be prevented and controlled by improving prenatal check-up and postpartum visiting, and increasing hospital delivery rate. Investigations conducted in some areas showed that the more education women received the more likely women would seek for prenatal check-up.

(4) Behavior factors

The behavior factors that influence women's health include smoking, drinking, behaviors of seeking doctors, sexual behaviors and reproductive behaviors, etc. The harm done to health by smoking has been proved for a long time. Smoking is not only the risk factor of many diseases such as lung cancer, but also will lead to the reduction of birth weight, intrauterine bradygenesis, the pregnant period shortening, the increase of spontaneous abortion, the increase of the pregnancy and delivery related complications, and the increase of perinatal ortality, and so on, if the pregnant smokes. According to the WHO report, in many countries the number of men smoking tends to reduce while that of women smoking tends to increase.

Bad sexual behavior possibly leads to STD, which does harm not only to women's health but also to children's health through vertical transmitting. Bad sexual behavior also possibly influences women's physical and mental health by destroying the structure and function of the family. Bad reproductive behavior can influence women's health, too. It is acceptable that these four kinds of situations will increase the probability for women's death, namely mother delivers baby too young or too late, the interval between pregnancies is too short or deliver so many babies. Therefore, family planning can improve women's health. Since the policy of family planning was carried out, the women's child-bearing age has been delayed and the birth rate has been reduced, women have been greatly relieved from the burden of pregnancy and suckling the baby, and the prevalence rate of the pregnancy related and delivery related diseases has also been reduced.

3. Community health measures for women

(1) Care the social problems influencing women's health

It needs the whole social participation to care all kinds of social problems influencing women's health and take social health measures to improve women's health. In order to improve the social status of women, esp. in rural areas, special attention should be paid to them to make girls and boys have equal educational opportunity; to provide more reproductive health service, in urban areas, this mission should be combined with social health service; in rural areas, the women's reproductive health service should be realized through further perfecting the original three-class MCH net.

(2) Focus on women's health problems and provide corresponding health care

Aim at the health status and existed health problems to provide corresponding health care. The service content is different in different communities, but the main content includes:

①Health education and consultation aims to disseminate the importance of women's health to the community residents, to make them, esp. women know the health problems in different periods and master the basic health care methods, and to reply the questions they care much.

②Reproductive health includes sexual health education, popularizing the knowledge of prepotency and good fosterage, carrying out the pre-gestational and gestational period education, etc. It also includes providing suitable prophylactic and contraceptive under the consent selection, providing suitable induced abortion technique and sterilization surgery and fallopian tube re-dredge, carrying out the quality management of birth control surgery, the treatment of surgery complication and the management of the complicated patients.

③Regular health examination mainly includes regular gynecological exam, cervical smear, leukorrhea exam and breast exam and other special exams.

(3) Emphasize the systematic management of gravidas and puerperants

The program of the systematic management of gravidas and puerperants refers to the program that during the first three months gravida should examine once and once per four weeks after that, and seven months later once per two weeks and nine months later once per week. The gravida should fill in the systematic management of gravidas and puerperants health handbook as soon as the pregnancy confirmed, and go to hospital or community health care facilities to receive pre-birth exam. After 36 weeks, the gravida should go to hospital to deliver her baby with health handbook. When discharged, mother and baby should go to the community health institute to carry out postpartum 3, 7, 14, 28, 42 day follow-up registry and settle the problems in time. If the high risk factors are detected, a special file of higher risk pregnancy should be set up.

Section 3 Social Medicine of the Aged

The book, *Aging Population and Its Economic and Social Significance*, published by UN in 1956, brought forward that 65 years should be the starting point of the aged. After the criterion of the aged that 60 years and above 60 years should be defined as the aged, in the world conference about aging problem held by UN in Vienna, many countries, including China, have adopted it. According to the regulation of UN, a society with people, 60 years and above, whose population accounts for more than 10% of the total, or people, 65 years and above, whose population accounts for more than 7% of the total, can be called aged society.

The fourth national census in 1990 showed that the aged population in our country, 60 years and above, was 97.39 million, and then our country had the largest aged population all over the world, which accounted for 8.59% of her total population. And according to the fifth national census in 2000, the aged population, 60 years and above, was approaching to about 129.97 million, 10.45% of the total, which symbolized our country's entering aged society. Therefore, more attention must be paid to aging problem and care for the aged.

1. The mental and physical characteristics and health problems of the aged

(1) Aging is an inevitable rule

The mature period of human is about 20 to 25 years, in which all kinds of physical functions reach to a climax in storage, vigor and potential state. With age increasing, the shapes and function of all systems and organs begin to degenerate at about 30 years, and accelerate to become aging at about 60 years. Aging is a natural process of life, which has 4 features: ①universality, which means aging will happen sooner or later, and no one is exception. ②internality, which means that aging is just the same as birth, growth and death to human, a connatural process, changed only by the internal bio-factors, such as heredity, not the external ones. ③ongoing, which means once aging emerges, it can never be restored, for its gradual irreversibility. ④danger, which means aging leads to the physical function's decline directly, then impacts physical and mental health, at last results in death.

(2) The physical and mental features of the aged

With the organism's caducity, the aged will change much in outlook, organ function and adjusting ability of the organism. In outlook, changes will take place, such as beard and hair whitening and falling, skin wrinkling, teeth shaking and falling, joints' inactivity. Organ functions decline mainly in eyesight, hearing, smell and taste, vital capacity and gastric juice secretion, heart-lung blood ejection, and immune function. With decline in adjusting ability of the organism, the movement and learning speed of the aged slow down and so do the operating ability and responding speed. And they will feel losing, lonely and being abandoned in psychology for lack of social contact.

(3) Health problems of the aged

Because of the decline in physical and immune function, the probability of disease of the aged increases, resulting in the the fact that disease prevalence of the aged is higher than that of other groups. According to survey data of national health service in 1996, the fortnight prevalence (250‰), chronic disease prevalence (540‰) and inpatient rate (61‰) of the aged, were all higher than those of other age groups. Furthermore, the aged are mainly suffering from chronic diseases and many of them are in a state with a long-term disease. At the same time many old people are suffering from multi-diseases as well. A home statistical data shows that the population of the aged who are inpatients suffered from two kinds of diseases or more accounted about to 85% of the total, and who suffered from four or five kinds of diseases was about 50%. Therefore the health demand of the aged is great, but the low rate of health service the aged actually received, for the factors of all aspects in society and economy, distinguishes the problem of deficient health service of the aged.

2. The social factors influence the aged's health

(1) Economic income

According to the national sampling survey in 1987, the increasing speed of the aged's income is lower than that of people on work, and the gap keeps on widening. Re-employment of the aged, the important measure to settle the economic shortage problem, can hardly be developed in today's society, with the rapid development of scientific technology. Therefore, the rate of reemployment keeps low. With the decreasing income, the economic status of urban old people in family drops, too. The low economic income problem of old people in rural areas is much sharper, for their income mainly comes from their own work and help from their family, instead of fixed guarantee. It is the low income that influences old people's nutrition, living condition, medical care and so on. According to a survey conducted by The Aged Institute of Beijing, in June,

1995, in Beijing urban areas, there are still 44.4% of the old people who found difficult to hospitalize, among which about 40% is related to economic factors.

(2) Marriage and family

When man is old, they will return to family from society. For the aged, family has three major functions, material support, mental comfort and life care. Therefore, it has become an important factor to their health. It will do good to old people's physical and mental health to possess a family with complete structure, harmonious atmosphere, good tradition of respecting the old and caring the young, or it will do great harm to health. Nowadays, the trend of family to change from big to small and nuclear families increases gradually. The national census in 2000 shows nuclear families account for 45.92%, single families account for 8.30%, adding up to over 50%. Although the increase of small families lows down the chance to family contradictions, it may impact the support and care, esp. mental care to the old.

(3) Social communication

After retirement, the contact between old people and their colleagues, or others related to work, is decreasing till entirely cutting-off, and they begin to communicate with their neighbors and relatives instead of their friends for their inconvenient movement. The previous requirement to exchange benefit with others, to communicate in work and to discuss for enterprise, is replaced by purpose of mutual comfort to communicate, to release depression and unpleasant feelings, or to share pleasure between each other. This kind of communication always conducts among their peers, who have much agreement in common and mutual communication. Comparatively, people who have higher education have a better social ability and more social communication, so they have a rich daily life, and feel pleasant in mind. A point deserving attention is that the urban old have a larger social communication circle, which is beyond the relatives' emotional relations and locational relations to beneficial relations. And the old male have more nonrelative and nonlocational relations than the old female.

(4) Social support

Many countries have established corresponding policy and countermeasures to settle aging problems, such as having set institutes and organizations to manage and serve for old people, increasing commodity and medical establishment for them. In 1996, our country established the *Guarantee Law of the Rights and Interests of the Aged of PRC*; in 1999, established National Aged Committee to set the foundation of the aged affairs. Because of the faultness of the social guarantee system of our country, insufficiency of the establishment for the old and influence of the traditional culture, about 95.3% of the old, when in difficulty, are attended by their offspring or spouses, and about 2.3% resort to relatives, and few resort to the society. Therefore, in order to make the aged gain necessary social support and improve their life quality, we should make full use of the community and society power, including medical care and other welfare.

3. Health care measures for the aged in community

(1) Establish and complete the healthy care net for the aged in community

The administering institutes for the aged health care in our country include: ① Aged Committee. All levels of agencies for the aged work were established from central government to province, city, county and township. ②Civil Administration Deptment. Including all levels of civil administration bureaus, from central government to province, city and county, and township civil. Administration staffs are in charge of the welfare of the aged. ③Health Department. From health restoring section of the medical department of central health dept. the medical sections of health offices and bureaus of province, city and county, to people in the township hospitals, are special in charge of the healthy care of the old. Although medical care net for the old has not formed throughout the country, in some cities, there are agedness disease hospitals and agedness disease sections in general hospitals. In order to carry out health care for the aged in community, we should bring the health care for the aged into community health service in urban areas, while in rural areas, we should bring the health care for the aged into health service based on the three classes of health care net.

(2) Manage the old systematically

Carry out the systematical management of agedness based on the establishing and perfecting of the health files of the aged, through the basic situation of agedness and resources in community. The contents include:

①Register the aged in community and set individual health file.

②Conduct regular health examination and quality of life, then classify the old to manage and provide corresponding service, according to the results.

A. Three classes medical care to the aged in community. Classify the aged into three types and to take corresponding care, according to their independent ability in life, age, illness state and so on.

B. Three periods service of the medical care to the aged in community. Provide different service to the sick aged, in different periods of disease; provide medical service to people suffering from both acute disease and recrudescent chronic one; provide restoring service to people who are in the restorement of disease, deferment of chronic disease and disabled; provide terminal care service to people who are in serious disease and aging multi-organ exhaustion.

C. We can also consult the foreign classification system (RUG), to classify the old into a sub-sectional types and then provide different service.

(3) Provide social service

In the world agedness conference held by UN, 1982, the conclusion pose that "the attention to the aged is not only lied in illness, but also must include the entire happy life of them. And the mutual relations between material, mental, social and environmental factors must be considered." Therefore, the community health care for the aged should not lied in health service, either, and other social services should be involved, such as attention, support, marriage introduction and entertainment for the aged.

4. Establish nonofficial support organization in community

Community nonofficial organization refers to some mass roots organizations to help and support the aged, and their names and practical forms may be various, such as the retired technical panel association, the aged association, lonely old group, physical association of the aged and reading association of the aged. Nonofficial support organizations play an important role in the community health care for the aged, through organizing them to join in all kinds of cultural and physical activities, which are good to their body and mind, and mutual help activities. Since our country is a developing country, with insufficiency in health resource and tight national finance, we should pay more attention to the nonofficial support organizations' function in the community health care of the aged. The basic management institutes of community are the nucleus force in the health care of the aged.

第三篇　社会卫生诊断

Part 3　Social Health Diagnosis

第八章 社会医学研究方法

第一节 社会医学研究原理

一、社会医学研究的目的

社会医学研究的主要目的是获得可靠的信息,用这些信息来解释、预测和理解我们打算研究的现象,同时根据这些信息来改造我们的环境。

社会医学研究要回答"为什么"的问题。例如,农村居民比城市居民看病次数少,有人解释成"农村人比城里人身体好"。也许外行听了不会说什么,但是社会科学家不能满足于这个解释,除非这个解释能够说明"为什么"。社会科学家在解释某种现象或者人类行为的时候,都要对一些可能造成这一现象或者行为发生的因素进行系统的、经验性的分析。

社会医学研究有的时候还要进行一些预测,而进行正确的预测,往往是所有科学分支领域最为重要的能力。没有足够的知识和信息,就无法进行预测。例如,如果我们了解到政府将实施对贫困地区转移支付的政策,我们就能够预测到将来农村居民看病的次数可能会有所增加。

社会医学研究的第三个内容是建立理解。理解这个词有截然相反的两种含义,一种是移情的理解,即允许社会科学家在进行研究的时候,对他们的研究对象注入情感;另一种是预测的理解,即要求社会科学家在社会环境中获得足够客观的知识,就如同他们研究自然现象一样。

二、社会科学方法论的作用

社会科学具有一套清晰的规则和程序,社会科学研究就是按照这套规则和程序进行的,也是按照这套规则和程序进行评价的,这些规则和程序就是方法论。不过这些规则并非僵化和一成不变的,相反,方法论在不断地完善,科学家也在不断地寻找新的研究方法,对社会现象和人类行为进行观察、推论、综合和分析。这些规则和程序是在研究中为所有研究人员所共通,它们用于三个目的:交流、推理和主体间一致性。

方法论的第一个用途是在科学家之间进行交流和沟通,以便他们能够共享某种经验。另外,通过把这些规则和程序搞得更加清晰、公开和方便,人们就可以重复这些研究,或者对这些研究进行评估。重复自己的或者他人的研究,能够消除一些偶然发生的错误,更能够避免欺骗性的研究结果得以哗众取宠。评估别人的研究,就是当某一个研究成果出现的时候,其他社会科学家都能够提出诸如"观察方法是否正确"、"使用的是什么研究方法"以及"检验是否有效"和"有没有什么别的因素干扰了结论"等问题。

社会科学方法论需要逻辑推理和分析。我们将分别讨论制定定义、分类、演绎和归纳推理的规则,概率理论,抽样程序以及测量的规则。

主体间一致性指的是研究所获得的知识和信息,以及所使用的科学研究方法是可以传递和共享的。所以,一位研究人员进行过调查和研究,另外一位研究人员就可以重复这项研究,并把其结果与之进行比较。如果方法学正确,研究情景没有变化的话,我们就可以预见,两者的研究结果应该是相似的。事实上,研究的情景往往会发生变化,所以就不断地会有新发现。不论如何,主体间一致性使得社会科学家能够理解和评价他人所使用的方法,开展类似研究,从而证实经验事实。

三、社会科学研究的一般步骤

科学知识应当是可以通过推理或者经验观察证实的知识,所以科学家往往运用逻辑有效性和经验可证实性作为评价一种新知识的标准。科学家通过研究的一般步骤,把这两个标准转化为研究活动。我们可以把研究过程看成是科学家产出研究成果的过程。

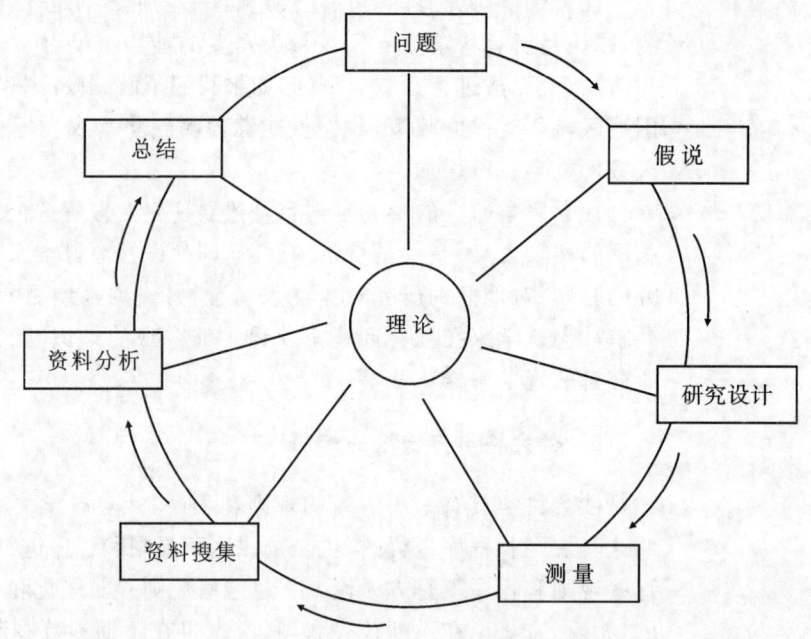

图 8-1 研究的主要步骤

如图 8-1 所示,研究过程包括七个主要步骤:问题的提出、假设的形成、研究设计、测量、资料搜集、资料分析和总结。每个步骤都会影响到理论的构架,而理论本身也会影响到每个研究步骤。本章将重点讨论其中几个步骤。

这七个步骤最主要的特征,是这些步骤本身的循环特征。一般来说,这些步骤从问题开始,至获得一个暂时性的经验总结结束。但是,这个暂时性的经验总结,仅仅是上一个循环的结束,它还预示着另外一个循环的开始。例如,一项研究结束的时候,往往留下更多的问题需要进一步的研究,所以这种循环往复的过程就是科学知识不断积累和认识不断深化的过程。

这个研究过程本身也是在不断地修正的,一个暂时性的经验总结往往需要通过逻辑推理和经验证实两项检验,如果这个暂时性的结论不能成立,研究者就会提出新的问题,研究进入新的一轮解决问题的过程。在这个新的过程中,每个步骤都要重新审视,因为上一个结论不能成立可能并非假设或者理论本身发生了错误,而可能是在解决问题的操作化过程中出现了误差。例如,有人作出了经济危机会导致政府增加投资的研究结论,如果这个结论不能通过逻辑检验和经验证实,这个结论显然是无法成立的。即使这个结论本身是正确的,但如果研究过程当中某个步骤出现了问题,也会导致这个结论无法成立,如样本缺乏代表性、测量误差或者数据分析过程有问题。

事实上,我们在图中所表示的研究过程是比较理想化的,在现实研究当中,可能出现如下几种情况:

(1) 研究进程有时候比较快,有时候比较慢;
(2) 有的研究设计严谨,有的研究相对不那么正式;
(3) 有时候很多研究人员介入,但通常是一个研究者完成所有研究工作;
(4) 有时候依靠研究者的想像,有时候依靠经验事实。

四、概念、定义、理论和模型

科学知识是需要经过逻辑和经验证实的,这意味着社会科学研究人员必须把两个层面——概念理论层面和经验观察层面的东西连接起来。社会科学研究就是这两个层面之间相互作用的结果。

(一) 概念

语言由一系列符号以及组合这些符号的规则构成。概念则是语言中最为重要的符号,在研究当中更是如此,科学研究就是从构架概念以便描述经验世界的行动开始的。所谓概念,就是对某些客观物体和现象的抽象表述。如"社会经济地位"、"贫困"和"信仰"都是社会医学当中常用的概念。

在社会医学研究当中,概念起四个方面的作用:作为交流的基础、介绍一种观点(即观察客观事物的方式)、作为分类和归纳的手段、构成理论的元素。

概念可以作为交流的基础。如果没有共同的概念,人们之间的相互交流就不可能实现。概念从物质的感官印象当中抽象出来,用于传递各种认同和信息。

概念用于介绍一种观点。通过形成科学的概念,我们所认识的感官世界才能充满秩序和联系,否则我们就无法正确认识我们周围的世界。

概念是分类和归纳的手段。科学家把他们的经验和观察用概念加以分类、组织和概括。例如,我们可以忽略桌子、椅子、床、柜子和沙发之间的区别,而把它们笼统地归纳为"家具"。"家具"是一个总体的概念,它让我们能够更好地理解丰富多彩的世界,把一些杂乱无章的事物在我们的头脑中加以归纳,赋予它们以规则。"家具"抽象出了桌子、椅子、床、柜子和沙发的共同特征,在概念抽象的过程中,这些家具失去了它们的特性。这个抽象和归纳的过程给科学家提供了描述现实世界的方便手段。但是,概念一旦形成,就很难再作为它所代表的对象的完美表述,因为抽象使得其本身的内容被抽掉了,只留下了科学家所认为重要的特征。

概念还能够作为理论的元素,从而用于解释和预测事物的发生。在任何理论当中概念都是至关重要的成分,因为概念构成了理论的雏形和内容。例如,"生活方式"这个概念构成了慢性病病因学理论的核心内容。

(二)定义

概念的作用是交流、感知、综合以及理论构建,所以概念必须是清楚的、准确的和为大家所认同的。我们日常生活当中所使用的语言往往是模糊的、模棱两可的、不准确的。所有学科都有自己的用语,社会医学也不例外。社会医学家根据社会科学的理论,建立了一系列定义,用于描述客观事物的特征。定义一般分为两种类型:一种是概念定义,一种是操作定义。

1. 概念定义。概念定义指的是用其他的概念来定义现有的概念。例如,"生活方式"可以用其他概念定义为"一群人所采取的集体行为",而"集体的"、"行为"又可以被其他概念所定义。如此下去,到最后总归会有一些概念无法找到其他概念来定义它们,这些概念就被称为原始概念。概念定义具有以下共同特征:

(1)必须说明它所定义的事物的共同特征;

(2)不能循环定义;

(3)定义的表述必须是肯定的而不是否定的;

(4)必须使用清晰的词语来下定义。

2. 操作定义。有一些概念所表述的事物和特征无法直接进行观察,在这种情况下,就需要制定操作定义。所谓操作定义,指的是采用一些办法和过程,根据概念,详细地描述一种现实现象的情形及其程度。操作定义多数情况下就是一系列实施的过程,通过这些过程,一个理论性的定义在现实当中被具体化了。如果概念形成过程是一个抽象的过程,那么操作化的过程正好与其相反。概念的操作化是理论转化为经验事实的桥梁,通过概念的操作化过程,人们知道应该采用什么规则、如何观察一个现象。

(三)一致性问题和理论的引入

从理论层面到操作层面的转换过程中有两个问题值得注意。一个问题是理论概念和操作定义之间的一致性,例如,"生活方式"如果被概念定义为"一群人所采取的集体行为",在操作化过程中,采用一个包含有关吸烟、饮酒、体育锻炼的问卷来测量这种集体性的行为,那么在这两个定义之间,一致性的程度如何?我们必须采用真实性(效度)测量的方法来衡量它们之间的一致程度。另一个问题是,有的时候如果不把概念放在一个理论框架内,就难以把概念恰当地进行操作化。科学概念能不能测量是一回事,是否符合一种理论假设则是另外一回事。也就是说,有一些概念必须在某种理论的支撑下才有意义,否则这种概念即使能够测量,也难以最终解释其测量结果。所以,概念操作化赋予概念以实际意义,而与理论相联系则赋予概念以理论意义。没有理论,概念就没有灵魂。正如我们在图 8-1 中所表述的那样,理论不仅用于总结问题、形成假设,还是关键概念的意义所在。

(四) 理论

对于不同的人,理论的意义不一样。有人认为理论就是经验现象的推理和抽象,另一些人则认为理论是哲学思想,还有一些人给理论下了一个比较狭义的定义:由一系列相互联系的概念经过逻辑推论形成的结论。由这个理论,可以产生一些能用于检验的命题。

理论没有一致的定义,社会科学家对其仁者见仁、智者见智。理论的定义之所以多种多样,主要是因为理论的种类本身多种多样,用于不同的目的。为了介绍方便,我们把理论划分成为三个层次:微观理论、中观理论和宏观理论。

微观理论是由一些经验事实归纳分类,简单地形成的。例如,病人满意度问卷中有一个问题"病人对医院提供的门诊服务是否满意"。我们可以把病人对这个问题的回答分为四种:很满意、满意、不满意和很不满意,这种分类就构成了一个微观理论。

中观理论包含着一系列的归纳分类,以及这些分类之间的相互关系,这些分类和关系可以用来解释和描述经验现象。这些分类之间也是相互联系的。

宏观理论包含着很多命题,这些命题之间以某种方式发生相互作用,一些命题产生自另外一些命题。一个宏观的理论能够对一个事物或者现象提供完满的解释。宏观理论的用途很广泛,不局限于某一个事物。

一般来说,宏观理论包括:①一系列概念和定义;②一系列以理论为基础的现象描述;③一些相互关系的陈述;④表述概念之间相互关系的逻辑推理。

(五) 模型

模型与理论的概念非常接近,也是一种系统化的概念组织。我们可以把一个模型看做为某种事物或者现象的近似。模型当中包括的是符号,而不是符号所代表的物质本身,所以模型当中包括的是某些经验现象的特征,包括这些现象的组成部分和各部分之间的关系,这些关系用概念之间的逻辑关系相联系。因此,模型的比较恰切的定义就是一种现实的抽象,其目的是把我们对现实世界的看法简单化、条理化,同时还能够让模型代表事物本身那些研究所必需的特征。

五、理论、模型和经验研究

社会科学建立在两个基础之上:理论和经验研究。研究者穿梭于两个世界——观察和经验的世界,以及思想、理论和模型的世界之间。在这两个世界之间建立一种系统化的联系,是社会科学研究的目的。那么,我们怎么才能建立这种联系呢?我们是应该先建立理论模型,然后再去观察经验世界,还是应该先去观察经验世界,而后建立理论呢?

1. 理论先于研究。这种研究一般采取四个步骤:①建立一个清晰的理论模型;②选择一个命题,进行经验研究;③设计一个研究项目检验这个命题;④如果来自理论的这个命题被经验数据所否定,修改理论或者研究项目,重复步骤②。

2. 研究先于理论。与理论先于研究截然相反,这种研究采取下面四个步骤:①调查某一个现象,详细描绘其特征;②测量其特征在不同情况下的变化;③分析研究的数据,从中发现变化的规律;④一旦发现系统性的规律,就可以建构理论。理论可以是我们讨论过的任何一种类型,如果能够建构宏观理论,则是最理想的。

六、研究的基本组成部分

在社会医学研究中,不管研究者采用的手法是先理论后研究、还是先研究后理论,有关研究问题、联系、假说的概念都会常常出现。这些概念就是研究的基本组成部分,有了它们,研究者才能把理论和设想付诸研究实践和操作化。

(一)研究问题

有时会问:"为什么农村人看病次数少?"或者问:"社会经济地位是否会影响卫生服务?"这些问题都可以转化为科学研究的问题。

不过,并非所有灵感都能够通过经验研究。有些问题无法具体化为一个实际问题,还有一些问题带有浓重的主观倾向、看法和价值观,也无法转化为实际问题。例如,"上帝是否存在"这类问题到现在也没有得到证实,而且永远得不到证实。

研究问题,除了必须能够经过实践检验之外,还需要表述得很清晰。例如,"人们节约能源的动机是什么"就太笼统太模糊,不同的人可能就会产生不同的理解。它既没有清晰地表明动机的类型(如经济学的、社会学的还是爱国主义的),也没有指明能源的来源(如石油、汽油、煤炭、天然气等),还没有能够区分清楚这种节约是家庭中的节省还是工业上的节约。缺乏清晰性和特异性,会使得研究结果混沌不清,无法应对别人的评价。

(二)变量

研究问题会转化成一系列概念,而这些概念是从经验事物或现象中抽象出来的。为了能够把这些抽象的概念转化为经验层次,以便测量,研究者一般把概念转换为变量。研究假设当中的概念就是用变量来表述的。

在把概念转化为变量前,要清晰描绘概念所代表的事物,然后给这个变量赋值。一般一个变量可以有若干个值,如性别可以有两个值:1=男,2=女。反过来我们也可以认为,如果一种事物可以被赋值、被分类的话,它就可以被看做一个变量。例如,"社会阶层"就是一个变量,因为至少可以把它分成五个类别:较低、中低、中等、中高和较高。当一个变量取值有两个的时候,我们称之为二分变量。为了研究方便,流行病学和统计专家区分了自变量、因变量和控制变量,还把变量分为连续和离散两类。这些内容请参阅流行病学和统计学书籍。

(三)联系

研究中的联系,往往指的是两个或者多个变量之间的关系。当我们说变量 X 与变量 Y 相关的时候,指的是这两个变量之间有着某种共性。通过研究建立一种相关关系的过程,指的是观察一个变量取值的变化如何导致其他变量的变化。

联系具备两个属性,它们是在经验研究中需要得到重视的。一个是联系的方向,另一个是联系的强度。联系的方向指的是两个变量之间的关系是正向的还是负向的;联系的强度指的是关联系数从 0 到 1 之间的取值大小。

(四)假说

假说以自变量和因变量之间关系的表述的面貌出现,是研究问题的暂时答案。之所以是暂时的,是因为它需要经过经验研究的证实。在提出研究假说的时候,研究者并不知道这个假说是否能够得到证实。提出假说之后,还要建构假说,随后对其进行检验,如果这个假说被否定了,就会提出另外一个假说;如果这个假说被证实了,它就能够成为科学知识的一部分。

假说的来源有以下几种:从理论当中演绎、从观察当中获得、来自直觉,或者来自以上方式的结合。不过,假说从何而来并不那么重要,重要的是如何接受或者拒绝这些假说。

研究假说有四个共同的特征:清晰、价值中立、特异,以及可以使用现成的科学研究方法在实践中得以证实。下面我们分别详述这些特征:

(1) 清晰。为了在实践中检验这些假说,研究者必须明确给假说当中的任何概念下定义,把它们转化为操作化的变量。在建构假说、定义变量的过程中,最好的办法就是查阅专业文献,请教该领域的专家。操作化的定义必须是特异的、准确的,不然的话就无法观察和进行重复观察。

(2) 价值中立。原则上,研究者在研究当中必须抛弃本人的价值、偏向和主观偏好。研究者一定要知道自己可能产生的价值是什么,这样才能彻底抛弃它们。

(3) 特异。研究者一定要指出研究变量之间的关系是什么,包括其方向和大小。

(4) 可以用现有方法进行检验。往往有一些研究假说很清晰,也是价值中立的,而且非常特异,但是找不到合适的方法来测量它们,这些假说也不能够最终成为研究假说。

第二节　调查研究的设计和结构

调查设计是指导研究者在收集、分析资料和解释观察结果的过程中总体的规划,是在调查的变量中进行因果关系推断的逻辑模型。调查设计要以普遍性为主,也就是说,得到的调查结果能被用来推断一个大的总体或者不同环境下的情况。

一、相关设计

相关设计通常也叫做横断面调查,是社会科学中占主导地位的一种研究设计方法。这种设计通常以调查研究为特征,是许多社会学领域常常用到的数据收集方法。调查研究通常包括向一个随机样本询问关于个人情况的一组问题,如生活背景、个人经历和态度。大多数情况下,调查研究可提供那些调查对象有关属性以及表达的数据资料;尽管众多的研究关注于调查对象属性以及表达之间的因果关系,其他的一个重要部分则是在这二者之间建立因果推断之前对它们之间的关系模式进行简单的描述。

相关分析的数据通常通过交叉表格和双变量百分比分析的方法进行分析。统计分析中的多变量方法在相关分析中是最常用的对照实验和推导因果关系的方法,如详尽的交叉表格和多元回归分析等。

但是要注意,在相关分析中不能通过统计分析建立变量之间的时间顺序。这种时间顺序只有通过研究者在有关理论指导下,结合具体情况并使用随机概率抽样的研究方法来获得。这样就能通过统计结果扩展到总体,并进而推及真实的生活情况,增加研究的外部效度。

二、测量方法

（一）抽样

抽样确保了一个有代表性的样本。在社会医学研究中，我们通常采用两种抽样方法：以现代抽样理论为基础的概率抽样和非概率抽样。概率抽样最显著的特征是可以确定包含抽样个体样本总体的每一个抽样个体的概率。在非概率抽样中，没有办法确定在样本中每个个体包含的概率，就不能保证每一个个体都有同等的机会被抽到。如果一批个体没有机会被选入样本，就意味着总体的精确度受到限制，也就是说，如果这批个体的特征是不可知的，那么总体的精确性也不可知。

一个好的抽样设计可以确保从所给总体中重复抽取大量不同样本时，结果与总体参数之间的差异不会大于一个特定的量。概率抽样设计可以估计抽样结果与对整个总体研究发现的结果之间的差异程度。在概率抽样设计中，样本统计量与总体参数的估计是紧密相连的。

虽然总体参数的精确度只有通过概率抽样的方法来计算，社会学家们使用非概率抽样的主要原因还是出于方便和经济。在许多特定的情况（比如探索研究）下使用非概率抽样要比使用概率抽样有更多的优点。非概率抽样也常用于一个抽样总体无法被精确定义时，再就是不能获得某一部分抽样总体时。

（二）非概率抽样

社会学家常常使用三种主要的非概率抽样方法：方便抽样、目的性抽样和定额抽样。

1. 方便抽样。就是研究者选择容易获得的抽样个体作为研究对象，比如，一个大学教授可以选择班里的学生作为研究对象，一个研究者可以选取在街上遇见的前200名愿意被采访的人作为研究对象。但是，方便抽样无法估计其代表性的好坏，也无法估计总体参数。

2. 目的性抽样。在目的性抽样（有时也叫做判断抽样）中，抽样个体被试图得到对总体代表性较好样本的研究者主观地选中。特定的抽样个体被选择的机会取决于研究者的主观判断。因为我们不清楚研究者是如何对他们选择的每一个抽样个体的代表性进行主观判断的，所以也不可能计算任一个特定的个体被抽中的概率。

3. 定额抽样。定额抽样的主要目的是选择一个与抽样总体尽可能相似的样本。比如，假使知道总体中男女人数是相等的，研究者就可以选择一个男女数量相同的样本。在定额抽样的访谈设计中，就是用性别、年龄和居住地之类的变量来具体指定定额分组的。

（三）概率抽样

这里给出四种常用的概率抽样方法：单纯随机抽样、系统抽样、分层抽样和整群抽样。

1. 单纯随机抽样。这是最基本的概率抽样方法。它给总体中 N 个抽样个体平等的、可知的非零概率的被选择的机会，所以它允许总体中的每个抽样个体有同等可知的概率被选入样本。

2. 系统抽样。在第一部分抽样个体从 K 个抽样单位中被随机选择出来后，再选择每个 K 抽样个体组成样本。例如，一个人想从10 000个人的总体中选取100人作为一个样本，他可以选择每一个100人的个体（$K=N/n=10\,000/100=100$），初次选择通过随机程序来决定,比如用随机数字表。假定第 14 个人被抽中,那么样本就由号码为 14,114, 214,314 依次类推的个体组成。

3. 分层抽样。它主要用于确保总体中不同组别平等的出现在样本中,以保证总体参数估计的精确度增加。而且,其他的特征是对等的,所以分层抽样大大地降低了运作成本。分层抽样的根本思想是:根据一个整体的总体信息来进行分组时,可以使各小组内的基本要素都尽量接近于总体,如果一系列的小组被这种方法抽到,当样本组合起来时,将组成一个更加异质的总体,就会产生更好的精度。对总体分层的必要前提是划分标准与所研究变量相关。第二点需要考虑的是划分标准不需要分太多的次级样本,那样会比简单随机抽样增加更大的样本量。

4. 整群抽样。它经常用于大规模的研究,因为它是最经济的抽样方法。整群抽样,首先划分成大的组,然后从组群中抽取样本个体,组群用简单随机抽样或者分层抽样来选取。组群中的所有抽样个体可以都包含在样本中,也可以用单纯随机抽样和分层抽样来从组群里选择一部分,这取决于所研究的问题。

我们介绍的这四种概率抽样方法并没有阐述详尽概率抽样方法的范围,建议参考另外的读本。然而,它们是在社会医学研究者中广泛应用的最基本的方法。

第三节 数据收集方法

社会医学中的数据是从正式或非正式渠道获得的,包括语言的(口头的和笔录的)和非语言的行为和反应。数据收集的这两种渠道和两类形式结合后产生了以下四种主要的数据收集方法:观察法、调查(个人访谈和调查问卷)、二手资料分析和定性研究。从方法学上可以大体分为定量方法和定性方法两种。

每种数据收集方法都有其各自的优点和局限性。研究结果在一定程度上受数据收集方法的影响。为将影响减至最少,研究者可以应用两种甚至两种以上数据收集方法来进行检验假设和测量变量。用不同数据收集方法得到相同的结果会增加研究结果的可信性。

在本节中,我们将以访谈调查为例介绍定量访谈调查与定性访谈调查的区别。然后通过说明如何开展问卷调查和个人采访(包括个人深入访谈和专题小组访谈)来介绍这两种方法。

一、定性方法与定量方法的区别

定性方法是一种灵活有效的方法,可以用来拓展许多新的研究领域。定性研究方法可以使临床医生日常工作中调查研究一些相关的问题,而其他方法难以解决。未经专业的训练,研究者很难从事一项新的研究技术,而访谈技巧的训练可以在一些大学和专业的研究机构里面获得。

定性研究与定量研究针对的问题不同。例如,在婴儿猝死综合征研究中使用的定量流行病学方法可以测量在国家和地区间发生率变异的统计学关联。定性方法研究可以通过采访不同社会经济阶层的新生儿的母亲,了解这些儿童养成的习惯,来发现引起某些地区婴儿猝死综合征的低发生率的原因。

定性研究调查者要尽可能在所使用的语言和观念上与被调查者很好地交流和理解，要尽量使议程灵活。他们致力于深入所调查问题中，对被调查者所谈话题尽可能详细地探索，揭示在研究开始时未预料的新的领域或想法。重要的是，采访者要确保能够理解回答者的意思而不是自己的猜测，以免发生明显的误解。

定性研究的调查者的目的是发现被采访者自己的意见，研究的任务就是尽可能地避免研究者的主观意见和假设。

访谈中结构化的程度越低，访谈前就有越少的问题被决定和标准化。大多数定性调查会有一系列涉及研究部分的核心问题。定性调查不像定量调查那样以高度结构化的调查问卷为基础，其问题的顺序将随着深入了解被调查者的某问题而发生变化。措辞也不能标准化，因为设计附加问题时调查者将会尽量使用个性化的词汇。同样，在定性研究过程中，采访者可以在他（她）对这个主题更加熟悉之后提出进一步的问题。

所有的定性调查都要考虑到被采访者以及访谈中观察到的阶级、种族、性别和社会差距等特征的影响。如果被采访者知道采访者也是医生，那么问题会更加严重。已经是病人或极可能成为病人的被采访者可能会为了取悦医生而给出他（她）认为医生想要得到的回答。为了达到研究目的，最好不要采访自己的病人，如果无法避免，应告诉他们说出其真实想法，而且如果所说内容医生认为不正确也不能修改（如抗生素适于治疗病毒性感染）。

采访过程中被采访者也很可能向采访者提问题。可能出现的问题是，回答这些问题时，临床研究者就可能把他们自己的观点强加于此次调查而使以前的努力白费。如果问题不被回答，就可能减弱被采访者回答后面问题的积极性。一个解决的方法是告诉他（她）采访结束时再回答这些问题，尽管这种回答也不是始终令人满意。

1. 研究员作为研究工具

定性访谈要求访谈者有很多技巧。有经验的医生可能认为已经具备了必要的技巧，的确许多技巧是相通的。为了完成从临床的问诊向研究性访谈的转换，临床研究者需要审查自己的访谈技术，批评性地审查他们自己所做的采访录音，并征求他人的意见。研究访谈的初学者应当清楚别人是怎样指导他（她）的，是否问了主要的问题，是否注意了或忽视了有关的线索，是否给了被采访者足够的时间以解释他们自己的意思。Whyte 设计了一个六点的趋势性量表来帮助初学者分析他们的访谈技术（表 8-1）。这并不是指没有趋向就是最好的，而是趋向的数量应适宜。一些回答者比其他人说得详细，控制访谈过程即显得非常重要。Patton 提供了控制访谈的三个策略：知道访谈的目的，正确地询问问题以得到需要的答案，恰当地给予口头的和非口头的回应。

表 8-1　Whyte's 访谈技术分析量表

1. 适当的鼓励性表示
2. 注意被访谈者的反应
3. 探究被访谈者的最终的意见
4. 探究被访谈者最终意见前的想法
5. 探究访谈初表达的观点
6. 引导新的话题（1＝最小的一级，6＝最大的一级）

表 8-2 保持对访谈的控制

1. 知道你想要发现的是什么
2. 询问恰当的问题以得到你要的信息
3. 给予适当的口头和非口头的回应

访谈者的一些共同的缺陷已经被 Field 和 Morse 证实，如外部的干扰、注意力不集中、怯场、尴尬的提问、主题的跳跃和诱导被访谈者（表 8-3）。意识到这些问题可以帮助访谈者发展一些克服的方法。

表 8-3 访谈的共同的缺陷

1. 外界干扰（如电话等）
2. 注意力不集中（如儿童等）
3. 访谈者或被访者的怯场
4. 向访谈对象问一些令人为难或尴尬的问题
5. 主题的跳跃
6. 教育（如向访谈对象提出医学建议）
7. 劝告（如过早地总结回答）
8. 提出自己的观点，从而使访谈产生潜在的偏倚
9. 访谈肤浅
10. 涉及隐私（如自杀威胁）
11. 翻译者的水平（如错误的翻译）

2. 确定访谈对象

抽样方法是由研究方案的目的决定的。定性研究通常不具有统计学代表性。同样，样本量不是由严格固定的标准所决定的，而是由其他因素决定，例如访谈的深度、持续的时间以及每个采访者的可行性。大规模的定性研究一般不超过 50～60 人，但也有例外。尽管对临床医生来说在他们自己的工作领域搞研究并不是问题，但是社会学家在设置医学研究时通常需要非常仔细的磋商。然而，研究者仍要接近可能的研究对象，解释研究目的，强调如果拒绝访谈并不会影响将来的治疗。还应有介绍信，说明访谈内容，访谈可能持续的时间和机密性的保证。采访也要考虑访谈对象的方便，对于那些白天工作的最好晚上去采访他们。访谈地点影响满意度，通常最好是在家里进行。

二、定量方法：调查问卷

（一）调查问卷的结构

问题是调查问卷的基础。调查问卷必须将研究目的转化为明确的问题；回答这些问题可以为我们的假设检验提供资料。问题必须能激发回答者，只有这样才能获得必要的信息。调查问卷的问题必须按照这两点来设置。明确叙述这些问题主要应考虑的是其内容、结构、形式和顺序。

调查的问题应该与事实、观点、态度、回答者的动机以及对某问题的认识水平有关。然而，绝大多数问题可分为两大类：①事实性的问题；②有关评价和态度的问题。

1. 事实性问题

设计事实性问题是为了引出回答者的客观信息，如与他们的背景、环境、习惯、爱好等有关的信息。事实性问题最常见的类型是背景问题，主要用于提供对回答者进行分类的信息，例如性别、年龄、婚姻状况、教育、收入等。相应的，这种分类可帮助解释行为和态度的差别。

通常认为这些类型的问题比其他类型的问题更容易设计。然而，即使是事实性问题也会给研究者带来困难。例如，在住房调查中，很多被调查者提供的卧室数比实际的要少，只是因为他们认为书房、娱乐室、客厅不是问题中所指的卧室。这个例子就说明了调查者与被调查者之间涉及的观点有可能不同。因此，需要明确定义概念以避免这种情况。

2. 有关评价的问题

"态度"的概念是指一个人对某种特定主题的倾向、偏见、想法、担心和确信的总和。另一方面，评价是态度的口头表达。

面对某种刺激时，态度能够以某种方式对其产生作用或反作用。只有当态度的对象被感觉到时，个体的态度才以言语或行为的方式表达出来。一个人可能强烈地赞同或反对某事，但只有在他们遇上与自身关系利害的事情时，这种态度才会被激发和表达出来。态度可以用内容（关于什么的态度）、趋向（对某物或某事的积极的、中立的或消极的感觉）以及强度（较强或较弱）来描述。

总的来说，我们对态度的测量很感兴趣，因为态度能说明被采访者总的倾向。评价性研究很重要，因为评价是态度的表达。询问评价和态度测量的主要区别是评价主要是通过估计同意某态度陈述的人在测量人群中的比例来测量的。态度量表是由 5~24，甚至更多的态度陈述组成，对每一个态度，回答者回答是否同意，然后测量态度。态度量表的一个本质要求是态度陈述要量化，即用某种技术将这些陈述从大量态度陈述中选出然后组合起来。

准确获取诸如某人婚否这类的信息要相对简单。对于回答者的评价和态度问题有时不容易获得。而且，考虑到很多态度都有不同的方面，回答者可能同意一方面而反对另一方面。这就是为什么态度不能用一个问题来测量的原因。用几种态度陈述可以减少片面反映的影响。

最后，回答评价和态度问题比事实性问题更容易受文字、侧重点和顺序等的影响。这将在某种意义上影响许多态度的多个方面。

三、定性方法：主要知情者的深入访谈和专题小组讨论

（一）主要知情者的深入访谈

（二）专题小组讨论（FGD）

专题小组讨论获得定性信息，而非定量信息。FGD 要获得的是每个人的态度、观点和感觉，并不是为了得到多数人的一致同意。

每个专题小组包括 6~12 个非随机选择的成员和一个主持人来引导整个交谈过程。

FGD通常包括三个重要步骤:计划、实施和分析。

1. 计划

(1) 确定研究目的。第一步是确定你要更透彻理解的问题。然后列一张你要在会上探讨的主要问题的清单。

(2) 选择12个人的样本。超过12个人的专题小组将难以控制。样本不需要随即选择,但应该是成年人,男女都有,熟悉卫生服务系统,并且愿意也能够对问题进行深入讨论。每个人将得到一个小礼物作为激励。

(3) 指定主持人。一个得力的主持人对专题小组是非常重要的。主持人必须具备良好的社交技巧,了解人的心理,对所讨论主题很有经验和丰富知识,并能够微妙的控制引导整个讨论。还要准备一个提纲以引导主持人按一般问题到特殊问题的顺序提问。

(4) 选择适宜的地点。选择的地点应有随便的和放松的氛围(如宾馆会议室或社区活动中心)。而不应当是像卫生局之类的官方的地方。应向每位成员提供点心。

(5) 发邀请函并给予提示。应提前邀请参与者,并得到明确回复。访谈前一天,应有人与他们联系并确定时间地点。

2. 实施

(1) 自我介绍,解释这个小组的情况,成员是如何选择的以及这次会议的目的。

(2) 询问成员的名字及相关情况,使他们感到轻松和舒适。

(3) 先询问一般性问题,然后向主题靠拢,最后是专业的问题。采取开放式的方法。如果感兴趣的部分肤浅了还可以再深入探讨。

(4) 展开讨论。不要让一两个人占据了大部分讨论时间。主持人的一个重要作用就是确保每个人有发言的机会。主持人应当使每一个成员都有表达他们感情的机会。有时某些人控制谈话太多,导致了只有他们的想法而其他人只是附和。这时主持人必须使他们安静下来,听一下其他人的想法,以防止产生潜在的结果偏倚。

3. 分析

详细笔录。如果可能的话可以录音。安排一个助手来做,这样主持人可以集中所有注意力以保证会议顺利进行。

会议结束后尽快转录。记下与主要观点有关的频率、相似点和趋势。总结出与访谈目的有关的主要问题,例如:①大多数人满意得到的卫生服务标准;②大多数人抱怨卫生服务的花费;③有些人说他们不能区分公家的和私人的提供者。

结论:FGD是一种用于收集深入观点、感觉和态度的有用工具。可以作为调查问卷所得的定量资料的补充。

Chapter 8 Research Methods in Social Medicine

Section 1 Principle Foundations of Research

1. Aims of social medical research

The ultimate goal of social medical research is to produce and accumulate a body of reliable knowledge. Such knowledge would enable *explanation*, *prediction*, and *understanding* of empirical phenomena of interest. In addition, a reliable body of knowledge can be used to improve the health conditions of all people.

Social medical research aims to provide a general explanation of "Why". For example, rural people visit doctors less frequently than urban people. "Because", some may respond, "rural people are healthier than urban people". Such an explanation might satisfy the layperson, but it would not satisfy social scientists unless they could employ the same reasoning to explain why rural people are less educated than urban people. When scientists ask for an explanation for why a given event or behavior has taken place, they ask for a systematic and empirical analysis of the antecedent factors that are responsible for the occurrence of the event or behavior.

Social medical research aims to provide prediction. The ability to make correct predictions is regarded as the foremost quality of science. If knowledge is deficient, prediction is impossible. If one knows the government will transfer payments to poor rural areas, one can predict that rural people may visit their doctors more often than before.

The third component of social medical knowledge is a sense of understanding. The meaning of the term understanding is used in two radically different aspects, empathetic understanding, which allows scientists to put themselves in the place of the subject of inquiry, and predictive understanding, which allows scientists to take a position from which they can attain objective knowledge in the study of the natural as well as the social world.

2. The role of social scientific methodology

Scientific methodology is a system with explicits rules and procedures on which research is based, and for which claims for knowledge are evaluated; this system is neither closed nor infallible. Rather, the rules and procedures are constantly being improved.

Scientists look for new means of observation, inference, generalization, and analysis. These rules are developed for communication, reasoning and inter-disciplines.

A major function of methodology is to facilitate communication between scientists who either share or want to share a common experience. Furthermore, by making the rules of methodology explicit, public, and accessible, the framework for replication and constructive criticism is set forth. Replication, the repetition of which is the same investigation in exactly the same way either by the same scientist or other scientists, is a safeguard against unintentional error or deception. Constructive criticism implies that as soon as one makes claims for knowledge, we can ask questions: "Are the observations correct?" "What are the methods of observation?" "Is the test valid?" "Do other factors interfere in drawing the conclusions?" "Should the findings be taken as evidence that can be used to prove another explanation is correct?"

The scientific methodology requires competence in logical reasoning and analysis. Rules for definition, classification, and form of deductive and probabilistic (inductive) inferences; theories of probability; sampling procedures; systems of calculus; and rules of measurement will be discussed later.

Inter-disciplines means that the knowledge in general or the scientific methodology in particular has to be transmissible. Thus if one scientist conducts an investigation, another scientist can replicate it and compare the two sets of findings. If the methodology is correct and the conditions have not changed, we would expect the findings to be similar. Indeed, conditions might change and new circumstances emerge. But the significance of inter-disciplines is that one scientist can understand and evaluate the methods of others and conduct similar observations so as to verify empirical facts. The methodological requirement for inter-disciplines is the evidence that empirical observations are uncontaminated by any factors common to all observers.

3. The research process of social science

Scientific knowledge is knowledge provable by both reason and experience (observation). Logical validity and empirical verification are the criteria employed by scientists to evaluate claims for knowledge. These two criteria are translated into the research activities of scientists through the research process. The research process can be viewed as the overall scheme of scientific activities in which scientists engage in order to produce knowledge; it is the paradigm of scientific inquiry.

As illustrated in Figure 8-1, the research process consists of seven main stages: *problem*, *hypothesis*, *research design*, *measurement*, *data collection*, *data analysis*, and *generalization*. Each stage affects theory and is affected as well. In this chapter, we will discuss extensively these several stages.

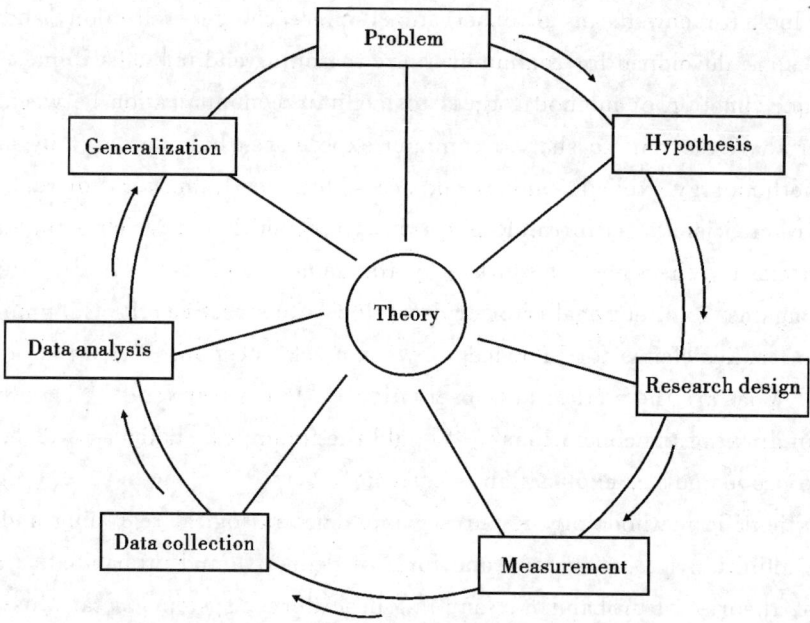

Figure 8-1   the main stages of the research procedure

The most characteristic feature of the research process is its cyclic nature. It usually starts with a problem and ends in a tentative empirical generalization. The generalization ending one cycle is the beginning of the next cycle. This cyclic process continues indefinitely, reflecting the process of the scientific discipline.

The research process is also self-correcting. Tentative generalizations to research problems are tested logically and empirically. If these generalizations are rejected, new ones are formulated and tested. In the process of reformulation, all the research operations are re-evaluated because the rejection of a tentative generalization might be due not to its invalidity but to errors in the research operations. For example, a generalization that economic crises lead to increased government expenditure will be rejected if it cannot be logically validated and empirically verified. But the generalization might also be rejected, even if it is true if procedures for validation and verification (for example, research design, measurement, or data analysis) are deficient. To minimize the risk of rejecting true generalization, one re-examining each of the stages in the research process should be prior to the formulation of new generalizations.

Finally, we should be aware that the research process as presented here is somewhat idealized, that is, it is a rational reconstruction of scientific practice.

In practice, the research process occurs: ①sometimes quickly, sometimes slowly; ②sometimes with a very high degree of formalization and vigor, sometimes quite informally, unconsciously, and intuitively; ③sometimes through the interaction of several scientists in distinct roles, sometimes through the efforts of a single scientist; ④sometimes only in the scientist's imagination, sometimes in actual fact.

Thus our idealized reconstruction of the research process is not intended to be rigid but rather to convey the underlying themes of social science research.

4. Concept, definition, theory and model

Scientific knowledge is provable by both reason and experience. This implies that social scientists operate at two distinct but interrelated levels, conceptual-theoretical and observational-empirical. Social science research is the outcome of the interaction between these two levels.

(1) Concept

Our language is a system of communication composed of symbols and a set of rules permitting various combinations of these symbols. Concept is the most significant symbol in language, especially as it relates to research. Science begins by forming concepts to describe the empirical world. A concept is an abstraction expression of an object, a property of an object, or a certain phenomenon. For example, "socio-economic status", "poverty", "norm", and "belief" are common concepts in social medicine.

Concept serves four main functions in social medicine research: concepts are the foundation of communication; concepts introduce a perspective, a way of looking at empirical phenomena; concepts are means for classification and generalization; concepts serve as components of theories and thus of explanations and predictions.

Concepts are the foundation of communication. Without a set of agreed-upon concepts, intersubjective communication is impossible. Concepts are abstracted from sense impressions and are used to convey and transmit perceptions and information.

Concepts introduce a perspective. Through scientific conceptualization, the perceptual world is given an order and coherence that could not be perceived before conceptualization.

Concepts are means for classification and generalization. Scientists categorize, structure, order, and generalize their experiences and observations in terms of concepts. For example, we can find the ways in which desks, chairs, beds, cupboards and settees differ from each other and grasp their generic resemblance via the concept "furniture". "Furniture" is the general concept that enables us to grasp a multiplicity of unique aspects and comprehend them within an order. "Furniture" is also an abstract concept in the sense that the unique attributes of desks, chairs, beds, cupboards and settees are lost in the conceptualization process. This process of abstraction and generalization enables scientists to delineate the essential attributes of empirical phenomena. However, once a concept is formed, it cannot be a perfect symbol of what it represents because its content is briefly reduced to the attributes that the scientist considers essential.

Concepts serve as components of theories and thus of explanations and predictions.

Concepts are the most critical elements in any theory because they define its shape and content. For example, the concept "lifestyle" defines the shape and content of theories of the causes of chronic diseases.

(2) Definition

If concepts are to serve the functions of communications, sensitization of experience, generalization, and theory construction, they have to be clear, precise and agreed-upon. The problem with everyday language is that it is often vague, ambiguous, and imprecise. Any scientific discipline is necessarily concerned with its vocabulary. Social medicine researches, based on the rule of social science, have attempted to establish a clear and precise body of concepts to characterize their subject matter. Two types of definitions are important: conceptual and operational.

①Conceptual definition

Definitions that describe concepts by using other concepts are conceptual definitions. For example, "lifestyle" has been conceptually defined as a selection of life behaviors, adopted by a collective population. And "behaviors", "collective" can be defined by still other concepts, and so on. At a certain point in this process, one encounters concepts that cannot be further defined. These are called primitive terms.

Conceptual definitions that enhance communication share the following essential attributes:

A definition must point out the unique attributes or qualities of whatever is defined.

A definition should not be circular.

A definition should be stated positively.

A definition should use clear terms.

②Operational definition

Often the empirical attributes or events which are represented by concepts cannot be observed directlfy. In this case, an operational definition is needed.

An operational definition is a set of procedures that describe the activities to perform, to establish empirically the existence or degree of existence of a phenomenon described by a concept. Operational definitions lay out the measuring procedures that provide criteria of the empirical application of concepts. Thus operational definitions are bridges between the conceptual-theoretical and empirical-observational levels. They tell what to do and what to observe in order to bring the phenomenon defined within the range of the researcher's experience.

(3) Congruence problem and theoretical import

Two important issues arise with the transition from the conceptual level to the empirical-observational level. The first is the degree of congruence between conceptual definitions and operational definitions. If "lifestyle" is defined conceptually as "a selection of life behaviors adopted by a collective of population" and operationally by a questionnaire which includes smoking, drinking, physical exercise, what is the degree of congruence between the two definitions? The degree of congruence can be evaluated with the aid of valid tests.

The second issue involved arises when concepts cannot be defined operationally, if not appropriately put into a theoretical framework. Scientific concepts should not be evaluated only in terms of their operability but also in terms of their theoretical import; that is, some concepts gain meaning only in the context of the theory in which they are introduced.

Concepts gain empirical meaning from operational definitions and gain theoretical meanings within the context of the theory within which they are employed. Theory plays a vital and central role in the research process, as indicated in Figure 8.1. It is not only an important source for the generation of problems and hypotheses, but the meaning and significance of key concepts are interpreted in the context of a theory.

(4) Theory

Theory means different things to different people. Somebody would identify theory with any kind of conceptualization, while others equate theory with the "history of ideas", and still others view theory in a narrow sense: a logical-deductive system consists of a set of interrelated concepts from which testable propositions can be deductively derived.

There is none simple definition of theory on which all social scientists would agree. This is because there are many different theories, serving different purposes. Generally, there are three levels of theory: micro-level theory, medium level theory and systematic theory.

Micro-level theory consists of arbitrary categories constructed to organize and summarize empirical observations. For example, the classification of individual patients' response to the questionnaire item "All patients are satisfied with the outpatient service which the hospital provided" into the four categories "Strongly Agree", "Agree", "Disagree" and "Strongly Disagree" constitutes an ad hoc classification.

Medium level theory consists of a system of categories constructed to fit the empirical observations so that relationships among categories can be described. Often the categories are interdependent.

Systematic theory consists of a system of propositions that are interrelated in a way that permits some to be derived from others. A theoretical system is one that provides a structure for a complete explanation of empirical phenomena; its scope is not limited to a particular aspect.

Usually one systematic theory should include: A set of concepts and definitions; A set of statements describing the situations in which the theory can be applied; A set of relational statements; A logical system employed to relate all concepts within statements.

(5) Model

Closely related to the idea of theory as a systematic conceptual organization is the notion of models. Conceptual organization is often attempted by model. A model can be viewed as a likeness of something. Models usually consist of symbols rather than physical matter; that is, the characteristics of some empirical phenomenon, including its components and the relationships between the components, are represented in logical arrangements among concepts. Thus we can more formally define a model as an abstraction from reality that serves as the purpose of ordering and simplifying our view of reality while still representing its essential characteristics.

5. Theory, models and empirical research

The research of social medicine rests includes two major components: theory and empirical research. Researchers operate in two "worlds" — the world of observation and experience, and the world of ideas, theories, and models. Establishing a systematic connection between these two worlds enhances the goals of the social sciences. But how should this connection be achieved? Should we first construct our theories and models and then move to the world of empirical research? Or should theory follow empirical research?

(1) Theory before research

This is often referred to as the theory-then-research strategy. It involves the following five stages: ①Construct an explicit theory or model; ②Select a proposition derived from the theory or model from empirical investigation; ③Design a research project to test the proposition; ④If the proposition derived from the theory is rejected by the empirical data, make changes in the theory or the research project and return to stage 2; ⑤If the proposition is not rejected, select other propositions for testing or attempt to improve the theory.

(2) Research before theory

In sharp contrast to the theory-then-research strategy, the procedures of the research-then-theory strategy are: ①Investigate a phenomenon and delineate its attributes; ②Measure the attributes in a variety of situations; ③Analyze the resulting data to determine if there are systematic patterns of variation; ④Once systematic patterns are discovered, construct a theory. The theory may be any of the types discussed earlier, although a systematic theory is preferable.

6. Basic elements of research

In social medicine research, whether carried out under the theory-then-research or the research-then-theory strategy, the terms research problem, variables, relation, and hypothesis crop up with great frequency. They are the basic elements of research; they help transform an idea into concrete research operations.

(1) Research problems

A research problem is an intellectual stimulus calling for an answer in the form of scientific inquiry. For example, "Why do rural people utilize less health service?" or "Does socio-economic status influence health care?" are both problems amenable to scientific research.

Not all intellectual stimuli can be studied empirically. Problems that cannot be empirically grounded or that are concerned with subjective preferences, beliefs, values, or tastes are not amenable to empirical research. For example, "Does God exist?" This kind of question is neither proven nor provable.

In addition to being empirically grounded, research problems have to be clearly and specifically articulated. For example, the problem "What incentives lead to energy conservation?" is too general and too ambiguous. It means different things to different people. It does not specify the types of incentives (e.g. economic, social, patriotic) or the source of energy (crude oil, gasoline, natural gas, coal). It also fails to distinguish between industrial and residential conservation. The lack of clarity and specificity may lead to ambiguous findings that can be interpreted in contradictory ways.

(2) Variables

Research problems are conveyed through a set of concepts. The concepts are abstractions representing empirical phenomena. In order to move from the conceptual level to the empirical level, concepts are converted into variables. It is variables that our concept will eventually appear in hypotheses and be tested.

Concepts are converted into variables by mapping them into a set of values. For example, assigning numbers (one type of value) to objects is a mapping of a set of objects into a set of numbers. A variable is an empirical property that takes two or more values. If a property can change in value or kind, it can be regarded as a variable. For example, "social class" is a variable because it can be differentiated by at least five distinct values: lower, lower middle, middle, upper middle, and upper. A variable that can have only two values is called a dichotomous variable. For reaching the purpose of research, it is important to make an analysis distinction among dependent, independent, and control variables between continuous and discrete variables. For more details about variables, please refer to the textbooks of statistics and epidemiology.

(3) Relations

A relation in research always means a relation between two or more variables. When we say that variable X and variable Y are related we mean there is something common in both variables. Establishing a relation in empirical research involves determining which value of one variable co-varies with values of one or more other variables.

Two properties of relations are concerned in empirical research: direction and magnitude. Direction of relation means that the relation between variables is either positive or negative. The magnitude of a relation is the extent to which variables co-vary positively or negatively. The relations studied in the social medicine are in magnitude between zero and perfect.

(4) Hypotheses

A hypothesis is a tentative answer to a research problem, expressed in the form of a relation between independent and dependent variables. Hypotheses are tentative answers because they can be verified only after they have been tested empirically. When proposing a hypothesis, the researcher does not know whether it will be verified or not. A hypothesis is constructed and tested; if it is rejected, another one is put forward; if it is accepted, it is incorporated into the scientific body of knowledge.

Hypotheses can be derived deductively from theories, directly from observations, intuitively, or form a combination of these approaches. The sources from which researchers derive their hypotheses are of little significance in comparison with the way in which they reject or fail to reject them.

Research hypotheses share four common characteristics. They are clear, value-free, specific, and amendable to empirical testing with the available research methods.

①Hypothesis must be clear. In order to test a hypothesis empirically, one has to define all the variables in the hypothesis operationally. The professional literature and experts' opinions can be of great help when constructing hypotheses and defining the variables. Operational definitions must be specific and so precise that observation and replication are made possible.

②Scientific hypotheses are value-free. In principle, the researcher's own values, biases, and subjective preferences have no place in the scientific approach. The researcher must be aware of personal biases and make them as explicit as possible.

③Hypotheses are specific. The investigator has to point out the expected relations among the variables in terms of direction and the conditions under which the relations will hold.

④Hypotheses are testable with available methods. One can arrive at clear, value-free, and specific hypotheses and find that there are no research methods to test them.

Section 2 Design and Structure of Research

A research design is the program that guides an investigator in the process of collecting, analyzing, and interpreting observations. It is a logical model of proof that allows the researcher to draw inferences concerning causal relations among the variables under investigation. The research design also defines the domain of generalization, that is, whether the obtained interpretations can be generalized to a larger population or to different situations.

1. Correlation design

Correlation design is often referred to as the cross-sectional study, perhaps the most predominant design employed in the social sciences. This design is often identified with survey research, and the method of data collection is common in many social science fields. Survey research usually involves asking a random sample of a set of questions to individuals about their backgrounds, experiences, and attitudes. In most cases, survey research yields to data that are used to examine relationships between property and dispositions; and although numerous studies are concerned with establishing causal relations between these properties and dispositions, an important component in many others is simply to describe the pattern of relation before any attempt of causal inference is made.

Data generated from correlation design is usually analyzed through techniques called cross-tabulation and bivariate percentage analysis. Multivariate method of statistical analysis is the most common alternative for experimental methods of control and the drawing of causal inference in correlation design, such as elaboration by cross-tabulation and multiple regression and so on.

Note, however, that in correlation design, one cannot establish the time order of the variables by performing statistical analysis. The time sequence has to be established by the researcher on the basis of theory and they are carried out in natural settings and permit the employment of random probability samples. This allows statistical inferences to be made to broader populations and permits generalization to real-life situations, thereby increasing the external validation of the study.

2. Measurement methods

(1) Sampling

Sampling secures a representative sample. In social medicinal research, we usually adopt two types of sampling method: probability and non-probability sampling, based on modern sampling theory. The distinguished characteristic of probability sampling is that one can specify the probability for each sampling unit of the population which the sampling unit will be included in the sample. In no probability sampling, there is no way of specifying the probability of each unit's inclusion in the sample, and there is no assurance that every unit has some chance of being included. If a set of units has no chance of being included in the sample, a restriction on the definition of the population is implied; that is, if the traits of this set of units are unknown, then the precise nature of the population also remains unknown.

A well-designed sample ensures that if a study were to be repeated on a number of different samples drawn from a given population, the findings would not differ from the population parameters by more than a specified amount. A probability sample design makes it possible to estimate the extent to which the findings based on one sample are likely to differ from what would have been found by studying the entire population. With a probability sample design, it is possible to attach estimates of the population's parameters to the sample statistics.

Although accurate estimates of the population's parameters can be made only with probability samples, social scientists do employ non-probability samples. The major reasons for this practice are convenience and economy, which under certain circumstances (e. g. exploratory research) may outweigh the advantages of using probability sampling. Non-probability samples are also used when a sampling population cannot be precisely defined and when a list of the sampling population is unavailable.

(2) Non-probability sample designs

Three major designs of non-probability samples have been used by social scientists: convenience samples, purposive samples, and quota samples.

①Convenience samples. A convenience sample is obtained when the researcher selects whatever sampling units conveniently available. Thus a college professor may select students in a class; or a researcher may take the first 200 people encountered on the street who are willing to be interviewed. There is no way of estimating the representativeness of convenient samples and of estimating the population's parameters.

②Purposive samples. In the purposive samples (occasionally referred to as judgment samples), the sampling units are subjectively selected by the researcher trying to obtain a sample that appears to be representative of the population. The chance that a particular sampling unit will be selected as the sample depends on the subjective judgment of the researcher. Because it is impossible to determine why different researchers judge each sampling unit they select to contribute to the representativeness of the sample, it is impossible to determine the probability of any specific sampling unit included in the sample.

③Quota samples. The chief aim of a quota sample is the selection of a sample that is as similar as possible to the sampling population. For example, if it is known that the population has equal numbers of males and females, the researcher selects an equal number of males and females as the sample. In quota sampling, interviewers are given an assignment of quota groups specified by variables such as gender, age, and place of residence.

(3) Probability sample designs

Here we present four common designs of probability samples: simple random sampling, systematic sampling, stratified sampling, and cluster sampling.

①Simple random sample. Simple random sampling is the basic probability sampling design. It gives each of the N sampling units of the population an equal and known non-zero probability of being selected, so that it allows every sampling unit of the population has an equal and known probability of being included in the sample.

②Systematic samples. It consists of selecting every "K" sampling unit of the population after the first sampling unit is selected at random from the first K sampling units. Thus if one desires to select a sample of 100 persons from a population of 10,000, one can take every hundredth individual ($K=N/n=10,000/100=100$). The first selection is determined by some random process, such as the use of a table of random digits. Suppose that the fourteenth person were selected, the sample would then consist of individuals numbered 14, 114, 214, 314, and so on.

③Stratified samples. It is used primarily to ensure that different groups of a population are adequately represented in the sample so that the level of accuracy in estimating parameters is increased. Furthermore, all other things being equal, stratified sampling reduces the cost of execution considerably. The underlying idea in stratified sampling is that available information of the population is used "to divide it into groups so that the elements within each group are more alike than that in the population as a whole." If a series of homogeneous groups can be sampled in such a way that when the samples are combined, they constitute a sample of a more heterogeneous population, and increased accuracy will result. The necessary condition for division into homogeneous strata is that the criteria for division are related to the variable being studied. A second consideration is that the criteria used do not require too many sub-samples, which would increase the size of the sample more than that required by a simple random sample.

④Cluster samples. It is frequently used in large-scale studies because it is the least expensive sample design. Cluster sampling involves selecting larger groupings called clusters, and the selecting the sampling units from the clusters. The clusters are selected by a simple random sample or a stratified sample. Depending on the research problem, all the sampling units in these clusters can be included in the sample, or a selection from the clusters can be made through simple or stratified sampling procedures.

The four designs of probability sampling which we have described do not exhaust the range of probability sampling procedures, and you are advised to consult the additional readings. However, these are the basic designs most commonly used by social medicinal researchers.

Section 3 Methods of Data Collection

Data in the social medicine are obtained in either formal or informal settings and involve either verbal (oral and written) or nonverbal acts or responses. A variety of combinations of these two settings for data collection and the two types of acts result in the four major forms of data collection: observational methods, survey research (personal interviews and questionnaires), secondary data analyses, and qualitative research. These are generally divided into two groups: quantitative and qualitative methods.

Each of these data collection methods has certain advantages and some inherent limitations. To certain degree, research findings are affected by the nature of the data collection method used. To minimize the effect, a researcher can use two or more methods of data collection to test hypotheses and measure variables. Consistent findings among different data collection methods increase the credibility of research findings.

In this section, as taking interview survey as an example, we attempt to introduce the differences between quantitative interview survey and qualitative interview survey methods, then try to exemplify these two methods through explaining how to carry out a questionnaire survey and personal interview (including in-depth personal interview and Focus Group Discussions).

1. The differences between quantitative and qualitative methods

Qualitative interviewing is a flexible and powerful tool, which can open up many new areas for research. It can enable practicing clinicians to investigate research questions of immediate relevance to their everyday work, which would otherwise be difficult to investigate. Few researchers would consider embarking on a new research technique without some form of training, and training in research interviewing skills is available from universities and specialist research organizations.

Qualitative studies address different questions from those addressed by quantitative research. For example, a quantitative epidemiological approach to the sudden infant death syndrome might measure statistical correlates of national and regional variations in incidence. In a qualitative study you might interview mothers of young babies in different socioeconomic groups to understand their child rearing practices and hence discover possible factors contributing to the low incidence of sudden infant death in some populations.

Qualitative interviewers try to be interactive and sensitive to the language and concepts used by the interviewee, and they try to keep the agenda flexible. They aim to go below the surface of the topic being discussed, explore what people say in as much detail as possible, and uncover new areas or ideas that were not anticipated at the outset of the research. It is vital that interviewers check that they have understood respondents' meanings instead of relying on their own assumptions. This is particularly important if there is obvious potential for misunderstanding.

A qualitative research interviewer aims to discover the interviewee's own framework of meanings; the research task is to avoid imposing the researcher's structures and assumptions as far as possible.

The less structured the interview, the less the questions are determined and standardized before the interview occurs. Most qualitative interviewers will have a list of core questions that define the areas to be covered. Unlike quantitative interviews based on highly structured questionnaires, the order in which questions are asked will vary, as will the questions designed to probe the interviewee's meanings. Wordings cannot be standardized because the interviewer will try to use the person's own vocabulary when framing supplementary questions. Also, during the course of a qualitative study, the interviewer may introduce further questions as he or she becomes more familiar with the topic being discussed.

All qualitative researchers need to consider how interviewees and the effects of characteristics such as class, race, sex, and social distance on the interview perceive them. This question becomes more acute if the interviewee knows that the interviewer is also a doctor. An interviewee who is already a patient or likely to become one may wish to please the doctor by giving the responses he or she thinks the doctor wants. It is best not to interview one's own patients for research purposes, but if this cannot be avoided, patients should be given permission to say what they really think, and they should not be corrected if they say things that doctors think are wrong (for example, that antibiotics are a suitable treatment for viral infections).

Interviewers are also likely to be asked questions by interviewees during the course of an interview. The problem with this is that in answering questions, clinical researchers may undo earlier efforts not to impose their own concepts on the interview. If questions are not answered, this may reduce the interviewee's willingness to answer the interviewer's subsequent questions. One solution is to say that such questions can be answered at the end of the interview, although this is not always a satisfactory response.

(1) Researcher as research instrument

Qualitative interviews require considerable skill on the part of the interviewer. Experienced doctors may feel that they already possess the necessary skills, and indeed many are transferable. To achieve the transition from consultation to research interview, clinical researchers need to monitor their own interviewing technique, critically appraising tape recordings of their interviews and asking others for their comments. The novice research interviewer needs to notice how he or she is being instructed, whether leading questions are being asked, whether cues are picked up or ignored, and whether interviewees are given enough time to explain what they mean. Whyte devised a six-point directiveness scale to help novice researchers analyse their own interviewing technique (Table 8-1). The point is not that non-directiveness is always best, but that the amount of directiveness should be appropriate. Some informants are more verbose than others, and it is vital that interviewers maintain control of the interview. Patton provided three strategies for maintaining control: knowing the purpose of the interview, asking the right questions to get the information needed, and giving appropriate verbal and non-verbal feedback (Table 8-2).

Table 8-1 Whyte's directiveness scale for analysing interviewing technique

1. Making encouraging noises
2. Reflecting on remarks made by the informant
3. Probing on the last remark by the informant
4. Probing an idea preceding the last remark by the informant
5. Probing an idea expressed earlier in the interview
6. Introducing a new topic (1=least directive, 6=most directive)

Table 8-2 Maintaining control of the interview

1. Knowing what you want to find out is
2. Asking the right questions to get the information you need
3. Giving appropriate verbal and non-verbal feedback

Some common pitfalls for interviewers that have been identified by Field and Morse include outside interruptions, competing distractions, stage fright, awkward questions, jumping from one subject to another, and the temptation to counsel interviewees (Table 8-3). Awareness of these pitfalls can help the interviewer to develop ways of overcoming them.

Table 8-3 Common pitfalls in interviewing

1. Interruptions from outside (telephone, etc.)
2. Competing distractions (children, etc.)
3. Stage fright for interviewer or interviewee
4. Asking interviewee embarrassing or awkward questions
5. Jumping from one subject to another
6. Teaching (for example, giving interviewee medical advice)
7. Counselling (for example, summarising responses too early)
8. Presenting one's own perspective, thus potentially biasing the interview
9. Superficial interviews
10. Receiving secret information (for example, suicide threats)
11. Translators (for example, inaccuracy)

(2) Identifying interviewees

Sampling strategies are determined by the purpose of the research project. Statistical representativeness is not normally sought in qualitative research. Similarly, sample sizes are not determined by hard and fast rules, but by other factors such as the depth and duration of the interview and what are feasible for a single interviewer. Large qualitative studies do not often interview more than 50 or 60 people, although there are exceptions. Sociologists conducting research in medical settings often have to negotiate access with great care, although this is unlikely to be a problem for clinicians conducting research in their own place of work. Nevertheless, the researcher still needs to approach the potential interviewee and explain the purpose of the research, emphasising that a refusal will not affect future treatment. An introductory letter should also explain what is involved and the likely duration of the interview and should give assurances about confidentiality. Interviews should always be conducted at interviewees' convenience, which for people who work during the day will often be in the evening. The setting of an interview affects the content, and it is usually preferable to interview people at home.

2. Quantitative method: questionnaire

(1) Questionnaire construction

The foundation of all questionnaires is the question. The questionnaire must translate the research objectives into specific questions; answers to such questions will provide the data for hypothesis testing. The question must also motivate the respondent so that the necessary information is obtained. It is to these two ends that the question becomes the focus around which the questionnaire is constructed. The major considerations involved in formulating the question are its content, structure, format, and sequence.

Survey questions may be concerned with facts, opinions, attitudes, respondents' motivation, and their level of familiarity with a certain subject. Most questions, however, can be classified into the two general categories of factual questions or opinion and attitude questions.

①Factual questions

Factual questions are designed to elicit objective information from the respondents regarding their background, their environment, their habits, and the like. The most common type of a factual question is the background questions, which is asked mainly to provide information by which respondents can be classified, such as sex, age, marital status, education, or income. Such classification, in turn, may aid in explaining differences in behaviors and attitudes.

These types of questions are thought to be easier to design than other types of questions. However, even factual questions can present the researcher with problems. For instance, in a housing survey, many respondents reported fewer bedrooms than their houses actually contained, simply because they did not think of a den, a playroom, or a guest room as "bedrooms" in the sense intended by the question. This example points to a possibly different frame of reference between the investigator and the respondents. A clear definition of what is meant by the concept is always required to avoid this.

②Opinion questions

The concept "attitude" refers to the sum total of a person's inclinations, prejudices, ideas, fears, and convictions about any specific topic. Opinions, on the other hand, are the verbal expression of attitudes.

An attitude can lead to a tendency to act or react in a certain manner when confronted with certain stimuli. The individual's attitudes are expressed, in speech or behavior, only when the object of the attitude is perceived. A person may have strong attitudes for or against something, but these are aroused and conveyed only when that person encounters some issue connected with the concern at hand. Attitudes can be described by their content (what the attitude is about), by their direction (positive, neutral, or negative feelings about the object or issue in question), and by their intensity (an attitude may be held with greater or lesser vehemence).

In general, we are interested in measuring attitudes because they account for the respondent's general inclination. The study of opinion is of interest only in so far as it is a symbol of an attitude. The main difference between asking for opinions and measuring attitudes is that an opinion is generally measured by estimating what proportion of the surveyed population say they agree with a single opinion statement. Attitude scales consisting of five to two dozen or more attitude statements, with which the respondent is asked to agree or disagree, measure attitudes. An essential requirement of attitude measurement is that such attitude statements be scaled; that is, that the statements be selected and put together from a much larger number of attitude statements according to certain techniques.

It is relatively simple to obtain accurate information on, for example, whether or not a person is married or single. With opinions or attitudes, the assumption that the respondents know cannot always be made. Moreover, given that many attitudes have various aspects or dimensions, the respondent may agree with one aspect and disagree with the other. This is why attitudes cannot be measured by a single question. By using several attitude statements, one can reduce the effects of one-sided responses.

Finally, answers to opinion and attitude questions are more sensitive to changes in wording, emphasis, and sequence than are those to factual questions. This reflects, in part, the multidimensionality of many attitudes.

3. Qualitative method: In-depth key informant interview and Focus Group discussions

(1) In-depth key informant interview

(2) Focus Group discussions (FGD's)

Focus Groups yield qualitative, not quantitative information. Focus Groups are designed to reveal individuals' inner attitudes, opinions and feelings. Reaching consensus is not its goal.

Focus Groups involve 6 – 12 participants, selected non-randomly, and a moderator who "guides" the conversation through the main issues to be addressed.

Usually FGD's include three important steps: plan, conduct, and analyze.

1) Plan

①Define research objectives. The first step is to define the issues that you would like to understand more thoroughly. Then make a list of the main questions you would like to probe during the session.

②Select sample of 12 people. Any number of people above 12 becomes hard to control in a focus group situation. The sample need not be randomly selected, but they should be adults, both male and female, who have experienced the health care system, and who are willing and able to discuss the issues in-depth. A small gift should be given to them as an incentive to participate.

③Appoint moderator. An effective moderator is the most important person in a focus group. He must have excellent communications skills, understand human psychology, have some experience and knowledge of the topic of interest, and must be able to lead and control the conversation in a subtle manner. A prepared script indicating the exact order of questioning, flowing from general issues to specific issues should guide him.

④Choose suitable site. The site chosen should have an informal and relaxing atmosphere (e.g. a meeting room in a hotel or a community center). It should not be an official place, like the Health Bureau. Refreshments should be provided for participants.

⑤Send invitation and reminder. Participants should be invited, and their availability confirmed, well ahead of time. One day before the focus group takes place, someone should contact them to confirm, and to remind them of the place and time.

2) Conduct

①Introduce yourself, explain what the group is about, how participants were chosen, and the purpose of the session.

②Ask names and information about the participants, make them feel relaxed and comfortable.

③Ask general questions first and move towards the issues, zeroing in on specific issues later. Ask in open-ended manner. Probe deeper if an interesting point surfaces.

④Spread discussion. Don't allow one or two persons to dominate the discussion. One of the most important roles of the moderator is to ensure that everybody has a chance to speak. The moderator should move the flow of conversation evenly around the group allowing everybody to express their feelings. In some occasions people dominate the conversation so much that only their thoughts are heard and everybody just agrees with them. These leaders must be quieted down and told to allow others to speak first, in order to eliminate a potential bias in the results.

3) Analysing

Keep detailed notes. Tape record if possible. An assistant should do this, so that the moderator's attention is focused entirely on keeping the discussion flowing in the right direction.

Transcribe the recording as soon as possible after the focus group. Note frequency, similarities and trends in relation to the main points raised. Summarize the main issues, in relation to the purpose of the focus group, e. g:

①Majority were happy with standard of health care received
②Majority complained about health care costs
③Some said they couldn't differentiate between public and private providers

Conclusion: Focus discussions are a useful tool to gather in-depth opinions, feelings and attitudes. They complement quantitative data derived from questionnaires.

第九章 健康危险因素评价

第一节 概述

健康危险因素评价(Health risk factors appraisal,HRFA)是20世纪60年代在美国产生并发展起来的一种研究危险因素与慢性病发病及死亡之间数量依存关系及其规律性的一种技术方法。其基本思想是研究人们生活在有危险因素的环境中发生死亡的概率,也就是研究在人们生产环境、生活方式和医疗卫生服务中存在的各种危险因素对疾病发生和发展的影响程度,以及当改变不良的生活行为方式,降低或消除可改变的危险因素时,可能延长的寿命。其主要目的是通过健康教育或咨询,促进人们自觉改变不良的生产和生活环境,改变不良的行为生活方式,自觉远离危险因素,从而达到减少疾病、提高健康水平的目的。

健康危险因素评价的产生和发展,与疾病谱的转变、医学模式的转变、人们健康观念的转变及对预防保健要求的提高等有关。

20世纪60年代以来,通过预防接种、杀菌灭虫、抗生素的使用使曾经严重危害人类健康的传染病在世界范围内日益得到控制,而慢性病逐渐成为人类最主要的死亡原因。由于慢性病的迁延性、难愈性、致残率及死亡率较高,不仅影响了个体的生命质量,而且对卫生资源造成了长久的消耗,因此预防和控制慢性病具有重要意义。美国大约在20世纪20年代慢性非传染性疾病死亡率超过传染病成为主要死亡原因。1900年传染病死亡率为650/10万人口,1970年为20/10万人口,70年间传染病死亡率下降了97%;1900年慢性非传染性疾病死亡率为350/10万人口,1970年增加到690/10万人口,70年增加了97%。我国20世纪50年代就消灭和基本消灭了天花、鼠疫、古典型霍乱等,1948年急性传染病的发病率为2万/10万,1985年下降为800/10万,下降了96%。

我国城市大约在50年代中期,农村大约在60年代初期慢性病死亡率超过了传染病而成为主要死因。根据国家卫生服务1998年调查结果,我国城乡居民的前五位死因都是慢性非传染性疾病。从我国死亡谱(前五位死因)的变化也可以看出这一点。

表 9-1 我国近 50 年的死亡谱

年份	前 五 位 死 因				
1957	呼吸系统疾病	传染病	消化系统疾病	心脏病	脑血管疾病
1963	呼吸系统疾病	传染病	恶性肿瘤	脑血管疾病	心脏病
1975	脑血管疾病	心脏病	恶性肿瘤	呼吸系统疾病	传染病
1985	心脏病	脑血管疾病	恶性肿瘤	呼吸系统疾病	消化系统疾病
2000	恶性肿瘤	脑血管疾病	心脏病	消化系统疾病	损伤和中毒
2002	恶性肿瘤	脑血管疾病	呼吸系统疾病	心脏病	损伤和中毒

慢性非传染性疾病是多种致病因素长期综合作用的结果。第二次世界大战后,各国均投入了大量人力、物力从事慢性非传染性疾病的研究及防治工作。经过长期的努力,在慢性非传染性疾病的病因学及流行病学研究方面取得了可喜的进展,如冠心病的发病,根据美国 6 个前瞻性调查的结果认为肥胖、高胆固醇、高血压和吸烟四个因素尤为重要,有上述四个因素者患冠心病的机会较无此四个因素者高 40 倍。恶性肿瘤发病也与行为生活方式、精神状况、环境、职业等有密切关系。慢性病的控制必须采取综合性措施,健康危险因素评价正是在这个背景下产生的。

健康危险因素评价的产生应归功于 L. Robbins,他通过对 10 多年死亡原因资料的分析、研究,制定了死亡率表,用这些死亡率表在 Temple 大学进行了健康危险因素评价的论证研究,但在这个研究中,危险因素没有被定量,仅用一般的描述表达。到 1967 年,与疾病有关的已确定的危险因素大多数都被定量,这个工作是由参加肿瘤、心血管疾病调查的专家根据较早的 Framingham 心脏病前瞻性研究的证据完成的。1970 年,L. Robbins 和 J. H. Hall 的 *How to practice prospective medicine*(《怎样从事医学前瞻》)系统论述了根据危险因素程度定量研究主要死亡原因发生概率的原理和方法,为健康危险因素评价的发展奠定了理论基础。

20 世纪 70 年代中期,又有许多学者将健康危险因素定量化,按其严重程度转化为危险分数。生物统计学家 H. Geller 和健康保险学家 N. Gesner 根据各种危险因素与相应慢性病之间联系的密切程度和作用强度,采用直接评分和多元回归分析等多种分析方法,将危险因素转换成危险分数,制成 Geller-Gesner 量表,健康危险因素评价方法臻于完善。

第二节 健康危险因素与慢性病的演变过程

一、健康危险因素

我们在健康危险因素评价中所讨论的健康危险因素主要是指在机体内外环境中存在的,与慢性病发生、发展及死亡有关的诱发因素。而慢性非传染性疾病的发生和发展及最终的预后与社会环境因素、行为因素、生物遗传因素以及医疗卫生服务有着密切的联系。我们可以通过对这些健康危险因素的评价,预测健康状况和疾病发生的概率,从而达到预防和控制慢性非传染性疾病的效果。

(一)环境危险因素

1. 自然环境危险因素。包括生物性危险因素和物理化学性危险因素。生物危险因素如细菌、病毒、寄生虫、生物毒物等。物理化学性危险因素包括各种噪声、振动、电离辐射、计算机以及某些精密仪器所发射的电磁辐射、生产性毒物、粉尘、交通工具排放的废气、农药,以及排放到河流中造成生活用水污染的废水等。

2. 社会环境危险因素。经济收入、营养状况、文化程度、社会制度等都对人群的健康起着重要的作用。其与健康的关系在"环境与健康"部分中已经详细介绍。

(二)行为危险因素

所谓行为危险因素,指的是个体所选择的生活方式所带来的危险因素,又称为自创性危险因素。据统计,前四位主要死因,即心脏病、肿瘤、脑血管病和意外伤害造成的死亡占总死亡数的70%以上,而这四类疾病都与行为生活方式密切相关。吸烟、酗酒、缺乏体育锻炼、静坐、饮食不合理等生活方式方面的危险因素对人的健康造成了不利的影响。

(三)生物遗传危险因素

有些疾病例如链状红细胞性贫血病、蚕豆病、血友病等都与遗传有关。生物遗传危险因素是一些传统的危险因素,但是随着医学科学技术的不断发展,也许在不久的将来,基因技术能够实现从基因水平上控制遗传物质,从而控制一些遗传性疾病的发生和发展。

(四)医疗卫生服务中的危险因素

医疗卫生服务的好坏直接影响着人群的健康水平。医疗质量、误诊漏诊、医院交叉感染、医疗卫生服务资源的合理布局、卫生保健网络的健全程度、人力资源的配备等都是影响健康的因素。目前由于资源配备的不合理,卫生资源主要集中在大城市,在农村以及偏远地区,卫生人员水平低、资源缺乏,这些地区居民健康状况较城市居民低下。

二、健康危险因素的特点

(一)潜伏期长

潜伏期长,指的是人们需要长时间反复接触这些危险因素后才会发病,并非像传染性疾病那样发病较快,而且潜伏期的长短因人而异。例如日本的夜班长途汽车司机通常在工作20年之后出现心血管系统的症状。吸烟者其吸烟史往往长达数十年之后才发生肺癌。潜伏期长既会使危险因素与疾病之间的联系不易确定,也容易使人们忽视这种联系,但同时又为卫生干预提供了时间。

(二)交互作用明显

当多种危险因素同时存在时,相互之间可以发生联合作用,而增强致病危险性。例如文献报道石棉接触与吸烟对肺癌的发病有联合作用,不吸烟与不接触石棉者的肺癌死亡率比值为1.0;不吸烟但有石棉接触史者肺癌死亡率比值为5.17;无石棉接触史有吸烟史者肺癌死亡率比值为10.85;同时有吸烟史和石棉接触史者肺癌死亡率比值为53.24。

(三)特异性弱

由于危险因素与疾病之间存在着单因多果、多因多果或多因单果的因果联系,使得危险因素的作用缺乏一定的特异性。如缺乏体育活动是冠心病的危险因素,而吸烟、肥胖等也是冠心病的危险因素。吸烟是肺癌的危险因素,也是心脑血管系统疾病和胃溃疡等多种疾病的危险因素。

由于潜伏期长而特异性又比较弱,这就更容易引起人们对危险因素的忽视。

(四)广泛存在

危险因素广泛存在于人们日常生活之中。社会环境因素、行为生活方式因素、医疗卫生服务因素等都与人们的生活联系密切。正因为其广泛存在,才更容易使人们忽视其存在,这就需要进行广泛的健康教育和健康宣传,使人们自觉地远离危险因素,而促进自身健康水平的提高。

三、慢性病的演变过程

随着医学科学技术的发展,人们对慢性病的演变过程有了一定的认识,对慢性病病程的了解更有利于我们对慢性病进行预防和治疗。根据 Robbins 和 Hall 的建议,可以把慢性病的自然过程划分为六个阶段。

(一)无危险阶段

在这一阶段,人们的周围环境和行为生活方式中不存在危险因素,可以通过保持良好的生活方式,选择良好的自然和社会环境,防止可能出现的危险因素。

(二)出现危险阶段

随着环境的改变、年龄的增加,人们的生产和生活环境中出现了危险因素,但是由于时间短暂、程度轻微,危险因素并没有产生明显的危害,或者对人体的危害还不易察觉。若此时进行行为生活方式调查或者是环境因素监测可发现危险因素。

(三)致病因素出现

随着危险因素数量增加及作用时间延长,危险因素转化为致病因素,对机体产生的危害作用逐渐显现。这一时期由于机体防御机制的作用及致病因素的弱化,疾病尚不足以形成。

(四)疾病征兆出现

疾病已经形成,症状开始出现,疾病形成可逆的形态功能损害,用生理和生化的诊断手段可以发现异常的变化。在此阶段用筛检的方法可以从正常人群中发现早期无症状患者,从而达到早发现,早治疗。

(五)体征出现

症状和体征可能并行也可能先后出现。患者常常因为自己感觉到形态和功能障碍而主动就医。在此阶段即使消除危险因素的作用,一般也不容易改变病程。

(六)劳动力丧失

此阶段是慢性病发展的最后阶段。由于症状加剧,病程继续发展,丧失生活和劳动能力。此阶段的主要措施是康复治疗。

健康危险评价是从慢性病病程的第一阶段开始,即在疾病尚未出现时就采取措施,通过评价危险因素对健康的影响,教育人们采取良好的行为生活方式,自觉地远离危险因素。在危险因素出现时,通过健康危险因素评价,计算它可能造成的危害,预测疾病发生的概率,从而达到了早期预防和控制慢性病的效果。因此,从疾病自然史的观点分析,健康危险因素评价是预防慢性病发生的一项有效措施。

第三节 健康危险因素评价的计算步骤

一、收集资料

(一)收集当地年龄别、性别、疾病别发病率或死亡率资料

患病率资料和死亡率资料可以通过登记报告、疾病检测、调查和死因登记资料等获得。在健康危险因素评价中,我们会用到死亡概率的资料,死亡率与死亡概率之间可以通过统计学公式进行换算。我们此处所指的死亡概率是指10年死亡概率。

通常我们选择当地危害健康比较严重的疾病,即前10~15位死因的疾病作为研究对象。这需要在收集到当地年龄别、性别、疾病别死亡率之后才能确定。需要注意的是我们所选择的是一种疾病,而不是一类或者一个系统的疾病。例如在健康危险因素评价中我们可以收集肺癌的资料,而不应该是肿瘤这一类疾病的发病和死亡资料。因为一种疾病的危险因素比较容易确定,而一类疾病由多种疾病构成,其危险因素更为复杂,难以确定而影响危险因素评价。

(二)收集危险因素资料

需要收集的危险因素资料,可以从影响健康和疾病的四个方面的因素来考虑。

1. 环境因素,如经济收入、居住条件、家庭关系、工作环境、心理刺激等。
2. 行为生活方式,如吸烟、饮酒、体力活动情况等。
3. 生物因素,如年龄、性别、种族、身高、体重、疾病遗传史等。
4. 卫生服务,如是否定期健康检查、直肠镜检查、阴道涂片等。

另外,应注意疾病史,需调查原有疾病史、婚姻生育史、家庭疾病史等。

目前,下列疾病与危险因素的关系已经明确。

表9-2 疾病与危险因素的关系

疾病	危险因素
冠心病	收缩压、舒张压、糖尿病史、体力活动、体重、血清胆固醇含量、家族遗传史
肺癌	吸烟、吸烟量、吸烟时间、开始吸烟年龄
乳腺癌	年龄、家庭史、哺乳史、有无定期自我检查乳房肿块
宫颈癌	年龄、社会经济状况、结婚与性生活开始年龄、生育胎数、有无定期阴道图片检查
子宫体癌	原因不明的不规则阴道流血
肠癌	肠息肉、肠出血、肠壁溃疡和肠炎、有无定期做直肠镜检查、是否有血吸虫病史
胃癌与食管癌	胃酸低、有无定期做胃液检查及钡餐检查
慢性风湿性心脏病	心脏杂音、风湿热及有关症状及体征
肝硬化	饮酒史(饮酒量、饮酒时间、饮酒种类)、肝炎史和血吸虫病感染史

(续表 9-2)

疾病	危险因素
糖尿病	体重、家庭史、高血压、血清胆固醇
肺气肿	吸烟、慢性气管炎
脑血管病	高血压、糖尿病、胆固醇高、吸烟、紧张忧虑
车祸	酒后驾车、服用兴奋剂和镇静剂史、平均驾车里程、安全带使用
自杀	饮酒量、家庭史、压抑、情绪紧张
其他意外伤害	饮酒、外出工作、犯罪记录、凶器制备、滥用药物、紧张、矛盾冲突和社会经济状况急剧变化

资料可以来自询问或自填式问卷调查，收集行为生活方式、环境危险因素和医疗卫生服务中的危险因素。通过病史询问、体格检查和实验室检查等，也可以获得重要的资料。

二、资料分析

(一)将危险因素转换成危险分数

我们只有将危险因素转换成危险分数才能将定性资料转化为定量资料，对危险因素进行定量分析。危险因素相当于当地死亡人群的平均水平时，危险分数定为 1.0，也就是说危险分数为 1.0 时，个体发生某种疾病死亡的概率相当于当地死亡概率的平均水平。危险分数大于 1.0 时，则个体发生疾病死亡的概率大于当地死亡概率的平均水平。危险分数小于 1.0 时，则个体发生疾病死亡的概率小于当地死亡概率的平均水平。危险分数越高，个体发生死亡的概率越大。危险因素与死亡概率之间的数量依存关系是通过危险分数转换来实现的。

危险分数转换有两种方法：①多元回归分析方法。这种方法的依据就是危险因素和死亡概率之间存在着函数关系，用数学公式确切地表达出危险因素严重程度与死亡概率之间的定量联系是在大量病因学和流行病学的研究成果基础之上进行的。②采用经验评估方法。邀请一部分有关专业的专家，根据前瞻性或者回顾性死因调查的结果，对危险因素与死亡概率之间联系的密切程度，提出危险因素严重程度的不同的赋值。在进行这项工作时，常常是以 Geller-Gesner 量表作为参考的。到目前为止还没有制定出一套适合我国具体情况的危险分数转换值供参考应用。目前在进行计算时可采用 Geller-Gesner 危险分数转换表，或者在 Geller-Gesner 表基础上结合我国的具体情况适当修改。表 9-3 列出了男性部分年龄组的危险因素与危险分数之间的转化。查表时需要注意，如果某人的危险因素指标值在表上查不到，可以选用相邻的两个指标值的危险分数来估计，或用内插法计算。如胆固醇值为 192 mg/dL，按表 9-3，40~44 岁男性危险分数转换表中没有 192 mg/dL 这一等级，根据规定 220 mg/dL 与 180 mg/dL 对应的危险分数分别为 1.0 与 0.5，用内插法计算出 192 mg/dL 的危险分数。

注意：血压一般将收缩压与舒张压分别考虑，如果两者中有一个或两个危险分数等于或小于 1.0，则仅用高的那个危险分数作为血压的危险分数，而不必分为收缩压、舒张压两项来记。例如一人的血压值为 16.0/9.3 kPa,从表 9-3 即危险分数转换表来看,16.0 kPa 的危险分数为 0.4,而 9.3 kPa 的危险分数小于 0.4,所以此人的血压这项危险因素的危险分数我们记为 0.4。

表 9-3　Geller-Gesner 危险分数转换表(男性,部分年龄组:40～44 岁)

死亡原因	危险指数	测量值	危险分数
冠心病	收缩压 kPa(mmHg)	26.6(200)	3.2
		23.9(180)	2.2
		21.3(160)	1.2
		18.6(140)	0.8
		16.0(120)	0.4
	舒张压 kPa(mmHg)	14.1(106)	3.7
		13.3(100)	2.0
		12.5(94)	1.3
		11.7(88)	0.8
		10.9(82)	0.4
	胆固醇(mg/dL)	280	1.5
		220	1.0
		180	0.5
	糖尿病史	有	3.0
		已控制	2.5
		无	1.0
	运动情况	坐着工作和娱乐	2.5
		有些活动的工作	1.0
		中度锻炼	0.6
		较强度锻炼	0.5
		坐着工作,有定期锻炼	1.0
		其他工作,有定期锻炼	0.5
	家庭史	父母二人 60 岁以前死于冠心病	1.4
		父母之一 60 岁以前死于冠心病	1.2
		父母健在(<60 岁)	1.0
		父母健在(≥60 岁)	0.9
	吸烟	≥10 支/日	1.5
		<10 支/日	1.1
		吸雪茄或烟斗	1.0
		戒烟(不足 10 年)	0.7
		不吸或戒烟 10 年以上	0.5
	体重	超重 75%	2.5

(续表 9-3)

死亡原因	危险指数	测量值	危险分数
		超重 50%	1.5
		超重 15%	1.0
		超重 10%以下	0.8
		降到平均体重	1.0
车祸	饮酒	频繁社交,明显无节制	5.0
		频繁社交,稍有节制	2.0
		适度和偶尔社交	1.0
		不饮	0.5
	使用安全带的时间	<10%	1.1
		10%~24%	1.0
		25%~74%	0.9
		75%~100%	0.8
	行车里程	每年行车里程/10 000＝危险分数	
自杀	抑郁	经常	2.5
		偶尔或没有	1.0
	家庭史	有	2.5
		无	1.0
肝硬化	饮酒	酗酒	12.5
		频繁社交,明显无节制	5.0
		频繁社交,稍有节制	2.0
		适度和偶尔社交	1.0
		极少社交	0.2
		在症状出现之前戒酒	0.2
		不饮	0.1
脑血管病	收缩压 kPa(mmHg)	26.6(200)	3.2
		23.9(180)	2.2
		21.3(160)	1.2
		18.6(140)	0.8
		16.0(120)	0.4
	舒张压 kPa(mmHg)	14.1(106)	3.7
		13.3(100)	2.0
		12.5(94)	1.3
		11.7(88)	0.8
		10.9(82)	0.4
	胆固醇(mg/dL)	280	1.5
		220	1.0
		180	0.5

(续表9-3)

死亡原因	危险指数	测量值	危险分数
	糖尿病史	有	3.0
		已控制	2.5
		无	1.0
	吸烟	吸香烟	1.2
		吸雪茄和烟斗	1.0
		戒烟	1.0
		不吸	0.8
肺癌	吸烟	40支/日	2.0
		20支/日	1.5
		10支/日	1.1
		<10支/日	0.8
		不吸	0.2
	雪茄和烟斗	≥5次/日,吸入	1.0
		<5次/日,不吸入	0.3
		戒烟	从原有危险分数中减去0.2,再减去戒烟年数乘0.1,但危险分数最小不能小于0.2
慢性风湿性心脏病	心脏杂音	有	10.0
		已用药	1.0
		无	1.0
	风湿热	有	10.0
		已用药	1.0
		无	1.0
	症状或体征	无	1.0
肺炎	饮酒	频繁社交活动	3.0
		适度或不饮酒	1.0
	肺气肿	有	2.0
		无	1.0
	吸烟	≥10支/日	1.2
		不吸	1.0
肠癌	肠息肉	有	2.5
		无	1.0
	原因不明的肛门出血	有	3.0
		无	1.0
	溃疡性结肠炎	≥10年	4.0

(续表 9-3)

死亡原因	危险指数	测量值	危险分数
		<10 年	2.0
		无	1.0
	每年直肠镜检	无	1.0
		有	0.3
胃癌、食道癌	胃酸过少	有	2.0
		每年用药	1.5
		无	1.0
高血压心脏病	收缩压 kPa(mmHg)	26.6(200)	3.2
		23.9(180)	2.2
		21.3(160)	1.2
		18.6(140)	0.8
		16.0(120)	0.4
	舒张压 kPa(mmHg)	14.1(106)	3.7
		13.3(100)	2.0
		12.5(94)	1.3
		11.7(88)	0.8
		10.9(82)	0.4
	体重	超重 75%	2.5
		超重 50%	1.5
		超重 15%	1.0
		超重 10% 以下	0.8
		降到平均体重	1.0
肺结核	X 线检查	未做	1.0
		阴性	0.2
	结核活动	有	5.0
		无	1.0

全表年龄 5 岁为一组,分性别各列出了 10~15 组主要疾病之间危险分数的转换。

(二)计算组合危险分数

前面已经提及因为多种危险因素同时对一种疾病起作用时,可能产生联合作用而增强致病性,所以数种危险因素并存时要计算组合危险分数。

计算组合危险分数时需注意:

1. 与疾病相关的危险因素只有一项时,组合危险分数即为此单项危险因素的危险分数。如肺癌的危险因素只有吸烟一项危险因素,则肺癌的组合危险分数即为吸烟单项危险因素的危险分数。

2. 与疾病有关的危险因素多项时,组合危险分数的计算步骤是:

(1) 将危险分数大于 1.0 的各项分别减去 1.0 后的余值作为相加项,1.0 作为相乘项。

(2) 危险分数小于或等于 1.0 的项作为相乘项。

(3) 相乘项之积和相加项之和相加,得到该疾病的组合危险分数。

例如表 9-4 中,冠心病的组合危险分数的计算为:①相加项:大于 1.0 的项有体力活动和体重,危险分数分别为 2.5 和 1.3,相加项为 $[(2.5-1.0)+(1.3-1.0)]\times 1.0=1.8$。②相乘项:小于等于 1.0 的项有血压、胆固醇、糖尿病史、家族史、吸烟,危险分数分别为 0.4,0.6,1.0,0.9 和 0.5,相乘项为 $0.4\times 0.6\times 1.0\times 0.9\times 0.5=0.108$。③组合危险分数为:$[(2.5-1.0)+(1.3-1.0)]\times 1.0+0.4\times 0.6\times 1.0\times 0.9\times 0.5=1.91$。

若无大于 1.0 的项,则组合危险分数为相乘项所计算得出的值;若无小于或等于 1.0 的项,则组合危险分数为相加项所计算得出的值。

(三) 存在死亡危险

存在死亡危险说明在危险分数单独或联合作用下,某种疾病可能发生死亡的危险程度。

计算公式:存在死亡危险=疾病别死亡概率×该疾病的组合危险分数。

如表 9-4 中,40～44 岁男子冠心病的存在死亡危险为:1 877/10 万人口×1.91=3 585/10 万人口。

表 9-4 列举了 11 种有明确危险因素的主要疾病,其余疾病都归并入其他一组,因为无明确危险因素可以评价,因此将其他疾病的组合危险分数用 1.0 表示,即用平均死亡概率表示其他一组的死亡概率。

(四) 计算评价年龄

评价年龄(appraisal age)是依据年龄和死亡概率之间的函数关系,从死亡概率水平推算得出的年龄值。15 岁及 15 岁以上人群中,年龄与死亡概率之间是存在正相关的;10～14 岁年龄组是死亡概率最低的一组;在小于 10 岁的人群中,年龄与死亡概率是存在负相关的。因此,在 15 岁及以上人群中,我们所得出的评价年龄越大,可以认为此人的存在死亡危险越大,也就是此人的健康状况越差。

评价年龄的计算方法:将各种死亡原因的存在死亡危险相加,得出总的存在死亡危险值。用总的存在死亡危险值查评价年龄表,可得出评价年龄值,表 9-5 为健康评价年龄表。

评价年龄表左边一列是男性合计的存在死亡危险值;右边一列是女性合计的存在死亡危险值;中间部分的上面一行数值是个体实际年龄的末位数,主体部分是评价年龄值。如表 9-4 列举 41 岁男子总的存在死亡危险为 7 167.45/10 万人口。查评价年龄表,在表左边一列接近这一数值在 6 830 和 7 570 之间。6 830 的评价年龄为 42 岁,7 570 的评价年龄为 43 岁,因此得出该男子的评价年龄为 42.5 岁。

(五) 计算增长年龄

增长年龄(achievable age)又称通过努力降低危险因素后可能达到的预期年龄,是根据存在的危险因素,提出可能降低危险因素的措施后预计的新的存在死亡危险,按与计算评价年龄相同步骤计算出的年龄。计算方法与计算评价年龄相似。

在所有的危险因素中,有些危险因素是较难改变的,例如疾病史、家族史等,但有些危险因素是可以改变的,例如行为生活方面的、卫生服务利用方面的。医生根据评价对象存在的可改变的危险因素的程度提出一定的建议,评价对象采取建议后其原来的危险因素的危险程度就会改变,因此我们查危险分数转换表也会得出一个新的危险分数。例如表9-4 中冠心病的危险因素"体力活动"一项原为坐着工作,危险分数为 2.5,而此人根据医生建议采取定期锻炼后,其危险程度减低了,新的危险分数为 1.0。我们根据新的危险分数就会算出新的组合危险分数,从而得出新的存在死亡危险,我们用新的存在死亡危险的合计值查评价年龄表,就会得出增长年龄。

表 9-4 中,新的总的存在死亡危险为 3 430.45/10 万人口,查表得增长年龄约为 36 岁。

(六)计算危险因素降低程度

危险因素降低程度表示被测试者接受医生建议后危险因素降低的程度,用存在死亡危险降低的百分比表示。

计算方法:(采取医生建议前的某死亡原因的存在死亡危险－采取医生建议后某死亡原因新的存在死亡危险)/原总的存在死亡危险。

例如表 9-4 自杀项中,抑郁危险因素降低程度＝(660.0－396.0)÷7 167.45×100%＝4%。

第四节 健康危险因素评价

健康危险因素评价既可用于个体评价,也可用于群体评价。

个体评价的结果可以作为健康教育的理论依据,并且可以促进个体自觉的远离危险因素,促进自身健康水平的提高。群体评价的结果,可以了解不同类型的危险因素在人群中的分布情况,从而确定不同人群的疾病防治工作重点。

一、个体评价

个体评价主要通过比较实际年龄、评价年龄和增长年龄之间的差距,了解危险因素对寿命可能影响的程度及降低危险因素之后寿命可能增长的年数,并确定此人的健康类型。

评价年龄大于实际年龄,说明被评价者存在的危险因素高于平均水平,即死亡概率可能高于当地同年龄性别组的平均水平。反之,危险因素低于平均水平,死亡概率水平亦可能低于当地同年龄性别组的平均水平。增长年龄与评价年龄之差值,说明被评价者接受医生降低危险因素的建议后,可能延长寿命的年数。

根据实际年龄、评价年龄和增长年龄三者的量值,将评价个体分为以下四种类型。

(一)健康型

特点:被评价者的评价年龄小于实际年龄。

如被评价者实际年龄 47 岁,评价年龄 43 岁,则此人属于健康型,即 47 岁的个体可能经历 43 岁年龄者的死亡历程。进一步降低危险因素不是没有可能,但降低的程度有限。

第九章 健康危险因素评价

表 9-4 某地 41 岁男性健康危险因素评价表

死亡原因	死亡概率 (1/10⁵)	疾病诱发因素	指标值	危险分数	组合危险分数	存在死亡危险	根据医生建议改变危险因素	新危险分数	新组合危险分数	新存在死亡危险	降低量	危险降低程度百分数
肺癌	202	吸烟	不吸	0.2	0.2	40.4	—	0.2	0.2	40.4	0	0
肝硬化	222	饮酒	不饮	0.1	0.1	22.2	—	0.1	0.1	22.2	0	0
车祸	285	饮酒	不饮	0.5			—	0.5				
		驾车里程	25 000 km	2.5	1.9	541.5	—	2.5	1.9	541.5	0	0
		安全带使用	90%	0.8			100%	0.8				
自杀	264	抑郁	经常	2.5	2.5	660.0	治疗抑郁	1.5	1.5	396.0	264.0	4%
		家族史	无	1.0			—	1.0				
冠心病	2 517	血压(kPa)	16.0/9.3	0.4			—	0.4				
		胆固醇	192	0.6			—	0.6				
		糖尿病史	无	1.0			—	1.0				
		体力活动	坐着工作	2.5	1.91	3 538.07	定期锻炼	1.0	0.11	206.47	3 378.6	47%
		家族史	无	0.5			—	0.5				
		吸烟	不吸	1.0			—	1.0				
		体重	超重30%	1.3			降到平均体重					
脑血管病	222	血压(kPa)	16.0/9.3	0.4			—	0.4				
		胆固醇	192	0.2	0.19	42.18	—	0.2	0.19	42.18	0	0
		糖尿病史	无	1.0			—	1.0				
		吸烟	不吸	0.8			—	0.8				

(续表9-4)

死亡原因	死亡概率(1/10³)	疾病诱发因素	指标值	危险分数	组合危险分数	存在死亡危险	根据医生建议改变危险因素	新危险分数	新组合危险分数	新存在死亡危险	降低量	危险降低程度百分数
慢性风湿性心脏病	167	心脏杂音	无	1.0				1.0				
		风湿热	无	1.0			—	1.0				
		症状体征	无	0.1	0.1	16.7	0.1	0.1	16.7	0	0
肺炎	111	饮酒	不饮	1.0				1.0				
		肺气肿	无	1.0	1.0	111.0	—	1.0	1.0	111.0	0	0
		吸烟	不吸	1.0				1.0				
肠癌	111	肠息肉	无	1.0				1.0				
		肛门出血	无	1.0	1.0	111.0		1.0	0.3	33.3	77.7	1%
		肠炎	无	1.0				1.0				
		直肠镜检查		0.3			每年一次	0.3				
高血压心脏病	56	血压(kPa)	16.6/9.3	0.4	0.7	39.2		0.4	0.4	22.4	16.8	0.2%
		体重	超重30%	1.3			降到平均体重	1.0				
肺结核	56	X线检查	阴性	0.2				0.2				
		结核活动	无	1.0	0.2	11.2	—	0.2	0.2	11.2	0	0
		经济和社会地位	中等	1.0			—	1.0				
其他	1987			1.0	1987		—	1.0	1.0	1987	0	0
合计	5560	—	—	—	7167.450		—	—	—	3430.35	3737.1	52.2%

表 9-5 健康评价年龄表

男性存在死亡危险	实际年龄最末一位数					女性存在死亡危险	男性存在死亡危险	实际年龄最末一位数					女性存在死亡危险
	0 5	1 6	2 7	3 8	4 9			0 5	1 6	2 7	3 8	4 9	
530	5	6	7	8	9	350	4 510	38	39	40	41	42	2 550
570	6	7	8	9	10	350	5 010	39	40	41	42	43	2 780
630	7	8	9	10	11	350	5 560	40	41	42	43	44	3 020
710	8	9	10	11	12	360	6 160	41	42	43	44	45	3 280
790	9	10	11	12	13	380	6 830	42	43	44	45	46	3 560
880	10	11	12	13	14	410	7 570	43	44	45	46	47	3 870
990	11	12	13	14	15	430	8 380	44	45	46	47	48	4 220
1 110	12	13	14	15	16	460	9 260	45	46	47	48	49	4 600
1 230	13	14	15	16	17	490	10 190	46	47	48	49	50	5 000
1 350	14	15	16	17	18	520	11 160	47	48	49	50	51	5 420
1 440	15	16	17	18	19	550	12 170	48	49	50	51	52	5 860
1 500	16	17	18	19	20	570	13 230	49	50	51	52	53	6 330
1 540	17	18	19	20	21	600	14 340	50	51	52	53	54	6 850
1 560	18	19	20	21	22	620	15 330	51	52	53	54	55	7 440
1 570	19	20	21	22	23	640	16 260	52	53	54	55	56	8 110
1 580	20	21	22	23	24	660	16 830	53	54	55	56	57	8 870
1 590	21	22	23	24	25	690	19 820	54	55	56	57	58	9 730
1 590	22	23	24	25	26	720	21 490	55	56	57	58	59	10 680
1 590	23	24	25	26	27	750	23 260	56	57	58	59	60	11 720
1 600	24	25	26	27	28	790	25 140	57	58	59	60	61	12 860
1 620	25	26	27	28	29	840	27 120	58	59	60	61	62	14 100
1 660	26	27	28	29	30	900	29 210	59	60	61	62	63	15 450
1 730	27	28	29	30	31	970	31 420	60	61	62	63	64	16 930
1 830	28	29	30	31	32	1 040	33 760	61	62	63	64	65	18 560
1 960	29	30	31	32	33	1 130	36 220	62	63	64	65	66	20 360
2 120	30	31	32	33	34	1 220	38 810	63	64	65	66	67	22 340
2 310	31	32	33	34	35	1 330	41 540	64	65	66	67	68	24 520
2 520	32	33	34	35	36	1 460	44 410	65	66	67	68	69	26 920
2 760	33	34	35	36	37	1 600	47 440	66	67	68	69	70	29 560
3 030	34	35	36	37	38	1 760	50 650	67	68	69	70	71	32 470
3 330	35	36	37	38	39	1 930	54 070	68	69	70	71	72	35 690
3 670	36	37	38	39	40	2 120	57 720	69	70	71	72	73	39 250
4 060	37	38	39	40	41	2 330	61 640	70	71	72	73	74	43 200

(二)自创性危险因素型

特点:被评价者的评价年龄大于实际年龄,并且评价年龄与增长年龄之差大。

如被评价者实际年龄41岁,评价年龄45岁,增长年龄36岁,则此人属于自创危险型。评价年龄大于实际年龄,说明危险因素高于平均水平;评价年龄与增长年龄之差较大,说明这些危险因素主要属于自身生活方式方面的,即自创性危险因素。采取医生建议后,可以延长预期寿命。

(三)难以改变的危险因素型

特点:被评价者的评价年龄大于实际年龄,但是评价年龄与增长年龄之差较小。

如被评价者实际年龄41岁,评价年龄47岁,增长年龄46岁,则此人属于难以改变的危险因素型,也称为历史危险因素型。评价年龄与增长年龄之差仅为1岁,说明个体的危险因素来自生物遗传因素与既往及目前疾病史,通常不易改变。因此,这类危险因素被降低的可能性较小,预期寿命延长的年数较少。

(四)一般性危险型

特点:评价年龄接近实际年龄,增长年龄和评价年龄接近。

被评价者的死亡概率或者说其预期死亡过程相当于当地平均水平,因此,危险因素接近于轻微危害程度,也称为少量危险型,降低危险因素的程度有限。

在个体评价中,我们还可以对某一种危险因素的严重程度进行进一步分析。例如,评价吸烟对健康影响的严重程度,我们可以计算在没有控制吸烟这个危险因素之前的评价年龄和控制这个危险因素之后的增长年龄,比较两者之间的差值,说明这种危险因素对个体预期寿命可能影响的程度。

危险因素对个体预期寿命影响的程度同样可以用改变危险因素后,危险因素降低的程度说明,例如表9-4中,被评价者听取医生建议,改变生活方式,总危险因素的降低程度为52.2%,冠心病的危险因素降低程度为47%,我们从危险因素降低程度这个指标可以看出生活方式这类危险因素对预期寿命的影响。

健康危险因素评价是预防慢性病的一种较为有效的方法,它可以在疾病尚未形成前评价危险因素对健康的影响,结果较为直观,人们易于接受,从而促进个人自觉改变或远离危险因素,促进自身健康水平的提高。

二、群体评价

群体评价是在个体评价的基础上进行的,一般可以进行以下几方面的分析。

(一)不同人群的危险程度

在个体评价中,根据实际年龄、评价年龄和增长年龄三者之间的关系将被评价者分为四种类型,即健康型、自创性危险因素类型、历史危险因素类型、少量危险型。在进行评价时,我们把健康型的个人归到健康组,把自创性和历史危险因素型归到危险组,把少量危险型归到一般组,这样我们就可以根据不同人群中各种类型的人所占比重来分析哪一种人群的危险水平高,以确定卫生防治重点。一般而言,某人群中危险组的人越多,这个人群的危险水平就越高。可以分析不同性别人群的危险水平(见表9-6),也可以分析不同职业、不同文化程度、不同经济状况人群的危险水平。从表9-6可以看出,上海市农村男性人群的危险水平远远高于女性,属于危险组的人占到近60%,应引起重视。

表9-6 上海市农村不同危险水平的人群构成

	男		女	
	人数	%	人数	%
危险组	40	59.70	3	30.75
一般组	24	35.82	17	21.25
健康组	3	4.48	60	75.00
合计	67	100.00	80	100.00

(二)危险因素的属性

大多数与人群疾病有关的危险因素属于行为生活方式方面,是人为因素造成的,也是可以人为控制的。可以计算生物遗传和疾病史等难以消除的危险因素与行为生活方面自创性危险因素之间的比例,分析健康教育或健康促进可能达到的预期效果。从表9-7可以看出成都市男性居民中生活方式方面的危险因素占的比重较大,而女性则主要是生物遗传疾病方面的,因此在成都市,男性应该是我们健康教育的重点。

表9-7 成都市不同性别人群危险因素的属性

	男		女	
	人数	%	人数	%
不易去除危险因素	15	13.51	78	70.27
可去除危险因素	96	86.49	33	29.73
合计	111	100.00	111	100.00

(三)单项危险因素对群体健康状况的影响

为了有针对性地制定预防措施,可以分析各种危险因素对群体健康的影响,看哪一种危险因素对当地人群影响最大,用危险程度来表示:危险程度=危险强度×危险频度,其中,危险强度为将各个体扣除某一项危险因素后所计算的增长年龄与评价年龄之差的均数,危险频度为这一单项危险因素在调查人群中所占的比重。从危险程度的计算公式中我们可以看出,单项危险因素对群体健康的影响,不仅与此项危险因素对个体影响的大小有关,还与它在人群中影响的范围有关。尽管有些因素虽然对个体影响很大,但在人群中的分布有限,它对整个人群来说影响并不严重。反之,有些因素对个体影响并不十分严重,但受其影响的人很多,它也值得注意。

例如表9-8中去除吸烟这一危险因素后,各个体的增长年龄与评价年龄之差的均数是1.74岁,而在被调查的人群中,吸烟者所占比重为85.07%,因而,吸烟的危险程度=1.74×85.07%=1.48岁。饮酒的危险强度是1.47岁,危险频度为41.49%,危险程度=1.47×41.49%=0.61岁,余类推,我们就可以得出吸烟较其他危险因素对人群的健康状况影响更大。

表9-8 单项危险因素对男性健康状况的影响

危险因素	危险强度(岁)	危险频度(%)	危险程度(岁)
吸　烟	1.74	85.07	1.48
饮　酒	1.47	41.49	0.61
接触农药	0.77	43.28	0.33
接触毒物	1.48	19.40	0.29
体重超重	0.23	16.42	0.04
肝　炎	0.28	8.96	0.03

总之,尽管健康危险因素评价目前有一定的局限性和缺点,如健康危险因素评价只注重生命数量而忽略了生命质量、评价所依据的完整的人口学资料和流行病学资料较难获得,目前一些疾病的危险因素还没有确定、有的危险因素很难定量化等,但是它仍然可以作为一种比较有效的预防疾病的技术,其方法简便易行,结果直观,有利于进行健康教育,对个体可以促使其改变不良行为和生活方式,对人群可以有针对性地倡导有利于健康的行为和生活方式,为消除各种危险因素提供科学依据。

练习题

调查某地41岁男性,其危险因素指标值见表9-9,请计算此人的评价年龄、增长年龄,评价此人的健康类型。

表9-9 某地41岁男性健康危险因素评价表

死亡原因	死亡概率 ($1/10^5$)	疾病诱发因素	指标值	危险分数	组合危险分数	存在死亡危险	根据医生建议改变危险因素	新危险分数	新组合危险分数	新存在死亡危险	降低量	危险降低程度百分数
肺癌	317	吸烟	20支/日	1.9			戒烟	1.7				
肝硬化	274	饮酒	6次/周	2.0			饮酒3次/周	1.2				
自杀	250	抑郁	无	1.0			—	1.0				
		家族史	无	1.0			—	1.0				
冠心病	1 355	血压	180/94 mmHg	2.2			血压<(140/88 mmHg)	0.8				
		胆固醇	220 mg/dL	1.0			—	1.0				
		糖尿病	无	1.0			—	1.0				
		体力活动	坐着工作,有定期锻炼	1.0			增加体力活动	1.0				
		家族史	无	0.9			—	0.9				
		吸烟	20支/日	1.5			戒烟	0.7				
		体重	增加15%	0.9			—	0.9				
车祸	255	饮酒	6次/周	2.0			饮酒3次/周	1.2				
		驾车里程	3 000 km/a					3.0				
		安全带使用情况	80%	0.8			100%	0.8				

(续表 9-9)

死亡原因	死亡概率 $(1/10^5)$	疾病诱发因素	指标值	危险分数	组合危险分数	存在死亡危险	根据医生建议改变危险因素	新危险分数	新组合危险分数	新存在死亡危险	降低量	危险降低程度百分数
脑血管病	142	高血压	180/94 mmHg	2.2			血压(140/88 mmHg)	0.8				
		胆固醇	220 mg/dL	1.0			—	1.0				
		糖尿病	无	1.0			—	1.0				
		吸烟	20 支/日	1.2			戒烟	1.0				
肠癌	78	肛门出血	有	3.0			—	3.0				
		息肉	无	1.0			—	1.0				
		肠炎	无	1.0			—	1.0				
		直肠镜检查	无	1.0			1 次/3 年	0.7				
肺炎	61	饮酒	6 次/周	3.0			饮酒 3 次/周	1.2				
		肺气肿	无	1.0			—	1.0				
		吸烟	20 支/日	1.3			戒烟	1.0				
其他				1.0			—	1.0				
合计	1 525											

Chapter 9   Health Risk Factors Appraisal

Section 1   Summary

    The technological method of Health Risk Factors Appraisal (HRFA) was developed in America in the 1960's and mainly studies the linear correlation of the conditional quantity and the rule between risk factors and the incidence of death due to chronic diseases. Basically the idea is to study the assumption that death probability is due to a person's living environment; that is, to study those risk factors that exist in people's work circumstances, life styles and health services, which have an effect on the incidence and development of disease, and as a result of the study, to prolong life through changing bad living and behavior habits which in turn will decrease or eliminate some changeable risk factors. The main purpose of the method is to decrease the incidence of diseases and improve a person's health level through health education or consulting, and to help them to avoid risk factors by changing work and livelihood circumstances and bad behaviors.

    The growth and development of HRFA is connected with the transition of diseases spectra, medicine model and people's views on health with the increasing requirement of prevention and health care services, etc.

    The infectious diseases of the 1960's that so seriously endangered health were controlled gradually throughout the world by vaccination, eradicating pathogens & killing parasites, and with antibiotics. Chronic diseases have become, step by step, the leading death-causation of man. Chronic diseases usually are continuous and are so hard to cure that the caused disability rate and death rate are very high, which not only affect the individual's life quality, but also cause the perennial consumption of health care resources, so it is most important to prevent and control all chronic diseases. In America during the 1920's chronic non-infectious diseases became the main reason for the high mortality rate and was higher than the rate for infectious diseases. In 1900, the mortality rate of infectious diseases was 650 per 100,000 people, and in 1970 declined by 97% over 70 years to 20 per 100,000 people, while chronic non-infectious disease rate was 350 per 100,000 people in 1900 and 690 per 100,000 people in 1970, an increase of 97 percent. In our country during the 1950's, diseases such as smallpox, plague, typical cholera, etc., were eliminated and nearly eradicated. The incidence rate of the rapid infectious diseases in 1948 was 20,000 per 100,000 and 800 per 100,000 in 1985, a decrease of 96 percent.

In the mid-1950's and early period of 1960, in the cities and rural areas of China, chronic diseases became the main cause of death due to the fact that the chronic disease mortality rate was higher than the infectious disease mortality rate. According to the results of the National Health Services Investigation in 1998, each of the five main causes of death of our national cities and rural dwellers was chronic non-infectious diseases. We could find this rule from the change of national death spectra (the five main causes of death).

Table 9-1 **The death spectra of our country in recent years**

Year	The Five Main Causes of Death				
1957	The respiratory system diseases	Infectious diseases	The digestive system diseases	Cardiac diseases	Cerebrovascular diseases
1963	The respiratory system diseases	Infectious diseases	Malignant tumors	Cerebrovascular diseases	Cardiac diseases
1975	Cerebrovascular diseases	Cardiac diseases	Malignant tumors	The respiratory system diseases	Infectious diseases
1985	Cardiac diseases	Cerebrovascular diseases	Malignant tumors	The respiratory system diseases	The digestive system diseases
2000	Malignant tumors	Cerebrovascular diseases	Cardiac diseases	The digestive system diseases	Injury and poison
2002	Malignant tumors	Cerebrovascular diseases	The respiratory system diseases	Cardiac diseases	Injury and poison

Chronic non-infectious diseases are caused by a variety of risk factors that influence the individual over all time. After World War II, many countries spent much and used a large number of people to undertake the study, control and cure of diseases. From these long-term efforts, there was gratifying progress in the study of etiology and epidemiology of chronic non-infectious diseases, such as the incidence of coronary heart disease. According to six prospective investigation results in America, the four factors of corpulence, high cholesterol, hypertension and smoking were so important that the probability of people being infected with coronary heart disease with these four factors is forty times greater than for people without the four factors. The incidence of malignant tumors is related with lifestyle, spirit conditions, environment and occupation. Thus, chronic disease must be controlled by synthetic methods. The HFRA came into being as a result of this background knowledge.

The growth of HFRA is due to L. Robbins who developed the mortality rate tables through studying and analyzing the death causation data of ten years at Temple University. However, in that study, risk factors were not quantified but were expressed by general descriptions. Prior to 1967 most of the definitive risk factors related with diseases were quantified by those specialists who joined in the investigation of tumors and disease of the heart and blood vessels on the grounds of the evidence of anterior prospective study on cardiac heart diseases by Framingham. In 1970, L. Robbins and J. H. Hall released the article *How to Practice Prospective Medicine*, which discussed systematically the principles and methods to study quantitatively the main death causation probability according to the degrees of risk factors, and provided the theoretical basis for the development of HFRA.

In the mid-1970's many other scholars quantified the health risk factors and transformed them to risk scores. Bio-statistician H. Geller and health-insurances N. Gesner took advantage of a variety of analysis methods such as direct scoring and multi-variable regression analysis to transform the risk factors to risk scores that made up the Geller-Genre table, in terms of the intense degree of correlation between the risk factors and corresponding chronic diseases, and the impact on them, and thus matured the methods of HFRA.

Section 2 The Evolving Process of Health Risk Factors and Chronic Diseases

1. Health risk factors

The health risk factors mentioned in HRFA are the inducing factors related to the happening, development and death of chronic diseases that exist both inside and outside the organisms. The occurrence, development and ultimate result of chronic non-contagious diseases are closely related to social environmental factors, behavior factors, biological heredity factors and medical health service factors. By appraising these health risk factors we can predict health conditions and genetic probability of many diseases and thus can better prevent and control chronic non-contagious disease.

(1) Environmental risk factors

①Natural environmental risk factors

These include biological risk factors, and physical and chemical factors. Biological risk factors include germs, viruses, parasites and biological toxins. Physical and chemical factors include various kinds of noise, vibration, electrical radiation, computers, electric and magnetic radiation from many intricate apparatus, productive toxins, dust, exhaust from transportation vehicles, pesticides and the wastes poured into the rivers, etc.

②Social environmental risk factors

Economic income, nutritional conditions, level of education and social systems all play an important part in the health condition of the public. Their relations with health have been discussed in passage "Environment and Health".

(2) Behavior risk factors

Behavior risk factors are risk factors resulting from the different lifestyles that people choose and are also called self-created risk factors. According to statistics, the four death reasons listed at the top are heart disease, cancer, brain and blood vessel diseases, and accidental injuries whose resulting deaths cover 70% of all the deaths while these four diseases are closely related to lifestyles. Risk factors like smoking, alcoholism, lack of exercise, prolonged sitting and irrational dieting habits do great harm to people's health.

(3) Biological heredity risk factors

Some diseases like chain-liked erythrocyte anemia, fauvism, haemophilia, all have much to do with heredity. Biological heredity risk factors are traditional risk factors. With the development of medical scientific technology it may be possible in the near future for genetic technology to control hereditary substances and thus control the occurrence and development of some hereditary diseases.

(4) Risk factors in medical health services

Medical health services directly influence the health level of the public, such as medical quality, mistreatment and lack of treatment, hospital cross infection, reasonable arrangement of medical service resources, level of hygiene, service networks and equipment of personnel resources, etc. At present due to the irrational equipment of resources, hygiene resources mainly concentrate in some big cities, while in the countryside and remote areas the low quality of medical staff and lack of medical resources contribute to inferior health conditions for countryside residents.

2. Characteristics of health risk factors

(1) Long incubation period

Long incubation period means that, unlike some contagious diseases, people catch diseases through repeatedly contacting these risk factors, while incubation period differs from person to person. For example, expressway drivers working at night in Japan usually begin to have the symptoms of blood vessel systems after 20 years while smokers with long smoking histories often catch lung cancers after 10 years. The irregularity of incubation period makes the relationship between risk factors and diseases uncertain and makes it easy for people to ignore this relationship, but at the same time provides enough time for medical intervention.

(2) Obviousness of cross effects

When many risk factors co-exist, a coalition effect may take place and the risk of catching some kind of disease may be enhanced. For example, it is reported there is a coalition effect between asbestos and smoking on lung cancer. The mortality ratio is 1.0

between no smoking and no asbestos contacting person. The mortality ratio between no smoking and asbestos contacting is 5.17, and it is 10.85 between no asbestos contacting and smoking, while the mortality ratio is 53.24 between smoking and asbestos contacting people.

(3) Feeble peculiarity

The relationship between risk factor and disease, such as single reason-many results, many reasons-single result and many reasons-many results, makes the effect of risk factors lack of peculiarity. For example, the lack of exercise is a dangerous factor to cardiac heart disease, while smoking and weight are both risk factors. Smoking is a risk factor to lung cancer and is also the risk factor to heart and brain blood vessel system diseases and peptic ulcer.

Because of their long incubation period and feeble peculiarity, it is easy for people to neglect their risk factors.

(4) Wide existence

Risk factors widely exist in people's daily lives. Social environmental factors, behavioral life factors and medical service factors are closely related to people's lives. Due to their wide existence it is easy for people to neglect them. We need to have wide health education and health propaganda, so that people can voluntarily distance themselves from these risk factors and enhance their health level.

3. Evolution progress of chronic disease

With the development of medical science technology, people have certain knowledge about the evolution progress of chronic disease. This is advantageous in prevention and cure. According to the advice of Robbins and Hall, the natural process of chronic disease can be divided into six phases:

(1) No risk phase

In this phase no risk factors exist in people's surrounding and behavioral living styles; we can prevent the advent of risk factors by maintaining better living styles and choosing good natural and social surroundings.

(2) Advent of risk factors

With the change of surroundings and the advent of age, the risk factors in procreation and living surrounding in the short term there is no conspicuous hazard observed or people are not aware of a hazard. In this period, we need investigate behaviors such as living styles or surveillance of surrounding factor.

(3) Appearance of pathogenic factors

Risk factors can be changed into pathogenic factors with the augment of quantity and longer action time and the appearance of hazard action. The disease cannot come into being for the body's defensive system and lower level of pathogenic factors.

(4) Appearance of symptoms of disease

When the disease has come into being and symptoms appear the reversible conformation damage is formed, we can observe these abnormal diversifications with physiological and biological diagnostic methods. In this period we can use screening methods to detect the non-symptom patients early from the normal cohort to achieve the aim of early detection and cure.

(5) Appearance of syndrome

Symptoms and syndrome may or may not appear at the same time. The patients will come to see a doctor for the disability of conformation and function. It is not easy to change the disease progress even though the risk factors are eliminated.

(6) Loss of manpower

This is the last period in the development of chronic disease, which will exacerbate symptoms, and the development of the disease affects the ability of living and working. Rehabilitation is the main method of medical intervention in this period.

Health risk appraisal begins from the first period of chronic disease, that is, steps are taken when the disease has not come into being, through the appraisal of risk factors on health. Educated people have a better behavior living style, far from risk factors. Before the risk factor's advent, through HRFA, calculating the possible danger, forecasting the incidence rate, so we can achieve the effectiveness of prevention and control of chronic disease in the early stages. Health risk factor appraisal therefore is an available method of prevention of chronic disease from an analysis of the natural history of the disease.

Section 3 The Calculation Stages of HRFA

1. Collection of data

(1) Collecting the data of the incidence and mortality rate of different age\sex\disease

Local data of the prevalence rate and mortality rate can be obtained through Register report and surveillance of disease and investigation and death causation registration. In the health risk factor appraisal, we will use the data of mortality probability; we can change mortality rate and death probability into each other through statistic formula. Here, the death probability we mentioned indicates is ten years death probability.

In general, we choose the severe disease that endangers local people's health, namely the 10 – 15 percentile death causation which is as our study target. This can be determined only when we finish collecting the local data of different age/sex/disease. At the same time, we should ensure the disease we need is a specific, not a species or a system. For example, in health risk factor appraisal, we can collect the data of lung cancer and should not collect the data of incidence rate mortality rate related to lung cancer. Because the risk factors of a species are easy to determine, however, a kind of disease is composed of many diseases, its risk factors are so complex and difficult to determine, this kind of characteristic can affect our risk factor appraisal.

(2) Collecting data of risk factors

We can think of the risk factors data we need to collect from four aspects that affect health and disease:

①Environmental factors, such as economic income, living condition, family relationships, working environment, mental stimulation, etc.

②Behavior and life styles, such as smoking, drinking, physical activity, etc.

③Biological factors, such as age, gender, race, height, weight, hereditary diseases, etc.

④Health services, such as whether a person comes to have a health examination, proctoscope examination, vagina smear test termly, etc.

Illness history should investigate illness history, marriage and procreation history, family disease history, etc.

At present the relationship between the following disease and risk factors is clear:

Table 9-2 Relationship between diseases and risk factors

Disease	Risk Factors
Coronary heart disease	contraction pressure, diastole pressure, diabetes history, physical activity, weight, content of cholesterin in serum, family heredity history
lung cancer	smoking, the amount of smoking, the smoking time, the age began smoking
galactophore tumor	age, family history, lactation history, the regimentation of whether or not regularly checking breast lump by oneself
womb neck tumor	age, social economic condition, marriage and the initial age of sex life, procreated fetus number, whether or not have the vaginal picture examination regularly
womb body tumor	Ill-defined causation, irregular blood shed from vagina
intestine tumor	intestinal polyps, intestinal haemorrhage, ulcer of intestinal inside and intestinia, whether or not have proctoscope examination regularly, whether or not have history of infecting schistosome
stomach and esophagus tumor	low stomach acid, whether or not examine regularly the stomach liquid and barium meal
chronic rheumatic heart disease	heart cacophony, rheumatic fever and related symptom and syndrome

(Table 9-2)

Disease	Risk Factors
hepatocirrhosis	libation history(drinking amount, libation time, types of libation), hepatitis history and infectious history of schistosomiasis
diabetes	weight, family history, hypertension, cholesterin in serum
emphysema	smoking, chronic tracheitis
Cerebrovascular diseases	hypertension, diabetes, high cholesterin, smoking, nervousness and anxiety
traffic accident	driving after drinking, history of taking excitant and ataraxic, average driving miles, usage of safety belt
suicide	the amount of drinking, family history, oppression, nervous emotion
other incident injury	drinking, out working, criminal record, criminal tools preparation, drug abuse, nervousness, contradiction and conflict and the intense change of social economic condition

The data can be obtained through inquiry and questionnaire which is completed by the individual; collect information on behaviour and life style\environment risk factors and health services risk factors, which is also available through inquiry on illness history, medical examination and laboratory examination, etc.

2. Analysis of data

(1) Transform risk factors into risk scores

We can carry out quantitative analysis on risk factors only when we change risk factors into risk scores, by this transform qualitative data into quantitative data. When the risk factor is equal to the local average level, we define the risk score is 1.0, that is to say, when the risk score is 1.0, the death probability of an individual for some disease is equal to the local average level. When risk score is greater than 1.0, the mortality probability of an individual for some disease is over the local average level, and the opposite is also correct. That is, the higher the risk scores, the more likely the death probability of an individual. The quantitative dependence relationship between risk factors and death probability can be implement by the risk scores transforming.

Two methods of risk score transformation:

①multiple regression analysis

According to the function relationship between risk factor and death probability and based on the research finding of a mass of etiology and epidemiology, this method uses mathematical formulae to express the quantity relationship between the degree of risk factor and death probability.

②adopting experience evaluation

To invite a specialist; announcing the different score of severe degree of risk factors according to the investigation result of prospective or historical death reason for estimating the close degree between the risk factor and death probability. When we carry out this sort of work, we often take the Geller-Genre table as a reference, for there is not a table of risk score transition that is fit for the concrete situation. At present, when there is a calculation we often adopt the Geller-Genre risk score transition table or make some propriety modification on the table on the basis of our country's concrete situation. Table 9-1 shows part of the males' transition between risk factors and risk scores. When we compare tables we can choose the two neighboring indices to assess if the risk score can't be found on the table, or use interpolation to calculate the figure. For example, if cholesterine is 192 mg, according to table 9-3, there isn't a corresponding figure to the 192 mg in the risk factor transition table of 40 - 44 year-old males. So we can use interpolation to calculate the risk score of 192 mg compared to the score of 1.0 and 0.5 of 220 mg and 180 mg.

Attention: we consider the blood pressure as contraction and diastole pressure respectively. If there is one or two risk scores equal or less than 1.0, then neglect the lower one, only use the higher as the risk score of blood pressure no longer to divide two parts to record. For example, if the value of a person's blood pressure is 16.0/9.3 kPa, from the table 9-3 that is risk score transition, we can see, the risk score of 16.0 kPa is 0.4, while 9.3 kPa is less than 0.4, so the risk score for blood pressure is 0.4.

Table 9-3 Geller-Gesner risk score transition table (male, part age group: 40 - 44 years)

Death reason	Risk index	Measurement value	Risk score
Cardiac heart disease	Contraction pressure kPa (mmHg)	26.6(200)	3.2
		23.9(180)	2.2
		21.3(160)	1.2
		18.6(140)	0.8
		16.0(120)	0.4
	Diastole kPa (mmHg)	14.1(106)	3.7
		13.3(100)	2.0
		12.5(94)	1.3
		11.7(88)	0.8
		10.9(82)	0.4
	Cholesterine(mg/dL)	280	1.5
		220	1.0
		180	0.5
	Diabetes history	Yes	3.0
		Under control	2.5
		No	1.0

(Table 9-3)

Death reason	Risk index	Measurement value	Risk score
	Exercise situation	Seated working and amusement	2.5
		A little activity work	1.0
		Middling degree training	0.6
		More intense training	0.5
		seated working, regular excises	1.0
		other job, regular excises	0.5
	Family history	Parents both die of Coronary heart disease before 60 years old	1.4
		One of parents die of Coronary heart disease before 60 years old	1.2
		parents being still living and in good health (less than sixty years old)	1.0
		parents being still living and in good health (more than or equal to sixty years old)	0.9
	Smoking	More than or equal to 10 pieces per day	1.5
		Less than 10 pieces per day	1.1
		Cigar or tobacco pipe	1.0
		give up smoking (less than 10 years)	0.7
		No smoking or smoking more than ten years	0.5
	Weight	Overweight 75 percent	2.5
		Overweight 50 percent	1.5
		Overweight 15 percent	1.0
		Overweight less than 10 percent	0.8
		Decline to average weight	1.0
Traffic accident	Drinking	Social affairs frequently without abstinence obviously	5.0
		Social affairs frequently with slight abstinence	2.0
		Moderate and occasional social affairs	1.0
		No drinking	0.5
	Usage of safety belt	Less than 10 percent of all the driving time	1.1
		From 10 percent to 24 percent	1.0
		From 25 percent to 74 percent	0.9
		From 75 percent to 100 percent	0.8

(Table 9-3)

Death reason	Risk index	Measurement value	Risk score
	Drive mileage	Drive mileage per year per 10,000 =risk score	
Suicide	Blues	Often	2.5
		Occasionally or never	1.0
	Family history	Yes	2.5
		No	1.0
Hepatocir-rhosis	Drinking	Tipple	12.5
		Social affairs frequently without abstinence obviously	5.0
		Social affairs frequently with slight abstinence	2.0
		Moderate and occasional social affairs	1.0
		Scintilla social affairs	0.2
		Abstinence before the emergency of symptom	0.2
		Not drinking	0.1
Cerebrovascular diseases	Contraction pressure kPa (mmHg)	26.6(200)	3.2
		23.9(180)	2.2
		21.3(160)	1.2
		18.6(140)	0.8
		16.0(120)	0.4
	Diastole kPa (mmHg)	14.1(106)	3.7
		13.3(100)	2.0
		12.5(94)	1.3
		11.7(88)	0.8
		10.9(82)	0.4
	Cholesterine(mg/dL)	280	1.5
		220	1.0
		180	0.5
	Diabetes history	Yes	3.0
		Under control	2.5
		No	1.0
	Smoking	Cigarette	1.2
		Cigar and tobacco pipe	1.0
		Giving up smoking	1.0
		No smoking	0.8
Lung cancer	Smoking	40 pieces per day	2.0
		20 pieces per day	1.5
		10 pieces per day	1.1
		Less than 10 pieces per day	0.8
		No smoking	0.2

(Table 9-3)

Death reason	Risk index	Measurement value	Risk score
	Cigar and tobacco pipe	Not less than 5 times per day and inhale	1.0
		Less than 5 times per day and no inhale	0.3
		Giving up smoking	Subtracted 0.2 from original risk scores, and subtracted the product of no-smoking years and 0.1, but the risk score not less than 0.2
Chronic rheumatic heart disease	Heart cacophony	Yes	1.0
		Medicine used	10.0
		No	1.0
	Rheumatic fever	Yes	10.0
		Medicine used	1.0
		No	1.0
	Symptom or syndrome	No	1.0
Pneumonia	Drinking	Frequent social affairs	3.0
		Moderate or never drinking	1.0
	Emphysema	Yes	2.0
		No	1.0
	Smoking	Not less than ten pieces	1.2
		No	1.0
Intestine tumor	Intestinal polyps	Yes	2.5
		No	1.0
	Anus haemorrhage without defined causations	Yes	3.0
		No	1.0
	Colonitis with ulcer	$\geqslant$10 years	4.0
		$<$10 years	2.0
		No	1.0
	Proctoscope examination per year	No	1.0
		Yes	0.3
Stomach and esophagus tumor	Low stomach acid	Yes	2.0
		Taking medicine per year	1.5
		No	1.0
Hypertension heart disease	Contraction pressure kPa (mmHg)	26.6(200)	3.2
		23.9(180)	2.2
		21.3(160)	1.2
		18.6(140)	0.8

Chapter 9 Health Risk Factors Appraisal

(Table 9-3)

Death reason	Risk index	Measurement value	Risk score
	Diastole pressure kPa (mmHg)	16.0(120)	0.4
		14.1(106)	3.7
		13.3(100)	2.0
		12.5(94)	1.3
		11.7(88)	1.3
		10.9(82)	0.4
	Weight	Overweight 75 percent	2.5
		Overweight 50 percent	1.5
		Overweight 15 percent	1.0
		Overweight less than 10 percent	0.8
		Declined to average weight	1.0
Tuberculosis	X-ray examine	No	1.0
		Negative	0.2
	Active	Yes	5.0
		No	1.0

The whole tabulation is classified by 5 years and gender, and 10 – 15 group of transform of risk score was ticked off among main diseases.

(2) Calculating the combined risk score

As mentioned above the pathogenic ability will be amplified for many risk factors to play a role to one disease at the same time. So we must calculate the united risk score when many kinds of risk factors coexist.

When calculating united risk score, we should pay more attention to the following aspects:

1) When only one risk factor is related to disease, the united score is the score of single risk factor. For example, when smoking is the single risk factor; also the united risk score to lung cancer namely is the single risk score of smoking.

2) When many risk factors are related to disease, the process of calculating the united risk score is:

①to add all the risk score which over 1.0 subtract 1.0, and 1.0 as the multiplier item.

②the risk score which less than or equal to 1.0 be the multiplier item.

③to add the results of the added one and the multiplier one, then we get the united risk score of this disease.

In table 9-4, for example, the united risk score of cardiac heart disease is calculated as follows:

①added item: the items over 1.0 are physical activity and weight, risk scores are 2.5 and 1.3 respectively, then the added one is $[(2.5-1.0)+(1.3-1.0)]\times 1.0=1.8$.

②multiplier item: the items less than or equal to 1.0 is blood pressure, cholesterine, diabetes history, family history, smoking, risk scores are 0.4, 0.6, 1.0, 0.9 and 0.5, then the multiplier one is $0.4 \times 0.6 \times 1.0 \times 0.9 \times 0.5 = 0.108$.

③the united risk score is $[(2.5-1.0)+(1.3-1.0)] \times 1.0 + 0.4 \times 0.6 \times 1.0 \times 0.9 \times 0.5 = 1.91$.

The united risk score is the result of multiplier item if there is no item over 1.0, also if there is no one under or equal to 1.0, the united risk score is the result of added item.

(3) Existence perish danger

Existence perish danger is used to demonstrate risk degree of some kind of disease that may happen when there is single or many risk scores existing.

Calculation formula: existence perish danger = death probability of different disease × united risk score of this disease.

In table 9-4, take cardiac heart disease as an example, the existence perish danger of 40 – 44-year-old of male is $1,877/100,000 \times 1.91 = 3,585/100,000$.

In table 9-4, it lists 11 kinds of main diseases with definite risk factors are illustrated, and all the other belong to another group; because there is no definite risk factor that can be appraised, the united risk score of the other diseases is indicated as 1.0, namely using the average death probability to indicate the death probability of the other group.

(4) Calculating appraisal age

Appraisal age is the age deduced from the death probability level according to the functional relationship between age and death probability. Among people that are 15 years old and above there is a positive correlation between age and death probability. The group among 10 to 14 years old have the lowest death probability; and among people below 10 years there is a negative correlation between age and death probability. Therefore, among the people that are 15 years old and above, we can conclude that the higher a person's appraisal age, the larger the existence of death risk, that is, heath conditions become worse.

The method to calculate appraisal age: Add all the existing death risks of various death reasons to get the whole death risk rate. Compare the whole existence death risk rate with the appraisal age table and get the appraisal age rate. Table three is the table for health appraisal age.

The left column of the table is the male's accumulated existence death risk value; the right column is the female's accumulated existence death risk value. The line of numbers above the middle part is the ending numbers of individual actual ages and the main part is the appraisal age value. As shown in table two, the whole existence death risk of 41-year-old males is $7,167.45/100,000$. According to the appraisal age table, the value on the left column of the table is between 6,830 and 7,570. The appraisal age for 6,830 is 41, and 42 is the appraisal age for 7,570. In this way we can conclude the male's appraisal age is 43.5.

(5) Calculating achievable age

Achievable age is the anticipated age after the risk factors are reduced. It is the new anticipated existence death risk after the reducing the possible risk factors according to the existing risk factors calculated in the same way as the appraisal age.

Among the risk factors some are hard to change, such as disease history, family history, etc. and some are changeable, such as factors related to life habits, behavior, and the use of health services, etc. Doctors can expound certain proposals according to the level of the existing changeable risk factors of the appraised object, and then the appraised object can change the level of his original risk factor after accepting the proposals. Therefore we can get a new risk score from the table for the transformed risk scores. In table 9-4, for example, cardiac heart disease risk factor for "physical activities" is sitting work, and its risk score is 2.5. After the person accepts the regular exercises proposed by the doctor, his risk level is greatly reduced and the new risk score is 1.0. According to the new risk scores, we can get the new united risk score and also the new existing death risks. Comparing the accumulated rate of the new existing risk factors to the table for appraisal age we can get the achievable age.

In table 9-4 the new existence death risk is 3,430.45/100,000, and the achievable age from the table is 36.

(6) Calculating reduced level of risk factors

Reduced level of risk factors is the level of risk factors reduced after the object accepts the doctor's proposals, and the reduced percentile of the existence death factors indicates that.

Calculating method: (the existence death risk of any death reason before accepting the doctor's proposal — the new existence death risk after accepting the doctor's proposal)/original whole existence death risk.

For example, in the items of suicide of table 9-4, the reduced level of depression risk factors=(660.0−396.0)/7,167.45×100%=4%.

Table 9-4 a man's HFRA table in an area

Death Causation	Mortality probability ($\times 10^{-5}$)	Malady's risk factors	Index value	Risk score	Fixed risk score	Existing death risks	Changing the risk factors according to the doctor	New risk score	New fixed risk score	New existing death risks	The declined amount	Declined percent of the risk
Lung cancer	202	Smoking	No	0.2	0.2	40.4	—	0.2	0.2	40.4	0	0
Hepatocirrhosis	222	Libation	No	0.1	0.1	22.2	—	0.1	0.1	22.2	0	0
Traffic accident	285	Libation	No	0.5			—	0.5				
		Drive mileage	25,000km	2.5	1.9	541.5	—	2.5	1.9	541.5	0	0
		Usage of safety belt	90%	0.8			100%	0.8				
Suicide	264	Blues	Often	2.5			Treatment of blues	1.5				
		Family	No	1.0	2.5	660.0	—	1.0	1.5	396.0	264.0	4%
Cardiac heart disease	2,517	Blood pressure (kPa)	16.0/9.3	0.4			—	0.4				
		Cholesterine	192	0.6			—	0.6				
		Diabetes history	No	1.0			—	1.0				
		Stamina activity	Sitting work	2.5	1.91	3,538.07	Exercise regularly	1.0	0.11	206.47	3,378.6	47%
		Family history	No	0.5			—	0.5				
		Smoking	No	1.3			—	1.0				
		Weight	Overweight 30 percent				Declined to average weight					
Brain vessel disease	222	Blood pressure (kPa)	16.0/9.3	0.4			—	0.4				
		Cholesterine	192	0.2			—	0.2				
		Diabetes history	No	1.0	0.19	42.18	—	1.0	0.19	42.18	0	0
		Smoking	No	0.8			—	0.8				

(Table 9-4)

Death Causation	Mortality probability ($\times 10^{-5}$)	Malady's risk factors	Index value	Risk score	Fixed risk score	Existing death risks	Changing the risk factors according to the doctor	New risk score	New fixed risk score	New existing death risks	The declined amount	Declined percent of the risk
Chronic rheumatic heart disease	167	Heart cacophony	No	1.0				1.0				
		Rheumatic fever	No	1.0				1.0				
		Symptom & syndrome	No	0.1	0.1	16.7	0.1	0.1	16.7	0	0	0
Pneumonia	111	Libation	No	1.0				1.0				
		Emphysema	No	1.0	1.0	111.0		1.0	1.0	111.0	0	0
		Smoking	No	1.0				1.0				
Intestine tumor	111	Intestine polyps	No	1.0				1.0				
		Haemorrhage from anus	No	1.0				1.0				
		Intestinia	No	1.0	1.0	111.0		1.0	0.3	33.3	77.7	
		Proctoscope exam	No	1.0				0.3				
Hypertension heart disease	56	Blood pressure (kPa)	16.6/9.3	0.4	0.7	39.2	Declined to average weight	0.4	0.4	22.4	16.8	0.2%
		Weight	Overweight 30 percent	1.3				1.0				
Tuberculosis	56	X-ray exam	Negative	0.2				0.2				
		Active	No	1.0				0.2				
		Economic and social status	middle	1.0	0.2	11.2		1.0	0.2	11.2	0	0
Other	1,987			1.0	1,987			1.0	1.0	1,987	0	0
Total	5,560			—	7,167.450			—	—	3,430.35	3,737.1	52.2%

Table 9-5 Health Appraisal Age

Male's existed death risk	The last number of the real age					Female's existed death risk	Male's existed death risk	The last number of the real age					Female's existed death risk
	0	1	2	3	4			0	1	2	3	4	
	5	6	7	8	9			5	6	7	8	9	
530	5	6	7	8	9	350	4,510	38	39	40	41	42	2,550
570	6	7	8	9	10	350	5,010	39	40	41	42	43	2,780
630	7	8	9	10	11	350	5,560	40	41	42	43	44	3,020
710	8	9	10	11	12	360	6,160	41	42	43	44	45	3,280
790	9	10	11	12	13	380	6,830	42	43	44	45	46	3,560
880	10	11	12	13	14	410	7,570	43	44	45	46	47	3,870
990	11	12	13	14	15	430	8,380	44	45	46	47	48	4,220
1,110	12	13	14	15	16	460	9,260	45	46	47	48	49	4,600
1,230	13	14	15	16	17	490	10,190	46	47	48	49	50	5,000
1,350	14	15	16	17	18	520	11,160	47	48	49	50	51	5,420
1,440	15	16	17	18	19	550	12,170	48	49	50	51	52	5,860
1,500	16	17	18	19	20	570	13,230	49	50	51	52	53	6,330
1,540	17	18	19	20	21	600	14,340	50	51	52	53	54	6,850
1,560	18	19	20	21	22	620	15,330	51	52	53	54	55	7,440
1,570	19	20	21	22	23	640	16,260	52	53	54	55	56	8,110
1,580	20	21	22	23	24	660	16,830	53	54	55	56	57	8,870
1,590	21	22	23	24	25	690	19,820	54	55	56	57	58	9,730
1,590	22	23	24	25	26	720	21,490	55	56	57	58	59	10,680
1,590	23	24	25	26	27	750	23,260	56	57	58	59	60	11,720
1,600	24	25	26	27	28	790	25,140	57	58	59	60	61	12,860
1,620	25	26	27	28	29	840	27,120	58	59	60	61	62	14,100
1,660	26	27	28	29	30	900	29,210	59	60	61	62	63	15,450
1,730	27	28	29	30	31	970	31,420	60	61	62	63	64	16,930
1,830	28	29	30	31	32	1040	33,760	61	62	63	64	65	18,560
1,960	29	30	31	32	33	1,130	36,220	62	63	64	65	66	20,360
2,120	30	31	32	33	34	1,220	38,810	63	64	65	66	67	22,340
2,310	31	32	33	34	35	1,330	41,540	64	65	66	67	68	24,520
2,520	32	33	34	35	36	1460	44,410	65	66	67	68	69	26,920
2,760	33	34	35	36	37	1,600	47,440	66	67	68	69	70	29,560
3,030	34	35	36	37	38	1760	50,650	67	68	69	70	71	32,470
3,330	35	36	37	38	39	1,930	54,070	68	69	70	71	72	35,690
3,670	36	37	38	39	40	2,120	57,720	69	70	71	72	73	39,250
4,060	37	38	39	40	41	2,330	61,640	70	71	72	73	74	43,200

Section 4 Health Risk Factors Appraisal

The HFRA can be applied to the evaluation of individual and the community.

The outcome of the individual evaluation can be used as the theoretical basis of health education and can urge the individual to keep off the risk factors self-consciously on his own and ensure the improving of health level. The outcome of the community evaluation can help us understand the different distributions of different types of risk factors in the population and then make sure the emphasis of work on disease prevention and cure of the certain different population.

1. Individual evaluation

The individual evaluation primarily indicates that by comparing the gap of actual age, evaluation age and growth age we can know to what possible degree risk factor affects life span and the probable years life span can be prolonged after we lower the risk factor and determine this person's health type.

If evaluation age is higher than actual age, it shows the risk factor of this person is higher than average level, namely, his death probability is higher than the average level of the local ground of an age and sex. Whereas, if the risk factor of this person is lower than average level, it indicates that his death probability is lower than the average level of the local ground of an age and sex. The difference between growth age and evaluation age means the probable years the life span of this person can be prolonged after he accepts the suggestion of the doctor to lower the risk factor.

According to the value of actual age, evaluation age and growth age, we can classify individual evaluation into four types as follows:

(1) Health type

Characteristics: The one who is evaluated has lower evaluation age than actual age.

For example, a person, with actual age, 47 years, and evaluation age, 43 years, belongs to the healthy type, namely the 47-year-old individual may experience the same death process of the 43-year-old person. There is some but just a little possibility to further lower the risk factor.

(2) Self-created risk factors type

Characteristics: The one who is evaluated has a higher evaluation age than actual age and the large difference between evaluation age and growth age.

For example, a person, with actual age, 41 years, evaluation age, 45 years, and growth age, 36 years, belongs to this type. That evaluation age is higher than actual age indicates his risk factor is higher than average level; the large difference between evaluation age and growth age explains that these risk factors primarily come from his private lifestyle, which is also called the self-created risk factor, and that we can prolong the expected life if we adopt the doctor's suggestion.

(3) The type of difficulty in changing risk factor (also called the type of historical risk factor)

Characteristics: The one who is evaluated has a higher evaluation age than actual age and the relatively lower difference between evaluation age and growth age.

For example, a person, with actual age, 41 years, evaluation age, 47 years, and growth age, 46 years, belongs to the type of difficulty in changing risk factor (also called the type of historical risk factor). The difference between evaluation age and growth age is only 1 year. This type indicates that the risk factor of individual originates from the inherent cause of living creature and former and current medical history and hardly change. So there is little possibility to lower it and the expected life can be only prolonged a little.

(4) The type of general dangerous (also called the type of a little amount of danger)

Characteristics: The one who is evaluated has evaluation age close to actual age, and growth age close to evaluation age.

This person's death rate, or expected death process is similar to the local average level. Therefore, the risk factor facing him is near the slight harm degree, and we have the limited degree to which we lower the risk factor.

In the process of the individual evaluation, we can also further analyze the serious degree of a certain risk factor. For example, taking our evaluation on the serious degree of smoking cigarette's affection on health, we can compute the evaluation age before we control smoke and the growth age after we control smoke and then by comparing them explain the probable influence of this kind of risk factor on individual's expected life.

The probable influence of risk factor on individual's expected life can also be explained by the lowed degree of risk factor after we change it. We can see in table 9-4 that after the person who is evaluated changes his lifestyle on doctor's suggestion, his degree of total risk factor is down to 52.2 percent, the risk degree of coronary heart disease down to 47 percent, from which we can make out the influence of this kind of risk factor, life style, on expected life.

The evaluation of risk factor on health is an effective method to prevent chronic disease, through which we can evaluate the influence of risk factor on health before the disease comes out. Owing to its relatively visual outcome, it is easy for people to accept it, and with it we can urge the individual to change or keep off the risk factor on his own to ensure his increase of health level.

2. Community evaluation

Community evaluation is conducted on the basis of the individual evaluation and generally includes the analysis of several aspects as follows:

(1) Degree of risk of different groups

In the process of the individual evaluation, according to the relation of actual age, evaluation age and growth age, we can divide the evaluation into four category types, namely, health type, the type of self-created risk factor, the type of historical risk factor and the type of a little amount of danger. In evaluating, we make those belonging to the health type come under the healthy group, those belonging to the type of self-created and historical risk factor under the danger group, and those belonging to the type of a little amount of danger under the average group. Thus according to the specific weight of different group accounting for in different crowd, we can analyze which kind of crowds possess a relatively high level of risk so as to place the emphasis of the work on prevention and cure. Generally speaking, the very group including the larger amount of dangerous group holds the higher dangerous level. By this way, we can analyze the dangerous level (see table 9-6) of different sex, and also of different occupation, culture degree and economic condition crowd. From table 9-6, we can see that the dangerous level of rural mankind group in Shanghai was far higher than that of womankind group, and that those belonging to the dangerous group near up to 60 percent, which should draw our attention.

Table 9-6 the crowd composition of different dangerous level in the rural of Shanghai City

	Male		Female	
	Quantity	Per cent	Quantity	Per cent
Dangerous group	40	59.70	3	30.75
Average group	24	35.82	17	21.25
Health group	3	4.48	60	75.00
Total amount	67	100.00	80	100.00

(2) Nature of risk factors

Most risk factors relevant to group disease come from behavior and lifestyle and are caused and also controlled by people themselves. We can calculate the proportion of those risk factors hard to eliminate such as heredity and disease history and those self-created such as behavior lifestyle to analyze the probably expected effect of health education and the health promotion. From table 5, we can see that the risk factor such as lifestyle took up a far larger percents in the male residents in Chengdu City, while in the female resident heredity and disease account for a large percent. Therefore, we should place the emphasis of health education on the male in Chengdu City.

The Social Medicine

Table 9-7 the nature of risk factor in different sex crowd in Chengdu City

	Male		Female	
	Quantity	Percent	Quantity	Percent
Risk factor hard to eliminate	15	13.51	78	70.27
Risk factor easy to eliminate	96	86.49	33	29.73
Total amount	111	100.00	111	100.00

(3) Influence of single-item risk factor on community health

For formulating effective preventive measures we can analyse the influence of all kinds of risk factors on community health, find out which kind of risk factor mostly influences the local resident and show its risk degree, which is calculated by the following equation: risk degree = risk strength × risk frequency. In this equation, risk strength means the average of evaluation age and growth age calculated after certain risk factor is taken out, and risk frequency means the proportion of this single-item risk factor in the inquired crowd. From the above calculation of risk degree, we can see that the influence of single-item risk factors on community health is not related to the same extent it affects the individual. Also with its large effect on the crowd, despite some factors having a strong effect on the individual and spreads quickly in the crowd, to the whole crowd is not serious. Whereas the effect of some factors on the individual is not quite so serious but it can influence a large crowd, so is also worth attention.

For example, in table 9-8, taking out the risk factor, smoking cigarette, each individual's average of growth age and evaluation age is 1.74 years, and in the inquired crowd, the specific weight of smoker is 85.07 percent. Therefore, the risk degree of smoking cigarette = 1.74 × 85.07 percent = 1.48 years. The risk strength of drinking is 1.47 years, and risk frequency is 41.49 percent, so its risk degree = 1.47 × 41.49 percent = 0.61 years, from which we can see that smoking has more effect on the health condition of the crowd than the other risk factors.

Table 9-8 influence of single-item risk factors on the male health condition

Risk factor	Risk strength(year)	Risk frequency (percent)	Risk degree(year)
Smoking	1.74	85.07	1.48
Drinking	1.47	41.49	0.61
Contact with pesticide	0.77	43.28	0.33
Contact with poison	1.48	19.40	0.29
Overweight	0.23	16.42	0.04
Hepatitis	0.28	8.96	0.03

Chapter 9 Health Risk Factors Appraisal

In a word there now are some limitations of the evaluation of risk factors of health. For example, it places emphasis only on life quantity but neglects life quality; it is difficult to acquire the complete demographic data and epidemic data on which evaluation can be conducted. At present the risk factors of some diseases are still uncertain; some risk factors are very difficult to get in the form of quantity, etc. However, it can still be used as a valid technique to prevent disease, is an easy and feasible method and visual outcomes are beneficial to health education, urging individuals to change bad behaviors and life styles and proposing crowd behaviors and life styles that are good for health, and a scientific basis to assist in eliminating all kinds of risk factors.

Exercises

To investigate a 41-year-old man at a certain area, his indicator of risk factor is as follows, please try to calculate the person's appraisal age and achievable age, appraise the health type (see table 9-9).

The Social Medicine

Table 9-9 HRFA table of a 41-years-old man in some area

Death Causation	Mortality probability ($\times 10^{-5}$)	Malady's inducement factors	Index value	Risk score	Fixed risk score	Existing death risks	Changing the risk factors according to the doctor	New fixing risk score	New existing death risks	Declined amount risk	Declined percent of the risk
Lung cancer	317	Smoking	20 pieces per day	1.9				1.7			
Hepatocirrhosis	274	Drinking	6 times per week	2.0							
Suicide	250	Blues	No	1.0			1.0				
		Family history	No	1.0			1.0				
Cardiac heart disease	1,355	Blood pressure	180/94mmHg	2.2			140/88mmHg	0.8			
		Cholesterine	220mg/dL	1.0			—	1.0			
		Diabetes history	No	1.0			—	1.0			
		Stamina activity	Sitting work	1.0			Exercise regularly	1.0			
		Family history	No	0.9			—	0.9			
		Smoking	20 pieces per day	1.5			—	0.7			
		Weight	Overweight 15 percent	0.9			—	0.9			
Traffic accident	255	Drinking	6 times per week	2.0			3 times per week	1.2			
		Drive mileage	3000km per year	3.0				3.0			
		Usage of safety belt	80%	0.8			100%	0.8			
Brain vessel disease	142	Blood pressure	180/94mmHg	2.2			<140/88mmHg	0.8			

(Table 9-9)

Death Causation	Mortality probability ($\times 10^{-5}$)	Malady's inducement factors	Index value	Risk score	Fixed risk score	Existing death risks	Changing the risk factors according to the doctor	New risk score	New fixing risk scoe	New existing death risks	The declined amount	Declined percent of the risk
		Cholesterine	220mg/dl	1.0			—	1.0				
		Diabetes history	No	1.0			—	1.0				
		Smoking	20 pieces per day	1.2			Giving up smoking	1.0				
Intestine tumor	78	Haemorrhage from anus	Yes	3.0			—	3.0				
		Intestine polyps	No	1.0			—	1.0				
		Intestinia	No	1.0			—	1.0				
		Proctoscope exam	No	1.0			One per three years	0.7				
Pneumonia	61	Drinking	6 times per week	3.0			3 times per week	1.2				
		Emphysema	No	1.0			—	1.0				
		Smoking	20 pieces per day	1.3			Giving up smoking	1.0				
Other	1,525			1.0			—	1.0				
Total												

第十章 生命质量评价

随着医学模式的转变、生活水平的提高和人类文明的进步,人们的健康意识在不断深化。健康不仅仅是没有疾病和病痛,而是生理、心理和社会的完好状态。人们已不满足于仅仅用生存率、发病率、患病率等指标来反应群体健康状况了。生命质量正是在这种客观健康水平提高和主观健康观念更新的背景下应运而生的一套评价健康水平的指标体系,它不仅有助于了解个体各系统的功能水平,还可以了解个体的心理状态、社会环境适应能力等,更全面地反映个体的健康状况,体现了积极的健康观。本章主要介绍生命质量评价的历史、发展、现状、评价工具及应用。

第一节 生命质量评价的发展

生命质量一词始于20世纪30年代,最初是一个社会指标,后来生命质量的理论和医学实践结合起来,就形成了健康相关的生命质量,在医学领域备受瞩目。目前生命质量评价被广泛地应用于医疗活动和预防医学领域。

(一)生命质量研究简史

生命质量一词是英文 Quality of life(QOL)的译文(也译为生存质量、生活质量、生命素质等),何时提出已不可考。实际上,人们一直在自觉地追寻生存质量的提高和生活水平的改善。在很大程度上说,人类整个的发展史就是不断地适应自然、改造自然,同时也完善自我、改善自我,从而提高生存质量的历史。但作为一个专门的术语并引出一片广阔的研究领域则始于20世纪30年代,兴起于50~60年代。70年代末期后在医学领域备受瞩目,并在80年代形成新的研究热潮,目前仍呈方兴未艾之势。总的说来,生存质量的研究可概括为三大时期。

1. 研究早期。生存质量的研究起源于20世纪30年代的美国,最先是作为一个社会指标来使用。当时经济复苏后的美国社会并未因经济的巨大增长而实现人们梦寐以求的生活安康、社会和谐,反而出现了世风日下、犯罪增加、社会动荡的局面。因此,人们要求建立除单纯经济指标外的其他社会指标,以便更全面地反映社会发展水平和人民生活好坏。在此前景下,开始了社会指标体系的研究,并逐渐发展成两大主流:社会指标研究和生活质量研究。

2. 成熟期。20世纪50~60年代是生活质量研究的成熟期。1957年,Guin等联合美国的几个大专院校进行了一次全国抽样调查,主要研究美国民众的精神健康和幸福感。进入60年代后,生活质量研究被政界承认,因而在全美各地蓬勃发展起来。

3. 分化期。随着社会领域生活质量研究的鼎盛以及医学本身的发展,20世纪70年代末医学领域广泛开展了生存质量的研究工作,并逐渐形成一个研究热潮。至今,与社会领域的研究并驾齐驱,且有超越或相互融合之势头。

实际上,医学界人士也一直在探讨生存质量测评问题。早在20世纪40年代末,Karnofsky就提出了著名的KPS量表。只是当时医学中尚以传染病较多,危害也较大,因而未引起足够重视。随着疾病谱的改变,威胁人类生存的主要疾病已不是传染病,而是难以治愈的癌症和心脑血管病等慢性病。对这些疾病很难用治愈率来评价治疗效果,生存率的作用也很有限,因此迫切需要综合的评价指标。

此外,疾病谱的改变和医学的发展引起了健康观和医学模式的转变,健康已不再是简单的没有疾病或虚弱状态,而是身体上、精神上和社会活动的完好状态。传统的仅关注生命的保存与局部躯体功能改善的一些方法和评价指标体系面临严重挑战:一则,未能表达健康的全部内涵;二则,未能体现具有生物、心理和社会属性的人的整体性和全面性;三则,未能反映现代人更看重活得好而不是活得长的积极心态。

鉴于此,广大的医学工作者进行了生存质量测评的探讨,并提出了与健康有关的生存质量概念HRQOL(health-related quality of life)。大体上说,70年代主要是引入和探索期,借用大量的一般人群评定量表来对病人的生存质量进行测定;80年代后则转向特定的肿瘤与慢性病的测评,并研制出大量的面向疾病的特异性测定量表。

(二)生命质量的概念及其发展

迄今为止对生存质量的内涵尚存很多争议。主要表现在:①生存质量的本质是什么?是否可测?②生存质量包括哪些方面?尤其,是否包括客观指标?

多年来,不少学者对此进行了探讨,但往往从自己的专业或好恶出发,因而各有不同的理解及回答,从而导致了生存质量的多义性并呈现出不同的层次。

首先,一些学者根本否定生存质量的测评。这主要是一些社会科学学者和泛政治主义者。在他们看来,生存质量的测评将不同人的质量分为高低,是对人人平等的社会价值观念的否定,因而是不道德的,也是不能被接受的。其次,有些人认为生存质量是一个虚无缥缈的、不可捉摸的概念,给生存质量下什么定义似乎完全取决于主观判断,因而生存质量是不可测的。甚至连在生存质量研究领域做出显著成绩的Aaronson也发出这样的感叹:"生存质量是个飘浮不定、难于捉摸的客观存在。"

值得庆幸的是,多数学者认为生存质量是可测的,而且很有必要进行测定。正因如此,大量学者投入了生存质量的研究,并提出了数以百计的生存质量概念。比如:

Andrews:良好的感觉。

Crib:对现实生活的满意程度。

Holmes:生存质量意味着一种幸福,是在生活中体现真正的自我,摆脱虚伪,泰然处世的状态。

Dubos:对自己每日生活活动有深切的满足感。

Levi：对由个人或群体所感受到躯体、心理、社会各方面的良好生活适应状态的一种综合测量，而测量结果是用幸福感、满意感或满足感来表示的。

Fayos：病人自我管理生活的能力。

Cella：生存质量是病人对现在的功能状态与其预期或认为可到达的功能状态相比时产生的赞同感和满足感。

Shumaker：个体对生活和个人良好状态的总体满足感。

Schipper：病人对疾病与治疗产生的躯体、心理和社会反应的一种实用的、日常的功能描述。

Hornquist：对特定生存需要（外界标准和个体感觉）的满意程度。

Calman：某一特定时间点个体期望与其现实体验的差别或距离，这种差别可随时间而改变，并可为个人成长所修正。改进生存质量包括改进有缺陷的生存方面（如疼痛）以及调整个体期望，使之与客观现实更为接近。

WHO生存质量研究组：不同文化和价值体系中的个体对与他们的目标、期望、标准以及所关心的事情有关的生存状况的体验。

由上可见，对生存质量的概念目前尚无公认的定义，争议颇多。本书主要侧重于与健康有关的生存质量，简称为生存质量。

(三) 生命质量的构成及其发展

对于生存质量的不同理解导致了对生存质量的构成有不同看法。这大体上分为三种情况。

1. "硬指标"。早期研究多局限于所谓"硬指标"范畴，如生存时间、人均收入、身体结构完整、受良好的教育、工作时间合理等客观指标。

2. 主观感觉指标为主。从20世纪60年代开始，生存质量的社会性在政治领域被接受。此时人们追求的是个体主观的幸福而不仅仅是生存的时间。故生存质量包括人的健康状态（生理状态、机能状态、心理健康、社会幸福感）和社会环境状态（经济来源、家庭生活、工作状况）。

Mesweeny认为生存质量的构成包括：①情绪功能，如精神症状的变化；②社会角色功能；③基本行为功能，如自我保健行为；④娱乐和享受。

Grogono将生存质量的构成分为10个部分：①工作；②娱乐；③躯体疾患；④心理疾患；⑤交往；⑥睡眠；⑦独立性；⑧饮食；⑨排泄；⑩性行为。

3. 主观感觉指标。20世纪80年代中期后，生存质量的界定及测量愈来愈趋向于仅测量主观感觉指标。虽然也涉及一些客观项目（如住房状况），但侧重于个体对住房状况的满意程度，而不是住房本身有多大、装备是否豪华等。

WHO的生存质量测定包括六个大方面（domain）：①身体机能；②心理状况；③独立能力；④社会关系；⑤生活环境；⑥宗教信仰与精神寄托。每个大方面又包含一些小方面（facet），共24个小方面。

总的说来，目前争议较大的是是否包括客观指标的问题，这源于对生存质量概念的不同认识。有学者认为应包括反映物质生活条件的客观指标，因为个体的生存条件如收入、住房、生态环境等无不与每天的生活息息相关，无不影响着个体的健康与疾病的发生发展。

从上面关于生命质量构成的各种观点看，WHO 的结构较全面，层次也比较分明。但全面性难免增加条目的长度，使得在临床上不一定实用。目前的趋势是逐步形成统一界定的 QOL 各个方面，并发展一个代表不同人群的生存质量，使得研究结果既可比性又有针对性。这就是所谓"共性"与"特异性"结合的研究模式。

综上所述，尽管对生存质量的概念与构成尚未达成共识，但以下几点是比较公认的：① 生存质量是一个多维的概念，包括身体机能、心理功能、社会功能等。② 生存质量是主观的评价指标（主观体验），应由被测者自己评价。③ 生存质量是有文化依赖的，必须建立在一定的文化价值体系下。

（四）我国生命质量研究状况

我国有关生命质量的研究工作从 20 世纪 80 年代中期开始，以社会学界开展的工作最多，在医学界开展较多的为生命质量调查及其评价指标的研究，一般多针对特殊人群，如老年人、肿瘤病人和精神病患者，如王蕾（1996）"社区精神分裂症病人生活质量对照研究"、颜丹红（1998）"278 例脑血管病患者生命质量评价"、刘红波（2002）"SF-36 问卷用于老年人群生命质量研究"等。近年来，我国生命质量研究较多，涉及多种疾病的生命质量评价（如糖尿病、心脑血管疾病、各种肿瘤、各种慢性疾病等）。生命质量的影响因素（行为因素、社会支持等）研究以及生命质量用于药效评价等研究都在蓬勃开展。

第二节　生命质量评价的主要指标

生命质量评价主要从躯体功能、心理功能、社会功能等方面进行综合评价，主要指标有以下几种。

（一）躯体功能 PH

反映个体生理功能的指标，包括疼痛与不适、精力与疲倦、睡眠与休息、行动能力、日常生活能力等躯体方面的状况。

（二）心理功能 PS

反映个体积极感受、消极感受、思想、学习、记忆、注意力及自尊、身材、相貌、精神支柱等心理方面的状况。

（三）社会功能 SO

反映个体个人关系、所需社会支持的满足程度、性生活等方面的状况。

（四）症状/副作用 ST

反映某种疾病相关的症状或者某种治疗所引起的不适感等。

（五）总生存质量

总的生存质量与健康状况又称健康指数，是工具表中所有项目评分之和，即生理功能、心理功能、社会功能和症状/副作用评分之和。

第三节　生命质量评价的相关工具

生存质量测定主要是量表测定，因此涌现出了大量的生存质量测定量表。根据使用目的、对象和排列方式等可对量表进行不同的归类。

一、生存质量测定表概况

(一)按照使用对象分

1. 普适性量表(generic scale)用于一般人群生存质量测定。如 SF-36,WHOQOL-100。

2. 疾病专表(disease-specific scale)用于特定人群(病人及某些特殊人群)。例如,用于癌症病人,有 FLIC,FACT-G,CARES,QLQ-C30 等;用于慢性病人,有糖尿病病人量表(DC-CT)、慢性阻塞性肺病病人量表(COPD)等。

3. 领域专表(domain-specific scale)侧重于测定生存质量的某一领域的量表。如 RCSL 侧重于疾病症状和治疗副作用的评定,KPS 侧重于行为表现功能的评定。

(二)按照应用目的分

1. 判别量表(discriminative)主要用于判别的量表,即用于区分不同的受试者。如说明治疗组与非治疗组、男性与女性间生存质量有无不同等,往往重视个体的判别。

2. 评定量表(evaluation scale)主要说明生存质量在时间上的变化。评定量表的目的不是区别不同的个体,因而不同个体间的差异并不太重要,而敏感性则更重要。

3. 预测量表(predictive scale)主要用于根据生存质量预测某些现象(如疾病复发、治疗反应)的发生。量表的使用价值主要取决于预测效度和校标效度。

目前的生存质量测定量表一般均具有前两个功能,而且常不加区别地都称为评定量表。至于预测作用还很少涉及。不过随着生存质量研究的深入,预测也将提上议事日程。量表的目的将是综合性的,尽管可以有所侧重。

(三)按照评分方式分

1. 线性评定量表(linear analog scale)通过在一条线段上定位来打分,如 LASA。

2. 等级描述评定量表(ordinal scale)通过在给定的几个等级中选择来打分,如 SF-36。

(四)按照评定者分

1. 自评量表(self-administered scale),即量表由被测者自己完成。

2. 他评量表(rater-administered),即量表由他人完成。有时既可由评定者完成,也可由代理者(家属、朋友)完成。

随着生存质量概念的深化,自评量表将逐渐取代他评量表。

二、常用生存质量测定表简介

目前已报道的生存质量测定量表有数百种,其适用的对象、范围和特点各异。这里按时间先后简介一些较有代表性的量表。

1. NHP:McEwen(1970)在英国诺丁汉市建立的诺丁汉健康调查表(Nottingham health profile,NHP)。设计的目的是评价个人对卫生保健的效果,共 45 条。内容包括 6 个方面(38 个条目)的个人体验(睡眠、身体活动、精力、疾病、情绪反应和社会孤独感)和 7 个方面(7 个条目)的日常生活活动(职业、家务、社会生活、家庭生活、性活动、嗜好和休假)。

2. SIP：Marilyn Bergner(1975)建立的疾病影响程度量表(sickness impact profile, SIP)。包括136个问题，测定身体、心理、社会健康状况、健康受损程度、健康的自我意识等。共分为12个大的方面，包括活动能力、自立能力、社会交往、情绪行为、警觉行为、饮食、工作、睡眠和休息、家务管理、文娱活动等。每个问题均经过专家讨论，给予权重。1981年作者又作了发展和最后修订。

3. LASA：Rrestman(1976)的线性模拟自我评价量表(linear analogue self-assessment, LASA)，包括10个项目，用于乳腺癌病人的生存质量测定。该量表具有两个特点：一是量表由病人对自己的行为、心理状态、健康状态等进行评分；二是量表采用线性计分法，即将量表中的每个问题分为两个极端状态(一端为0分，另一端为10分)，中间连上10厘米的线，病人根据自己对该问题的感受程度在直线上画记。

4. QWB：Kaplan等(1976)的生存质量指数(quality of well being index, QWB)，包括有关病人日常生活活动的内容，移动、生理活动和社会活动三方面，每个方面下设3～5个等级描述；由21个症状及健康问题的条目构成。QWB以指标定义清楚和权重合理而广为应用。

5. FLIC：Schipper(1984)的癌症病人生活功能指标(the functional living index-cancer, FLIC)，包括22个条目，用于癌症病人生存质量的自我测试，也可用作鉴定特异性功能障碍的筛选工具。它比较全面地描述了病人的活动能力、执行角色功能的能力、社会交往能力、情绪状态、症状和主观感受等，较适宜预后较好的癌症病人，如乳腺癌患者。每个条目的回答均在一条1～7的线段上作标记。

6. MOS SF-36：该量表是美国医学结局研究(medical outcomes study, MOS)组开发的一个普适性测定量表。该工作开始于20世纪80年代初期，形成了不同的条目、不同语言背景的多种版本。1990～1992年，含有36个条目的健康调查问卷简化版SF-36的不同语种版本相继问世。其中用得较多的是英国发展版和美国标准版，均包含躯体功能、躯体角色(role-physical)、机体疼痛、总的健康状况、活力(vitality)、社会功能、情绪角色(role emotional)和心理卫生8个领域。中山医科大学方积乾教授已得到该机构授权并研制了中国版SF-36。

7. CARES：Schag(1990)的癌症康复评价系统(cancer rehabilitation evaluation system, CARES)，包括139个项目，用于全面评价癌症病人生存质量。1991年作者又简化为含59个项目的简表(CARES-SF)，包含躯体、心理、医患关系、婚姻和性功能五个主要方面。

8. EORTCC QLQ-C30：欧洲癌症研究与治疗组织(European Organizaion for Research and Treatment)的生存质量核心量表。该组织于1986年开始研制面向癌症病人的核心量表(共性量表)，在此基础上增加不同的特异性条目(模块)即构成不同的特异量表。1987年，含26个条目的第一代核心量表QLQ-C36开发出来。20世纪90年代初，含30个条目的第二代QLQ-C30第一、二版相继问世。后者由5个功能子量表(躯体、角色、认知、情绪和社会功能)、3个症状子量表(疲劳、疼痛、恶心呕吐)、一个体健康状况子量表和一些单一条目构成。目前已开发出肺癌、乳腺癌、头颈部癌、直肠癌等多个特异性模块。

9. WHOQOL-100：该量表是世界卫生组织20余个国家和地区共同研制的跨国家、

跨文化并适用于一般人群的普适性量表。1991年开始研制,经几年的探索,1995年从236条构成的条目池中选出100条,形成WHOQOL-100。该量表由6个领域的24个小方面外加一个总的健康状况小方面构成。每个小方面由4个条目构成,分别从强度、频度、能力、评价四方面反映同一特质。同时,还研制了含26个条目的简表WHOQOL-BREF,便于操作。由中山医科大学生存质量课题组主持研制的WHOQOL中文版已经通过专家鉴定,被确认为我国医药卫生行业标准。

第四节 生命质量评价量表的设计

前面已经谈到,目前的生存质量测定主要是量表测定。因此,量表成为测定的重要一环。本节从分析量表的构成入手,全面介绍量表的设计方法及步骤。

一、量表的构成元素及层次结构

根据测定的对象和目的不同,生存质量测定量表的构成略异,但一般均含条目(item)、方面(facet)和领域(domain)。方面由若干条目组成,领域由若干方面组成,量表由若干领域组成。领域又常称为子量表或亚量表。以下着重介绍有关条目的内容。

条目是量表的最基本构成元素,是不能再分割的最小构成单位。所有备选的有关条目的集合称为条目池(item pool)。一个量表的好坏在很大程度上取决于条目的选择。

(一)条目的形式

主要有六种类型的条目:

1. 线性条目。被测者在有一定刻度(如0~10)的线段上画记,答案的选择项为整个线段。

2. 等距等级条目。被测者在等距离的一些程度语词(选择项)间选择答案。如很差、差、中等、好、很好。这由Likert于1932年所创立,故常称为Likert法,形式有3点法、5点法和7点法,但以5点法最为常用。

3. 不等距等级条目。同上,但语词间不完全等距。

4. 两分类条目。回答仅在两项中选择,如是、否。

5. 累积型条目。由Guttman于20世纪40年代提出并用于心理评定,后来用于生存质量评定。其一个条目反映的内容按难度或数量分成小项回答。如:

您的健康影响您的行动吗?
A. 能步行约1 500米的路程(是 否);
B. 能步行约500米的路程(是 否);
C. 能步行约100米的路程(是 否)。

这种条目的回答存在明显的逻辑关系,而且可用于分析同质性。如在A上回答"是"的,则在B和C上也应回答"是",否则其回答就有问题。

6. 描述性条目。每个条目的各种答案均作较详细的描述,以便被测者选择。如反映活动能力及范围的条目,回答选项可为:

0 整天卧床,不能走;

1 只能在室内做些轻微活动；
2 能在住宅周围活动；
3 可任意自由活动。

那么，以哪种条目为好呢？这很难进行评价，可以说各有所长。一般说来，线性条目比较精确，较易分析，但文化程度低者不易理解；等级条目较易理解和回答，但在程度语词的设置及结果的分析上都有诸多不便，需采取一定的方法处理；两分类条目较简单，但包含的信息少。因此，很多量表常兼有多种条目，起到取长补短之效，如 MOS SF-36。但也有的量表只有一种条目，如 FLIC。总的说来。线性条目和等距等级条目最常用，而且二者很可能长期并存。

(二) 条目的语义

可分为下述四种条目：

(1) 评价性条目(evaluation)，如：好，差。
(2) 强度性条目(intensity)，如：重，极重。
(3) 频度性条目(frequency)，如：很少，经常。
(4) 能力性条目(capacity)，如：能，完全能。

这是根据 Osgood 等在语义心理学研究的基础上提出的，后在 WHO 的生存质量评定中广为采用。

(三) 条目的性质

可分为两种条目：

(1) 可知觉的客观性条目(perceived objective)。
(2) 自我报告的主观性条目(self-reported subjective)。

二、量表的制定方法及步骤

(一) 制定方法

生存质量量表的制定是一个复杂的系统工程，包括从测定概念的确立及操作化定义、条目的形成及筛选、量表的考评及修订等一系列过程中涉及的各种方法。但狭义而言仅指明确制定概念并形成条目的方法，也就是从测量学原理出发，提出条目形成条目池的方法。从具体的实施过程来说，最好采用结构化的决策方法(programmed decision)来制定量表，即通过议题小组(nominal group)和选题小组(focus group)又称核心工作组的交互工作方式来完成。

(二) 制定步骤

1. 明确研究对象及目的。确定所测的人群；针对一般人群制定普适性量表还是针对某一特殊人群（如老年人、肺癌病人等）的特殊量表；量表今后的应用是侧重于判别还是评价等。

2. 设立研究工作组。在医学领域，一般是测定某些疾病患者（如癌症病人）及一些特殊人群（如老年人）的生存质量，因此需由医学专家、医生、护士、病人以及其他正常人等多种层次人员组成议题小组和核心工作组负责量表的制定与考核。其中，议题小组的成员应广泛一些，主要负责条目的提出；核心工作组则专业化和精干一些，负责具体的研究工作。

3. 测定概念的定义及分解。由核心小组给出所测概念的可操作化定义及构成。如所测生存质量指什么,包括哪些领域和小方面以及其含义是什么等。

4. 提出量表条目形成条目池。由核心小组将上述第 3 步的内容向议题小组详细介绍和说明(最好召集一个会议),然后由议题小组成员分别独立地根据专业知识和个人经验等写出与上述概念有关的条目。严格说,应分别按每个领域或小方面来写,这样会层次分明。但如觉麻烦,也可笼统地写出整个量表的条目。将各成员提出的条目收回并进行整理分析,对含义相同但表达不同者进行统一描述形成一个条目,所有不同的条目构成条目池。

5. 确定条目的形式及答案选项。多半采用线性和等级方式。对于前者,只要给出一定长度(通常为 10 cm)的线段,并定出两个端点的选项即可。如是等级形式,则各答案选项原则上应通过反应尺度(response scale)分析来确定。

反应尺度分析的目的就是对可作答案选项的各种程度副词进行定位分析。具体说来,就是先对同一种类型的条目提出 10~15 个可能的答案,如反映频度的可有总是、经常、很少、偶尔、几乎不、从来不等;然后请被试者分别在一段确定了两端点的线段上(10 cm)一一标上这些词,再对这些词的位置(均数或众数)进行分析,从而选出有关的词。比如按 5 点法,因为两个端点的词已固定,只需取位置大约定在 2.5 cm,5.0 cm 和 7.5 cm 处的三个词。这样做的目的是使得每个选项间等距离,从而方便评分(比如分别取为 1,2,…,5 分)及统计分析。

当然,也有量表在事先设计时,未作定位分析,各条目按习惯上的排列给出几个选项词,这时各选项间不一定等距。分析时,严格说来应再作各词的定位试验及分析,以便对各选项的得分进行调整。

6. 指标分析及筛选。对条目池的各条目用统计学方法进行分析及筛选,以筛出的指标构成初步量表。

7. 预调查及量表考评。用上述形成的初步量表进行预调查,由此对量表的信度、效度、反应度等特性进行考评。

8. 修改完善。在上述基础上进行修改完善,形成最终的测定量表。

以上简要介绍了量表制定的方法和步骤。对于已经研制出的大量的西文量表,对其进行汉化、研制成中国版的量表不失为量表开发中的一大捷径。其方法或步骤与上述不尽相同。

三、条目分析及筛选方法

(一)条目分析

对已提出的条目池中的各条目进行考察及必要的预试验,并根据其反应结果的统计分析来进行条目的选择和改良,这一系列的手续称为条目分析。简单地说,就是从不同角度来说明条目的好坏,从而为选择条目提供依据。它包括考察条目的困难度、反应度、辨别力、代表性和独立性等。

困难度分析可用条目的通过率来反映。如某个条目很多人都未回答,则说明条目不适宜或难以理解。

反应度分析就是考察被测者对各条目如何进行回答。这主要是考察选择项的有效性。回答集中于特定选择或者某个选择项完全没人问津都是不适宜的。

(二)条目筛选方法

生存质量测定量表制定中的一个关键问题就是条目(指标)筛选。专门谈及生存质量测定指标筛选方法的文章尚未见报道。张罗漫等曾报道用"老手"评判法、变异系数法、相关系数法、聚类分析法和主成分分析法来筛选医院评价指标。这些方法无疑可用于生存质量测定指标的筛选。

条目筛选应遵循重要性大、敏感性高、独立性强、代表性好、确定性好的原则,并兼顾可操作性及可接受性。

下面介绍的一些方法,分别从不同的角度和目的来进行条目筛选。除方法1和方法6外,其他方法均需按备选条目进行预调查,得到各条目的一批实测值,从而进行分析。预调查的样本含量最好在100例以上。

1. 主观评价法。这是从重要性和确定性角度筛选指标。方法是由医生或病人独立地对所提出的各个备选指标根据自己认为的对健康的重要程度按百分制进行打分(项目少时也可进行排序),从而根据各指标的重要性得分(平均分)来挑选指标,舍去得分较低的指标。平均分的计算与重要性得分的分布有关,若为正态分布用算术均数,否则用中位数。在求算术均数时为了避免极端值的影响,也可先弃掉一个最大值和最小值后再求平均。此外,医生的重要性评价与病人的往往不相同,应分别进行并兼顾两者的评价来挑选指标。

2. 离散趋势法。这是从敏感性角度挑选指标。指标的离散趋势小,用于评价时区别能力就差。因此应选离散趋势较大的指标。很多情况下可直接用标准差来反映离散趋势。但应注意若干条目的计分值不呈正态分布则应先作变量变换使之成为正态分布。

3. 相关系数法。这是从代表性与独立性角度挑选指标。计算任何两个指标间的相关系数并作统计检验,以与之相关的指标个数较多和较少者作为被选指标。因为前者有代表性,可提供较多的信息;后者有独立性,为其他指标所不能代替。采用什么相关系数视资料特性而定。

4. 主成分分析与因子分析法。这是从代表性角度筛选指标。从各指标的相关矩阵出发进行主成分分析,根据量表的设想结构及贡献率的大小确定所需的主成分数,然后根据各主成分与各指标的相关性大小分别考虑各个主成分主要由哪些指标决定,选择系数较大的指标。比如根据设想,生存质量量表应包括五个主要方面(身体机能、精神心理、社会关系、症状及毒副作用、环境),则可考虑取五个主成分。若作因子分析则根据因子负荷的大小来挑选指标,留下载荷较大者。

5. 聚类分析法。这也是从代表性角度筛选指标。先采用一个聚分类方法(一般用系统聚类法)对各指标进行聚类分析(R型聚类分析)把指标聚为一定数目的类别,然后选择每一类中的代表指标为入选指标。按相关系数的平方来选择代表指标,原则是:①以每类中平均而言与其他指标相关性最好的指标作为代表指标;②以类内平均相关性较好而类间平均相关性较差的指标为代表指标。

6. 基于重要性评价逐步筛选。该法是方法1的直接推广,类似于美国Rand公司提出的德尔斐(Delphi)预测法。即先用方法 1 选择出一些得分较高或位次排前的指标(一轮筛选),将选出的指标反馈给评价者,再用方法 1 进行第二轮筛选……逐步进行下去即可得到较公认的重要指标。

7. 逐步回归分析法。此方法是通过预调查得到一批人数据,并要求被调查者对其总的生存质量进行总的评分,将总的评分作为因变量 Y,然后用 Y 与各指标($X_1, X_2, \cdots, X_n$)进行多重逐步回归分析,筛选出对 Y 影响较大的指标。取不同的检验水准 α 即可得到不同数目的重要指标,以供进一步选择。该法也可设计为生存质量结构,以每个方面总评分为因变量 Y,与相应的指标进行逐步回归分析,选出对每一个方面影响较大的指标。但调查时应对被调查者讲清生存质量的含义,否则总的评分很难代表其生存质量。

8. 逐步判别分析。生存质量测定的目的之一就是要评价不同的疗法或措施的效果,因此不同的人群(如病人与正常人)其生存质量应该不同,好的量表应具有这种区分能力。基于此,在预调查中可设计包括不同的人群(不失一般性,假定有病人和正常人两类),用逐步判别分析即可筛选出对于判别这两类人贡献较大的指标。由这些指标构成的量表就具有较好的区别能力。

附:世界卫生组织生命质量测定量表中文版的研制

中山医科大学卫生统计学教研室方积乾教授作为世界卫生组织生命质量测定量表中文版研制小组负责人,受世界卫生组织和中华人民共和国卫生部的委托,在世界卫生组织生命质量测定量表 WHOQOL-100 和 WHOQOL-BREF 的基础上,结合中国国情,遵照世界卫生组织推荐的程序,已经制定了上述两种量表的中文版。

(一)WHOQOL-100 广东版本的制作

将 WHOQOL-100 量表英文版翻译改造成中文版的工作是从 1995 年开始的。根据世界卫生组织生命质量研究中心的工作纲要,中山医科大学卫生统计学教研室负责全部的工作。

研制步骤如下:

(1) 两位公共卫生专家独立地将量表从英文翻译成中文,第三位专家对翻译稿进行总结,形成量表的第一稿。

(2) 两个核心工作组分别就第一稿进行讨论。一个核心工作组由医生、护士和医科大学学生组成,另一个核心工作组由病人组成。经过讨论,对第一稿进行修改,形成第二稿。

(3) 将第二稿寄给世界卫生组织总部,同时请一位英语教师把第二稿逆向翻译成英文。

(4) 核心工作组对逆向翻译稿和英文原版进行比较,修改第二稿,形成第三稿。

(5) 请一组病人和医科大学学生做反应尺度练习,根据结果修改反应尺度,形成第四稿。

(6) 在广东省的东、西、南、北和中部各选一个地区进行预实验(每个地区调查约 100 名对象),选中的 5 个地区分别是湛江、梅州、韶关、中山和广州。

(7) 根据调查所得资料分析量表的信度、效度和反应度等计量心理指标,同时根据结果制定了一个含有较少条目的简表。

(8) 根据预实验结果对第四稿进行修改,最后形成 WHOQOL-100 广东版。广东版是在广东省卫生厅的指导下,在广东地区完成的。量表的语言是标准汉语(普通话)。

(二)国内合作研究

国内合作研究组织会议在卫生部高教司标准办公室的指导下,于 1996 年 4 月 17 日至 19 日在北京召开,与会者 13 人。会上交流了各自在生命质量研究方面所做的工作、所取得的经验及信息,中山医科大学报告了 WHOQOL-100 广东版制定过程,介绍了"WHOQOL-100 中文版的制定及相关研究"的计划。与会者对 WHOQOL-100 广东版进行了逐字逐句的讨论和修改,并把修订稿称为"96 中文版"在全国 6 个城市进行现场试验。

现场试验在广州、北京、上海、成都、西安、沈阳等 6 个城市进行。每地调查 300 人,样本中注意病人与非病人、男与女、年龄结构等因素的均衡。病种主要有年轻人中的慢性肝炎、胃溃疡、慢性支气管炎、抑郁症等,中年人中的高血压、冠心病、糖尿病、关节炎等,老年人中的癌症、心血管疾病、糖尿病和骨折等。另外还考察了 50 名病人治疗前后生命质量的变化。6 城市现场试验的资料于 1997 年 2 月汇总到中山医科大学卫生统计学教研室,并寄给世界卫生组织总部。

由另外两位英语教师独立完成了 96 中文版的逆向翻译工作。通过比较逆向翻译稿和原文,参考 6 城市现场试验的结果,对 96 中文版进行了微小的改动,形成了"97 中文版"。相应地,对之进行了逆向翻译。"97 中文版"及其逆向翻译稿连同中文版研制和现场考核报告一并报请世界卫生组织生命质量研究协作组审核。协作组于同年正式接受"97 中文版"为世界卫生组织生命质量测定量表的中文版。

中山医科大学卫生统计学教研室的教师和研究生们除了研制 WHOQOL-100 普适性量表外,还研制了适用于戒毒者、肝癌患者和糖尿病患者的特殊量表,作为 WHOQOL-100 普适性量表的补充。

第五节 生命质量评价在卫生领域中的应用

生存质量测评目前已广泛应用于社会各领域,成为不可或缺的重要指标和评定工具。在医学领域主要有 4 个方面的应用:①人群健康状况的测量;②资源利用的效益评价;③临床疗法及干预措施的比较;④治疗方法的选择与决策。

一、一般及特殊人群健康状况评定

一些普适性的生存质量测定量表并不针对某一种疾病病人,测评的目的不在于评价治疗效果,而在于了解一般人群的综合健康状况,甚至作为一种综合的社会经济和医疗卫生指标,以便比较不同国家、不同地区、不同民族人民的生存质量和发展水平以及对其影响因素的研究。这在早期的生存质量评定中较为常见。如 GHO,NHP,MHIQ(McMaster health index questionnaire)以及 20 世纪 80 年代初开始研制的 MOS SF-36 和目前正在进行的 WHOQOL 跨文化跨国家量表都主要用于一般人群的生存质量评定。

在国内,林南等根据千户抽样调查资料研究了天津市市民的生活质量;王滨燕等对北京中年知识分子的健康和生活质量进行了综合分析;李凌江等以湖南省城乡家庭为抽样框架,对社会人群的生活质量及其影响因素进行了分析。

有时,生存质量的评定仅限于某些特殊人群,以了解其健康状况及其影响因素,并解决某些相关的问题。比如,随着人口老龄化的发展老年人问题愈显重要。老年人都有不同程度的健康受损,但如果没有引起功能障碍则不算严重威胁,更重要的是日常生活自理能力和在功能减退情况下生活需要帮助的程度。因此老年人生存质量及相关问题有其特殊性,引起了广泛的关注和研究。如 Katz 等对老年人的功能状况等进行了评定并引进积极健康寿命(active life expectancy,ALE)这一概念来反映考虑生存质量后的期望寿命;Pearlman 专为测定老年人机能状况而建立了老人综合评价量表(COPE);许淑莲对离退休老干部的生存质量与自觉幸福度及其影响因素进行了研究。

此外,Longabaugh 等人对酒精滥用者的生存质量进行了研究;万崇华等对吸毒者的生存质量及其影响因素进行了分析。

二、肿瘤及慢性病患者生存质量测评

肿瘤与慢性病患者的生存质量测评是医学领域生存质量研究的主流。目前,每年有数百篇文章涉及肿瘤与慢性病的生存质量测定,而且正呈方兴未艾之势。

(一)癌症患者的测评

早在 1980 年,欧洲癌症治疗研究组织创立了有 7 个国家参加的生存质量研究组,从较大的规模上进行癌症生存质量测评的协作研究。目前,欧洲 16 个国家和澳大利亚、加拿大、美国均参加了该研究组,并已制定出一个反映癌症病人共性的核心量表 QLQ-C30,以及很多具体癌症的特异量表,如肺癌 QLQ-LC13、乳腺癌 QLQ-BR24、头颈部癌症 QLQ-H&N37、食道癌 QLQ-OES24 和直肠结肠癌 QLQ-CR38 等。美国癌症研究所已在六个社区临床肿瘤计划地区和得克萨斯大学的 Anderson 医院及肿瘤研究所开展生存质量评价研究,主要目标是探明与癌症临床试验同时进行的生存质量研究的有关问题并提出解决方法。芝加哥的 Rush-Presbyterian-St. Luke 医学中心研制出了癌症治疗功能评价系统 FACT(functional assessment of cancer therapy),该系统由一个测量癌症病人生存质量共性部分的一般量表 FACT-G 和一些特定癌症的子量表构成。此外,尚有 CARES 及 CARES-SF 的开发及应用。

比较著名的量表几乎均出自在癌症领域。近 20 年来,生存质量测评在抗癌药物疗效评价、治疗方案选择等方面得到了广泛应用。比如,许多学者对乳腺治疗方案用生存质量进行了评定,使得其治疗从全切除转向部分切除。Gelber 等用生存质量与生存时间结合的方法综合分析了乳腺癌手术后是否进行辅助治疗以及选何种治疗。Mcneil 等对喉癌病人是采用手术还是放疗以及要活得长还是要保持正常说话能力从生存质量角度进行了综合评定。在国内,已有人开展了乳腺癌、肝癌、鼻咽癌等癌症病人的测定工作。从病种上看,以乳腺癌和肺癌研究较多,原因是这两种癌症在欧美较高发。

(二)慢性病测评

近 20 年来,国外对心血管系统疾病、慢性阻塞性肺病、风湿性疾病、泌尿系统以及内分泌系统疾病等慢性病进行了大量的生存质量研究。Fletcher 研究了心绞痛病人治疗前后生存质量的变化规律。Spertus 等制定了西雅图心绞痛量表 SAQ(seattle angina questionnaire)并用于相应患者的测定。Bernie 等通过生存质量与生存分析对心脏移植项目的效果进行了评价。Evans等对进行肾移植和血液透析的晚期肾病患者生存质量进行了分析,发现前者的生存质量高于后者。

在国内,目前已有人作了高血压、糖尿病、哮喘、肾虚症、脑卒中等患者的生存质量评定。

(三)临床治疗方案的评价与选择

前面谈到生存质量已广泛用于临床上癌症和慢性病患者的测评。测评的目的,除了反映综合健康状况外,更重要的是用于药物疗效和治疗方案的评价与选择,即通过对患者在不同疗法或措施中生存质量的测定与评价,为治疗与康复措施的比较提供新的结局指标。如Willians等通过对低位直肠癌患者直肠切除术后生存质量的考察,发现低位括约肌保留切除术的病人在饮食、性功能、情绪等方面均优于传统的经腹会阴切除术,从而说明这一方法优于传统方法。Sugarbaker的研究或许可以作为一个典型范例:在临床上,对于肢体肉瘤的治疗方法通常有两种:一是截肢,二是保留疗法并辅以大剂量的放射治疗。按传统观点,认为能不截肢则尽量不截。Sugarbaker对两疗法患者的生存质量评价发现总的生存质量无统计学差异,但截肢组在情绪行为、自我照顾、性行为等方面优于保留疗法组。据此得出结论:从生存质量观点看,保留疗法并不优于截肢疗法;从减少复发的愿望出发,应考虑截肢。王伟等(2000)用多因素分析的方法对绝育、上环和药具组妇女的生命质量影响因素进行了分析,发现影响妇女生命质量的主要因素是生活满意度和心理状况,而影响生活满意度的主要因素是家庭物质生活条件,影响心理状况的因素主要是健康状况,也就是说物质生活条件的改善和身心的完好状况将直接影响妇女的生活质量,而不同的避孕方式对妇女生活质量无显著的影响。有关这方面的应用还很多。

(四)预防性干预及保健措施的效果评价

预防性干预及保健措施是面向社区一般人群的,随着预防医学和初级卫生保健的发展,对其措施的效果评价日益重视。对其效果进行综合评价可借助生存质量这一高度概括的指标来进行。这通常需要进行干预前后的生存质量对比才能进行评价。Brook等通过生存质量来评价实行共同保险措施对成年人健康状况的影响。吕维善探讨了健康教育对提高老年人生存质量的作用。

(五)卫生资源配置和利用的决策

卫生资源配置和利用决策分析的主要任务是选择投资重点,合理分配和利用卫生资源并产生最大的收益。随着生存质量研究的广泛开展和深入,人们越来越倾向用质量调整生存年QALYs(quality adjusted life years)这一指标来综合反映投资的效益。因为QALYs综合考虑了生存时间和生存质量,克服了以前将健康人生存时间和病人生存时间同等看待的不足。因此生存质量指标可用于卫生立法、卫生政策的制定、卫生资源分配等。

(六)探讨健康影响因素与防治重点

目前生存质量已作为一个健康与生活水平的综合指标,而且已经或正在成为医学或社会发展的目标,对生存质量影响因素的探讨有利于找出防治重点,从而促进整体健康水平的提高。万崇华对吸毒者生存质量的影响因素进行了分析。

Chapter 10 The Evaluation of Quality of Life

With the transformation of medical model, improvement of living condition and the advancement of human civilization, people's health consciousness keeps on deepening. Health is a state of complete physical, mental and social well-being and not merely an absence of disease or infirmity. It is not enough to reflect group's health situation merely with such indicators as survival rate, incidence rate and prevalence rate, etc. Quality of life (QOL), emerging with the background that the improvement of objective health situation and update of subjective health conception, is such an indicator system to evaluate health situation. It helps to find out not only the system function level but also psychology and ability to adapt to social environment of individual, which comprehensively reflect individual health situation and active health view. This chapter mainly introduces the QOL in terms of its history, development, current status, evaluating instrument and application.

Section 1 Development of Quality of Life Evaluation

QOL is first introduced in the 1930s, which was originally a social indicator, and is defined as health-related QOL when combining with QOL theory and medical practice. It attracts most attention in medical realm and the evaluation of QOL has been widely used in health service and preventive medicine at present.

1. History of QOL research

QOL has several kinds of translations in Chinese and it was impossible to research when it was brought forward. Actually, human beings are consciously pursuing the improvement of living quality and condition. To a large extent, the whole development history of human beings is such a history that people keep on adapting and rebuilding the nature; meanwhile perfecting and improving ourselves as well as improving quality of life sequentially. But it was in the 1930s that QOL became a special term and exploited a wide research realm. It rose in the 1950-60s', attracted most attention in medical realm at the end of the 1970's, became a new pop issue in the 1980's and is still in the ascendant at present. In a word, the research process of QOL can be divided into three main periods.

(1) Early stage

The research of QOL started in the USA in the 1930s and was used as a social indicator initially. At that time following the post-war economic revival in USA was not the dreaming well-off society, but unsteady society with increasing criminals. Therefore, besides simple economic indicators people need develop other social ones in order to reflect the development of society and people's living condition more comprehensively. Based on this situation, the research about social indicator system was started and gradually divided into two main parts: research of social indicator and research of QOL.

(2) Stabilization stage

1950 – 60s was the stabilization stage of the research about QOL. In 1957, Guin associating with several main universities in USA carried out a national sampling survey, which focused on investigating the mental health and happiness. When it entered the 1960s the research of QOL was accepted by political circles and thus it flourished in the whole USA.

(3) Differentiation stage

With the flourishment of study about QOL in social realm and the self-development of medicine, such studies were widely carried out in medical realm and gradually became a pop issue at the end of the 1970s. Up to the present, they have kept the same pace with those carried out in social realm and have the tendency to surpass them and to merge each other.

Actually the medical scholars are exploring the measurement and evaluation of QOL all the times. Karnofsky had put forward the famous KPS scale as early as the 1940s. But it wasn't paid more attention to because at that time the prior diseases were infectious diseases, which did great harm to people. With the transformation of medical model, the prior diseases, which threaten the survival of human being are not infectious diseases any more but such chronic diseases as cancer, cardiovascular and cerebralvascular diseases which are difficult to treat. It is hard to evaluate the effect of treatment with cure rate and survival rate. So it is urgent to develop comprehensive evaluation indicators.

Furthermore, the development in the spectrum of disease and in the whole medicine resulted in the relative transformation in view of health and in the medical model. Health is a state of complete physical, mental and social well-being and not merely an absence of disease or infirmity. The traditional evaluating methods and indicator system, which merely pay attention to saving life and improving partial function of the body, face a great challenge: first, they haven't covered the entire meaning of the health; second, they haven't reflected the integrity of human beings which possess biologic, psychological and social character; third, they haven't reflected the active psychology of modern generation which values not the quantity but the quality of the life.

Therefore, numerous health professionals have explored the measurement and evaluation of QOL, based on the concept of HRQOL (health-related QOL) which they brought forward. By and large, the whole 70s' was the period of introducing and exploring the HRQOL, during which the patients' QOL were measured through applying a large numbers of scales fit for common people; when it entered the 80s' the measurement and evaluation on certain cancer and chronic diseases were carried out and plenty of distinctive disease-oriented scales were established sequentially.

2. The concept and its development of QOL

So far, there have been many debates about the meaning of QOL. The main list is as follows:

(1) What is the essence of the QOL, What if can be measured?

(2) What aspects are included in the QOL? If there is any objective indicator especially?

Quite a few scholars have studied those problems for a long time based on their own professional knowledge and taste. So they got different understandings and answers, which accordingly resulted in the multi-meaning and multi-stratification of QOL.

Firstly, some scholars deny the measurement and evaluation of QOL completely. Most of them are scholars in social science. In their opinions people are ranked in the quality by measuring and evaluating their QOL, which is a denial to the social value that everyone is equal, so its immoral and shouldn't be accepted. Secondly, some people consider the QOL an abstract concept and it completely according to personal opinion to define the QOL, so it can't be measured. Even Aaronson, who has obtained great achievements in the research of QOL, pointed out that QOL's objective was difficult to master.

Fortunately, most scholars think the QOL can be and is necessary to be measured. Therefore large numbers of scholars devoted to the research and have developed hundreds of concepts about QOL. For example:

Andrews: Nice feeling.

Crib: Degree of optimism towards life.

Holmes: QOL means a kind of happiness, which is such a state to really express oneself in life, get rid of false thought and live calmly.

Dubos: One has great satisfaction to the activities in daily life.

Levi: It's a kind of comprehensive measure to the well adaptation of individual or group to the whole physical, psychological and social factors. The result is expressed by blessedness, satisfaction or contentment.

Fayos: QOL is that the patient has the ability to manage one's life.

Cella: QOL is the agreement and satisfaction reached when patient compares the current functions and status with the expected ones.

Shumaker: QOL is the individual's general satisfaction to life and personal well-being.

Schipper: QOL is practical and daily functional description about the patients' response to the diseases and treatment physically, mentally and socially.

Hornquist: QOL is the extent of satisfaction to certain survival demands (exterior standards and individual feeling).

Calman: QOL is the gap between individual expectations and his/her real experiences at a certain time, which changes as the time goes by and can be adjusted when he/she grows up. The improvement of QOL includes improving the defective life (such as pain) and adjusting individual expectation, thus making it more practical.

QOL research group of WHO: QOL is the individual's experiences to living status related to their aims, expectations, standards and issues they concerned about, who live in different culture and value systems.

It's obvious that there are many disputes about QOL at present and has been no accepted concept yet. This text focuses on the HRQOL, abbreviated as QOL.

3. The constitution and development of QOL

The different comprehensions to the QOL lead to the different opinions to its constitution. There are three kinds of indicators:

(1) "Hard indicators"

The early studies were limited in the category of so called "hard indicators", such as life time, average income, the integrity of body, well education and proper working time, all of which were objective indicators.

(2) The indicators of subjective feeling account for the main part

Since the 1960s the sociality of QOL has been accepted in political domain. At that time people sought for the subjective blessedness of individual instead of the lifetime. So QOL included people's health situation (physical fettle, function fettle, mental health and feeling of social blessedness) and social environment (economic source, family life and working condition).

Mesweeny thought that the constitution of QOL should include those listed as follows: ①Mood function, such as the change of spirit signs; ②Function of social role; ③Function of basic behavior, such as behaviors of self health care; ④Entertainment and enjoyment.

Grogono divided the constitution of QOL into 10 parts: ① Working; ②Entertainment; ③physical diseases; ④Mental diseases; ⑤Association; ⑥Sleeping; ⑦Independency; ⑧Diet; ⑨Excretion; ⑩Sexual behavior.

(3) The indicators of subjective feeling

After the middle of the 1980s the definition and measurement of QOL increasingly tended to focus on the indicators of subjective feeling merely. Although some objective items (such as living conditions) were included, it emphasized individual contentment to the living conditions instead of how big the house or if it's equipped luxuriously.

Based on the definition from WHO, the measurement of QOL includes six key domains: ①Body function; ②Psychological fettle; ③Independent ability; ④Social relationship; ⑤Living environment; ⑥Faith and mental consolation. Each domain includes several facets and there are 24 facets totally.

In a word, the current main dispute is whether the objective indicators should be included in the constitution of QOL, which result from the different comprehension to the concept of QOL. Some scholars think that those objective indicators reflecting substantial living conditions should be included in it, for all such individual living conditions as income, housing and environment are closely linked with life and influence the individual health and disease.

According to the different opinions on the constitution of QOL cited before, the one from WHO is more comprehensive in the frame and more clear between different levels, which increases the length of the item unavoidable that it's not necessarily practical in clinic. The current tendency is to gradually form a uniform definition to different domains of QOL, and develop such a QOL that can represent different groups to guarantee the comparability and pertinence. This is the research model called the combination of "commonness" and "specificity".

To sum up, there has been no common understanding on the concept and constitution of QOL yet. However, those points are acknowledged:

(1) QOL is a multidimensional concept including body function, psychological function and social function.

(2) QOL is a subjective evaluating indicator (subjective experiences), which should be evaluated by oneself.

(3) QOL relies on certain culture and must be set up in such culture-value system.

4. The current satatus of QOL-study in China

The QOL-related studies started in the mid-1980s in China, most of which were carried out in sociology domain. Those carried out in medical domain focused on the study of QOL survey and its evaluating indicators, which aimed at special groups such as senior citizens, patients of tumor and psychopath. For example, Wang Lei (1996) "QOL control study on schizophrenic in communities"; Yan Danhong (1998) "QOL evaluation to 278 cases of cerebralvascular diseases"; Liu Hongbo (2002) "QOL study on the old person with SF-36 scale", etc. There are more studies about QOL recent years, and the QOL evaluation has involved various diseases (such as diabetes, cardiovascular and cerebralvascular diseases, various tumors and chronic diseases, etc.). The studies on the influence factors of QOL (behavior and social support, etc.) and drug effect evaluating with QOL have been carried out flourishly.

Section 2 Indicator for HRQOL

HRQOL evaluate systematically from PH, PS and SO, etc. There are the main indicators:

1. PH

The indicators reflecting PH include the situation of physical body, for example, pain and unwell, energy and weariness, sleep and rest, ability to action, and ability to daily life.

2. PS

The indicators reacting the individual psychological situation include positive and pessimistic precept, ideology, study, memory, attention, and self-respect, body figure, appearance, and spiritual support as well.

3. SO

Including the indicators reflecting individual relationships, the degree of satisfaction about social support of need, sexual life and so on.

4. ST

It reflects the relative symptom to certain disease or the unwell sense caused by certain therapy.

5. General QOL

The general QOL and healthy situation are called health index, too, which equal the sum of the scores of all items in the instrument sheet, namely the sum of PH, PS, SO and ST.

Section 3 The Relative Instruments of QOL Evaluation

It usually uses various scales to measure QOL so that there emerge large numbers of scales on QOL. Those scales can be classified into different categories according to the aims, objects and forms.

1. The general situation of QOL scales

(1) Classified according to the objects

Generic scale: which is used to measure the QOL of general population, such as SF-36 and WHOQOL-100, etc.

Disease-specific scald: which is used to measure the QOL of specific groups (patients or some specific groups), such as FLIC,FACT-G,CARES,QLQ-C30, which suit patients of tumor; DC-CT is suitable for diabetes patients and for patients of COPD, both of which are chronic diseases.

Domain-specific scale: which emphasizes particularly on one certain domain of QOL. For example, RCSL evaluates the symptoms of the disease and side effect of the treatment; KPS pays more attention to the evaluation of behavior function.

(2) Classified according to the aim

Discriminative scale: its main function is to categorize patients. For example, using it we can make out if there is any difference in QOL between treated group and non-treated group, male group and female group. It pays more attention to individualization.

Evaluation scale: the main function of which is to find the change of QOL in terms of the time. It doesn't aim at discriminating different individuals. So the most important is not the difference but the sensitivity.

Predictive scale: which is used to predict the occurrence of some phenomena (such as the relapse of disease and the responses of treatment). The value mainly lies in the validity of the prediction and adjustment of the scale.

Generally speaking, the present scales of QOL have two main functions and both are called evaluation scales without any distinction. The function of prediction seldom comes down. However, as the result of the gradual in-depth study of QOL, the function of prediction will be listed in the schedule of study. The aim of the scale will be comprehensive while it can have certain emphasis.

(3) Classified according to the mode of grade

Linear analog scale: which is scored by locating on a line. Such as LASA.

Ordinal scale: which is scored by making choice in given grades. Such as SF-36.

(4) Classified according to the person to evaluate

Self-administered scale: the one who received the test will accomplish the scale.

Rater-administered: the scale will be accomplished by other persons. It can be accomplished by the evaluator and succedaneum (relatives or friends).

With the deepening of the concept of QOL, the self-administered scale will replace the rater-administered scale gradually.

2. The brief introduction of QOL scales in common use

Hundreds of QOL scales have been reported, which vary in objects, ranges and characteristics. We just introduce some representative scales according to the order of the time.

Chapter 10 The Evaluation of Quality of Life

(1) NHP

McEwen(1970) developed the Nottingham health profile (NHP) in Nottingham, England, the aim of which is to evaluate the effect of health care on individuals. There are 45 items totally and cover individual experiences in 38 entries of 6 domains (sleep, body activity, energy, disease, emotional response and feeling of loneliness in society) and daily activities in 7 entries of 7 domains (occupation, housework, social life, sexual life, hobby and vacation).

(2) SIP

Marilyn Bergner(1975) developed the sickness impact profile (SIP), which includes 136 questions to evaluate physical, mental and social health situation, the extent of health harm, and the self-awareness of health. It is divided into 12 main domains, which involve activity ability, self-help ability, social intercourse, emotional behavior, alertness, diet, working, rest, household management and entertainment. Each question has been discussed and assigned certain weight by experts. The author developed it and accomplished the last emendation in 1981.

(3) LASA

Rrestman(1976) developed the linear analogue self-assessment (LASA), which involves 10 items and is used to evaluate the QOL of breast cancer patient. This scale has two characteristics: one is that the patient evaluates his/her own behavior, psychological fettle and health situation; the other is that the scale uses the linear scoring method, namely each answer of the question shows two extreme conditions (one end is scored 0 point and another is 10 points), which are jointed by a line. The patient will score on the line according to his/her own feeling about the question.

(4) QWB

Kaplan. etc. (1976) developed the quality of well being index (QWB), in which three domains related with the patient's daily activities are included; they are motion, physiological activities and social activities. There are 3 - 5 grade descriptions under each domain, which include 21 items of symptoms and health problems. QWB is widely used for its clearly-defined indicators and proper weight.

(5) FLIC

Schipper(1984) developed the functional living index-cancer (FLIC), which involves 22 items. It is used as instrument of QOL self-evaluation by cancer patient as well as filtering instrument of appraisal to special functional handicap. It comprehensively describes the patient from his/her activity ability, ability of performing role function, ability of social intercourse, emotion fettle, symptom and subjective feeling. So it is suitable for those cancer patients with benign prognosis, such as patient of breast cancer. Each item will be answered by marking on a line, the two ends of which are 1 and 7.

(6) MOS SF-36

It is a generic scale developed by the group of medical outcomes study (MOS). This research started in the early 1980s and several versions with different items and different lingual background were developed. From 1990 to 1992, the predigested versions of health survey questionnaire SF-36 containing 36 items in various languages were published one after another, among which the British expanding version and the USA standard version were in common use. Both of them cover 8 domains of the body function, role-physical, body ache, general health situation, vitality, social function, emotional role and mental health. Professor Fang Jiqian in Zhongshan Medical University was selected for this work to develop Chinese version of SF-36.

(7) CARES

Schag (1990) developed the cancer rehabilitation evaluation system (CARES), which involves 139 items and is used to comprehensively evaluate the QOL of cancer patient. In 1991, the author developed the predigested version, CARES-SF, which contains 59 items and covers 5 domains of body, mentality, the relationship between doctor and patient, marriage and sexual function.

(8) EORTCC QLQ-C30

It's just the core scale of QOL developed by European Organization for Research and Treatment. The organization started to develop the core scale (commonness scale) targeting to cancer patient in 1986 and based on which various special scales were formed by adding relative special items (modules). The first generation of core scale QLQ-C36 which contains 26 items was developed in 1987. The first and second version of the second generation of core scale QLQ-C30 was developed one after another in the early, 1990s The latter consists five functional sub-scales (body, role, perception, emotion and social function), three symptom sub-scales (fatigue, ache and vomit), one health situation sub-scale and some single items. Various special modules have been developed at present, which is targetted to cure lung cancer, breast cancer, head and cervix cancer and recta cancer.

(9) WHOQOL-100

It is a generic scale developed by more than 20 countries and regions of WHO, and is cross-nation and cross-culture for ordinary people. The research started in 1991, and after years of exploration selecting 100 items from the item pool containing 236 items of 1995 formed the WHOQOL-100. The scale consists 24 sub-domains of 6 domains and 1 sub-domain of general health situation. Each sub-domain consists of 4 items and reflects the same speciality from intensity, frequency, capacity and evaluation. At the same time, the predigested scale WHOQOL-BREFwhich contains 26 items also has been developed for easy operation. The Chinese version of WHOQOL developed by QOL research group of Zhongshan Medical University has been appraised by experts and affirmed as the criterion of the medicine in China.

Chapter 10 The Evaluation of Quality of Life

Section 4 Design for Profile of QOL

As mentioned above, at present, measuring HQOL was often done through profile. Therefore, profile becomes an important part in the measurement of QOL. This section introduces the methods and procedures for design profile of HQOL, beginning with analyzing the components of the profile.

1. The component and hierarchy

The components of profile for QOL are slightly different according to the different subjects and objects, but they all include items, facets and domains. Facets are made up of many items, and domains are made up of many facets, profiles are made up of many domains. So, domains also are called sub-profiles. The content of relative items is introduced as follows:

Item is the most basic element, which can't be divided any more. A group of relative items is called an item pool. The quality of a profile is decided by the choice of items to a great degree.

(1) The form of item

There are six main kinds of forms:

①Linearity items: The testers make marks on the line with scale (for example 0 – 10), the choices of answer distribute on the whole line.

②Equal interval and equal class items: The testers are asked to select answer from the equal interval degree phrases, such as, worse, bad, moderate, good and better. These kinds of items were founded by Likert in 1932, so it is called Likert method too, in form, there are three points method, five points method and seven points method, among which the five points method is often used.

③Unequal interval but equal class item: almost the same as ②, but only the interval between these degree phrases is not equal.

④Bi-classified items: The answers are only two kinds, for example, yes or no.

⑤Cumulative items: They are made out and used for psychological evaluation in the 1940s, later it was used to evaluate QOL. The content of each item is divided into several sub-items to be answered according to its difficulty and amount. Taking the question does your health influence your action for example:

(a) Can you walk about 1,500 meters on foot (yes or no)?

(b) Can you walk about 500 meters on foot (yes or no)?

(c) Can you walk about 100 meters on foot (yes or no)?

Therefore, there is obvious logic relationship between the answers for these kinds of items, what's more, they can be used to analyse homogeneity. For example, if the answer to (a) is yes, the answers to (b) and (c) should also be yes, otherwise, the answers are wrong.

⑥Descriptive items: Every alternative answer for each item is described in detail so that it could be convenient for testers to choose. For example, for the item reflecting the ability to action and the scope of movement, the alternative answers are:

0   lies in bed all day, unable to walk;
1   can only do little action in house;
2   can only move around in house;
3   can freely move around.

However, which item is the best one? It is very difficult to properly evaluate. Each has strong points and weak points at the same time. Generally speaking, the linearity items are more accurate and easier to analyze, but people with low education have difficulty to understand them. The degree of items is easily to be understood, but it is inconvenient for designing the choices and analyzing the result. So it need to adopt some methods to deal with the inconvenience. The bi-classified items are simpler, but the information contained is too little. So, many profiles include several kinds of items at the same time. In this way, every item can use others' strong points to offset its own weakness, like MOS SF-36. Meanwhile, some profiles only include one kind of item, like FLIC. Generally speaking, the linearity items and the equal interval and class items are most often used. Furthermore, they two are more likely to exist for long.

(2) Implication of items

Items can be classified into four kinds according to the implication of items as follows:

①Items for evaluation, such as good or bad.
②Intensity of items, such as heavy and heavier.
③Frequency of items, such as rare and often.
④Capacity items, such as capable and absolutely capable.

These items are put forward according to the result of meaning-psychology study by Osgood, etc., and later are widely utilized in evaluation for HQOL by WHO.

(3) Feature of items

Items can be divided into two kinds as follows:

①Perceived objective items.
②Self-reported subjective items.

2. The methods and procedure for profile design

(1) Methods

The methods for profiles are a very complicated systematic project, including all the methods involved in the process from deciding conception of measurement, developing and selecting items, to evaluating and modifying profile. However, in a narrow sense, the methods only refer to the methods for defining conception and developing items. That is to say, beginning with the principles of measurement, the methods are used to bring out items and develop into item pool. As far as the process of implementation is concerned, it is best to adopt the programmed decision methods to set up profile. Namely profile is set up through the joint work of nominal group and focus group (core work group).

(2) Procedures

①Decide subject and object for study

The testers need be decided first. There is a need to decide what profile should be used and set up. For example, general profiles suit for ordinary people, special profiles for the special crowd (the old people or lung cancer patients). The role of the profile should be decided. For example, it focuses on judgment or evaluation and so on.

②Set up research group

In medical area, it is necessary to measure the QOL for patients with certain disease (cancer) and the special group (the old people). So the topic discussion group and core work group, who are responsible for making and modifying profile, should be made up of the relative members of each level, suchas medical experts, doctors, nurses, patients and other relative normal people. Among them, the topic discussion group should involve a wider range of people and are mainly in charge of putting forward items. And the core work group should be made up of more professional members and elites, who are responsible for specific research work.

③Defining the conception for measurement and deciding its components

The core work group decides practicable conception for the items, and their elements. For example, what does the QOL refer to? What field and sub-facet does it include? And what does the each sub-facet mean?

④Bring out items and make into item pool

The content of③should be introduced and explained to the topic discussion group in detail by the core work group (it is best to hold a meeting for that), then the items related to above definition are worked out by the members of topic discussion group respectively according to their professional knowledge and experiences. Strictly, the items might be more clearly if they work out them according to the content of each field and sub-facet. If the work is too difficult in this way, they can only work out the items for the whole profile generally. Then all of the items are collected and analyzed, the items that only have different forms but have similar meanings should be made into one item, and all of the different items make up one item pool.

⑤Decide the style of items and alternative answer

The linearity and degree methods are widely utilized, and the former need a line with certain length (often 0 – 10cm) and the alternatives for the two ends of the line need be given. In this way, the linearity one is formed. As to the latter one, in principle, each alternative answer should be decided through analysis of response scale.

The purpose of analysis of response scale is orientation analysis for all kinds of degree adverbs that may be the alternative answer. Firstly, 10 - 15 possible answers for the same kind items need to be worked out, such as frequency adverb: always, often, rarely, occasionally, seldom, never and so on. Secondly, let a tester mark these words on a line with two ends (0 - 10cm), then analyze the place of each word (average and) and select the relative words from them. Take the five points method for example, because the words for two ends are decided, only the words for the place of 2.5cm, 5.0cm and 7.5cm need be decided.

Equal interval between each alternative can be attained in this way, and in this way it is very convenient to rank (it can be ranked 1, 2, ... ,5) and statistically analyze.

Of course, some profiles are designed in advance and there isn't orientation analysis, and each item is often followed by several alternatives and maybe the interval between each choice isn't equal. Strictly speaking, the orientation test and analysis for each word should be done in the process of analysis. If so, it might be convenient to adjust the score of each alternative.

⑥Analyze and screen indicators

Each item of item pool should be statistically analyzed and screened, and the indicators attained through screening make up the pilot profile.

⑦Pre-survey and evaluation for profile

The above pilot profile is used to do pre-survey, and thus the reliability, validity and responsibility of the profile are evaluated.

⑧Modifying and perfecting

The final profile can be achieved through modifying and perfecting based on the above process.

The methods and procedures for developing profile are briefly introduced above. It is also a shortcut method for developing new profile that the Chinese profiles are achieved through translating and studying the ready western profiles, but the methods and procedures are not completely same.

3. Analysis of items and method of screening

(1) Analysis for item

Inspection and carrying out pre-trail for each item of the item pool that has been worked out, and selection and perfection of the items according to statistic analysis about the result of pre-trail are required. All of these processes are called analysis of item. In brief, analysis of item refers to explaining the strong points and weak points from every aspect and providing evidence for selecting items. It includes evaluating the difficulty, responsibility discretion, representativeness and independence.

Analysis for difficulty can be reflected through pass rate of items. The item isn't proper or is too difficult to understand, if many testers can't answer it.

Analysis for responsibility is to find out the way that the testers answer the items. The main purpose is to learn about the reliability of items. It isn't proper that all testers only focus on some special items or some items aren't answered by anybody

(2) Method for item screening

It is a key step in the process of developing QOL to screen the items (indicators). There isn't yet any special book that involves method about screening items for QOL. Zhang Luoman once reported that the indicators for evaluating hospital can be selected through old hand evaluation method, coefficient of variation method, coefficient of correlation, cluster analysis method, and principle component analysis method. No doubt, these ways can be used to select the indicators for QOL.

The principles, which should be followed in the process of selecting indicators, should be with great importance, high sensitivity, strong independence, good representativeness, good certainty, appliance and acceptability as well.

There are some methods introduced as follows. They are used to select items from different angles and purposes. Apart from the first and the sixth methods, these methods all need to carry out pre-survey according to the ready items. So a series of true values from measurement can be achieved, and then researcher can carry out analysis. The sample size had better be more than 100.

①Subjective evaluation

This means to select indicators from importance and certainty. The method is that doctors and patients mark the ready indicators according to the importance for health in their minds (the full scores are one hundred). Then the researchers can select indicators according to the scores (average) and give up the indicators with low scores. There is a relationship between the method for calculation of average and the distribution of scores, if the distribution is normal distribution and the average should be arithmetic mean, otherwise the average should be median. When we calculate average, the maximum and minimum should be cancelled in order to avoid the influence of the extreme value on the average. In addition, the evaluation of importance by doctors is often different from that by patients. So selecting indicators should carry out respectively, at the same time should jointly concern both of them.

②Tendency of dispersion method

This is the method to select indicators from the aspect of sensitivity. If the tendency of dispersion of indicators isn't so remarkable, the ability to find out difference is weak. Therefore, the indicators with obvious tendency of dispersion should be selected. The standard deviation is often used to reflect tendency of dispersion directly. If the scores of each item do not assume normal distribution, researchers should transform the variables and make them assume normal distribution.

③Correlation coefficient method

This is the method for selecting indicators from the angle of representativeness and independency. According to calculating the coefficient of each of two indicators and carrying out statistic test, the indicators should be selected which have more and less correlative indicators. Because the former can provide more information and the latter has strong independency, both of them can't be substituted for by any others. Correlative coefficient should be decided according to the feature of the data.

④Principle component analysis and factors analysis method

It is the method to select indicators from aspect of representativeness. Principle component analysis begins with the correlative matrix of each indicator. Principle component should be decided according to the assumed structure and contribution rate of the profile, then the main indicators made up of the principle component analysis are decided according to the correlativity of the principle component and indicators (select the indicators with large correlative coefficient). For example, according to the assumption, the profile for HQOL should include five main parts (PH, PS, SO, St and environment), and there are five main elements that should be concerned. Factor analysis selects indicators according to the burden of element and selects the indicators with great burden.

⑤Cluster analysis method

It is also the methods that are used to select indicators from representativeness. First it uses one kind of clustering method (often hierarchical clustering method was used) to do cluster analysis for each indicator (often R cluster analysis). Thus, indicators can be clustered into number of sorts. Then the representative indicators of every sort are the needed indicators. The representative indicators are selected according to the square of coefficient of correlation, and the rule is: (a) The representative indicator of each sort is the one that has the best average correlation to other indicators. (b) The representative indicator is the one that has good average correlation to the indicators of the same sort but has bad average correlation to the indicators of other sorts.

⑥Stepwise selection based on evaluation of importance

It is generalization of the first method and similar to the Delphi forecast method that was worked out by the American Rand Company. That is to say, first of all, select the indicators with higher scores and former place through the first method (selection for the first time), feedback these indicators to the valuators, then go on selecting for the second time. In this way, step by step, the acceptable important indicators can be achieved.

⑦Stepwise regression analysis method

This method needs get a series of data through pre-survey, let the participants for pre-survey wholly grade their own HQOL, take the scores of Y as the function of X, then use Y and each indicator($X_1, X_2, \ldots, X_n$) to do gradual regression analysis and find out the indicators which can greatly influence every aspect. However, the meaning of HQOL should be explained in detail to the participants in the pre-survey, otherwise, the total scores can't reflect HQOL.

⑧Stepwise discriminant analysis

One purpose of HQOL is to evaluate the effect of different therapies and measures. So different population have different HQOL, and a good profile should be with the ability to differentiate the difference. Thus, in the pre-survey, researcher can select different population (assuming there are patients and normal people), the indicators which greatly attribute to differentiate the two groups can be found through gradual discriminant analysis method. So the profile made up by these indicators has strong ability to differentiate difference.

Appendix:
Development of Chinese version about the profile of WHOHQOL

Professor Fang Jiqian, from the statistic staff room of Zhongshan Medical University, is the principal of development group for Chinese version of the profile of WHOHQOL. Under the trust of WHO and the national Health Ministry of the People's Republic of China, based on WHO's profile for HQOL — WHOQOL-100 and WHOQOL-BREF, and concerned the situation of China, the Chinese version for the above two profiles has been developed, which followed the procedures recommended by WHO.

(1) The development of the Guangdong version of WHOQOL-100

It started from 1995 to translate and develop the profile WHOQOL-100 into Chinese version. The statistic staff room of Zhongshan Medical University was in charge of the whole work according the program for research center of QOL made by WHO.

The procedure of development is as follows:

①Two experts for public health independently translated the profile into Chinese; the third expert checked and summarized the transcripts, then made it into the first draft of profile.

②Two core work groups carried out discussion respectively. One core work group was made up of doctors, nurses, and students from medical university, the other one was made up of patients. After discussion and modification the first draft became the second draft.

③Posted the second draft to the headquarters of WHO, and at the same time, invited an English teacher to translate the second draft from Chinese into English.

④The core work groups compared the English version of the second draft with the original English version, then modified it and made it into the third draft.

⑤Invited a group of patients and students of medical university to practice the reaction scale, then modified the reaction scale according to the result of this practice and made it into the fourth draft.

⑥Respectively selected one region from the east, west, south, north and middle of Guangdong Province and carried out pre-test (in every place survey 100 subjects), the five regions selected are Zhanjiang, Meizhou, Shaoguan, Zhongshan, and Guangzhou.

⑦Analysed the quantitative psychic indicators, such as reliability, validity, response and so on according to the data from survey. Meanwhile, made a simple sheet including less items according to the result of analysis.

⑧Modified the fourth draft according to the result of pre-test and finally developed into the Guangdong version, which was finished in Guangdong district and directed by Health Bureau of Guangdong province. The language of this profile is standard Chinese.

(2) Domestic cooperation study

The organization meeting for domestic cooperation study was held in Beijing from April 17th to 19th in 1996, which was directed by the Standard Office of Higher Education Department of Health Ministry and thirteen people participated this meeting. They talked about the work relative to QOL and exchanged the personal experience and information in the study of QOL. Zhongshan Medical University reported the process of development of the Gangdong version WHOQOL-100, and introduced the plan about the development of Chinese version WHOQOL-100 and relative study. The participants modified the Guangdong version WHOQOL-100 word by word after they attentively discussed it. What's more, they named the modified one as **96 Chinese version** and carried out field trial in six cities across China.

The field trials were carried out in six cities, namely, Guangzhou, Beijing, Shanghai, Chengdu, Xi'an, and Shenyang. In every place, 300 people were surveyed, and the researchers noticed the balance of patients and inpatients, male and female, structure of ages in the process of sampling. Among young people the diseases include chronic hepatitis, gastric ulcer, chronic bronchitis, depressed disease, among middle-aged people there are high blood pressure, coronary heart disease, diabetes, arthritis and so on, and among the old people the diseases mainly are cancer, cardiovascular disease, fracture. In addition, learned about the change in QOL of 50 patients before and after treatment was inspected. The data of the field survey in six cities were collected to the Statistic Staff Room of Zhongshan Medical University, and posted to the headquarters of WHO in February, 1997.

The translation of the **96 Chinese Version** was done independently by two English teachers. The **96 Chinese Version** was slightly modified and made into **97 Chinese Version**. After that the translation one compared with the original one and the result of the field survey of the six cities was studied carefully. Accordingly, the **97 Chinese Version** was translated into English. The **97 Chinese Version**, and its English transcript, together with the reports about the study of Chinese and field survey were reported to cooperation team of WHOQOL for auditing. In this year, the cooperation team also formally accepted the *97 Chinese Version* as the Chinese version for the profile of WHOQOL.

In addition, the colleagues and postgraduate students of the Statistic Staff Room in Zhongshan Medical University developed the general profile WHOQOL-100. They developed the special profile for the denoting people, liver cancer patients and diabetics as well and took it as a supplement for the profile WHOQOL.

Section 5 The Application of QOL Evaluation in Health Domain

The QOL evaluation has been widely used in various domains in the society and has become a necessary indicator and evaluating instrument. It is used in 4 fields in health domains: ①To evaluate the health situation of population; ②Benefit-evaluating to the resource utilization; ③The comparison of clinical treatment and intervening measures; ④The choosing and decision-making of treatment.

1. The health situation evaluating to common and special population

Some kinds of generic QOL scales do not aim at the patient of certain disease, and the purpose of QOL evaluation is not to appraise the treatment effect but try to know the comprehensive health situation of ordinary people. It is even regarded as a kind of general indicator of social economy and medicine so that the comparison of QOL and its developing level in different countries, different regions and different nationality as well as the research on its influencing factors can be carried out, which is familiar in the QOL evaluation in early. As for GHO, NHP, MHIQ (McMaster health index questionnaire), MOS-36 developed from the early 1980s and the cross-nation and cross-culture WHOQOL which is being developed at present, all of which are used to evaluate QOL of ordinary people.

At home, Lin Nan studied the residents' QOL of Tianjin according to the data of sampling survey of 1,000 families. Wang Bingyan, etc. comprehensively analyzed the health situation and QOL of the middle-aged intellectuals in Beijing. Li Lingjiang chose the families in towns and countries in Hunan Province as sampling frame, and analyzed the QOL of those people and its influencing factors.

Sometimes the QOL evaluation just aims at some special populations to try to know their health situation and its influencing factors as well as solving the relative problems. For example, the issue of senior citizens has become more and more significant with the aging of the society. All the old have health damage with different extent; however, it's not serious if without functional obstacle. The most concerned is the ability of self-provision in normal life and the extent of demanding help for old people in the circumstance of function drop. Hence the QOL and its relative problems of the old people are so special that have attracted the extensive attentions and related studies have been carried out. For example, Katz etc. evaluated the function fettle of the old and introduced the concept of active life expectancy(ALE) into the consideration the life expectancy after QOL. Pearlman established the COPE, which is only for senior citizens, to evaluate their function. Xu Shulian carried out the research on the QOL, self-blessedness degree and its influencing factors of the retired cadres.

Furthermore, Longabaugh etc. have studied the QOL of alcohol abusers; Wan Chonghua etc. have analysed the QOL and its influencing factors of junkies.

2. The QOL evaluation to patients of cancer and chronic disease

The study of the QOL evaluation to patients of cancer and chronic diseases is the mainstream of QOL study in medical field. There are hundreds of articles talking about it every year, which are in the ascendant.

(1) The evaluation to cancer patient

At the early 80s' last century the QOL Research Group was established by European Cancer Treatment and Research Organization. Seven countries joined it and carried out collaborative study on the QOL evaluation of cancer patients in a larger scale. Now Australia, Canada and USA along with other 16 European countries have joined this group. They have developed a core scale QLQ-C30, which reflects the commonness of cancer patients, and some other special scales for certain cancers, such as QLQ-LC13 for lung cancer, QLQ-BR24 for breast cancer, QLQ-H&N37 for head and cervix cancer, QLQ-OES24 for gullet cancer and QLQ-CR38 for recta and colon cancer. The USA Cancer Academy has carried out the study of QOL evaluation in 6 communities, which implemented the clinical tumor plan, Anderson Hospital in Texas University and the Tumor Academy. The study aimed at exploring the relative problems of QOL study, which was carried out contemporarily with the clinical trial on cancer, and putting forward the solutions. Rush-Presbyterian-St. Luke Medical Center in Chicago developed the FACT(functional assessment of cancer therapy), which consists of FACT-G, evaluating the commonness of QOL of cancer patients, and some other sub-scales to evaluate certain cancers. Furthermore, CARES and CARES-SF are being developed and applied.

Most of the famous scales were developed in domain of cancer. In the recent twenty years the QOL evaluation has been widely used in treating effect evaluation of antitumor drugs and in choosing treatment regimes. For example, many scholars evaluated the treatment regime of breast cancer with method of QOL, and then improved it from total resecting to partial resecting. With the method of combining QOL and survival time, Gelber etc. comprehensively analyzed whether it's necessary to conduct supplementary treatment to the patient after she got the breast cancer operation and what treatment should be selected. Mcneil etc. conducted comprehensive QOL evaluation on the treatment to larynx cancer patient on those points: do operation or use radiotherapy, aim at allowing the patient to live longer or maintaining the natural ability to speak. In China, the evaluations on breast cancer, lung cancer and nasopharyngeal carcinoma have been carried out. As for the disease category, most of the evaluations were about breast and lung cancer, for they have high prevalence rate in Europe and USA.

(2) The evaluation to chronic disease

In recent twenty years, a large number of QOL evaluations have been conducted abroad, which were about such chronic diseases as cardiovascular and cerebralvascular disease, COPD, rheumatism, urological diseases and endocrine diseases. Fletcher et al. studied the changing rules on QOL of the angina pectoris patients before and after they got the treatment. Spertus et al. developed the SAQ(Seattle angina questionnaire) and applied it to evaluate the relevant patients. Bernie et al. evaluated the effect of heart implantation with the method of QOL and survival analysis. Evans et al. conducted the QOL evaluation to those patients who were carried out kidney implantation and nephritic disease patients at later period who were conducted the hemodialysis, and got the result that the QOL of the former was better than that of the latter.

In China, QOL evaluations have been carried out on HBP, DM, asthma, nephritic diseases and stroke.

(3) Evaluating and choosing clinical treatment regime

QOL has been widely used in clinical evaluation on patients of cancer and chronic diseases. The evaluation targets to not only reflect the general health status but evaluate the treating effect and choose treatment regime, and the latter is more important. Through monitoring and evaluating the patient's QOL under different regimes and measures, provide new outcome indicators for the comparison of treatment and recovery measures. Through studying the QOL of low rectal cancer patients after they got the rectectomy, Williams et al. found that in terms of diet, sexual function and emotion, those patients that got operation maintaining rectal sphincter were superior to those that got abdominoperineal resection of rectum, thus proved that the former method was better than the latter. Sugarbaker provided a typical example: there are two common treatments to body tumor, one is amputation and the other is retaining the body but supplementing vast-dose radiotherapy. Based on the traditional opinion the body won't be amputated until there is no other choice. Sugarbaker evaluated the QOL of the patients who treated by these two ways and found that there was no significant difference in statistic, but in terms of emotion, self-care and sexual behavior, the amputation group was better than the group that retained the body. According to this, he drew the conclusion that the treatment of retaining was not necessarily better than amputation; in order to reduce the relapse amputation should be conducted. With the multi-factors analysis method, Wangwei etc. (2000) analyzed the influence factors of QOL of three kinds of women who were conducted sterilization, conception control with instruments or with drugs. They found that the life satisfactory and psychological fettle were the main factors that influence women's QOL, material condition was the key point that influence the life satisfactory and health status was the main factor to the psychological fettle. That means women's QOL were directly influenced by the improvement of material condition and the perfection of physical and psychological fettle. However, different ways of conception control had no significant influence on women's QOL. There are many related studies.

(4) Evaluating the effect of preventive interventions and health care measures

Preventive interventions and health care measures are oriented to ordinary people. With the development of preventive medicine and PHC, more and more attentions have been paid to the effect evaluation to the relative measures, and this comprehensive evaluation can be conducted with the indicator of QOL and has to compare the QOL before and after the intervene. Using QOL, Brook et al. evaluated the influence of mutual insurance on the health status of adult. Weishan Lv explored the role that health education played to old people's QOL.

(5) Policy decision on health resources allocation and utilization

The main target of policy decision analysis to health resource allocation and utilization is to choose the priority of the investment, properly allocate and utilize health resources to maximize the profit. With the wide conducting and deepening of QOL research, people tend to adopt the indicator of QALYs (quality adjusted life years) to comprehensively reflect the investment benefit, for QALYs combines the survival time and life quality, and overcomes the weakness of the former indicators, which ignored the differences of survival time between healthy people and patients. Hence indicators of QOL can be used in legislation for health care, making health policies and allocating health resources.

(6) Explore the influence factors of health and priorities of diseases prevention and treatment

Nowadays QOL has been regarded as a comprehensive indictor of health and living standard, and has been or is being the target of medical and social development. It's helpful to find the priorities of diseases prevention and treatment through exploring the influence factors of QOL, thus accelerating the improvement of integrated health level. Chonghua Wan et al. analyzed the influence factors on QOL of drug addicts.

第四篇 社会卫生处方

Part 4 Social Health Prescription

第十一章 社会卫生策略

社会医学的根本目的就是通过社会学的视角来认识健康问题，借鉴社会学的知识来分析健康问题。因此我们应该学会利用综合的社会手段来解决健康问题，这种处理卫生问题的方法主要依靠政府的社会卫生策略来实现。

WHO明确指出："政府对人民健康负有责任。"政府责任的落实主要依靠政策的作用，通过制定、执行、评估一系列的卫生政策，最终达到保护公民健康的目的。

卫生政策(health policy)是指社会为了满足人们的医疗卫生需要而采取的行动方案和行为依据。卫生政策其目的是研究社会如何以合理的方法，在能承担的成本(一定资源条件)下达到高质量和高数量满意服务所需的各种方法，属公共政策的一个范畴。

卫生策略(health strategy)是指为实现既定目标采取的手段与方法，是执行政策所要采取的行动要点和选择合适的行动路线。

确定卫生目标，并为保证其顺利实现制定相应的政策措施，是各国政府的一项基本职责。追求卫生服务的公平性和效率，提高全体人民的健康水平一直是各国政府长期努力的主要目标。

下面我们对现有的主要卫生策略简单地加以介绍。

第一节 初级卫生保健

初级卫生保健(primary health care, PHC)是世界卫生组织提出的一项全球性战略目标，它得到了联合国和世界多数国家政府的认同和承诺，是全世界人民健康的必要保障，为人类的健康事业作出了重要贡献。

一、初级卫生保健的提出

世界卫生组织(WHO)与联合国儿童基金会(UNICEF)于1978年9月6～12日在前苏联的阿拉木图主持召开了国际初级卫生保健大会，会上发表了《阿拉木图宣言》和一份世界健康报告，提出了"人人享有卫生保健"策略，明确指出初级卫生保健是实现人人享有卫生保健的关键。会议确定了初级卫生保健的概念，交流了初级卫生保健工作的经验，明确了初级卫生保健的原则和实施方法，解决了实施初级卫生保健中的一些实际问题。希望通过开展初级卫生保健活动来提高广大人群的保健水平。

1979年的联合国大会和1980年的联合国特别会议,分别表示了对《阿拉木图宣言》的赞同,使初级卫生保健活动得到了联合国的承诺。我国政府分别于1983年、1986年、1988年明确表示了对"2000年人人享有卫生保健"战略目标的承诺。

二、初级卫生保健的基本概念

《阿拉木图宣言》的定义:初级卫生保健是一种基本的卫生保健。它是由社区通过个人和家庭的积极参与,依靠科学的、又受社会欢迎的方法和技术,费用也是社区或国家在各个发展时期依靠自力更生和自觉精神能够负担得起的,普遍能够享受的卫生保健;是国家卫生系统的中心职能和主要要素;是国家卫生系统和社区经济发展的组成部分;是个人、家庭和社区同国家系统保持接触,使卫生保健深入居民生活与劳动的第一环节,能使卫生保健尽可能接近于人们居住及工作的场所;它还是卫生保健持续进程的起始一级。

我国政府五部(委、局、会)(卫医字〔90〕第1号)文件把它概括为:初级卫生保健是指最基本的、人人都能得到的、体现社会平等权利的、人民群众和政府都能负担得起的卫生保健服务。

三、初级卫生保健的基本原则

1. 预防为主。初级卫生保健实施的最根本目的就是保护和促进人们的健康,尽量做到少得病。减少疾病伤害最经济、有效的方法就是预防。许多疾病到了晚期将难以治愈,而且费用昂贵,此时传统的治疗手段将难以达到预期的效果。初级卫生保健重视综合性的致病因素对健康的影响。因为人们的健康受到多方面因素的影响,自然环境、社会环境、行为生活方式、生物遗传因素、心理因素等对健康产生直接或间接的影响,因此必须采取措施加以预防控制。

2. 社区参与。社区广泛参与到对疾病的预防和救助的活动中去,对特殊人群、脆弱人群提供帮助,利用社区资源做到互助共济,开展宣传教育,改善生活环境,改变人们不良生活方式,执行各种有益的卫生保健策略,达到保护和促进健康的目的。

3. 适宜技术。开展初级卫生保健采用的手段应该是技术可靠的、方法简便的、人们能够接受的、经济上能负担得起的。

4. 政府支持。初级卫生保健工作单靠卫生部门难以落实,它需要全社会共同参与,因此需要政府协调各部门之间的利益关系,组织财力物力支持这项工作。政府应该对人们的健康负有责任。

四、初级卫生保健的基本内容

初级卫生保健的目标是要使全世界人民达到尽可能高的健康水平,即人人享有卫生保健。根据《阿拉木图宣言》初级卫生保健工作可为四个方面任务、八项内容。

(一)初级卫生保健的基本任务

1. 促进健康。包括健康教育,保护环境,合理营养,饮用安全卫生水,改善卫生设施,开展体育锻炼,促进心理卫生,养成良好生活方式等。

2. 预防保健。在研究社会人群健康和疾病的客观规律及它们和人群所处的内外环境、人类社会活动的相互关系的基础上,采取积极有效的措施,预防各种疾病的发生、发展和流行。

3. 合理治疗。及时发现疾病,及时提供医疗服务和有效药品,以避免疾病的发展与恶化,促使早日好转痊愈,防止带菌(虫)和向慢性发展。

4. 社区康复。对丧失了正常功能或功能上有缺陷的残疾者,通过医学的、教育的、职业的和社会的措施,尽量恢复其功能,使他们重新获得生活、学习和参加社会活动的能力。

(二)初级卫生保健的基本要素

1. 对当前主要卫生问题及其预防和控制方法的健康教育。
2. 改善食品供应和合理营养。
3. 供应足够的安全卫生水和基本环境卫生设施。
4. 妇幼保健和计划生育。
5. 主要传染病的预防接种。
6. 预防和控制地方病。
7. 常见病和外伤的合理治疗。
8. 提供基本药物。

1981年第34届世界卫生大会上,除上述八项内容外,又增加了"使用一切可能的方法,通过影响生活方式、控制自然和社会心理环境来预防和控制非传染疾病和促进精神卫生"一项内容。

五、初级卫生保健的特点

初级卫生保健具有社会性、群众性、艰巨性和长期性等特点。

1. 社会性。健康不仅是指没有疾病或虚弱,而是指生物、心理、社会的完好状态。健康是每个人的基本权利。初级卫生保健就是通过全社会的参与,控制或消除各种健康危险因素,使所有人达到尽可能高的健康水平。因此,初级卫生保健具有广泛的社会性。

2. 群众性。初级卫生保健的服务对象是全体人群。初级卫生保健关系到每个人的身体健康,居民不仅有享有卫生保健的权利,同时有参与实施初级卫生保健的义务。因此初级卫生保健具有广泛的群众性。初级卫生保健需要社会广大群众广泛参与,只有人们共同努力才能实现预期的目标。健康教育的开展、生活方式的改变、环境的改善等等都需要群众参与。

3. 艰巨性。初级卫生保健的内容涉及卫生工作的方方面面,结合我国的卫生状况来看,初级卫生保健的任务是相当艰巨的。近年来,我国卫生事业取得了巨大的成就,农村初级卫生保健取得了阶段性成就,但是,医疗卫生事业还满足不了人民群众对医疗保健日益增长的需要。同时发展不平衡,城乡之间、东部与西部地区之间差距很大。许多农村地区生活卫生条件很差,远没有达到初级卫生保健的最低标准。在相当多的地区,传染病、地方病还严重威胁着人们的健康。心血管疾病、恶性肿瘤等慢性非传染性疾病不断上升已经成为人们健康的主要威胁。

4. 连续性。我国农村已基本实现了1990～2000年初保阶段性目标,但初级卫生保健又面临许多新情况、新挑战。首先,随着社会的发展和居民生活条件、认识水平的不断提高,必然会对健康提出越来越高的要求;其次,人口的老龄化、新的疾病的出现、医学模式的转变都要求初级卫生保健的内容和水平不断提高;最后,任何一个国家都没有足够的财力来保证居民的所有健康问题,因此初级卫生保健在不同时期都会有强大的生命力。由此可以看出,初级卫生保健政策是一个长期、连续的政策。

第二节 健康教育与健康促进

一、健康教育与健康促进的概念及意义

初级卫生保健策略的第一条内容就是"对当前主要卫生问题及其预防和控制方法的健康教育"。初级卫生保健需要全社会参与,要通过改变人们自身的行为方式来完成,因此必须通过健康教育来统一行动。健康促进是"人人享有卫生保健"全球战略的关键要素。健康教育学是研究健康促进与健康教育的理论、方法和实践的科学,其知识体系和研究内容涉及医学、行为学、教育学、心理学、人类学、社会学、传播学、经济学、管理学、政策学等有关学科领域。

(一)健康教育

健康教育(health education)通过有计划、有组织、有系统的社会和教育活动,促使人们自觉地采纳有益于健康的行为和生活方式,消除或减轻影响健康的危险因素,预防疾病,促进健康和提高生活质量。

健康教育的核心问题是促使个体或群体改变不健康的行为和生活方式,尤其是组织行为改变。诚然,改变行为与生活方式是艰巨的、复杂的过程。许多不良行为并非属于个人责任,也不是有了个人的愿望就可以改变的,因为许多不良行为或生活方式受社会习俗、文化背景、经济条件、卫生服务等影响,更广泛的行为涉及生活状况,如居住条件、饮食习惯、工作条件、市场供应、社会规范、环境状况等。因此,要改变行为必须增进有利健康的相关因素,如获得充足的资源、有效的社区领导和社会的支持以及自我帮助的技能等,此外还要采取各种方法帮助群众了解他们自己的健康状况并作出自己的选择以改善他们的健康,而不是强迫他们改变某种行为,所以健康教育必须是有计划、有组织、有系统的教育过程,才能达到预期的目的。

(二)健康促进

健康促进(health promotion)的概念比健康教育更为广义。1986年在加拿大渥太华召开的第一届国际健康促进大会发表的《渥太华宪章》中指出:"健康促进是促使人们提高、维护和改善他们自身健康的过程。"这一定义表达了健康促进的目的和哲理,也强调了范围和方法。《渥太华宪章》还提出了健康促进的五点策略。

1. 制定健康的公共政策。健康促进超越了保健范畴,它把健康问题提到了各个部门、各级领导的议事日程上,使他们了解他们的决策对健康后果的影响并承担健康的责任。健康促进的政策由多样且互补的各方面综合而成,它包括政策、法规、财政、税收和组织改变等。

2. 创造支持性环境。人类与其生存的环境是密不可分的,这是对健康采取社会-生

态学方法的基础。健康促进在于创造一种安全、舒适、满意、愉悦的生活和工作条件。任何健康促进策略必须保护自然、创造良好的环境以及保护自然资源。

3. 强化社区性行动。健康促进工作是通过具体和有效的社区行动,包括确定需优先解决的健康问题,作出决策,设计策略及其执行,以达到促进健康的目标。在这一过程中,核心问题是赋予社区以当家作主、积极参与和主宰自己命运的权利。

4. 发展个人技能。健康促进通过提供信息、健康教育和提高生活技能以支持个人和社会的发展,这样做的目的是使群众能更有效地维护自身的健康和他们的生存环境,并作出有利于健康的选择。

5. 调整卫生服务方向。卫生部门的作用不仅仅是提供临床与治疗服务而必须坚持健康促进的方向。调整卫生服务方向也要求更重视卫生研究及专业教育与培训的转变,并立足于把一个完整的人的总需求作为服务对象。

综上所述,健康促进的概念比健康教育更为完整,因为健康促进涵盖了健康教育和生态学因素(环境因素和行政手段)。健康促进是指一切能促使行为和生活条件向有益于健康改变的教育与生态学支持的综合体。健康促进是健康教育发展的结果。健康促进是"人人享有卫生保健"全球战略的关键要素。

(三)健康相关行为

健康相关行为(health related behavior)指人类个体和群体与健康和疾病有关的行为。按其对行为者自身和他人的影响,可分为健康行为(health behavior)和危险行为(risk behavior)。

根据哈律士(Harris)和顾坦(Guten)的建议,健康行为可分为五类。

1. 基本健康行为。即一系列日常生活中基本的健康行为,如积极的休息和睡眠等。

2. 预警行为。预防事故发生以及事故发生后如何处置的行为,如驾车系安全带、地震后的自救行为等。

3. 保健行为。即合理、正确行使医疗保健服务以维护自身健康的行为,如预防接种等。

4. 避开环境危害行为。环境危害包括对身体有害的自然环境、社会环境和生活事件。

5. 戒除不良嗜好行为。不良嗜好主要指吸烟、酗酒和吸毒等。

健康教育的目的就是使人们消除或远离危险行为,培养或保持健康行为,最终达到保护、提高健康的目的。

二、健康教育的途径——传播活动

从20世纪60年代起将传播学的概念引入健康教育领域,并逐渐形成了健康传播学,极大地丰富了健康教育的策略方法和理论宝库,有效地指导着健康教育的实践。

(一)传播概念

传播(communication)是一种社会性传递信息的行为,是个人之间和集体之间以及集体与个人之间交换、传递新闻、事实、意见等信息的过程。

（二）传播模式

美国著名社会学家、政治学家哈罗德·拉斯韦尔提出了一个被誉为传播学研究经典的传播过程的文字模式，即"一个描述传播行为的简便方法，就是回答下列 5 个问题：①谁（who）？②说了什么（says what）？③通过什么渠道（through what channel）？④对谁（to whom）？⑤取得什么效果（with what effect）?"拉斯韦尔五因素传播模式（又称5W模式）具体地说是：谁、说什么、通过什么渠道、对谁、取得什么效果；或者是：传者、信息、传播途径、受者、效果。

健康传播的效果可分为四个层次。

1．知晓健康信息。这是传播效果中的最低层次。通过信息的共享，使公众的医药卫生知识水平不断提高，为其自身保健技能的提高打下良好的基础。

2．健康信念认同。受者接受所传播的健康信息，并对信息中倡导的健康信念认同一致，自觉或不自觉地依照这样的信念进行对健康的追求与选择。

3．态度转变。即人们对特定对象的认知、情感和意向的比较持久的内在意识。态度的形成既有社会交往过程的影响，又有心理过程的作用。态度一旦形成就成为一种心理定势。一般来说态度是行为改变的先导，先有态度，才会有行为的改变。

4．采纳健康的行为。这是传播效果的最高层次。受者接受健康信息后，在知识增加、信念认同、态度转变的基础上，改变其原有的不利于健康的行为和生活方式。这是健康传播的最终目标。

三、健康促进规划

健康促进是一项涉及面广泛而艰巨的任务，直接作用于影响健康的各种危险因素或病因；涉及社会的诸多方面及生命的各个阶段；综合使用各种教育手段与传播方式；而且涵盖了多学科的知识。因此，健康促进工作的开展必须有一个科学、周密的规划，才能很好地发挥作用。

任何一项健康促进规划由设计、实施和评价三部分组成。三者构成相互制约、密不可分的整体。

（一）规划的设计

1．概念：规划的设计是基于研究目标人群有关健康问题及其特征，并形成该问题的理论假设，提出解决的目标以及实现目标所采取的一系列具体方法、步骤和策略，为规划实施奠定基础，同时又为科学的评价提供量化指标。

2．RECEDE-PROCEED 模式：健康教育和健康促进规划设计的模式有多种，但在众多模式中，应用最广泛、最具生命力的首推美国著名学者劳伦斯·格林（Lawrence W. Green）提出的 PRECEDE-PROCEED 模式。该模式的特点是从"结果"入手，用演绎的方式进行思考，即从最终的结果追溯到最初的起因。PRECEDE-PROCEED 模式前后相互呼应，为规划设计、执行及评价提供一个连续的步骤或阶段。实际上可将上述模式分为两个阶段：

第一个阶段为诊断阶段（或称需求评估），即 PRECEDE 阶段（predisposing, reinforcing and enabling constructs in educational/environmental diagnosis and evaluation），指

在教育/环境诊断和评价中应用倾向、促成及强化因素；

第二阶段为执行阶段，即 PRECEDE 阶段(policy,regulatory and organizational constructs in educational and environmental development)，执行教育/环境干预中应用政策、法规和组织的手段。

3. 规划设计的基本步骤：根据 PRECEDE-PROCEED 模式的程序，将规划设计分成 9 个基本步骤，即从最终的结果追溯到最初的起因，用演绎的方式逐步推进。

(1) 社会诊断。从评估目标人群的生活质量入手，评估他们的需求和健康问题。最好有目标人群的亲自参与。

(2) 流行病学诊断。通过流行病学和医学调查确认健康问题和目标。

(3) 行为与环境诊断。确认与上述健康相关的行为和环境。

(4) 教育与组织诊断。制定教育与组织策略，应从影响行为和环境的因素入手。这些因素可归纳为三大类，即倾向因素、促成因素和强化因素。研究这三类因素的主要目的在于正确地制定教育策略，即根据各种因素的相对重要性及资源情况确定干预重点。

(5) 管理与政策诊断。评估组织与管理能力及在计划执行中资源、政策、人员能力和时间安排。通过社区开发、协调、完善组织与政策，以便规划的顺利开展。

(6) 执行阶段。相当于健康促进规划的实施阶段。

(7) 评估阶段(步骤 7～9)。评价不是 PRECEDE 模式的最后步骤，评价工作贯穿于整个模式始终。

(二)规划的实施

规划的实施是按照规划去实现目标，获得效果的过程，也是体现规划根本思想的具体活动和行动。没有有效的实施工作，再好的规划也只能是一纸空文。因此，在健康教育和健康促进活动中，实施规划是主体工作部分，也是重点和关键。实施工作包括建立反馈信息系统、建立执行计划程序、组织协调与质量控制等。健康促进规划实施中的主要任务有：

1. 社区开发。社区开发的目标主要包括建立领导机构、积极动员靶人群参与、加强网络建设和部门间的协调以及制定政策支持项目的开展。

2. 项目培训。项目培训是为达到项目目标而建立与维持一支高效工作队伍的活动。

3. 社区为基础的干预。社区为基础的健康促进干预是多种干预活动的整合，领导机构的建立、政策的支持、多部门的参与、干预管理人员的培训都是干预的重要因素，也是社区干预成功的前提。

4. 项目执行的监测与质量控制。无论是规划的设计还是规划的执行和评价，建立监测与质量控制体系对健康促进规划的开展有着十分重要的意义。

(三)规划的评价

评价是评估规划所规定的目标是否达到以及达到的程度。评价工作是健康促进规划设计的重要组成部分，贯彻于整个课题设计、实施、评价的始终，而不是完成整个规划后再考虑评价问题。规划评价是全面检测、控制、保证规划方案设计先进、实施成功并取得应有效果的关键性措施。是否执行严密的规划评价已成为衡量一项规划是否成功、是否科学的重要标志。

完整的规划评价包括 4 个类型。

1. 形成评价。形成评价(formative evaluation)是在规划执行前或执行早期对规划内容所作的评价。包括为制定干预规划所作的需求评估及为规划设计和执行提供所需的基础资料。

2. 过程评价。过程评价(process evaluation)是规划实施过程中监测规划各项工作的进展,了解并保证规划的各项活动能按规划的程序发展,即对各项活动的跟踪过程。过程评价是了解是否按规划的程序进行,规划活动中存在什么缺陷,应如何改进等,常规地监测、反馈各项活动的进展情况以期及时地调整规划的不合适部分。

3. 效果评价。效果评价(effectiveness evaluation)的目的是确定干预的效果,包括近期、中期和远期效果评价,其中远期效果评价又称为结局评价。

4. 总结评价。总结评价(summative evaluation)是综合形成评价、过程评价、效果评价以及各方面资料作出总结性的概括。综合性指标更能全面地反映规划的成败。总结评价从规划的成本-效益、各项活动的完成情况作出判断,以期作出该规划是否有必要重复或扩大或终止的决定。

第三节 全球卫生策略

一、20世纪全球卫生策略的历史回顾

(一) 2000年人人享有卫生保健战略的提出

WHO《组织法》明确规定:"健康是人类的一项基本权利,各国政府应对其人民的健康负责。"但是,由于社会制度、经济、文化等条件的不同,人类健康权利的平等和卫生服务之间差异的矛盾日益尖锐,1977年第30届世界卫生大会,提出了"2000年人人享有卫生保健"的全球战略。

(二) 2000年人人享有卫生保健的基本思想

1. 健康是人类的基本权利,居民享有卫生保健的机遇是均等的,不论是城市居民还是农村居民都应如此。

2. 卫生服务的重点应从侧重城市转向农村,从重视高技术治疗转向预防保健的普及,努力提高居民的文化教育水平、营养水平和生活条件。

3. 打破卫生事业狭隘的部门封闭状态,动员社会各部门积极参与实现"人人健康"的战略目标。

(三) 2000年人人享有卫生保健的具体含义

1. 人们在工作和生活场所都能保持健康。

2. 人们将运用更有效的办法去预防疾病,减轻不可避免的疾病和伤残带来的痛苦,并且通过更好的途径进入成年、老年,健康地度过一生。

3. 在全体社会成员中均匀地分配一切卫生资源。

4. 所有个人和家庭,通过自身充分的参与将享受到初级卫生保健。

5. 人们将懂得疾病不是不可避免的,人类有力量摆脱可以避免的疾病。

(四)人人健康战略的主要障碍

1. 实施人人健康的政治承诺不力;
2. 在获得基本医疗卫生服务的所有要素方面未能体现公平;
3. 妇女社会地位继续低下;
4. 社会经济发展缓慢;
5. 实现跨部门卫生行动陷入困境;
6. 人力资源分布不均以及对其支持力度薄弱;
7. 促进健康活动普遍不足;
8. 卫生信息系统薄弱,并缺少基线数据;
9. 环境污染,缺少安全饮用水供应和环境卫生设施;
10. 人口和流行病学方面的迅速变化;
11. 昂贵技术不适当的利用和资源分配不合理;
12. 自然和人为灾害。

只要上述障碍没有消除,人人健康就无从谈起。鉴于新的世界政治、经济、社会和环境状况,重新修订人人健康的全球战略,并制定各国适宜的行动计划,面对21世纪的挑战,势在必行。

二、新时期全球卫生策略

(一)21世纪人人享有卫生保健战略的提出

1995年5月第48届世界卫生大会决议(WHA48-16号)要求总干事为修订人人健康战略,强调个人、家庭和社区对健康应尽的责任,并将健康列为总体发展的核心,在协商一致的基础上最终形成新的全球健康发展政策。

21世纪人人健康全球战略,是"2000年人人健康"发展过程的延续,是指导各级(国际、区域、国家和地方)卫生行动的战略性文件,是21世纪全球卫生可持续发展的行动纲领。

(二)21世纪影响人类健康的新趋势

1. 广泛的绝对和相对贫困。贫困是导致营养不良和不健康的主要原因,它加剧疾病的传播、削弱卫生服务的有效性和减缓对人口的控制。

2. 人口的变化。老龄化导致慢性非传染性疾病、伤残和精神病例的增加;城市化超越了卫生基础设施满足人群需求的承受能力,过度拥挤和恶劣的工作环境导致焦虑、抑郁和慢性紧张状态,对家庭和社区的生活质量造成不利影响。

3. 流行病学变化。传染病的持续高发病率,新老传染病仍然对21世纪的全球卫生发展造成严重威胁;慢性非传染性疾病已经成为全世界人口死亡、疾病和残障的主要原因;暴力、车祸等损伤的增加,已经成为人类健康的重要威胁。

4. 全球环境威胁着人类的生存。全球环境的恶化,如空气污染、臭氧枯竭、气候改变、生物多样性的丧失,以及有害物品和废物跨越国界的运输都对健康产生极为不利的影响。

5. 新技术的发展。信息技术(包括远程医疗服务)和生物技术的发展将有助于发现、预防和减轻疾病的暴发,使更多的人获得卫生服务和健康教育。

6. 私营和公立部门以及公共社会各部门之间的卫生合作伙伴关系。为了适应新的形势,有必要考虑一些因素给卫生系统带来的机遇和压力,包括权力下放并将职责移交给地方政府和社会各机构,增加私营部门对卫生的参与以及居民参与卫生保健的决策,发展彼此之间的卫生合作伙伴关系。

7. 贸易、旅行、价值和思想传播的全球化。贸易、旅行和移民的急剧增加以及通讯与市场营销的发展威胁着人民的健康,尤其是食品跨越国界的运输和人口大规模的流动导致对健康的全球威胁。

(三) 21世纪全球卫生发展战略的行动基础

开展人人享有卫生保健战略的关键在于强化人民大众和社区参与健康活动。其行动基础为:

1. 承认获取最大可能的健康水平是一项基本人权;
2. 继续并加强伦理对卫生政策研究和服务提供的适用性;
3. 实施面向公平的政策和战略,以激励团结;
4. 将性别观体现于卫生政策和战略。

(四) 21世纪人人享有卫生保健战略的总目标

1. 提高全体人民的期望寿命和生活质量;
2. 改善国家间和国家内部的健康公平;
3. 建立和完善使人人享有可持续发展的卫生保健体制与服务。

(五) 截至2020年全球人人健康的具体指标

1. 健康公平。到2005年,将在国家内和国家间利用健康公平指数作为促进和监测健康公平的基础。最初以测定儿童发育为基础来评价公平,到2020年,在所有国家内的特定人群中5岁以下儿童发育不良(指年龄与身高相称程度在参考值以下超过两个标准差)的百分比应低于20%。

2. 生存。孕产妇死亡率(MMR)为每10万活产100以下;5岁以下儿童死亡率(CMR)为每1 000活产45以下;所有国家出生期望寿命均在70岁以上。

3. 采取措施。扭转全球5大疾病(结核、HIV/艾滋病、疟疾、烟草相关疾病和暴力/损伤)导致的发病率和伤残率上升趋势。

4. 根除和消灭某些疾病。到2020年,麻疹将得到根除,淋巴丝虫病、沙眼将被消灭;到2010年,恰加斯病传播将被阻断,麻风病将被消灭(每个县、区患病率为万分之一以下);到2005年,麦地那龙线虫病的传播将被阻断;预期到2000年脊髓灰质炎将被根除。

5. 改善人人享有的水、环境卫生、食品和住房条件。到2020年,所有国家将通过部门间行动在提供安全饮用水、适宜的环境卫生、数量充足和质量可靠的食物和住房条件方面取得重大进展。

6. 促进健康的举措。到2020年,所有国家将通过管理、经济、教育、组织和以社区为基础的综合规划,采取通过积极管理和监测以求巩固和增进健康的生活方式,减少有损健康的生活方式的战略。

7. 制定、实施和监测人人健康的国家政策。到2005年,所有国家都将制定、实施和监测与人人健康相配套的各项政策的运行机制。

8. 改善人人可获得的综合性的基本医疗卫生服务质量。到 2010 年，全体人民将在其整个生命过程中获得由基础公共卫生功能支撑的综合、基本、有质量的医疗保健。

9. 实施全球和国家卫生信息系统与监控系统。到 2010 年将建成适宜的全球和国家的卫生信息、监控和警报系统。

10. 支持卫生研究。到 2010 年，研究政策和体制运行机制将在全球、区域和国家各级水平上予以推行。

(六)政府在全球卫生战略中的责任

1. 全体人民在其整个生命过程中都能获得优质的卫生保健；
2. 预防和控制疾病以及保护健康；
3. 促进支持建立可持续的卫生保健体制和及其发展的法规；
4. 开发卫生信息系统，确保积极有效的监测；
5. 促进研究，激励卫生科学与技术的应用和创新；
6. 建设和维持卫生人力资源；
7. 获得适当的可持续资金的供给。

(七)行动准则

1. 与贫困作斗争。贫困是影响健康的重要因素。加速人类发展和经济增长，使贫困人口摆脱贫困，需要各国政府以及国际社会共同努力。同时，卫生干预措施有利于打破贫困与不健康的恶性循环。

2. 在一切环境中促进健康。包括生活、工作、娱乐和学习等所有与人类接触的自然、社会、生活环境。这需要个人、家庭、社会的共同努力。

3. 调整部门的卫生政策。保护人类健康仅仅依靠卫生部门的努力是远远不够的，政府的各个部门都可能对卫生产生影响，同时一项卫生政策的落实需要所有部门的共同努力，因此要求社会各个部门协调一致，共同维护和促进健康状况。

4. 将健康纳入可持续发展计划。要使健康成为发展的中心，健康必须在可持续发展计划中获得最优先考虑。首先，社会事业的发展必须以有利于或不危害人们的健康为重要依据；其次，在保护人类健康的活动中，必然消耗大量的资源，由于资源的有限性和需求的无限性的矛盾，要求卫生系统自身的发展也要有可持续性。

第四节　中国卫生策略

一、中国卫生工作方针

卫生工作的指导方针是指政府领导卫生工作的基本指导思想。

(一)卫生工作方针的历史沿革

1949 年 9 月第一届全国卫生会议确定了全国卫生工作的总方针为："预防为主，卫生工作的重点应放在保证生产建设和国防方面，面向农村、工矿，依靠群众，开展卫生保健工作。"

1950 年 9 月 8 日中央人民政府政务院正式批准了卫生工作的三大原则"面向工农兵、预防为主、团结中西医"。1952 年 12 月第二届全国卫生会议总结了爱国卫生运动的实践经验,周总理提出"增加卫生工作与群众运动相结合"的原则,从此以后统称为中国卫生工作的"四大方针",即"面向工农兵"、"预防为主"、"团结中西医"、"卫生工作与群众运动相结合"。50余年来,"四大方针"指引着我国卫生事业逐步兴旺昌盛,取得了举世瞩目的成就。

回顾过去,在贯彻预防为主方面仍存在一些不足。1991年4月9日七届全国人大四次会议批准的《国民经济和社会发展十年规划和第八个五年计划纲要》中,明确提出卫生事业贯彻"预防为主、依靠科技进步、动员全社会参与、中西医并重、为人民健康服务"的方针。1996年调整为"以农村为重点、预防为主、中西医并重、依靠科技与教育、动员全社会参与、为人民健康服务、为社会主义现在化建设服务"。此新时期卫生工作方针,指明了我国卫生工作的发展方向和重点,也为我们的医学教育和学习指明了方向。

(二)新时期卫生工作方针的主要内容

1. 以农村为重点。农村人口占我国总人口的绝大部分,农村人口的健康水平决定着全国总体健康水平。农村卫生关系到保护农民健康和振兴农村经济大局。医疗保健网在广大农村有了一定的基础.乡村医生队伍已有一定的规模,初级卫生保健工作取得了较大进展,农村人口的健康水平逐步提高。但是,从全国情况来看,农村医疗卫生工作薄弱的状况仍未根本改变,一部分农民因贫困看不起病,一部分农民因病致贫、因病返贫,疾病已成为农民脱贫致富的主要制约因素。另外,城乡之间及不同地区医疗卫生条件和人民健康水平差距有进一步扩大的趋势。这是一个十分值得重视、需要解决的问题。

2. 预防为主。坚持预防为主的方针,是因为预防保健费用低、效果好,是卫生工作低投入、高效益的关键所在。无论是传染病、地方病或慢性非传染性疾病中任何一个或几个病种的大面积发生,对我国这样一个发展中的人口大国来说,其卫生资源等消耗和经济上的损失都将是灾难性的。

建国以来,我们在儿童计划免疫接种、传染病的控制、地方病的预防等方面取得了重大的成就。我国政府积极参与国际卫生活动,并作出庄严承诺,先后制定了消灭脊髓灰质炎、消除新生儿破伤风、基本消灭麻风的规划、《九十年代中国儿童发展规划纲要》、《妇女发展规划纲要》、《中国九十年代营养行动计划》、《中国2000年消除碘缺乏病规划纲要》、《中国儿童发展纲要(2001~2010)》、《中国妇女发展纲要(2001~2010)》以及控制艾滋病规划等等。

目前我国多种传染病传播流行的各种因素依然存在,随着商品、人口和运载工具的大流动,有可能使一些局部地区发生的传染病扩散蔓延;对外开放也可能带来某些新病种传播,或已被控制、消灭的疾病又死灰复燃。同时,随疾病谱的变化,高血压、心脑血管疾病、肿瘤、糖尿病等慢性病,不仅在城市成为预防工作的重点,而且在农村也出现类似的趋势。按照各项预防保健规划的要求,要达到预期的目标,实现我国政府对国际社会的承诺,任务重,时间紧,必须加倍努力。

3. 中西医并重。中华民族在长期同疾病作斗争的实践中,创造了独具特色的中医药体系,是中华民族传统文化的瑰宝,在世界医药学发展史上独树一帜。党和政府历来重视中医药事业,毛泽东同志在建国初期就指出:"中国医药学是一个伟大的宝库,应当努力发掘,加以提高。"国家为发展中医药事业制定了一系列方针政策,经过广大中医药工作者的勤奋工作,中医药事业得到迅速恢复和发展。1978年,在医治"文革"创伤、国民经济还比较困难的状况下,邓小平同志明确要求各级党委和政府"要为中医创造良好的发展与提高的物质条件",使中医药事业获得长足发展。随着改革开放的进展,中西方文化交流日益频繁,江泽民同志强调指出"弘扬民族优秀文化,振兴中医中药事业"。我们要认真贯彻党中央三代领导人关于扶持、发展中医药事业的指示精神,并促进中西医结合,在继承中医特色和优势的基础上,积极利用先进科学技术和现代化手段发展中医药。

4. 依靠科技和教育。社会经济的发展和人民健康需求的增长,对科技进步提出了更为迫切的要求。医疗卫生是科技密集型、知识分子比较集中的行业,防治各种疾病,提高医疗卫生服务的质量,都离不开医学科技的发展和医学人才的培养,党中央和国务院确立了"科教兴国"的战略,关于科技和教育的发展都已有了明确的方针政策,医药科技与医学教育必须结合自身特点,认真贯彻落实这些方针。

5. 动员全社会参与。爱国卫生运动是全社会广泛参与的最好例证,爱国卫生运动是具有中国特色的一大创举。群众性的爱国卫生运动,从初期的除"四害"、打扫卫生,发展到今天党政军民共同创建卫生城市、卫生村镇,发生了质的飞跃。爱国卫生运动在实践中积累了丰富的经验,可以概括为:政府组织,地方负责,部门协调,群众动手,科学治理,社会监督。在创建卫生城市中,由于重视城市卫生基础设施建设、卫生文明管理制度建设和市民文明素质的提高,日益得到群众的信任和拥护,也成为党和政府为人民办实事、办好事的德政之一,对全国城镇两个文明建设起到推动作用,这项适合中国国情的把群众运动同经常性卫生基础建设结合在一起的创举,也得到国际赞许。

6. 为人民健康服务,为社会主义现代化服务。为人民健康服务,为社会主义现代化建设服务是卫生方针的核心,所有的一切都是围绕这个目的进行的。它既是卫生工作的出发点,又是落脚点,体现了全心全意为人民服务的宗旨。

卫生工作为社会主义现代化建设服务,是把卫生工作明确地纳入社会经济发展的总规划体系,并要求卫生事业发展与国家经济和社会发展相协调;卫生事业与社会经济发展是互相促进和互相制约的,卫生事业发展既是经济发展的前提和保证,也是经济发展的直接体现。卫生事业只有通过为人民健康服务才能保护好社会生产力,为社会主义现代化建设服务。

二、卫生发展总目标

到 2000 年,初步建立起具有中国特色的包括卫生服务、医疗保障、卫生执法监督的卫生体系,基本实现人人享有初级卫生保健,国民健康水平进一步提高;到 2010 年,在全国建立起适应社会主义市场经济体制和人民健康需要的、比较完善的卫生体系,国民健康的主要指标,经济较发达地区达到或接近世界中等发达国家的平均水平,使发达地区达到发展中国家的先进水平。

三、卫生工作的基本任务

1. 积极推行区域卫生规划,改革城市卫生服务体系,发展社区卫生服务,深入开展农村初级卫生保健,逐步形成不同层次、布局合理、具有综合功能的卫生服务网络,缩小地区之间卫生服务的差异。

2. 建立和完善适合我国国情的、多种形式的医疗保险制度。加快公费、劳保医疗制度改革,建立城镇职工基本医疗保险制度;扩大合作医疗和健康保险等多种形式的农村医疗保障制度覆盖面,使绝大多数居民都能得到基本的卫生服务。

3. 基本控制已有有效预防和治疗手段的疾病。进一步降低传染病、寄生虫病、地方病对人民健康的威胁,对慢性非传染性疾病逐步开展针对危险因素的综合防治。

4. 加强妇幼保健工作。提高妇幼保健工作水平,做好婚前保健服务,基本普及妇女和儿童系统保健管理。

5. 建立和完善包括食品、饮用水、化妆品、儿童用品、生活日用化学品、消毒器械、置入人体内的特殊装置(人造器官等)等制品以及生产、生活、学习、娱乐等场所以及医疗服务等的综合卫生执法监督体系,保障人民的健康权利。

6. 大力开展健康教育,普及基本卫生知识,使城乡居民逐步养成良好的卫生习惯;继续改善饮水卫生和环卫设备。

7. 积极推进医疗机构的配套改革,严格管理,促进医疗服务质量与效率的提高。

8. 建立起以政府负责、群众参与、部门协调、法制保障为基本特征的卫生工作体系,建立与社会主义市场经济体制相适应的筹资和运行机制。

四、卫生发展战略

以满足人们的健康需求为导向,以提高人民健康水平为中心,突出农村卫生、预防保健和中医药三个战略重点,按照公平与效率兼顾的原则,强化基本卫生服务和卫生监督管理工作,推行区域卫生规划,走以内涵发展为主、内涵与外延发展相结合的道路。

案例

中国农村初级卫生保健

农村初级卫生保健是农村居民应该人人享有的,与农村经济社会发展相适应的基本卫生保健服务。实施农村初级卫生保健是我国社会经济发展总体目标的组成部分,是各级政府的重要职责。

(一)中国农村初级卫生保健的提出与发展

"2000年人人享有卫生保健",是世界卫生组织提出的全球战略目标。对此,我国政府已作了承诺。1989年8月卫生部主持召开了第一次全国初级卫生保健试点工作会议,会议讨论了《我国农村实现"2000年人人享有卫生保健"的规划目标》、《初级卫生保健工作管理程序》、《初级卫生保健工作评价指标》。这次会议在中国农村初级卫生保健事业的发展中具有里程碑的意义。

国家计委、农业部、国家环境保护局、全国爱国卫生运动委员会和卫生部等部委于1990年3月下发并实施《我国农村实现"2000年人人享有卫生保健"的规划目标》,全国农村实现"2000年人人享有卫生保健"规划目标大致分两步走。第一步,1995年以前50%的县达标;第二步,到2000年再有50%的县达标。具体分为以下3个实施阶段:

第一个阶段(1989~1990年)为试点阶段。主要任务是:①全面进行初级卫生保健的宣传教育,重点是开发领导层,培训管理干部、技术队伍和群众卫生骨干;②健全农村三级医疗卫生网,改革与完善医疗保健制度,完成实施初级卫生保健的组织准备;③通过调查研究,在搞清各项规划指标本底情况基础上,以"最低限标准"为依据,提出本县预定值,制订相应的实施办法;④选择条件适宜的县作为实施初级卫生保健的试点,建立在本地区具有典型意义的示范县。力争全国有10%的县首先达到规划目标的最低限标准(其中婴儿死亡率、孕产妇死亡率和法定报告传染病发病率1990年应较1988年分别降低5%,4%,15%)。力争全国有10%的县首先达到规划目标的最低标准。

第二个阶段(1991~1995年)为全面普及阶段。主要任务是在当地政府领导下,通过政府各职能部门的协同,群众的充分参与,全面实施"人人享有卫生保健"发展规划。各省、自治区、直辖市至少有50%的县达到"最低限标准"。

第三阶段(1996~2000年)为加速发展、全面达标阶段。主要任务是:①在社会经济条件进一步发展的基础上,完善发展初级卫生保健的内部机制,加快步伐,使所有的县都能达到初级卫生保健最低限标准,完成第二个50%;②第二阶段已达标的县,要在新的基础上继续努力,以更丰富的内涵和更高的标准,向新的目标前进;③全国范围的检查考核,总结验收,使所有的县都能达到最低限标准。

"2000年人人享有卫生保健"最低限标准(以县为单位)

初级卫生保健指标	不同经济地区的最低限标准			
	贫困	温饱	宽裕	小康
1.把初级卫生保健纳入县、乡(镇)政府工作目标和当地社会经济发展规划(%)	100	100	100	100
2.县、乡政府年度卫生事业拨款占两级财政支出的比例(%)①	8	8	8	8
3.健康教育普及率(%)	50	65	80	90
4. A.行政村卫生室覆盖率(%)	90	95	100	100
B.甲级卫生室占村卫生室比例(%)	30	50	70	90
5.集资医疗保健覆盖率(%)	50	50	60	60
6."安全卫生水"普及率(%)	60	70	80	90
7."卫生厕所"普及率(%)	35	45	70	80
8.食品卫生合格率(%)	80	80	85	85
9.婴儿死亡率每五年递降百分比(%)	20	15	8	5
10.孕产妇死亡率每五年递降百分比(%)	30	25	20	15
11.儿童"四苗"单苗接种率(%)	85	85	90	95
12.法定报告传染病发病率每五年递降百分比(%)	15	10	10	10
地方病病区特定指标②:地方病患病率每5年递降百分比(%)	10	10	5	5

注:①根据我国现行财政体制,该项指标由各级地方政府审定。
②为地方病病区"2000年人人享有卫生保健"规划目标的必列指标,其他地区不作要求。

(二)新时期的农村初级卫生保健

经过努力,我国农村已基本实现了1990~2000年初级卫生保健阶段性目标。在过去的10年中,广大农民的健康水平和生活质量已得到明显提高。为不断提高初级卫生保健水平,开创新世纪初级卫生保健工作的新局面,卫生部、国家计委等七部委公布了《中国农村初级卫生保健发展纲要(2001~2010年)》。

《中国农村初级卫生保健发展纲要(2001~2010年)》的参考指标,其中涉及政府支持、农村医疗卫生机构与人员建设、基本医疗管理规范率、疾病预防保健服务、卫生监督、妇幼保健、环境卫生、健康教育、医疗保障、居民健康水平共10个方面的29项指标,并根据东部、中部、西部地区农村现有医疗卫生水平的不同,制定出了相应的参考指标。例如,该纲要提出了到2010年应实现的指标:乡村医疗机构的覆盖率(居民步行或乘车30分钟能够达到医疗机构的村所占比例)东部地区为100%,中部地区为90%,西部地区为85%。

1. 总目标

通过深化改革,健全农村卫生服务体系,完善服务功能,实行多种形式的农民医疗保障制度,解决农民基本医疗和预防保健问题,努力控制危害严重的传染病、地方病,使广大农村居民享受到与经济社会发展相适应的基本卫生保健服务,不断提高农民的健康水平和生活质量。到2010年,孕产妇死亡率、婴儿死亡率以2000年为基数分别下降1/4和1/5,平均期望寿命在2000年基础上增加1~2岁。

2. 主要任务

(1) 落实疾病预防控制措施,重点控制传染病、地方病、寄生虫病、职业病和其他重大疾病,加强精神卫生工作,防止各种意外伤害。稳定计划免疫接种率,提高现代结核病控制策略的人口覆盖率。预防、管理慢性非传染性疾病,做好老年保健。

(2) 提高乡、村卫生机构常见病、多发病的诊疗水平,规范医疗服务行为,为农村居民提供安全有效的基本医疗服务。

(3) 加强对孕产妇和儿童的管理,提高农村孕产妇住院分娩率,稳步降低孕产妇死亡率和婴儿死亡率,改善儿童营养状况,不断提高妇女、儿童健康水平。

(4) 加大农村改水、改厕力度,提高农村自来水及农村卫生厕所普及率,结合小城镇和文明乡镇建设,创建卫生乡镇,改善农村居民的劳动和生活环境。

(5) 开展健康教育和健康促进,积极推进"全国亿万农民健康促进行动"(原"全国九亿农民健康教育行动"),提高农村居民基本卫生知识知晓率和中小学健康教育开课率,倡导文明健康的生活方式,增强农村居民的健康意识和自我保健能力,促进人群健康相关行为的形成。

(6) 依法加大对公共卫生、药品和健康相关产品的监督力度,控制危害农村居民健康的主要公共卫生问题,努力抓好食品卫生、公共场所卫生和劳动卫生。

(7) 充分利用中医药资源,发挥中医药的特点与优势,不断提高农村中医药服务水平。

(8) 完善和发展农村合作医疗,探索实行区域性大病统筹,逐步建立贫困家庭医疗救助制度,积极实行多种形式的农民医疗保障制度。

思考1. 农村初级卫生保健的必要性和重要性如何?

思考2. 健康教育如何在农村初级卫生保健中发挥作用?

思考3. 如何在农村地区开展初级卫生保健工作?

Chapter 11 The Social Health Strategy

The basic aim of social medicine is to understand health problems from the view of sociology, analyze them relying on the knowledge of sociology and solve them through methods of sociology. So we must depend on social health policy and strategy.

WHO said: "Governments should be responsible for civil health." The extent of governmental responsibility mainly depends on the operation of policy. In order to protect civil health, the government should establish, implement and evaluate a series of health policies.

Health policy means the plans and basic policies adopted by society whose goal is to satisfy the medical demands of its citizens. The aim of health policy is to study how to use reasonable methods to acquire qualitative and quantitative achievement.

Other experts define health policy as the methods through which goals and emphasis of improving social health status could be accomplished. For example, "Everyone enjoys health care in 2000" is the overall target of improving the status and state of social health. The main way to attain the target is by primary health care.

Health strategy is the last resort and measure used to realize pre-determined goals. It is the essential starting point and responsible way to implement health policy.

It is a basic responsibility of all governments to determine health goals and establish corresponding strategic measures that guarantee the attainment of health goals. Every government always works hard to obtain the justice and efficiency of medical service and to improve the health level of the population.

Section 1 Primary Health Care

"Primary Health Care (PHC)" is a global strategic goal put forward by WHO approved by the UN and most countries. PHC is a necessary guarantee that protects people's health worldwide and makes an important contribution to their health service.

1. Presentation of PHC

From the sixth to twelfth September, 1978, WHO and UNICEF presided over the international PHC convention in Alma Ata, former Soviet Union, and came out with the *Declaration of Alma Ata* and a world health report that put forward the strategy "Health for All". This defined the role of PHC as basis to realize health for all. The convention defined the concept of PHC, communicating the experience of PHC, and defined the principles and implementation strategy to solve practical problems in the hope to improve the level of people's health through PHC activities.

The 1979 UN convention and the 1980 UN special convention respectively expressed consent to the *Declaration of Alma Ata* and received promises from the UN. Our government showed promises to the strategic goal "Health For All By 2000" in 1983,1986 and 1988.

2. The concept of PHC

According to *Declaration of Alma Ata*, PHC is a primary health care. It refers to communities depending on scientific and popular methods and technologies, with people and families' active participation.

PHC is the key function and main factor of national health system, and a component of national health system and social economy. It connects individual, family and community with national health system, and it is the first step that makes health care go deep into people's lives and labor, and it can provide health care for people on their working spots, which is also a primary procedure of health care sustaining process.

The document of five departments generalized: PHC refers to the most radical health care service that everybody can access, embodies equal social right, and can be afforded by both the people and government.

3. The principles of PHC

(1) Giving priority to prevention: The essential goal of PHC is to protect and promote human health, and try to reduce the incidence of disease. The most economic and effective way to decrease damage is prevention. Many diseases in late period are difficult to cure, and the expenditures are high, and in this phase the traditional treatment is difficult to reach as expected. PHC synthetically emphasizes on pathogenic factors, which influence health. Because human health can be influenced by many factors, such as natural and social environment, behavior-life style, biogenetic and mental factors, etc., they can influence health directly or indirectly. So, we must take some measures to prevent and control them.

(2) The participation of community: The community should broadly participate in disease prevention and relieving activity, provide help to special, weak public. Using community resources, community should do self-help, carry out health education, improve living environment, change the harmful life style, implement kinds of helpful health care strategies, thus could achieve the goal of preventing and promoting health.

(3) Suitable technologies: The methods, which are used for dealing in health care, should be reliable, simple, acceptable, and affordable.

(4) Government supports: PHC cannot simply be accomplished by only depending

on health section, but also needs social participation. So, government is required to coordinate different benefit of different sections, and organize financial and material resources to support this work. Government should be responsible for people's health.

4. The contents of PHC

The goal of PHC is to make people attain the best health level throughout the world, which is healthy for all. According to *Declaration of Alma Ata*, PHC contains four tasks, eight contents.

(1) The tasks of PHC

①Health promotion: They are health education, environment protection, sound nutrition, having safe drinking water, improved health facilities, developing physical exercise, promoting mental health, and building up better life style, etc.

②Preventive care: On the basis of studying the objective rules of social public health and disease with the relation between the rules and the internal and external environment in which people are, as well as human social activities, people adopt positive and effective measures to prevent disease from occurring, developing, and spreading.

③Favorable treatment: It contains discovering disease early, providing medical service and effective medicine in time, so preventing disease from developing and worsening, making people recover early.

④Community healing: It means disabled people who lose normal performance or have disabilities, through medical, educational, occupational, and social measures, could recover their performance as best as they can, re-gain living, developing learning abilities and participating in social activities.

(2) The elements of PHC

①The education of main current health issues as well as the preventive and restraining methods.

②Improvements on food supply and sound nutrition.

③Providing enough safe water and basic environmental health facilities.

④Woman and child care, family planning.

⑤The vaccinations against primary infectious diseases.

⑥The prevention and control of endemic diseases.

⑦Favorable treatment of familiar disease and trauma.

⑧Providing essential medicine.

Besides the eight contents, the thirty-fourth World Health Convention in 1981 added "using every possible method, by influencing the lifestyle, controlling natural and social mental environment to prevent and control non-infectious disease and promote mental health."

5. The characteristics of PHC

PHC has some characteristics, such as sociality, the mass character, hardness, and long-term character.

(1) The sociality

Being healthy is not only without disease or weakness, but also to be in perfect physical, mental and social condition. Health is the primary right of human. PHC is to make all the people achieve the best health level through social participation, controlling and eliminating all kinds of risk factors. Therefore, PHC is broadly the characteristic of sociality.

(2) The mass character

The service object of PHC is the whole public. PHC is related to everyone's health. People have not only the health right, but also the obligation of participation in the implementation of PHC; thus, PHC is of the mass character. PHC needs large participation of social public. Only with the common effort, can the expected be achieved. The development of health education, the change of life style, and the improvement of environment, etc., all need public participation.

(3) The hardness

The contents of PHC come down to every aspect of health, associated with our health situation; the task of PHC is very tough. Recently, our health service has achieved large success, and rural PHC has gained phase accomplishment. But overall, the medical service can not meet the increasing need of people. At the same time, the imbalances between urban and rural area, east and west, are large. The living condition of some rural areas is poor, and there are large discrepancies from the lowest standard of PHC. In many areas, infectious and endemic diseases are still threatening people's health. Cardiovascular disease and malignant tumor, etc., chronic non-contagious diseases are now the main threats.

(4) Continuity

In our country, the rural area basically achieved the 1990 – 2000 goals of PHC, but PHC will face many new situations and challenges. First, with the development of society and the improvement of public living condition and cognitive level, there are higher health demands; second, the aging population, the appearance of new diseases and the change of medical model, all these are needs of the improvement in PHC contents and level; finally, no country has enough finance to insure public health issue. Therefore, PHC has strong life in different periods. We can see that PHC strategy is a long-term continuous policy.

Section 2 Health Education and Health Promotion

1. Conception and significance of health education and health promotion

The first piece of content of primary health care (PHC) strategy is health education aiming at main health problems and the measures to prevention and control. PHC needs the participation of all society. It should be accomplished through the change of behavior mode. So, the activities must be united with health education. The essence of new public health method is health promotion and it is the key factor of worldwide strategy "Health for all". Health education is a science of researching theories, methods and practices of health education and health promotion. Its knowledge system and research content involves medicine, behavior science, pedagogic, psychology, anthropology, sociology, communication science, economics, management science and policy science, etc.

(1) Health education

Health education is to urge people to consciously adopt sanative mode of behavior and daily life, to annihilate or alleviate risk factors damaging health and to prevent diseases, promote health and improve life quality via planed, organized and systematic action of society and education.

The core of health education is to make individual and colony change unhealthy mode of behavior and daily life, especially of organizational action. It is true that the change of behavior mode is a formidable and complicated course. The responsibility of many bad behaviors does not belong to individuals and they are cannot be changed by individual wish because they are influenced by social conventions, cultural background, economic condition and medical service and so on. Most of the behaviors involve life condition such as residential condition, diet habit, working condition, market supply, social criterion and environment, etc. Thereby, for changing behaviors factors, benefiting influence, such as gaining ample resource, effective community leadings, social supports and self-help technology, must be enforced. Besides, all kinds of methods must be adopted to make people understand their health status and do their own choice for sake of improving health instead of forcing people to change their behaviors. So, the anticipated goal of health education could be obtained only if it is planned, organized and systematic.

(2) Education promotion

The definition of education promotion is broader than that of health promotion. The first international conference of health promotion that was held in Ottawa, Canada in 1986 published *Ottawa Constitution*. The constitution said that health promotion is a course in which people are motivated to elevate, maintain and improve their own health.

This definition expresses the goal and philosophy of health promotion, and emphasizes the range and methods at the same time.

Ottawa Constitution put forward five strategies of health promotion. They are as follows:

①Establishing public health policy: Health promotion transcends the scope of health care and brings health problems into the agenda of every department and leaders of all levels. It lets them understand the sequence of their decision-making and charge them with responsibility. Health promotion policy is synthesized by multiple and mutual-reinforced aspects. It includes policy, rule of law, finance, revenue and organic alteration.

②Creating supportive environment: Human beings' inseparable existence with environment is the basis of society-ecologic methods. Health promotion is to create safe, comfortable, satisfying and delighting working and living conditions. Any health promotion strategy must protect nature, create favorable natural conditions and protect natural resources.

③Strengthening community action: Health promotion obtains the goal of improving health through idiographic and effective community action including determining health problems requiring precedence, decision-making, devising and implementing strategies in order to promote health. During this course, the core is endowing right to the community to be host, actively participate and control their own destiny.

④Developing individual skills: Health promotion supports the development of individuals and society by the way of supplying data, health education and improving life skills. These actions make mass maintain their own health, existing in environment more effectively and making sanitary selections.

⑤Modulating the direction of health service: The function of health departments is both supplying clinical service and insisting on the direction of health promotion. Modulating the direction also requires more attention to health research and the transition between professional education and training. At the same time, it regards the overall demands of a person as service target.

In a conclusion, the definition of health promotion is more integrated than health education because it contains health education and ecologic factors-environment and administrative means. Health promotion is the synthesis of all behaviors and life conditions that benefit health education and ecologic support. It is the result of the development of health education, the essence of new public health policy and key factor of the worldwide strategy "Health for all".

(3) Making related health behavior

Making related health behaviors mean behaviors of individual and colony related to health and diseases. Including to their effect to doers and others, related health behaviors are classified into health behaviors and risk behaviors. According to the advice of Harris and Guten, health behaviors are sorted to five kinds.

①Basic health behavior. This means a series of basic health behavior in daily life such as positive relaxation and dormancy, etc.

②Warning behavior. This is defined as the behavior, preventing accidents and teaching how to deal with accidents, such as tying safety belt when driving and saving oneself after earthquake.

③Health protection behavior. It is the reasonable behavior of making the proper use of medical care service to maintain health such as vaccination.

④Avoiding-behavior. During environment endanger including natural and social environment and life affairs that harm body.

⑤Behavior refraining from ill addiction. Ill addiction mainly includes smoking, drinking and freaking-out.

The goal of health education is annihilating risk behaviors or keeping people away from risk behaviors, cultivating or holding health behaviors, and ultimately protecting and improving health.

2. The ways of health education — communication movement

From the 1960s, when the concept of communication was introduced in the field of health education, it grew up as health communication. It enriches the policy methods and theory of health education enormously, and instructs the practice of health education effectively.

(1) The concept of communication

Communication is a social action of transferring information. It is a process of changing, transferring the news, fact, opinions, etc. information between individual-collectively and group-individually.

(2) The model of communication

The famous USA sociologist, politician Harold Laswill brought forward a character mode which was a praised research standard of communication. That is, "a simple way of describing communication behavior, also answer five questions such as: who, say what, through what channel, to whom, with what effect?" Laswill's five factor communication mode (5W mode) explained concretely: who, say what, through what channel, to whom, with what effect. Or, it represents communicator, information, and the way of communication, recipient, and effect.

The effect of health communication could be divided in 4 levels:

①Knowing the information of health. This is the lowest level in the communication effect. Through sharing information, public knowledge level of medicine and sanitation can be improved continualy, and a good foundation can be made to improve their health care skill.

②Identity of health faith. The receivers receive the health information, and believe it through the spark plug of faith called health faith. Being conscious or unconscious according to faith, they pursue and choose health.

③The attitude change. It means people have relative long-term adherent consciousness to special object's perception, sensibility, and intent. The form of attitude is not only affected by social assortment, but also affected by mental course. Once attitudes are formed, they become mentally fixed. Commonly, attitude is the forerunner of changing of behavior; you must first change the attitude, and then can only change the behavior.

④To accept health behavior. It is the highest level of communication effect. When a person receives health information, on the basis of increasing knowledge, identification with faith, changing attitude, shift their intrinsic unhealthy behavior and lifestyle; this is the last goal of health communication.

3. The programming of health improvement

Health improvement is an arduous task, which relates to many factors. It depends on the unhealthful factors and the cause of illness directly. It involves much with a good social aspect and each phase of life. It must use all kinds of education methods and communication mode, and it covers many subjects' knowledge. Therefore, the work of health improvement must have a scientific and thorough program. Any health improvement program must be composed of design, implementation, and evaluation. These three parts restrict each other, and cannot be divided.

(1) Design of program

①Concept: The design of program is based on the investigation of target crowd about their health problem and its character. This is done by forming the theoretic supposition of the problem, putting forward a series of ways, steps, and tactics which would be taken for realizing the aim, establishing the foundation of the program, offering the quantitative target to scientific evaluation simultaneously.

②PRECEDE-PROCEED model

There are many models of health education and health improvement program. In such models, the PRECEDE-PROCEED model, which was put forward by US famous scholar Lawrence W. Green, is applied abroad mostly. This pattern's character is "begin from an end", using the deductive way of thinking, that is, ascending from the final result to the origin. In the PRECEDE-PROCEED model, back and forth echo each other, offering a continuous process for phases for the program's design, implications and evaluation.

First phase: Predisposing phase, namely PROCEED. Reinforcing and suggesting factors in educational/environmental diagnosis and evaluation.

Second phase: implication phase, namely PRECEDE. Making policy, using policy, stabilizing, and organizing way in educational and environmental development.

③The basic process of program design

Based on the process of PRECEDE-PROCEED model, we can divide the program design into 9 basic steps. That is from the final ending trace back to the initial origin, using the deductive way in progress.

A. Social diagnoses: It is done beginning from the evaluation of the target crowd's life quality, evaluating their demand and health problem. The target crowd may take part as well.

B. Epidemiological diagnoses: This is done through the epidemiological and medical investigation, affirming the health problem and aim.

C. Behavior and environmental diagnoses: This is done through affirming the behavior and environment related with health.

D. Educational and organizational diagnoses: Setting up the strategy of educating and organizing does, this is started with the factor which is most influenced by behavior and environment. These factor can be reduced to three kinds, that is incline factor, procure factor and intensity factor. The main aim of these factors is to establish the educating strategy correctly, that is according to all sorts of factors' relatively significant to resource condition confirming the interferences.

E. Management and policy diagnoses: Evaluation of the capability of organizing and managing, and how to arrange the time, resource, policy, and personnel when executing the plan. Through exposure and harmonizing community, perfecting the organization and policy, we can develop the program smoothly.

F. Implementation phase: Corresponding the implementation phase of health promotion program.

G. Evaluation phase (step G, H, I): Evaluation is not the last phase of the PRECEDE model. The work of evaluation runs through the entire model.

(2) Implementation of the program

Implementation is a course of the program to realizing the aim, gaining the effect. It is also the movement and the action that embodies the main thought of the program. If we don't have an effective implementation in work, the best program is nothing; it can't produce any social effect and economic benefit. So, in a course of health education and health promotion program, implementation of program is the main part of work, is also emphases and key. Implementation includes setting up feedback information system, founding up implementing program process, organizing and harmonizing, controlling the quality, etc. The main mission of health promotion program is as follows:

①Community exposure

The main aim of community exposure includes establishing leader organ, mobilizing active participation of crowd in realizing the aim, enforcing the construction of network and harmonizing each department, and framing the item on which policy sustains.

②Item training

Item training is to achieve the item goal, establish and maintain a troop that has power and efficiency.

③The interface based on community

The health interface programs based on community are the whole of many programmed movements such as establishing of leader organ, policy implementation, participations of various departments, the training of program management personnel are all the important factor, promising the of success of the community based programs.

④Monitoring of the item implementation and quality control

In program's design, implementation and evaluation, establishing the supervision system and quality control system is very important to developing health promotion program.

(3) Evaluation of program

Evaluation is to assess whether the program has attained its aims and to what degree. Evaluation is the important part of health promotion program; it is run throughout the entire task from its design, control, and evaluation. If the entire program cannot accomplish the aim, then evaluation should be done. Program evaluation is the key measure of checking, controlling, guaranteeing the program's design in advance, and implementation success, and to gain the effect.

The whole program evaluation should include 4 styles:

①Formative evaluation

Formative evaluation is the evaluation to the program contents before the program implementation or the beginning stage of implementation. It includes on-demand evaluation of establishing the interface program and offering basic data to the design and implementation of programs.

②Process evaluation

Process evaluation is a process following each activity; it supervises the course of implementation of program, finding out and guaranteeing that each activity of the program can be developed through its course. Process evaluation should have the mechanism to detect whether it is on the course or not, and if there are some deficiency in the program, ways to fill them, etc. The program should be routinely supervised, feedback should be provided on each activity's evolving conditions so as to adjust the unfit part of the program in time.

③Effectiveness of evaluation

Effective evaluation's goal is to confirm the effect of the interference, which includes the effect of evaluation in the near future, metaphase effect, and long-term effect.

④Summative evaluation

Summative evaluation is a summarizing concept of forming evaluation, processing evaluation, and many data. Synthetic target can reflect the program's success or failure roundly. Summative evaluation makes the judge by the program's cost-benefit, completes condition of each activity, and then makes the decision that the program should be repeated or enlarged or washed-up.

Section 3 The Global Health Strategy

1. **The history of the global health strategy "Health For All By 2000"**

(1) The outcomes of the global strategic goal "Health For All By 2000"

The Organization Laws of WHO say, "Health is a basic benefit of human beings, and the government has a duty to the people's health of his country". But because of the difference of the regime economy and culture, the conflict of humanity health right and sanitation service is acutely increasing; the thirtieth fall due world health congress in 1997 brought forward a global health strategy "Health For All By 2000".

(2) The basic ideology of the global health strategy "Health For All By 2000"

①The health is the basic right of human beings, and the opportunity of sharing in the health service is equal, either in rural or in city.

②The health service's emphases should transfer from city to rural area, from high tech therapy to prevention, enhance the dweller's knowledge of health, nutrition standard and living condition.

③Breaking sanitation career's narrow section state, and mobilising all branches of society to take part in the overall health strategy.

(3) The significance of the global health strategy "Health For All By 2000"

①People can keep healthy at work and in living.

②People will use more effective measures to prevent disease that will alleviate the pain of unavoidable disease and disablement and mature from a better path to attain a healthy lifestyle.

③Distribute all health resources equally to all members of society.

④All of individuals in the family will share in the primary health.

⑤People will know diseases are unavoidable, and have the strength to get rid of diseases.

(4) The main obstacle of health for all

①The political promise of health for all isn't its best.

②All elements of attaining basic medical health service are not equal.

③The social class of femininity continually drops.

④Society economy develops slowly.

⑤The actions of all departments are a serious problem.

⑥The distribution of manpower resource is odd and the support is weak.

⑦The action of advancing health is insufficient.

⑧Health information systems are weak and lack baseline data.

⑨Environment pollution, lacking safe drinking water provision and environment health establishment.

⑩The aspect of population and epidemiological changes rapidly.

⑪Expensive technique is used unsuitably of and the resource is distributed unreasonably.

⑫Disaster from nature and human being.

If these problems are not resolved, we cannot achieve the aim of Health for All. It is necessary to put forward a new global strategy about health for all in the 20th century in order to adapt for the changing situation of politics, economy, society and environment.

2. The Global Health Strategy in the New Period

(1) The coming of the strategy about "Health For All in the 21st century"

The decision was brought forward at the 48th world health congress in May, 1995, the "Health for All" strategy that emphasizes the duty of individual, family and community for health. They take health as the center of their work and draft a new world health plan based on common opinion.

The 21st century health strategy is development of "health for all by 2000", which is a guidelines for the health service everywhere.

(2) The new trend of factors affecting the people's health

①Absolute or relative poverty: The poverty is the main cause of hypo alimentation and ill health, which picks up the spread of disease and weakens the efficiency of health service. In the poor area, the population always increases quickly.

②The change of population: Aging leads to more diseases such as chronic non-contagious disease, disability and mental illness. Urbanization causes people need more and more health service. However, the output of health service can't meet it. At the same time, excessive crowd and abominable work condition lead to anxiety, blues and stress, which are harmful to their living quality in family and community.

③The changes of Epidemiology: The incidence of infectious diseases is still high; those diseases are dangerous to the world health in the 21st century. Chronic non-contagious diseases become the most important factor that causes death, disease and disability. Violence and traffic accident has become the main danger to our health.

④The global environment is threatening the human being: The global environment destruction such as air pollution, ozone drying up, climate changing, the losing of diversity of biology and insurant and rubbish's transportation overseas, and so on, is very harmful to our health.

⑤The development of new techniques: The advancement of information technology (for example long-distance medical treatment) and biotechnology helps people find, prevent and lighten disease, which also helps people get more health services and health education.

⑥The cooperation among private sectors, public sectors and social departments: In order to fit the new position, we should notice those factors which give our health system chances and challenges. For instance, central government gives some of its functions to local governments and social departments, prompts private sectors to join in health services, and lets inhabitants participate in health policy. In this way, they can cooperate easily.

⑦The globalization of commerce, travels, and transmission of values and ideas: The rush of increasing commerce and travels, as well as transmigration, and the development of communication and market are dangerous to people's health. Moreover, transporting food abroad and large-scale population travel cause the effects on health worldwide.

(3) Action basis of the 21st century global health development stratagem

The key of developing PHC is to mobilize the masses and the community to participate in health action. The basis of action is:

Firstly, acknowledging that attaining most possible health level is the basic human rights.

Secondly, strengthening the applicability of ethics continually that act on health policy research and health service supply.

Thirdly, carrying the policies and stratagem, which face the equity into execution, in order to inspire the community.

Finally, health policy and stratagem should embody the difference of sex.

(4) The general goal: Health For All By 2000

①Enhance expectation life and life quality.

②Improvement of the health level within the country and outside.

③To establish the consummate system of health care and health service for all which can be sustaining.

(5) General index of Health For All by the year 2020

①Health equality: by the year of 2005, the index of health equality will be used as a basic index to promote and surveillance health between countries and interior. In the beginning, evaluating equality was based on index of child growth. By the year of 2020, the percent of hypo genesis of children under five years old (that's age and height below the reference value exceeding two standard deviation) must be below 20 percent.

②Survival: MMR should be under 100 per 100 thousand. CMR that under 5 years old children should be under 45 per 1,000 birth survival. The life expectation must be over 70 years old in all the countries.

③Take measures: changing the rising trend of incidence rate and disability rate that result in five global diseases (tuberculosis, HIV, AIDS, malaria, diseases related to tobacco, violence and damning).

④Root up and perish of some diseases: by the year of 2020, measles will be rooted up and filariasis and trachoma will be perished; by the year of 2010, chagas disease will be eradicated; Hansen's disease will be perished (the prevalence rate below 1/10,000 in every county).

⑤Improve the condition of water, environment sanitation, food and housing situation: by the year of 2020, all the countries will make great progress in some aspects, such as supplying safe water, suitable environment sanitation, sufficient and top quality food, good housing situation.

⑥Promoting health measure: by the year of 2020, all the countries will take measures to decrease some health risk factors, which impair people's health; the measures include administration, economy, education, organization, synthetic scheme. On the other hand, such measures can be taken as positive administration and surveillance to promote health life.

⑦Constitute health policy, put it into practice and supervise it: by the year of 2005, all the countries will establish action mechanism, which accord with all the health policy.

⑧Improve the quality of synthetic and basic medical service that can be attained by all: by the year of 2010, all the people can attain synthetic and basic medical service and top-quality health care in the whole life.

⑨Establish global and national health information system and supervise system: by the year of 2010, suitable health information supervision and alarm system will be established in the world.

⑩Sustaining health research: by the year of 2010, policy and system action mechanism research will be brought into effect at different levels in the seven seas, some regions and countries.

(6) The role of government in global health stratagem

①People can attain top quality health care in the whole life.

②Prevent and control disease, protection of health.

③Promote establishment of sustainable health care system.

④Exploitation of health information system, insure positive and effective surveillance.

⑤Promote research: application and innovation of health science and technique.
⑥Establish and maintain health manpower resource.
⑦Obtain appropriate sustainable fund supplement.

(7) The rule of action

①Fight against poverty. Poverty is an important factor that has impact on health. Accelerating the development of human beings with an the increase of economy needs great effort made by all nations and the international society. At the same time, the health intervention measures the favor of breaking the vicious cycle between health and poverty.

②Promotion of health in every environment: This includes life, work, entertainment and study and all other natural, social, life environment that are in touch with people.

③Adjust departmental health policy. Protecting health of human beings depends on not only the health department but also the other government departments, because all the social departments must make efforts together in order to put a health policy in practice. So, all the governments must assort with each other to protect and promote people's health.

④Bring health promotion into sustainable development scheme. If health promotion will be the center of development we must give priority to health in the sustainable development scheme. First, social cause must be in favor of people's health; secondly, in the course of protecting people's health we must consume plenty of resource, but the resource is finite. So there is a contradiction between finite resource and infinite demand. In order to settle the contradiction, the health system itself must be sustainable.

Section 4 Health Strategy of China

1. The health guideline of China

Health guideline is the primary directive idea of government.

(1) The history of the health guideline of China

The first health convention in Sep. 1949 defined our health guideline as "giving priority to prevention, paying more attention to insuring production and national defense, facing the country, factory and mine, depending on the mass, developing health care service".

On September 8th, 1950, the State Department of center government authorized three principles of health care, "facing the worker, peasant and soldier, giving priority to prevention, drawing Chinese medicine and west medicine together". In December 1952, the second health convention summarized the experiences of patriotic health movement, and Prime Minister Zhou put forward the principle that "to enhance the combination of health service and the mass movement". From then on, all these were called "the four guidelines" of Chinese health service, namely that, "to face the worker, peasant and soldier", "to give priority to prevention", "to draw Chinese medicine and west medicine together", "to combine health service and the mass movement". In the past fifty years, the four guidelines steered our health service to prosperity and achieving notable success.

In retrospect, there are some deficiencies in the implementation of giving priority to prevention. On April 9th, 1991, the seventh convention of the National People's Congress presented that... in "the national economy and social development ten-year program and the eighth five-year planning design" ... the health service should carry out the guidelines, "to give priority to prevention, to depend on technology development, to mobilize the whole population to participate in, to stress on the Chinese medicine and west medicine, to serve people's health".

In 1996, the guidelines were adjusted as "to emphasize the rural areas, to give priority to prevention, to stress on the Chinese medicine and west medicine, to depend on technology and education, to mobilize the whole population to participate in, to serve people's health, to serve socialist modernization construction". These health guidelines in the new period will direct the development and emphases of our health service, and at the same time, demonstrate the medical education direction.

(2) The health guideline of China in new days

1) To emphasize the rural areas

Rural population is a majority of our country, so the level of their health decides the whole health standard. The rural health service is connected with people's health and economy in rural areas. The medical treatment system has been based in rural areas, and there are quite a lot of rural doctors. We have got a great success at PHC, and the health level is enhanced in rural areas. However, the rural health service is still very poor. There are many persons who have not enough money to see doctor. Moreover, many countrymen reach or return poverty for disease. In addition, there are absolute difference in health service and health levels between city and rural areas. We must regard for and solve it.

2) To give priority to prevention

Sticking to the policy that prevention is mainly. The reason is low expense of prevention health and good effect. It is the crucial place of the health services with low input and high benefit. No matter in infectious disease, local disease or chronic non-infectious disease, any kind of disease occurring in large-scale will be disastrous in the consumptions such as its health resource and the loss on economy in our developing country with such a large population.

At present, international community shows great concern over the control and prevention of disease. The world Declaration of Children's Survival, Protection and Development and The Action Program during the 1990s were passed in the conference attended by all the heads of states in 1990, and The Paris Declaration of Preventing AIDS of Heads of Governments was also passed in 1994. The Chinese government made positive efforts to participate in these international activities and made a solemn pledge, and developed the projects of eradicating poliomyelitis and newborn infant tetanus and eradicating basically leprosy. *Chinese Children's Development Projects Program in the 1990s*, *Women Development Projects Program*, *Chinese Nutrition Action Plan in the 1990s*, *Chinese Eradicating Iodine Shortage Disease Projects Program in 2000*, *Chinese Children's Development Program (2001 – 2010)*, *Chinese Women's Development Program (2001 – 2010)*, and the projects of controlling AIDS were passed. The goals are specific, and the task is heavy.

Nowadays, there are still varieties of factors causing the transmission of communicable diseases. The move of transportation presumably causes the diffusion of the communicable diseases occurring in local areas. For instance, there are risks of outbreak of the plague, cholera, hepatitis and so on. Opening to the rest of the world possibly leads to the transmission of new types of diseases, or the diseases that have been brought under control or eradicated appear again. In these aspects, there are profound lessons home and abroad. So, lots of energies and money still need to be spent in carrying out surveillance for the diseases eradicated basically in our country, except for the diseases such as smallpox announced to have been eradicated in the whole world. Otherwise, the accomplishments made in the prevention and treatment of disease will be meaningless. Meanwhile, with the change of cause of disease, some chronic diseases, including hypertension, cardiovascular and cerebrovascular diseases, tumor, diabetes and so on, have become the major objects of prevention in urban areas, and there is similar tendency in rural areas. Due to heavy task and less time, we must make double efforts in order to attain expectant aims and carry out the promises of Chinese government to international community, according to the requirements of disease prevention and health care planning.

3) To stress the Chinese medicine and west medicine

In long-term practice of struggling with diseases, the Chinese nation created characteristic Chinese traditional medicine and pharmacy system, which is the gem of traditional culture of the Chinese nation and is unique in the fields of world medicine and pharmacy. The Party and government always put emphasis on Chinese traditional medicine and pharmacy cause. "Chinese traditional medicine and pharmacy is a great treasury, and we should make more efforts to dig something useful in it and develop it," Comrade Mao Zedong pointed out when the People's Republic of China was founded. A series of principles and policies were worked out to develop Chinese traditional medicine and pharmacy, and hard work of a great mass of Chinese traditional medicine and pharmacy workers rapidly recovered and developed them. In the situations of more troublesome national economy and vast damage caused by the Cultural Revolution, Comrade Deng Xiaoping required clearly that the the Party Committees and governments of all the levels create good material conditions for the development of Chinese traditional medicine in 1978, which boosted greatly the development of Chinese traditional medicine and pharmacy. With the development of reform and opening and more frequent cultural communication of China and the West, General Secretary Jiang Zemin emphasized Promoting Excellent Culture of the Chinese Nation and Developing Chinese Traditional Medicine and Pharmacy. We must implement seriously the directions of the leaders of three generations of the CPC Central Committee concerning supporting and developing Chinese traditional medicine and pharmacy, promote the integration of Chinese traditional medicine and western medicine, and apply actively advanced sciences and technologies and modernization methods to develop them on the basis of inheriting the characteristics and advantages of Chinese traditional medicine and pharmacy.

4) To depend on technology and education

The development of social economy and increasing demand for health care bring more urgent requirements to the advance of science and technology. Science and technology-densified medical practice gather more intellectual. Both the prevention and treatment of diseases and improvement of the quality of health service rely on the development of medical science and technology and training of medical talents. The CPC Central Committee and State Council established the strategy of Developing the Country Depending on Science and Technology and Education. And clear-cut principles and policies on the development of science and technology and education have been worked out. These principles and policies must be implemented earnestly in the fields of medical and pharmaceutical science and technology and medical education.

5) To mobilize the whole population to participate

Patriotic Campaign for Better Sanitation is a creative action with Chinese characteristics and the best proof of all walks of life widely participating. The primary stage of Patriotic Campaign for Better Sanitation was to eradicate four kinds of pests and do some sweeping. Nowadays, it is that all walks of life commonly create health city, town, and countryside. It has had a qualitative leap. Abundant experience have been accumulated in the practice of Patriotic Campaign for Better Sanitation which can be summarized as follows: ①the central government should organize it; ②the local authorities should be in charge of it; ③the department should coordinate it; ④the masses should participate it actively; ⑤ the government should operate it with scientific methods; ⑥ and all walks of life should monitor it. Due to emphasis put on health infrastructure construction, the establishment of civilized rules and regulations of health, and the improvement of citizens' civilization quality, the activities of creating health city have acquired the support and trust of the masses, become one of good political measures serving the people truly, and boosted the development of two civilization construction of national town. The activities integrate the mass campaign with constant health infrastructure construction, which accords with Chinese realities. The creative activities are acclaimed by international community.

6) To serve people's health, to serve socialism modernization construction

Serving people's health and socialist modernization program is the core of health guidelines. Thus all the work revolves around it. As the starting point and final aims of health work, it embodies the concept of serving the people heart and soul.

Serving socialist modernization program requires that health work be brought into general socio-economic development projects system and the development of health services parallel national socio-economic development that are mutually promoted and restricted. The development of health services is not only the precondition and guarantee of economic development, but also the direct reflection of economic development. Only by serving people's health can health service protect social productivity and serve socialist modernization program.

2. The general goals of health development

By 2000, a health system having Chinese characteristic that includes health service, medical insurance, and health law-surveillance should be established, and it should realize health for all. The civil health level should also increase more; by 2010, a more perfect health system adapted to socialist economic system will be set up, and the main indexes of civil health in developed areas will achieve or be close to middle income country, in developing area and will reach to the highest level in developing country.

3. The primary tasks of health service

(1) To push regional program of health activity, reform urban health service system, develop community health service, carry out country PHC deeply, gradually form the health service net that has different levels, reasonable arrangement, and synthetic function, to shorten the regional difference of health service.

(2) To establish and perfect the medical insurance system adapted to our country's situation and having different forms. To quicken the socialized medicine and labor medicine system reform, setting up city employee basic medical insurance system, expanding different rural medical insurance system's coverage, such as the cooperative medicine and health insurance, etc., to make most resident obtain primary health service.

(3) To basically control the diseases that can be prevented and treated effectively.

Reduction of the threat of contagious diseases, and verminosis, and endemic diseases. Aiming at the risk factors, to gradually develop the synthetic prevention and treatment of the non-contagious diseases.

(4) To strengthen maternal and child care. To increase maternal and child health care level, better premarital health care service should be provided, basically popularize woman and child systemic care management.

(5) To establish and perfect the synthetic health law-surveillance system including food, drinking-water, cosmetic, children's articles, daily life chemical, disinfectants, special facilities arranged in human body (man-made organs, etc.), etc., and the sites of production, life, learning, entertainment, as well as medical service, etc., to guarantee people's health right.

(6) To develop health education and popularize primary health knowledge, help urban and rural people have better health habits step by step, and continuously improve drinking water and environmental facilities.

(7) To actively advance medical institutions set reform, manage strictly, and improve the medical service quality and efficiency.

(8) To establish a health service system characteristic of government responsibility, mass participations, sections correspondence, law insurance, and set up a financing and running mechanism.

4. Health development strategies

Follow the direction in satisfying people's health demands, focusing on improving people's health level, giving prominence to the three strategic emphases, the country health service, prevention care, and Chinese medicine, in the light of the principle — giving attention to fairness and efficiency, intensifying primary health service and surveillance, advancing regional program of health, health service should be steered to a path focusing on meaning of development and combining intension and extension development.

Case Example

Primary Health Care in Chinese Rural Areas

The rural primary health care is a basic health service, which should be accessible to each rural resident, compatible with the development of rural economic society.

And its performance is a part of the overall target of Chinese social and economic development, and a cardinal job of the government of all levels.

1. Bringing it forward and its development

"Health care for everyone by 2000", is a world strategic target produced by the World Health Organization, on which Chinese government made the commitment.

In August, 1989, the Chinese health department convened the first conference about the experimental work of nationwide primary health care, discussing *The Programming Target of Realizing "Health Care for Everyone by 2000" in Chinese Rural Areas* and *The Managing Program of Primary Health Care Work*, evaluating *index of primary health care work*, which set a milestone in the development of Chinese rural primary health care.

In March, 1990, National Family Planning Committee, Department of Agriculture, National Environmental Protection Committee and the Health Department issued *The Programming Target of Realizing "Health Care for Everyone by 2000" in Chinese Rural Areas*, covering and realizing the programming target by two steps: firstly 50 percent counties attained the target by 1995; secondly, the other 50 percent counties attain the target by 2000. Concrete performance stage we will go through as follows:

The first stage (1989 – 1990) is an experimental stage in which the cardinal mission is:

(1) Carry out the publicity and education on primary health care, with the emphasis on developing the leaders, training the leading cadres, technical manpower and the key member;

(2) Improve the tertiary-level health net in the rural areas, reform and perfect the medical care system and complete the organizational preparation to perform the primary health care;

(3) Through investigation and research and on the basis of attaining the basic index of variety of programs as well as in accordance with The Lowest Standard, each county should bring up the pre-arranged value and establish the performance method accordingly;

(4) Choose the suited county as the experimental area to carry out the primary health care, and establish the typical county in the local region.

Strive to attain 10 percent of counties, which firstly achieve the lowest standards of the programmed targets (among them infant's death rate, the maternal mortality rate and the incidence of the legally reported infectious disease should be respectively down by 5 percent, 4 percent and 15 percent).

The second stage (1991 – 1995) is an all-round popularization stage in which the cardinal missions are as follows:

Under the leadership of the local government, through the cooperation among each functional agents of the government and the full participation of the multitude, to completely carry out the program of "the health care for everyone".

At least 50 percent of all the counties in each province, autonomous region and municipality directly under the Central Government attain the target of the lowest standard.

The third stage (1996 – 2000) is a stage to accelerate the performance and completely reach the standard, in which the cardinal missions are as follows.

(1) On the basis of the further development of social and economic term, better the internal mechanism of the primary health care and quickening the pace to make all counties attain the lowest standard of primary health care and complete the second 50 percent;

(2) The county having attained the lowest standard in the second stage should continue to attain the new target on the new basis, with more abundant content and higher standard;

(3) The examination, evaluation, summarization and acceptance check throughout the country.

To make all counties attain the lowest standard. The lowest standard of "the health care for everyone by 2000" (county as unit)

Index of the primary health care	The lowest standard in different economic regions			
	Poverty	Enough to live	Affluence	Well-being
1. Get the primary health care under the coverage of the work target of the county and village government and the development program of the local society and economy. (%)	100	100	100	100
2. The percent of health appropriation of county and town government accounting for their fiscal expenditure (%)①	8	8	8	8
3. Popularization rate of health education	50	65	80	90
4. A. The coverage of administrative village (%)	90	95	100	100
B. The percentage of grade A health center accounting for the village health center (%)	30	50	70	90
5. The coverage of fund raising health medicine (%)	50	50	60	60
6. Popularization rate of "secure and healthy water" (%)	60	70	80	90
7. Popularization rate of "healthy toilet" (%)	35	45	70	80
8. The quality rate of food health (%)	80	80	85	85
9. The percentage of decrease of infant's death rate per five years (%)	20	15	8	5
10. The percentage of decrease of maternal death rate per five years (%)	30	25	20	15
11. Children's inoculation rate of the single one of "four vaccine" (%)	85	85	90	95

(Table)

Index of the primary health care	The lowest standard in different economic regions			
	Poverty	Enough to live	Affluence	Well-being
12. The percentage of decrease of incidence rate of legally reported infectious disease per five years (%)	15	15	10	10
13. The specific index of endemic region②: the percentage of decrease of prevalence rate of endemic disease per five years (%)	10	10	5	5

Notes:

①according to the current public finance system, the index should be approved officially by local government of all levels.

②means a endemic district where the required index for the program "the health care for everyone by 2000", with which other regions is not required.

2. The rural primary health care in new period

Our countryside has already basically realized the stepped target of 1990-2000. In the past decade, the health level and living quality of the farmers have already got an obvious exaltation. In order to enhance the level of the primary health care and create its new situation in the 21st century, health bureau and so on under the different commissions and ministries produced *The Development Outline of Chinese Rural Primary Health Care (2001 - 2010)*.

In the book the index refers to 29 items including governmental support, development of rural health constitution and manpower, norm rate of basic health administration, service for the prevention and health care, sanitary control, maternal and child health care, environmental hygiene, health education, medical safeguard, the health level of residents. Some relevant index was established according to the different levels of current health care in the eastern, centra and western regions.

For example, *The Outline* brings forward the referential index which should realized by 2010. They are, in the main, as follows: The coverage of the rural medical institution (the percent of the village in which the residents can reach the medical organization within 30 minutes on foot or by bike): the eastern region should reach up to 100 percent, central region 90 percent, and western region 85 percent.

(1) Total targets

Through further reform, perfect the rural health care system, improve the function of health service, perform varieties of medical insurance system for farmers, cope with the basic medical and prevention health care confronting the farmer, endeavor to control the seriously dangerous infectious disease, endemic disease to enable the multitude farmers to enjoy the basic health care service compatible with the social and economic development and enhance the farmer's health level and living quality. By 2010, the maternal mortality, infant's death rate will respectively go down by one fourth and one fifth on the basis of that of 2000, average expectation life will increase 1 − 2 years on the basis of that of 2000.

(2) Cardinal tasks

①Put into effect the preventive and controlling measures of disease, with the emphasis of controlling infectious disease, endemic disease, parasitic disease, occupational disease and other serious disease, and heighten the mental health work and prevent varieties of accidental injuries. Stabilize the planning vaccination rate, and increase the coverage of the modern control strategy of tuberculosis. Prevent and manage the chronic and noninfectious disease and perform perfectly the health care for the aged.

②Increase the diagnosis and treatment levels of the town and village medical organization for the common and frequent disease, standardize the offering of the medical service and provide the secure and effective basic medical service for the rural residents.

③Strengthen the management of the mother and child, increase the rate of the village materials being delivered in the hospital, steadily lower the maternal mortality rate and the infant's death rate, improve children's nourishment condition, and continuously increase the health level of the women and children.

④Emphasizing the reform of the rural water and toilet, increasing the popularization rate of the rural tap-water and health toilet, creating healthy town together with the instruction of small towns and civilized towns and villages and better the labor and living conditions of the rural residents.

⑤Carry out the health education and health promotion, positively advance "the health promotion for national farmers of hundreds of millions" (formerly "the health education for national farmers of nine hundred millions"), increase the understanding rate of basic health knowledge among rural residents and giving-a-course rate of health education among primary and junior schools, advocate a healthy and civilized life style, enhancing the health perception on the self-cared ability of the rural residents and urge the formation of the health-related behavior of the crowd.

⑥Follow the law to strengthen the supervision over public health, drug and health-related product, control the cardinal public health problems endangering the rural residents, endeavor to better public health and labor health.

⑦Make full use of the Chinese medicine resources, develop its advantages and service level.

⑧Perfect and improve the rural cooperative health care, make experiments to carry out territorial plans and control big diseases, gradually establish the medical aids system for poor family and perform the medical guarantee system in various forms for farmers.

Consideration and Discussion:

1. What's the necessity and importance of the rural primary health care?

2. How to perform function of health education in the rural primary health care?

3. How to carry out the work of primary health care in the rural areas?

第十二章 城市与农村社会医学

第一节 城乡社会结构对卫生发展的影响

一、城乡二元制社会结构

在计划经济时期,我国实行了对城乡分别治理的管理政策,"分灶吃饭"形成了所谓的城乡二元制社会结构。早在20世纪80年代,中国社会学界就展开了对城乡二元社会格局(结构)的研究,认为它是我国城乡之间因人口流动受到严格约束而出现的一种分割状态,是我国50年代在户口管理、粮油供应、就业安置、社会保障等各方面实施城乡区别对待的政策基础上形成的。

我国的城市结构特点:一是城市规模过大,大城市过多,中小城市发展不够。二是地域分布欠均衡,主要集中在东部沿海地区,西部地区城市发展严重滞后。三是城市产业结构失衡,主要集中在工业,第三产业发展严重滞后,特别是交通运输业和市政基础设施发展不够。

城市化滞后是中国非典型化工业化发展的一个严重缺陷,使得中国经济发展面临许多矛盾和问题。首先,城市化滞后使二元经济矛盾不断拉大。改革以前,中国重工业超前发展和城乡隔绝制度下的城市化进程,造就了十分悬殊的二元经济结构。1985年以来,由于农业劳动力向非农产业转移缓慢,使二元经济矛盾又进一步拉大。特别是近几年,由于大量劳动力滞留在比重不断下降的农业上,导致农民收入下降,农民与非农民的收入差距迅速扩大。城乡二元经济矛盾不断拉大。

二元制社会结构不仅限制了城乡之间人口的社会流动,也使得城乡差别加大。我国城乡二元制社会结构形成了城乡不同的社会结构。在政治上,城市各种社会组织更紧密,而农村相对松散。在人口特征上,农村人口的同质性较强,文化程度相对偏低,而城镇人口的异质性较强,文化程度相对偏高;农村社区联系比较紧密,城市社区联系比较松散。农村人口的社会保障水平低,而城镇人口的社会保障水平相对较高。在经济上,农村经营的个体化强,而城市经营的社会化程度高。从所有制结构看,过去农村多属于集体经济成分,而城市多属于国家所有制成分,当然随着改革开放、社会主义市场经济的建立,这种状况有所改变。从社会的开放程度看,城镇的社会开放程度高,而农村的社会开放程度相对较低。

二、城乡二元制社会结构对卫生发展公平性的影响

城乡二元社会结构对我国的卫生事业发展的公平性产生很大的影响。所谓的卫生保健公平"一般包括健康公平、卫生服务的可及性公平、实际服务利用公平和筹资公平"。健康公平是指人群的健康状况基本相似。卫生服务的可及性是指保障人们都能得到最基本的卫生服务。实际卫生服务利用公平是指有相同医疗需求的人可以得到相同的医疗服务。筹资公平是指按支付能力大小支付费用。2000年,世界卫生组织对191个会员国的卫生系统分三个方面进行了绩效评估,在卫生负担公平性方面,中国被排列在第188位。我国卫生保健方面的公平性主要表现在地区差距、城乡差距和阶层差距三个方面,而城乡差距是二元制社会结构在卫生领域中的体现。

在卫生改革方面政府的"良治"体现为应当向全体居民提供基本公共卫生服务,将有限的公共卫生资源投入到对农村居民传染病、地方病、营养不良症以及妇幼疾病等方面的防治和初级卫生保健的提供。农村初级卫生保健中坚持"预防为先"的方针,把对疾病的预防摆在优先位置,减少疾病的发病率和治疗成本;政府应该在建立适合现阶段农村发展的医疗保障制度中发挥主导作用;改变城乡社会结构,改善农民的待遇,实现城乡公平卫生发展。

第二节 城市和农村的主要社会卫生问题

一、我国人口基数大、人口的社会流动引发大量社会卫生问题

世界人口自1960年以来翻了一番,达到61亿,主要增长在一些较穷的国家。预计到2050年将增加到93亿,较多的人口需要使用更多的资源。"我国人口多,底子薄"是国情之一。2000年全国第五次人口普查资料显示,祖国大陆的人口中,居住在城镇的人口为45 594万,占总人口的36.09%;居住在乡村的人口为80 739万人,占总人口的63.91%。同1990年第四次全国人口普查相比,城镇人口占总人口的比重上升了9.86个百分点。从总体看,其趋势是农村人口向城市转移。城市化也称都市化,是以集居在城市地区的人口占总人口的比重来衡量。在城市化过程中,必然伴随着农村人口向城市的转移,但在这种转移过程中也增加了城市的社会卫生问题。社会流动是指人们在社会关系空间从一个地位向另一个地位的移动。由于社会关系与地理空间具有密切的联系,因此,一般人们在地理空间的流动也归于社会流动。民工进城是一种地理空间位置上的流动,同时,也是社会身份的一种变动。社会学家称农民向城市的大量流动为"民工潮",称民工为"流民",带有一定的贬意。而农民的流动对推动社会的进步,推动我国的城市化步伐具有积极的意义。他们为我国的现代化建设作出了积极的贡献。但同时应当看到农民进城对城市就业带来了一定的压力,也引发了一些安全问题和卫生问题:一是增加了城市的就业难度,造成了城市人口的贫困化,影响了人群的健康,就业压力的增加也对人们的社会心理产生一定的影响,带来一些社会病。二是人口大量流动带来的安全问题、卫生问题。

有资料表明,城镇实际失业人口突破2 000万。2001年上半年,中国的城镇登记失业率是3.3%,登记失业人口是619万;下岗人员是632万,两者相加为1251万人。有的专家估计城镇实际失业率应该是10%左右。从农村向城市流动的剩余劳动力有6 000万。中国的农业问题和农民问题自20世纪90年代以来也日益突出。中国的耕地面积人均仅有1.2亩,劳均4.1亩。中国已有1/3的省(直辖市、自治区)人均土地面积小于1亩,1/3的县(市)人均小于0.8亩,低于联合国确定的土地对人口的最低生存保障线。中国农村的土地正在逐渐丧失其作为生产资料的功能,而蜕变为对农民的"最后的保障"。人地关系的紧张使中国农村产生了大量的剩余劳动力,专家们估计在2亿左右。其中,乡镇企业吸纳了将近1.2亿(包括本地的和外来的),大约有7 000多万已经向城市或者已经城市化的富裕地区(如珠江三角洲地区、长江三角洲地区)流动。实际上至少还有6 000万农村劳动力需要工作岗位。

由于就业岗位不足,城乡居民一部分成了贫困者,这一部分人中有的缺乏起码的健康保障,患病时无力支付医疗费用,从和谐论的观点看,这打破了人与社会的和谐。这一次"非典"的爆发流行,天津某医院的一个老年"非典"患者,造成上百人感染。有的患病后缺乏基本的医疗保障,其住院费完全由政府承担。因此,我们应当充分地认识到我国就业问题所引发的社会卫生问题。

我国农民进城工作带来的问题很多,据1994年11月10日北京市的一次定时普查资料显示,北京的流动人口已达到329.5万人,这些人已成为北京人生活中不可或缺的一部分。保姆、清洁工、蹬三轮车的、炸油条开餐馆的,凡是脏活累活,北京人不干的,外地人都干。有关统计表明,北京市环卫、纺织、矿山、煤炭等脏、重、累行业中,总共雇用24万民工。80多万外地建筑工人,是北京建筑工劳动市场的主力军。

外地民工除了帮助北京市的建设外,身上有许多缺点:随意遗污,破坏市容卫生;刺激消费,拉动物价上涨;商贩们缺斤少两,粗制滥造,所制作的大饼、油条据说极不卫生,让人不敢吃等等。最严重的问题是大批外地人员进京带来的治安问题。北京警方公布,在违法犯罪案件中,不少是外地民工所为,以1994年为例,刑事案件中,有46%是外来民工所为。为数众多的盲流,抢劫偷盗,杀人越货,无所不为。特别是团伙犯罪相当严重。近30个外地人聚居地,如新疆村、浙江村等,成了藏垢纳污之所、吸毒贩毒的基地。

流动人口的计划生育和优生优育在管理上也存在较多问题,有的形成管理的盲点,有的强行检查,重收费,忽视管理的实效。这些问题大都是由于人口流动所引发的。随着交通工具的发展,人口的流动速度加快,对传染病的迅速流行提供了特殊的外部条件。因此,在现代社会中人口流动的负性健康影响也应当引起高度的重视。

二、人口素质亟待提高

我国不仅人口数量多,而且人口的素质也是一个问题。从文化素质上看,2000年全国人口普查资料显示,中国大陆的人口中,接受大学(指大专以上)教育的4 571万人;接受高中(含中专)教育的14 109万人;接受初中教育的42 989万人;接受小学教育的45 191万人(以上各种受教育程度的人包括各类学校的毕业生、肄业生和在校生)。与1990年第四次全国人口普查情况相比,人口的文化素质有了一定的提高,但总体上并不乐观。接受高等教育的比重不高,另外,文盲和小学文化程度人口占的比重较大,文化程度总体水平不高,不仅制约经济的发展,同时也影响人们的保健意识、保健行为,进而对健康产生一定的影响。

随着我国实行计划生育的基本国策的实施,不仅对人口数量进行了控制,人口的生理素质也有了很大的提高。婚姻法的修订,优生优育政策的落实,使得遗传病大大降低。但有些人口政策的实施对人口质量的提高产生了负面影响,如提倡一对夫妇生一个孩子,而第一胎出现某些疾病的,可以生第二胎,这样做是尊重了群众的需要,但在客观上却造成了人口素质的下降,毕竟第一胎生理素质不高,第二胎生理素质偏低的风险性也很大。另一项政策是城市实行一对夫妇一个孩子的生育政策,而农村第一胎是女孩的可以生第二胎,这一政策是从满足农村对劳动力的需求出发而制定的,但客观上导致了人口的逆淘汰,即人口素质高的少生,而人口素质低的多生,最后的结果是降低了人口的素质。

再一个问题是人口的结构变化带来的社会卫生问题不容忽视。根据2002年我国权威人士透露,中国大陆60岁以上人口已经达1.32亿,并以每年3.2%的速度急剧增长。老龄化社会的到来,使得城乡老年人的社会卫生问题非常突出,老年人的卫生保健应当提到议事议程(参见老年社会医学部分)。

三、环境卫生问题突出

经济的飞速发展,同时要付出了高昂的代价,从环境卫生问题看,出现了如下特点:

一是污染从发达国家向发展中国家转移。这种转移,是在发达国家经历了环境卫生问题的一系列经验教训后,环境保护意识增强,逐步采取了对环境的综合性控制措施,这些措施包括对污染企业的严格治理,综合性的措施初见成效。但是,这些污染企业也从发达国家和地区转移到了欠发达国家和地区。随着城市工业生产交通运输事业的发展,煤炭、石油等能源利用的不断增长,燃料的大量燃烧,各种生产废气的排放,生活灶与采暖锅炉大量使用,水资源的减少与枯竭,绿化面积减少,农村过度开垦,对森林、植被的破坏,造成沙漠化,使得空气中颗粒物和有害物质的浓度急剧升高。工业化较早的国家最初是以煤烟污染为主,如1956年的英国伦敦的烟雾事件。20世纪60年代以后,随着石油取代煤成为主要的燃料,使二氧化硫成为城市的主要污染物。交通运输业的发展,城市汽车的发展,汽车尾气的排放,光化学烟雾(大气中存在的烃类物质和氮氧化物在强烈的阳光照作用下,经过一系列光化学反应而生成的二次污染物蓄积于大气中形成的一种浅蓝色烟雾,这种二次污染主要是臭氧、过氧酰基硝酸酯、过氧化氢、酮类、醛类,以及盐酸盐和某些高分子有机化合物所形成的气溶胶颗粒等)成为大气污染城市的主要罪魁。像美国洛杉矶曾多次发生的光化学烟雾事件。大气污染引发许多健康问题,首先对身体体表有一定的刺激作用,其次会引起许多呼吸道疾病,还会引起急性或慢性中毒,甚至会有致癌作用。此外,水源污染、噪声污染等危害也很严重。

二是城市污染向农村转移。城市环境保护意识增强后,将一些污染严重的小企业搬到农村发展,造成了农村的环境污染。有的个体经营者在不具备生产条件的情况下,单纯地追求利润,违法经营,造成工人的中毒。据2002年30个省、自治区、直辖市(缺西藏)统计,各类职业病发病14 821例,其中尘肺12 248例、慢性职业中毒1 300例、急性职业中毒590例、职业性眼病159例、职业性耳鼻喉疾病206例,其中有一部分发生在农村。环境卫生问题不能再走发达国家先污染后治理的老路子,要未雨绸缪,防患于未然。

四、慢性病是危害城乡居民健康的主要卫生问题

20世纪70年代疾病谱和死因谱发生了很大的变化,慢性病都排在了前几位。卫生部卫生统计信息中心的统计资料显示:城乡居民主要死亡原因(ICD-10),2002年30个市和78个县(县级市)死因统计,城市居民前十位死因为:①恶性肿瘤$135.4/10^5$,②脑血管病$100.6/10^5$,③呼吸系病$89.9/10^5$,④心脏病$84.1/10^5$,⑤损伤和中毒$50.4/10^5$,⑥消化系病$19.6/10^5$,⑦内分泌、营养和代谢及免疫疾病$14.1/10^5$,⑧泌尿、生殖系病$9.7/10^5$,⑨神经系病$5.2/10^5$,⑩围生期病$4.9/10^5$,前十位死因合计占死亡总数的89%;农村居民前十位死因为:①恶性肿瘤$84.3/10^5$,②脑血管病$70.6/10^5$,③呼吸系病$63.8/10^5$,④心脏病$58.5/10^5$,⑤损伤和中毒$41.5/10^5$,⑥消化系病$14.5/10^5$,⑦泌尿、生殖系病$5.9/10^5$,⑧内分泌、营养、代谢及免疫疾病$4.9/10^5$,⑨围生期病$4.4/10^5$,⑩肺结核$4.3/10^5$,前十位死因合计占死亡总数的87%(注:由于首次采用ICD-10疾病分类标准,农村地区死因谱发生变化,故死亡率偏低)。

可以看出慢性病引起的主要死亡原因,城乡基本上一致,只有很小的差异。过去由于城乡生活条件差异较大,死亡原因也有较大的差异。而农村地区由于自然条件的原因,地方病明显比城市多。

慢性病的大量增加,折射出我国城乡居民随着生活条件的提高,生活方式的改变,营养过剩比较普遍,城乡生活节奏都有所加快,饮食过量,但活动比较少,引起肥胖、高血压、心脏病、恶性肿瘤、糖尿病等大量增加。

另一方面,应当看到城乡的差异性。城市居民随着社会转型,竞争非常激烈,但社会保障工作做得好,幼儿园等社会化服务非常有效,促进了儿童的身心健康,但部分农村地区的儿童就没有这么幸运。在实行联产承包责任制以后,农村改变了过去以生产队为单位的经营模式,形成了以家庭为单位的生产方式。这种生产方式,确实调动了农民的生产积极性,比生产队为单位的经营模式有了很大的发展,但同时也应当看到,由于农村相应的社会化服务比较差,家政服务等社会化程度比较低,在夫妇都致力于农业、林业或水产业等生产的家庭,对学龄前儿童大都放任自流,这些儿童无人照看,其生长发育受到了很大的影响,有的甚至出现严重的营养不良等疾病。这些问题应当引起关注。在一些落后的农村地区,营养不良、地方病仍然非常突出。

在城市化过程中,由于机动车辆的大量增加,车祸不断增加,从以上数据可以看出,城市和农村都是排在死因的第五位,但城市略高些。城市化的发展确实会付出沉重的代价,城市由于人口密度大,交通拥挤,发生事故率也偏高。农村地区虽然车辆密度较小,但随着农业的机械化程度提高,农用机械的大量增加,有的农民未经正式培训就驾驶机动车辆,有的机动车辆不上牌照,驾驶者无驾驶执照,加上农村地区对机动车辆疏于管理,有的造成严重的恶性事故。这些问题应当引起重视。另外,农村地区对农药的管理、使用等环节都存在一定的漏洞,造成中毒卫生问题非常突出。

五、城乡卫生资源分布不均衡，农村卫生服务问题尤为突出

改革开放以来，我国卫生事业发展速度很快。卫生总费用持续增加，据测算，2001年卫生总费用达5 150.3亿元，比2000年增长386.3亿元。卫生总费用构成：政府预算卫生支出800.6亿元，占15.5%；社会卫生支出1 236.4亿元，占24.0%；居民个人卫生支出3 113.3亿元，占60.5%。2001年人均卫生费用403.6元，比2000年增加27.2元。

从卫生资源的分布看，仍然是城乡之间的剪刀差加大，分布更加失衡。2002年末，全国医疗机构床位311.3万张，其中，非营利性医疗机构295.3万张，占94.9%；营利性医疗机构8.5万张，占2.7%。医疗机构中：医院床位222.2万张，占71.4%；卫生院床位68.5万张，占22.0%。与上年比较，医院床位增加3.4万张，卫生院床位减少6.1万张。2002年每千人口医院和卫生院床位2.32张。农村卫生院经营状况不佳，其床位仍有下降的趋势。这种情况在1982年以后就出现了，医疗卫生工作的重点从那时就转向了城市。1982~2001年间，我国医院床位从205.4万张增加到297.6万张，涨幅为44.9%，在此期间，城镇医院床位数从83.2万张增加到195.9万张，涨幅为135.3%，而农村医院床位不但没有增加反而下降到101.7万张，降幅为16.7%。农村医院床位数占床位总数的比重从1982年的60%跌至2001年的34.2%。

2002年新法接生率97.2%，其中市98.8%、县96.0%；住院分娩率达78.8%，其中市87.0%，县69.0%。与上年比较，住院分娩率增加2.8个百分点。据2001年妇幼卫生监测地区统计，孕产妇死亡率50.2/10^5，新生儿死亡率21.4‰，婴儿死亡率30.0‰，5岁以下儿童死亡率35.9‰。统计资料表明，孕产妇和儿童死亡率城乡差异明显（见表12-1）。

表12-1 监测地区孕产妇和儿童死亡率

	合计		城市		农村	
年份	2000	2001	2000	2001	2000	2001
孕产妇死亡率(1/10^5)	53.0	50.2	29.3	33.1	69.6	61.9
新生儿死亡率(‰)	22.8	21.4	9.5	10.6	25.8	23.9
婴儿死亡率(‰)	32.2	30.0	11.8	13.6	37.0	33.8
5岁以下儿童死亡率(‰)	39.7	35.9	13.8	16.3	45.7	40.4

资料引自中华人民共和国卫生部网站信息统计资料。

基层卫生组织的发展面临空前的挑战，有的乡镇医务人员只能发基本工资，而没有奖金，有的连基本工资也不能按时发放，挫伤了医务人员的积极性，造成了乡镇医院恶性运行；有的地方政府甚至将乡镇医院一卖了之，使农村三级卫生网受到了很大的冲击。在村一级，有的村办卫生室解体，有的个体医生水平差，医疗市场秩序混乱，个别地区无证行医者泛滥。直接后果是农村看病难，对孕产妇死亡率、婴儿死亡率和儿童死亡率的影响充分说明了这一点。可见在农村不管卫生资源的配置，还是卫生服务的组织管理和实施，都存在一定的问题。

不仅卫生资源的配置存较多的问题，农村卫生组织的防保功能发挥较差，在市场经济的条件下，防保人员追求的利益与人民群众不一致，有的防保机构是健全的，但由于防保

机构单纯追求经济利益,放松了疾病的防治,结果导致传染病和寄生虫病在局部地区的暴发流行,教训是深刻的。防保机构的任务艰巨,不能以赢利为目的,政府应加强管理,对防保部门要进行准确定位,同时要对防保机构增加投入。

目前,中国的医疗保险占卫生总费用的1/4左右,中国现行的医疗保险制度也存在着严重的城乡不公。以前城镇从业人员享受公费医疗或劳保医疗,现在他们享受到了社会医疗保险。2000年,企业职工医疗保障费约为600亿元,行政和事业单位职工医疗保障费也在600亿元左右,两者相加总共为1 168亿元,但是这笔保障费只有大约7 000万城镇居民分享,还占不到全国13亿人口的6%,而绝大部分农村居民没有任何社会医疗保险,卫生保障完全靠自费。这种不公平影响到农民的健康水平,也制约着农村经济的进一步发展。

第三节 城乡居民保健的社会医学措施

经过几十年的卫生实践,我国城乡人群的卫生保健得到了很大的发展,积累了许多宝贵的经验。中共十六大提出的全面建设小康社会的发展目标其核心在于促进"人"的全面发展,改善人民福利。而健康是人民福利的核心要素,应当成为"全面小康"的重要组成部分。联合国首脑论坛提出的千年发展目标中,卫生发展目标占有重要地位,报告首次提出并确立了"福利优先"的思想。政府应当制定新的卫生政策,致力于提高群众的健康水平,并且重新界定政府在卫生领域的职能,调整卫生投入方向,形成政府新的管理模式。

一、针对城市居民的社会卫生措施

首先,进一步开展社区卫生服务,真正实现医疗、预防、保健、康复、健康教育、计划生育六位一体的卫生服务。这是实现城市人口人人享有基本卫生保健的重要环节。其次,进一步完善职工医疗保险,扩大医疗保险的覆盖面。第三,建立科学的城市卫生运行机制,试行将医疗保险同社区卫生服务结合起来的机制,使得防保效果同医疗机构的利益结合起来,促进卫生事业的有序、协调发展,形成卫生事业良性运行的机制。第四,加快对城市医疗、防保机构改革的步伐,实行科学的绩效评价,加速人事制度改革的步伐,注重调整不同群体的利益关系,做到自由与契约的平衡、公平与效率的平衡。

二、针对农村居民的社会卫生措施

(一)加强农村三级医疗预防保健网的建设

农村三级医疗预防保健网,是指以村卫生所为前哨、乡卫生院为枢纽、县级医疗卫生机构为中心,把预防、保健、医疗工作联结在一起,在全县范围内组成一个完整的医疗预防体系,为广大农民提供医疗预防保健服务。县、乡、村三级医疗卫生组织的关系是:各有分工,相互协作,上下支援,逐级指导。县级医疗卫生机构有责任对乡卫生院,特别是中心卫生院的工作给予指导;乡卫生院有责任对村卫生所实行业务指导和支援。农村三级医疗预防保健网在20世纪60年代已基本形成,改革开放以来,更加趋于完善。有关资料显示,进入90年代,国家计委、财政部、农业部和卫生部联合开展了农村"三项建设"工作,对乡镇卫生院、县防疫站和县妇幼保健机构进行重点建设,更加促进农村三级医疗预防保健网的发展与完善。仅1991～1994年间全国农村卫生"三项建设"的投资即达59.6亿元，使13 635所卫生院、716所防疫站和730所妇幼保健站改变了落后面貌。至1994年，全国已有县医院2 062所，县妇幼保健所、站1 625所，县卫生防疫站1 777所，乡卫生院5.19万个，有医疗点的行政村为65万个，占行政村数的88%。有的省、市进行了乡村一体化管理，取得了明显的成效。

但应当看到，在新形势下，农村医疗预防三级保健网的建设也遇到了新的挑战。正如上面提到的，一是乡镇卫生院经营状况堪忧，有的地区把乡镇卫生院作为包袱甩给了社会，使三级医疗预防保健网遭到了破坏。二是村级卫生室有的已经变成了个体医疗诊所，其完全变成了赢利组织，影响了其功能的发挥。

首先，要根据农村卫生需求的特点，重新整合基层卫生组织，乡村实行一体化管理是一条出路，但要注意乡村医生整合到乡镇卫生组织以后要解决他们的养老保险、医疗保险等后顾之忧，真正做到"一体"。对于功能重叠的卫生组织应当进行撤并。其次，政府对农村卫生应当承担更多的责任，进一步加大投入，使农村卫生事业与社会经济发展相协调。再次，制定优惠的政策，吸引优秀卫生人才到农村去工作。还有，加强乡村医生的培训，在农村开展社区卫生服务，严格进行执法监督，控制无证行医，保证农民享受安全、可靠的基本卫生服务。

(二) 完善和创新农村医疗保障体系

我国农村合作医疗是农民群众创造的适合我国农村的医疗保障制度。党和政府多年来予以关注和支持，对于保证农民获得基本医疗服务、落实预防保健任务、防止农民因病致贫具有重要作用，受到广大农民的欢迎和支持。但是，由于认识上的不尽一致，相关的政策、措施不配套，致使这个制度发生了很大波折，而在农村经济体制变化中，合作医疗制度又陷入了低谷，近来虽有所恢复，也仅有10%左右的行政村实行这个制度。农村再次出现看病难、医疗负担重的状况。

建设中国特色的农村医疗保障体系，是完成"人人享有卫生保健"的要求，更是发展生产，摆脱"因病致贫"、"因病返贫"的需要。从1990年到1999年，农民平均纯收入增长了2.2倍；但同期卫生部门统计的每人次平均门诊费用和住院费用，则分别增长了6.2倍和5.1倍。医疗费用的大幅度上升，给农民造成了沉重的经济负担。据调查，农民生病无钱就诊的比例由1985年的4%上升到1993年的7%，需住院而无钱未住院的比例由13.4%上升到24.5%。越来越多的农民无力承受日益增长的医疗费用，成为当前农村医疗卫生保障的突出矛盾。受人口老龄化等因素的影响，农民的两周患病率、慢性病患病率、因病休工天数、因病卧床天数等指标都有明显增加，农村居民因病休工和卧床天数高于城市。有的出现因病致贫。他们迫切需要一定程度的医疗保障，以保证最基本的卫生健康。

有的学者提出，在城镇职工"基本医疗保险"制度改革的经验和基础上建立农民基本医疗保障制度，要坚持以下几个基本原则：第一，坚持国家支持的原则。要建立国家与农户共同投入、风险共担的机制，可以借鉴城镇职工医疗个人账户的形式，建立农户家庭医疗保障账户，促进农户节约资金，提高抵御疾病风险的能力。同时，要强调多元投入的机制，引导社区经济、企业、慈善机构、外资机构及个人等方面的捐助，充实农民医疗保障基金。第二，坚持因地制宜的原则。由于我国幅员辽阔，各地经济、社会发展水平差异很大，应当允许各地区从自己的实际情况出发，因地制宜地积极探索适合农村特点的多形式、多层次的医疗保险制度尤其是合作医疗保险制度。第三,坚持社会化的原则。应当以县级区域(而不是以村或乡)为基础,通过国家立法(而不仅仅是"自愿参加")促使农户参加进来。第四,坚持保重大疾病的原则。农民的疾病威胁主要是重大疾病,这是他们无力承担的风险。应当为农民建立"最基本重大疾病保障"制度,把有限的资金用于最急需的地方。通过完善和创新农民医疗保障体系,促进农民健康水平的提高。第五,坚持分类实施的原则。我国经济发展很不平衡,在经济发达地区、经济中等地区以及经济欠发达地区应当分类实施不同的医疗保障制度。

(三)发展农村初级卫生保健

在农村发展初级卫生保健是我国卫生事业发展的基本经验之一。"2000年人人享有卫生保健",是世界卫生组织提出的全球战略目标。对此,我国政府已作了承诺。当时,为了实现"2000年人人享有卫生保健"的目标,在全国农村分地区、分阶段、分层次地实施全面初级卫生保健。从此,我国农村的初级卫生保健,成为农村卫生工作的"龙头",牵动着农村卫生工作向纵深发展。

发展农村卫生工作,首先,要树立社会大卫生观,最根本的是要根据农村存在的主要社会卫生问题,有针对性地解决农村的卫生饮用水问题、农药安全管理问题、慢性病的健康教育问题等。其次,要形成发展农村初级卫生保健同社会经济协调发展的机制,通过立法的形式规定下来,通过建立行政管理上的激励机制,强化农村初级卫生保健工作。第三,将初级卫生保健工作同社区卫生服务工作有机地结合起来,形成改善环境条件与医疗、预防、保健、康复、健康教育密切结合的局面。第四,加强对农村环境的监测,对"三小"企业、排污超标的企业进行严格的控制,防止污染企业向农村的转移。

案例

洛杉矶光学烟雾事件

20世纪40年代初发生于美国洛杉矶市,主要是汽车排放的废气在日光作用下形成毒雾,对人体造成危害。

滨海城市洛杉矶,背山临海,风景优美。1936年开发石油以来,飞机制造和军事工业迅速发展,成为美国西部的重要海港。

当时,洛杉矶有250万辆汽车,每天有1000千多吨碳氢化合物、石油废气、一氧化碳和氧化氮、铅烟等进入大气中。汽车废气在阳光作用下与空气中其他化学成分发生化学反应,产生一种浅蓝色烟雾,其中含有臭氧、氧化氮、乙醛及其他氧化剂。这是一种刺激性很强的化学烟雾。

洛杉矶处于三面环山一面临海的口袋形地势,50千米长的盆地中,一年有300天的逆温层,因而光学烟雾扩散不出去,长期停滞在市内,毒化空气,形成污染。洛杉矶烟雾,主要刺激眼、鼻、喉,引起眼病、喉头炎和不同程度的头痛,严重的能造成死亡。同时,也能使家畜患病,妨碍农作物和植物生长,腐蚀材料和建筑物,使橡胶制品老化。由于烟雾使大气浑浊,降低了大气的能见度,影响了汽车和飞机的安全,造成车祸和飞机坠毁事件增多等危害。

思考1. 从这起环境事件中应当吸取什么教训?

思考 2. 城市环境卫生问题的社会性体现在哪些方面？

湖北宜城农村卫生院公开拍卖

阳春三月，正是犁耙水响闹春耕的时节。湖北省宜城市，一场农村卫生院产权制度改革在全市 40 万农民、1 200 多名卫生工作者中掀起阵阵波澜。将企业改革的成功经验导入事业单位改革，把全市 16 家农村卫生院全部公开向社会拍卖，这在全国还是首家。截至 4 月 25 日，宜城市已有 6 家农村卫生院通过公开拍卖，由"官"办转为"民"办。对于这场改革几乎所有的人都说，宜城人在"吃螃蟹"。

宜城市的乡镇卫生院大多是建国初期在联合诊所的基础上建立起来的。全市有农村卫生院 16 家，按照编制应配人员 580 人，而现有人员 1 282 人，且每年按政策必须接收的人员还在不断增加；卫生院资产总额 2 371 万元，负债 2 811 万元。2001 年，全市农村卫生院亏损面 100%；卫生院职工个人收入低微，2001 年人均月工资 240 元左右，而效益较差的只能勉强发放职工最低生活费，人均仅 120 元左右；投入机制不畅，近几年农民收入增长缓慢，农民减负导致乡镇财政普遍困难，根本无力对卫生院投入。2001 年，宜城市卫生院财政拨款实际到位仅 29.6 万元，比 2000 年减少 90 万元。与此同时，医药体制改革致使传统的以药养医体制难以为继。全市工业企业产权制度改革的成功使得市领导在农村卫生院改革上得到了启发、产生了想法。而全国卫生工作会议文件又使这种想法找到了"依据"：要通过体制创新，建立权责明晰、富有生机的医疗机构管理体制，使医疗机构真正成为自主管理、自我发展、自我约束的法人实体。鼓励营利性与非营利性医疗机构之间展开竞争，促进民营医疗机构的发展。2 月 21 日，宜城市召开农村卫生院产权制度改革动员大会，拉开改革的序幕。

宜城市认准了改革的核心是引入竞争，并迅速作出抉择：拍卖。接着，宜城市确定了"保证一头"（防疫保健）、"放开一片"（将医疗服务推向市场）的指导思想。按照"防、治分离"的原则，将原卫生院的防疫保健职能剥离出来，在镇（街道办事处）设立独立的卫生防疫保健机构，承担卫生防疫、妇幼保健和基层卫生管理职能。

产权改革，公开拍卖，意味着要彻底打破原有的利益格局，随之而来的职工安置是人们关注的焦点。

农村卫生院产权卖断后，按民有营利性医疗机构管理，原卫生院干部职工身份随即终止，其经费与政府财政脱钩，其人事档案交由市人才交流中心保管；以其拍卖所得对在职正式职工一次性发给安置费；一次性补齐所欠的养老保险金，其原有退休人员由社会保险机构发给退休费，确无能力补齐养老保险金的，由社会保险机构按有关政策酌情发给生活费；离休人员交地方政府管理，其离休工资、医疗费等福利待遇由政府负责落实。

据了解，我国 5 万多个农村卫生院，有 2/3 遇到经济困难。以企业改革闻名的湖北省宜城市，今年 2 月开始，将企业改革的成功经验导入事业单位改革，把全市 16 家农村卫生院全部公开向社会拍卖，这在全国还是首家，十分引人关注。

思考 1. 你是否同意乡镇卫生院拍卖？

思考 2. 乡镇卫生院拍卖与农村三级医疗预防保健网的建设是否存在矛盾，你认为如何解决这个矛盾？

Chapter 12　Urban and Rural Social Medicine

Section 1　The Influence of the Urban and Rural Social Structure on Health Development

1. Dual social structure in the city and countryside

During the time of planned economy in our country, the government carried out a managerial policy in which urban and rural areas were administered separately. It is called "having a meal on different cooking stoves", the so-called urban and rural dual social structure. The sociology circles of China have launched research on the urban and rural dual social structure since the 1980s. It was thought that it was in a separated state because the population was strictly controlled in moving between urban and rural areas. It was formed on the basis of a different policy in urban and rural areas covering resident control, food and oil supply, employment arrangements, social insurance.

There were three characteristics of this urban structure. First, the urban scale was too large with too many large cities and there was not enough development in the middle- and small-sized cities.

Secondly, it was not evenly distributed in the regions. The cities were mainly situated in the eastern coastal areas of China and urban development in the western areas was seriously behind.

Thirdly, the urban industrial structure was imbalanced; industry took the leading part of the national economy and thus the development of tertiary industry seriously fell behind especially for transportation and basic municipal facilities. The backwardness of urbanization was a serious shortcoming for the development of atypical industrialization in China and created many contradictions and problems for the Chinese economy. Under the previous system of development heavy industry cut off in urban and rural areas, and urbanization produced a very different dual economic structure. The contradictions of the dual economy became worse because since 1985 farm laborers slowly marched to non-farming industry. Especially in recent years a large number of farm labors declined constantly which made farmers' incomes decline and differences in the income rapidly expanded.

The dual social structure not only limited the population to move in society but also expanded the gap between the urban and rural areas and formed a different structure in each of these areas. Politically, there were closer relations for the various urban organizations, which were relatively loose in the rural areas. In respect to features of the population, there was more consistency for the rural population than for the urban population. There was a lower level of education for the rural population than for urban population; there were closer relationships in rural communities than in urban communities, and there was a lower level of social insurance for the rural population than for the urban population. In respect to the economy, the individual led the rural economy. The socialization level of the urban economy was higher. On ownership, in the past the rural economy mainly belonged to the collective ownership, and the urban economy was mainly state-ownership. With reform and establishment of the socialist market economy, the situation has been changed. And the level of social change is higher in urban areas than that in rural areas.

2. The influence of the urban and rural dual social structure on the equity of health development

The urban and rural dual social structure has greatly influenced the equity of health development in China. The so-called equity of health care normally includes health equity, attainable equity of medical services, equity of utilization on practical services and equity on collecting funds. Health equity means that the health situation of the population basically is similar. The accessibility of health services means people have access to the most basic health services. Equity of utilization on practical services means people who have the same requirements can get the same medical service. Equity on collecting funds means paying health care expenses according to the ability to pay. In 2000, WHO appraised the performance of health systems in three aspects of the 191 member Countries. On the equity of medical burden, China was listed at 188. Equity on health care is mainly shown in three aspects. There is difference in region, difference between city and countryside and difference on the social stratum. In respect to the differences between city and countryside there were some relationships between the influence of the dual social structure and marketing reform. The right administration of government on medical reform showed that basic public health service should be provided to all residents, the limited public medical resource should be put into the prevention and cure of infectious disease, endemic disease, and malnutrition disease to the rural residents, and diseases for women and children and primary health care. For the rural primary health care, the government should insist on a policy of prevention as a priority to reduce the incidence of diseases and treatment costs. The government should play the leading role to establish a system of medical insurance that meets the rural requirements of the present time and it should change the situation of carrying out two separate systems to improve the national treatment of farmers and realize the urban and rural equity of health development.

Section 2　The Major Problems of Urban and Rural Social Health

1. China's large population and frequent movements of people have led to creating many social health problems

The global population has doubled since 1960 to reach 6.1 billion with the increase mainly in some poor countries. It will reach 9.3 billion in 2050 according to predicted data, and obviously the larger population will consume more resources. It is the situation of the state that there is a large population with a poor foundation in China. According to data of the Fifth National Census in 2000, there was an urban population of 455 million. And 36.9 percent of the general population is in 31 provinces, autonomous regions and municipalities directly under the central government on the mainland, and there are 807.39 million rural population sharing 63.91 percent. Compared with the Fourth National Census in 1990 the proportion of the urban population has risen 9.86 percent. In general, the trend was rural population transferring to the cities. During urbanization, the transfer of the rural population to the cities is bound to continue.

Because of this, social health problems increased in the cities. The social movement means that people moved from one position to another in the social relation space. Because there is a close relationship between social position and geographical space, so the movement of people on the geographical space belongs also to the social movement. A movement on the geographical position of farmers moving to cities is also a movement on the social position. The movement of large numbers of farmers to the cities was called "a tide of farming laborers" by sociologists. There is some derogatory sense in calling farm laborers a floating population, but it still has a positive meaning in promoting social progress and increasing urbanization in China. The floating population has made a significant contribution in modernization, but at the same time has brought some pressure on employment and also caused some safety and health problems.

First, the tide of farm laborers increased the difficulty of employment arrangements, reduced the general living standards of the urban population and influenced the health of the population. The increasing pressure on employment has made some influence on people's psychology to cause some diseases.

Secondly, the large floating population caused some problems with safety and health. Relevant data showed that more than 20 million of the population were unemployed. In the first half of 2001, the registered rate of unemployment was 3.3 percent in the urban areas in China and the registered population of unemployment 6.19 million.

There were 6.32 million personnel going off sentry duty, a total of 12.51. Some specialists estimate that the practical rate of unemployment should be about 10 percent in urban areas. There were 60 million surplus laborers entering the cities from the countryside. The problems of agriculture and farmers in China have become increasingly prominent since the nineteen nineties. Per capita cultivated area in China is only 1.2 Mu, and the per capita cultivated area is 4.1 for laborers. The per capita cultivated area is less than 1 Mu in one third of the provinces of China, and there are one-third of the counties with the per capita cultivated area less than 0.8 Mu. Those quantities of cultivated area are lower than the last support line for existence stipulated by UN The rural land of China is gradually losing its function as a producer of material to transform the last support of farmers. Large numbers of surplus laborers have been produced because of the strained relations between the population and cultivated land. Specialists estimate there are about 200 million surplus laborers. Among them 120 million surplus laborers were accepted by township enterprises (including local and external surplus laborers). There are about 70 million surplus laborers who have moved to urban or urbanized and rich areas, such as Zhujiang River Triangular Area, Changjiang River Triangular area. There are at least 60 million farm laborers needing jobs.

Because of a shortage of jobs, a proportion of urban and rural residents become poor people. These people are short of the minimum health insurance; they are unable to pay for medical treatment when required. This situation has broken the harmony of mankind and society. At the time when SARS broke out in Tianjin, a victim of SARS in a hospital infected more than one hundred people. Some sufferers were short of the basic medical insurance. The government paid all hospitalized expenses for them. So we should fully realize the problems on social health in China caused by the problems of unemployment. It brings many problems when farmers enter the cities to look for jobs. According to the census material of Beijing on November 10, 1994, the floating population in Beijing reached 3.295 million. They have become a necessary part of the people living in Beijing. They work as child nurses, housekeepers, cleaners, drivers of three-wheel vehicles, and as workers in restaurants. They do all the dirty and heavy jobs which local people do not want to do. The relevant statistics show there were 240,000 rural employees doing dirty, heavy jobs in cleaning, textile, mining and coal industries. There were more than 800,000 construction workers who were not local and were the main force of construction in Beijing. The rural laborers have a lot of shortcomings. They throw rubbish in a mess to damage the urban appearance. They stimulate consumption, which causes the price of goods to rise. Some peddlers do cheating business and make products in a rough and slipshod way. It was said that the food made by them was very dirty. The most serious problem was the safety problems brought to Beijing by the large floating population. The Police Bureau of Beijing announced that among illegal works and crime, most of them were committed by the floating population. For example, in 1994, 46 percent of crime was found in the floating population. The large number of the floating population robbed, stole, killed a person, robbed his goods and stopped at nothing, especially the group committing very serious crimes. There were nearly 30 areas where the floating population lived in compact communities, such as Xinjiang Village and Zhejiang Village, which became a sink of iniquity, a base of drug abuse and trafficking narcotics.

There are many problems on the managements of family planning, giving good birth and good care to the floating population. Some of them have formed managerial blind spots. Some members of the floating population were forced to do body examinations. Some management only laid stress on collecting fees and ignored the managerial effectiveness. The floating population was the root of almost all of the problems. The traffic and transportation developed with the floating populations. It provided the external conditions in which infectious diseases can spread rapidly. So in modern society, we should pay great attention to the negative effects of the floating population.

2. There was urgent demand to the quality of the population

In China, not only is there a large population, but also there is a problem of the quality of the population. On education quality, according to the census material in 2000 there were 45.71 million population with college degrees, 141.09 million population with senior middle school degree, 429.89 million with junior middle school degree, 451.96 million population with primary school degree (population above with various education degree included graduates from all kind of colleges and school, students among of the population of the mainland and army serviceman). Compared with the Fourth National Census in 1990, the quality of population has slightly improved. But in general it is not optimistic. The proportion of the population with a university education is low. In addition, the population of illiteracy and primary degree occupied larger proportion. With poor education in general, it not only restricts economic development but also affects people's consciousness on health care and taking action, which in turn affects health of people to greater degree. With carrying out the basic national policy of family planning in China, not only the amount of the population was controlled, but also the physiological quality of the population was greatly improved. Revised marriage law and policy of giving good birth and care significantly reduced hereditary diseases. But some policies of population have produced a negative effect on improving the quality of the population, such as advocating a married couple to only bear one child and if there is some disease with that child, they will be allowed to bear a second child. This policy met the requirement of the masses. On objectivity, it reduced the quality of the population. After all the physiological quality of the first child is not high, and also the second child takes a greater risk of physiological quality. Another policy carried out in the city is that a married couple is allowed to bear only one child but in the countryside if the first child is a girl, then a second child will be allowed. This policy was formulated to meet the demand for laborers in the countryside. But, this policy has led to a contrary elimination of population. Thus, the population with quality is little and the population without quality is less. The final result is a reduction in the quality of the population. Another point is that we cannot neglect the social health problems with the different composition on the population. It was revealed by authoritative person in 2002 that the aged population above 60 years old has reached 132 million and will rapidly increase at a rate of 3.2 percent per year. With the arrival of an old-aged society, the social health problems of urban and rural old people have become very conspicuous. The medical care for old people should be put on the agenda. (See the part of social medical science on aged people)

3. The prominent environmental sanitation

With the economic development at full speed a high cost has been paid to the environmental sanitation. The following are features of environmental sanitation. The problems on environmental sanitation have been transferred to the developing countries from the developed countries. The synthetic measurement gradually has been done to protect environment with strengthening consciousness on environmental protection after the developed countries have undergone a series of lessons on environmental sanitation. These measurements include the strict treatment of pollution enterprises. The synthetic measurement has won initial success, but these pollution enterprises have been transferred to developing countries from the developed countries and regions.

With the development of industry and transportation in the cities, growing use of energy resources, various waste gases into air, widespread use of cooking stove and heating boiler, the decrease and drying in water resources, the decrease in numbers of green areas, excessive opening up of wasteland, destroying forest and vegetation which makes more desert areas, there is an overall increase in the density of particles and harmful matter going up into the air. The main pollution was smoke at the beginning of industrialization in some countries, such as the smoke incident in London in 1956. Petroleum replaced coal to become the main fuel after the 1960s. Sulfur dioxide has become the main pollutant in cities. With the development of traffic and transportation, the exhaust gas of automobiles and photochemical smoke has become the chief criminal of air pollution in urban areas. Hydrocarbon matter and nitrogen oxide existing in air has become secondary pollutant after a series of photochemical reactions under strong sunlight action to be stored up in air and forms a smoke with light blue color. The main compositions of the secondary pollutant are ozone, perhydrol, ketone, aldehyde, the aerosol particulate formed by hydrochloric acid and some macromolecular organic compounds, etc.

Many photochemical smoke incidents occurred in Los Angeles where air pollution caused many health problems. At first, it caused irritation to the skin and then caused many kinds of diseases of the respiratory system and also led to acute and chronic poisoning. It went so far as to cause cancer. In addition, it caused the pollution of water source. Secondly, the urban pollution began to transfer to the countryside. With a strengthening of the consciousness on environmental protection in the city, some small-sized enterprises with heavy pollution in the city were transferred to countryside for development and that polluted the rural environment. Some private enterprises merely were after profits to do illegal business without safe producing conditions, which led to poisoning of the workers. According to the statistics of the entire country, with the exception of Tibet and Taiwan, in 2002, among 14,821 various occupational diseases, there are 12,248 cases of pneumoconiosis, 1,300 cases for chronic occupational poisoning, 590 cases for acute occupational poisoning, 159 cases for occupational ophthalmic disease and 206 cases for occupational otolaryngological disease. Some diseases occur in the countryside. China must not make the mistakes that some developed countries have made in treating the environment after creating pollution, but rather take precautions and preventative measures to protect the environment.

4. Chronic diseases are major problems and do harm to the health of urban and rural residents

The reasons for disease and death have changed very much since the 1970s. All chronic diseases are listed in the front positions. The statistics from the information center of the Health Ministry showed that the main reasons for deaths of urban and rural residents (ICD-10: ten leading causes of death) are as follows: ①135.4/100 thousand for malignant neoplasms, ②100.6/100 thousand for cerebrovascular, ③ 89.9/100 thousand for diseases of respiratory system, ④ 84.1/100 thousand for heart diseases, ⑤ 50.4/100 thousand for injury & poisoning, ⑥ 19.6/100 thousand for diseases of the digestive system, ⑦ 14.1/100 thousand for diseases of the endocrine, nutritional & metabolic diseases, ⑧ 9.7/100 thousand for diseases of the genitourinary system,. ⑨ 5.2/100 thousand for diseases of the nervous system, ⑩ 4.9/100 thousand for diseases originating in the prenatal period, and the total amount of the first ten reasons causing deaths took 89 percent of the total number; the first ten reasons causing deaths for rural residents as follows: ①81.3/100 thousand for malignant neoplasms, ②70.6/100 thousand for cerebrovascular, ③ 63.8/100 thousand for diseases of respiratory system, ④ 58.5/100 thousand for heart diseases, ⑤ 41.5/100 thousand for injury & poisoning, ⑥ 14.5/100 thousand for diseases of the digestive system, ⑦5.9/100 thousand for diseases of the genitourinary system, ⑧4.9/100 thousand for diseases of the endocrine, nutritional & metabolic diseases, ⑨ 4.4/100 thousand for diseases originating in the prenatal period, ⑩ 4.3/100 thousand for disease of pulmonary tuberculosis. The total number of reasons took 87 percent of the total number of deaths. (Note: because it was the first time to adopt ICD-10 classified standard for diseases, the list of reasons causing deaths in the countryside has changed. So the rate of death is on the low side.)

The data above show that the main reasons for deaths caused by chronic diseases showed nearly no difference between city and countryside. There was very little difference. But in the past, there was a big difference in living condition between city and countryside. So there was a big difference in the reasons causing deaths, and there was obviously a higher rate of endemic disease in the countryside than in the city because of natural conditions.

The large increase of chronic disease reflected that the urban and the rural living condition and style and nutrition have been improved. Now the urban and rural life rhythm has quickened with eating and drinking too much and less exercise and this way of life causes an increase in obesity, hypertension, heart disease, malignant neoplasms and diabetes.

On the other hand, we should keep sight of the difference between city and countryside. With social reform, the competition becomes sharp for urban residents, but they have good social insurance. The social services of kindergarten are very effective in promoting the children's health of body and mind. But some rural children are not so lucky.

After reform, the production team as a production unit has changed into a form of a family as a production unit. This production style really aroused the enthusiasm of farmers. There was great progress compared with the style of taking a production team as a production unit. But meanwhile, we should keep insight of the fact that rural social service was rather poor.

The social service level for family service is rather low. For some families in which the couple run farming, forestry and aquatic products, there is nobody to look after preschool children. Their growth was deeply affected, even some children suffering from serious malnutrition, diseases, etc. We should pay close attention to these problems.

During the course of urbanization, traffic accidents consistently increased with the large increase in the number of automobiles. According to the data above, it shows this reason as the fifth both in city and in countryside, and is a little higher in the city. It is a heavy cost to pay for urbanization. Because there is a high density of population and therefore traffic problems in the city are great, the rate of accidents is higher. Although the density of automobiles was lower in the countryside some serious accidents still occurred because the number of agricultural machines largely increased with the improvement of the level of agricultural mechanization, and some farmers drive vehicles without training. Attention should be paid to all these problems.

In addition, there are some loopholes in the management and usage of pesticides in the countryside. The problem of poisoning is very conspicuous.

5. The distribution of rural health resource is imbalanced

The problems of rural health service were particularly conspicuous. Improved health undertakings were quickly developed since the reform and opening up policy of China. Medical expenses have continued to increase. According to statistics the total medical expenses reached 515.03 billion RMB in 2001 and increased by 38.63 billion RMB in 2002.

The total amount of medical expenses was composed of 80.06 billion RMB budgetary outlays from government, taking 15.5 percent of the total expense; 123.64 billion RMB from the social medical outlays, taking 24.0 percent; 311.33 billion RMB from the individual outlays of the population, taking 60.5 percent. The per capita medical expense was 403.6 RMB, which meaned a 27.2 RMB increase compared with that in 2000.

The distribution of medical resources widened the gap between the city and the countryside. The distribution became even more imbalanced. There were 3.113 million beds in the medical facilities throughout the country at the end of 2002. Among these were 2.953 million beds in non-profitable medical institutes, taking 94.9 percent, and 85 thousand beds in the profitable medical institutes, taking 2.7 percent. Among the medical institutes, there were 2.222 million beds in the hospitals, taking 71.7 percent, 0.685 million beds in the community hospitals, taking 22 percent. Compared with last year there was a an increase of 34,000 beds in hospitals and a decrease of 61,000 beds in community hospitals. There were 2.32 beds per thousand people both in hospitals and community hospitals in 2002. The running situation of the community hospitals was poor in the countryside, and still there is a declining trend for the number of beds they keep. This situation has occurred since 1982. The stress in medical and health work began to transfer to urban areas from that time. In the whole country, the beds kept in hospitals have increased to 2.976 million from 2.054 million between 1982 and 2001. The increase reached 44.9 percent. During this period, the number of beds kept in urban hospitals has increased to 1.959 million from 0.832 million. The increase reached 135.3 percent. But in rural community hospitals, not only was there no increase but also there was a 16.7 percent decrease to 1.017 million beds. The proportion of the number of beds kept in the rural hospitals took the total number of beds kept in all hospitals has decreased to 31.2 percent in 2001 from 60 percent in 1982.

The rate of delivering children with the new way reached 97.2 percent in 2002. Of this percentage, 98.8 percent was in the city and 96.0 percent in the country. The hospitalization rate for childbirth reached 78.8 percent. Of this figure, the rate reached 87 percent in the city and 69 percent in the country. The hospitalization rate for childbirth increased 2.8 percent. According to statistics for women and children health in some monitored regions in 2001, the death rate of pregnant and lying-in woman was 50.2/100,000. The death rate of newborn baby was 21.4‰. The death rate of baby was 30‰. The death rate of children under 5 years old was 35.9‰. Statistics show that the difference of death rate for pregnant and lying-in women and children between city and countryside was obvious. (see Table 12-1)

Table 12-1. The Death Rate For Pregnant, Lying-in Women and Children in Monitored Regions

	Total Amount		In the City		In the Countryside	
	2000	2001	2000	2001	2000	2001
The death rate for pregnant (1/100 thousand)	53.0	50.2	29.3	33.1	69.6	61.9
The death rate of newborn baby (‰)	22.8	21.4	9.5	10.6	25.8	23.9
The death rate of baby (‰)	32.2	30.0	11.8	13.6	37.0	33.8
The death rate of children under 5 years old (‰)	39.7	35.9	13.8	16.3	45.7	40.4

In extract, compared with last year from the website of the Health Ministry of China, there is unprecedented challenge to the development of medical organization at the basic level. In some towns, medical personnel can only be paid the basic wage without bonus, and some basic wage cannot be paid in time and so dampens the enthusiasm of the medical personnel. This leads to a vicious circle in the township hospitals; even there were some township hospitals, which were sold out by the government to heavily pound at the rural three-level medical network. In the village level, some clinics owned by the village were disintegrated, the skill of some individual doctors was poor, and the medical workers were not in order; in some regions some people were practicing medicine without a license. The direct result was that it was becoming difficult to see a doctor in the countryside. This influenced the death rate of pregnant, lying-in women, babies and children. The rate of death in the countryside obviously was higher than that in the city. This shows there are some problems in the disposition of medical resources, management and implementation of medical services.

Not only were there some problems on the disposition of the medical resources, but also the preventive and health functions of the medical organization in the countryside were relatively poor. Under conditions of the market economy there is different interest between the prevention, health personnel and masses. Some preventive and health institutes with complete function related to the prevention and treatment of diseases to seek economic interest alone and as a result it causes infectious and parasitic diseases break out in some areas. The lessons are profound. There are arduous tasks for the preventive and health institutes. They cannot make profit-making their sole purpose. Government should strengthen their management and accurately define their work and meanwhile should increase input to them.

At present, medical insurance only takes about one quarter of the total medical expenses in China and there is serious unfairness under the current system of medical insurance between the countryside and the city. Previously, urban employees enjoyed free medical service or labor insurance on medical treatment. Now they enjoy the same social medical insurance.

There were about 60 billion RMB for the medical insurance expenses of employees working for enterprises in 2000 and about 60 billion RMB for the medical insurance expenses of employees working in administrative units and institutions, a total of 116.8 billion RMB. The expenses were only enjoyed by 70 million urban residents, per capita 1,670 RMB, taking less than 6% of the total population, and there is no social medical insurance for most rural residents who pay for all medical expenses by themselves. The unfair treatment has affected the health level of farmers and restricted the further development of the rural economy.

Section 3 The Social Medical Measurement on Health Care for Urban and Rural Residents

After ten years of medical practice in China, a lot of valuable experiences on the development of health care for the urban and rural masses have been accumulated. The Sixteenth National Congress of CPC put forward the developing goal to build the overall comfortable society with its core of developing mankind in an all-round way and improving people's welfare, and regarding the health as the key element of people's welfare and the important part of the overall comfort of society. Among the developing goals of thousand years advanced by the Forum of Heads of UN for first time, the developing goal for health is the most important. The Forum advanced and established the priority of welfare. The government should establish new health policies to improve the health level of the masses, redefine the function of government in areas of health, adjust the input direction on health and form a new model of government management policies.

1. The social medical measurement for urban residents

Firstly, development of health services in communities to integrate medical treatment, prevention, health care, recovery, education about health and family planning.

This is a key step to ensure that everybody in the urban population enjoys basic health care. Secondly, devising medical insurance for employees, and enlarging the range of medical insurance. Thirdly, establishing scientific operating systems for urban health, trying out the system to join medical insurance with health service for communities, joining the effects of prevention and health care with the interests of medical institutes to promote the development of health undertakings and creating good operating systems for undertaking health services. Fourthly, quickening the reform to the medical, preventive and health institutes, carrying out scientific appraisal on performance, quickening the reform of human resource systems, paying particular attention to the relationship between different mass groups to achieve a balance on freedom and contract that is fair and efficient.

2. The social health measurement for rural residents

(1) Strengthen the rural prevention and health network on three-level

The health network means that the village clinic is the advance guard, the commune hospital is the pivot, the medical institute on the county-level is the center to link up the prevention, health care, medical work and forms a complete system of medical prevention in the county to serve all farmers. The relationships between the medical health organizations on the three levels are cooperating with each other, guiding level by level. The medical institute has the responsibility to give guidance to the township commune hospitals and especially to the central commune hospital. The township commune hospitals also have responsibility to guide and help the village clinics. The rural medical preventive and health care network in three-level was basically built up during the nineteen sixties. It gradually perfected this model since reform and opening up. The relevant material shows that the Planning Committee of State, Financial Ministry, Agricultural Ministry and Health Ministry jointly launched the construction of the rural three projects to put stress on building the township commune hospitals, the epidemic prevention station and the health care center for women and children since the early nineties of last century. These measurements became even better developed and completed the rural medical prevention and health networks in three-level. Between 1991 and 1994, 5.96 billion RMB was invested in building the rural three projects for health to put an end of the backwardness in 13,635 commune hospitals, 716 epidemic prevention stations and 730 health care centers for women and children throughout the country. In 1994 there were 2,026 hospitals, 1,625 health care centers for women and children, 1,777 health epidemic stations in county-level and 51.9 thousand-township commune hospitals all over the country. There are 0.65 million administrative villages with clinics in the whole country to take 88% of the total administrative villages. In some provinces and cities, the integrated management to towns and villages has been conducted and has gained marked effect.

Under this new situation, we should notice that there is some new challenge to the construction of the rural medical preventive network for health care in three-level. Just like the problems mentioned above, the running situation of the township commune hospitals was very worrisome. Some hospitals were cast off as a burden to society. In some areas the rural medical preventive health networks were destroyedin three-level and some village clinics has changed into individual medical clinics and become a profitable organization to lower its function. At first, according to the feature of the rural health requirement we should reorganize basic health organizations. It is a way to carry out integrated management in towns and villages, but it needs paying attention to eliminate the fear for their old-aged and medical insurances after village doctors were reorganized into the township commune hospitals. It is really done as an integrated whole. Health organizations with overlapping functions should be cancelled or combined. Secondly, the government should bear more responsibility for rural health to further increase input in order to develop the rural health undertakings and social economy in coordination. Thirdly, favorable policies should be formulated to attract outstanding medical personnel to work in the countryside. Even more, training for village doctors should be strengthened, the medical services in rural communities should be provided, strictly supervised to prevent practicing medicine without license in order to ensure all farmers can enjoy safety and reliable basic medical services.

(2) Completing the rural medical insurance system and blazing new trails in the rural medical insurance system

The cooperative medical service is the medical insurance system, which was created by the rural masses and suited to the countryside of China. The government has paid close attention to this service and supported it for many years. The systems were well received by farmers and important action to ensure that farmers could get basic medical services, and the prevention and health care tasks were fulfilled to prevent farmers becoming poor from diseases. But the system has taken an unexpected turn because of differences of understanding as there is no relative policy and measurement. The system became unpopular again during the transformation of the rural economic system. Although there was something to return, it only took 10% of total administrative villages conducting the system. In the countryside, seeing a doctor with trouble was a heavy medical burden. Establishing the rural medical insurance system with the special characteristics of China is the requirement of realizing that everybody enjoys health care. Even more it is a requirement to develop production, to free from poverty and returning from disease. The average net income of farmers increased 2.2 times from 1990 to 1999. But at the same time, the average outpatient and hospitalized expense for each person increased each time by 6.2 times and 5.1 times according to the statistics from the medical department. With this large increase for the medical expenses, it became a heavy financial burden for farmers to see a doctor. The proportion of farmers who do not have money to see a doctor has risen 7% in 1993 from 4% in 1985.

Meanwhile the proportion of farmers who do not have money for hospitalization has risen to 24.5% from 13.4% according to the rural survey. More and more farmers do not have the ability to bear the increasing medical expenses, and this has become the marked contradiction of the rural medical insurance at present. With the influence of an aging population there is an obvious increase in the rate, of which farmers suffer from illness every two weeks, chronic disease and the days having to rest and stay in bed for illness. There were more days having to rest and stay in bed for illness in the countryside than in the city. Some farmers developed poverty from diseases. There is an urgent need for medical insurance at a fairly high level for them to ensure basic medical care.

Some scholars advanced several principles to establish a new-style system for medical insurance in the countryside. It is that the basic system for rural medical insurance should be established on the experience and basis of reforming basic medical insurance for urban employees. There are several principles as follows:

Adhere to the principles supported by the state: We should establish a system in which the state and farmers share a common input and risk, establish the medical insurance that accounts for rural family, drawing on the experience of urban employees in order to save money for the rural family to raise capabilities against disease and risk. Meanwhile, emphasis must be placed on the system of multiple inputs in order to guide contributions coming from the community's economy, from enterprise and the charitable institution to replenish funds for rural medical insurance.

Adhere to the principle of measures to suit local conditions: With a vast territory in China, there are big differences on the local economy and social development level. The multi-style, multi-level system for medical insurance, especially for the cooperative medical insurance system should be allowed to positively seek local conditions and rural features.

Adhere to the principle of socialization: This should be on the basis of county range (not in village and small town range) to urge the rural family to join in through the legislation of the state (not only of their own free will).

Adhere to the principle of insurance against heavy diseases: The main threat of disease for farmers is the heavy diseases. It is impossible for farmers to bear the risk of heavy diseases and a system of insurance covering basic heavy diseases should be established for farmers. The limited capital should be used in the most necessary need to improve the heath level of farmers through completing the system of the rural medical insurance and creating new and improved systems.

Adhere to the principle of classified implementation: The economy of China was not developed in balance. A classified system of medical insurance should be implemented according to the different economic conditions.

(3) Developing rural primary health care

It is one of the basic experiences in our country to develop primary health care. It is the strategic goal advanced by the WHO that everybody enjoys health care in 2000. The government of China has made a promise to do this. At that time, overall primary health care was implemented in different areas, stage and level to realize the goal that everybody enjoys health care in 2000. From then on, the rural primary health care in our country became the leading work in the countryside and will lead to the rural health work developing in depth.

In order to develop rural health undertakings, the health viewpoint on general society should be set up at first. The most essential work is to settle the problems of sanitary drinking water, safety control of pesticide, and health education about chronic diseases in accordance with major social health problems existing in the countryside. Second, the system should be set up to develop the rural primary health care in coordination with the social economy. The system should be stipulated by the law for strengthening the rural primary health care through establishing the system of inspiration on the administrative management. Third, primary health work should be organically combined with the health services in communities to form a situation which closely combines improving surrounding conditions with the education of medical treatment, prevention, health care and health recovery. Fourth, the rural environmental monitor should be strengthened and should be strictly controlled for the small enterprise in three aspects to stop any pollution enterprises and enterprises with drain pollutant above standard being transferred to the countryside.

Case Example

The Photochemical Smoke Incident in Los Angeles

This happened in Los Angeles, USA at the beginning of the 1940s. It mainly concerns the poisonous fog formed by exhaust gas from vehicles under action of sunlight, and does harm to people's health. Los Angeles is a coastal city with hills behind and the sea in front and scenic beauty. The airplane and military industry have been developing rapidly since petroleum was exploited in 1936. Los Angeles has become an important harbor in the western coast of the United States of America. At that time there were 2.50 million automobiles in Los Angeles. There was more than one thousand tons of hydrocarbon gas, carbon monoxide and carbon oxide and lead smoke discharged into the air every day. The exhaust gas of motor vehicles had a chemical reaction with other chemical compositions of the air under the action of sunlight and formed a smoke with light blue color containing ozone, carbon oxide, acetaldehyde and other oxidants. This chemical smoke caused a strong irritation. In Los Angeles, the terrain is bag shape surrounded by mountains on three sides and with a border to the sea on one side. There are three hundred days with inversion layer weather per year in a basin that is fifty kilometers long. It is difficult for photochemical smoke to diffuse. The smoke stagnates in the city to poison the air and forms pollution. In Los Angeles, the smoke mainly irritates the eyes, nose and throat leading to ophthalmic diseases, laryngitis and headache of different degrees. It can lead to death with serious irritation. Meanwhile it can cause diseases to poultry, hamper and obstruct the growth of crops and plants, corrode material and building, age rubber products, and the smoke makes the air murky thus reducing visibility and influencing the safety of automobiles and planes which increases a the risk of accidents.

Discussions:

1. What lessons should be drawn from this environmental incident?

2. Which aspects do these social expressions of urban environmental problems show?

Rural Commune Hospital Publicly Auctioned in yicheng, Hubei Province

According to a report on the People's Daily website on April 29, 2002, Beijing

The Rural Commune Hospital was publicly auctioned off in Yicheng, Hubei Province. March of Spring is the right season for the spring plough with the water sounds of the plough and harrow. In Yicheng City, Hubei Province, the reform of the property rights of the rural commune hospitals created great excitement among 0.4 million farmers and 1,200 medical personnel. The successful experience of enterprise reform was introduced into institutional reform. Sixteen rural commune hospitals throughout the city, which were publicly owned rural commune hospitals have been publicly auctioned in Yicheng City to transfer the office to be privately operated. Almost everyone said that the people of Yicheng were eating crab. Most commune hospitals of Yicheng were set up on the basis of the combined clinic at the beginning of the founding of the People's Republic of China. There are sixteen rural commune hospitals in the city in which 580 staff should be provided according to their authorized size. But there were in fact 1,282 staff as a result of a policy that more personnel must be accepted each year thus continuously increasing the numbers. There is 23.71 million RMB of total assets with 28.11 million RMB of liabilities. All rural commune hospitals of the city were unprofitable in 2001. The individual income of staff was low. The per capita wage monthly was about 240 RMB. In some rural commune hospitals with low profits, the staff received the lowest living expenses per capita, about 120 RMB. The system of input was blocked. In recent years, the farmer's income increased slowly. Lightening the burden on farmers led to general financial difficulties for villages and towns. There was no ability to invest in the commune hospitals at all. There was only 296,000 RMB of financial allocation in the hands of the rural commune hospitals, which was decreased to 900,000 yuan RMB in the year 2000. At the same time, reform of medical systems caused the traditional system of supporting hospitals by selling medicine was difficult to maintain. The municipal leaders were inspired by the success achieved in reforming the property rights system of industrial enterprises and had the idea of reforming the rural commune hospitals. The national conference document about health work provided the basis for this idea. We should establish the management system of medical institute with clear rights, responsibility and vitality through creating systems, and each medical institute must become a legal entity, which is managed, developed and controlled independently. In order to encourage competition between the medical institutes of profitability and non-profitability and to develop the privately owned medical institutes, Yicheng municipality convened a mobilization meeting on reforming the property rights system of the rural commune hospitals to begin the reforming process, on January 21. Yicheng municipality had a clear understanding of the reform required to introduce the competition system and quickly made the decision to go to auction. After that the municipality determined a guiding thought that one function was reserved (epidemic health care), others were opened (the medical service was pushed to the market). According to the principle of separating prevention from treatment, the function of epidemic care in the original commune hospitals was scrapped. The independent health epidemic care institutes were established in the town (in a residential district office) to carry out the management function on health epidemic, prevention, health care for women and children and basic level health. Reforming property rights and the public auction meant that the original interest structure was completely changed. The people paid close attention to the focal problem on arrangements of staff as a result of the auction. After the rural commune hospitals were sold, they were managed according to the privately owned profitable medical institutes. The status of staff in original commune hospitals ended immediately. Their outlay was separated from government finance. The personal files of staff were kept in the Exchange Center for Qualified Personnel. The former staffs were paid an arrangement allowance of a lump sum and old-age insurance pension, which was not paid previously. The social insurance institute should pay the former retired staff. For some, the old-age insurance pension could not be paid by the former commune hospitals, which lacked the capacity to do so; the social insurance in-

Chapter 12 Urban and Rural Social Medicine

stitute had paid living expenses to them at their discretion according to relevant policy. Personnel who retired with honour were handed over to local government for management. The government is responsible for settling their wages, medical expenses, etc.

It was found that there are more than 50,000 rural commune hospitals in the whole country, and two thirds of them face economic difficulty. Yicheng municipality is famous for enterprise reform which began by introducing the successful experience on enterprise reform into institutions in January this year. Sixteen rural commune hospitals throughout the city were publicly auctioned. This is the first time this has occurred in the whole country. It is very spectacular. (An extract from the Website of the People's Daily)

Discussions:

1. Do you agree that the rural commune hospitals should be auctioned?

2. Is there a contradiction between auctioning the rural commune hospitals and establishing networks of rural medical treatment, prevention and health care? How would you resolve this contradiction?

第十三章 卫生服务研究

第一节 概述

卫生服务研究(health services research)是20世纪80年代以来在我国卫生领域中发展起来的一门新兴学科,成为社会医学与卫生事业管理方面的一个分支学科。卫生服务是卫生部门通过一定的方法与途径向居民提供适宜的医疗、预防、保健、康复等服务的过程。由于世界各国的社会经济发展水平、文化背景、卫生服务体系、医疗保健制度、生活方式等不同,卫生服务所面临的问题也不一样,国内外至今还没有对卫生服务研究形成一个明确、统一的定义。世界卫生组织(WHO)顾问委员会提出,卫生服务研究是系统开发和分析各种影响卫生服务利用的因素,重点研究覆盖面(coverage)和服务可及性(accessibility)、医疗需求、卫生资源和服务利用等因素之间的相互关系,研究这些因素对卫生服务系统的影响。一般认为,卫生服务研究是从卫生服务的供方(provider)、需方(consumer)和第三方(third party,如医疗保险公司)及其相互之间的关系出发,研究卫生服务组织、实施及其影响因素以及与居民健康状况的关系,探索改善卫生服务系统的功能以及提高卫生资源使用效益的途径。卫生服务的研究范畴包括理论研究、发展研究、卫生服务计划、分析和评价以及政策分析,为制定卫生政策提供依据;具体研究内容涵盖卫生服务的计划、组织、管理、实施、控制、评价、服务利用及费用、效益、效果分析等方面。基本程序由卫生服务计划、实施与评价三个互相衔接、循环发展的环节组成。

一、卫生服务研究的目的及意义

在医学模式的转变以及卫生服务日趋社会化和现代化的形势下,单纯依靠生物医学成就、先进的疾病防治技术和方法,并不能保证取得满意的防治效果和提高人群健康水平,还必须相应地调整、改进卫生服务系统的组织结构、功能及工作方式和方法,采用适宜的卫生服务计划、实施与评价管理技术,合理分配与使用卫生资源,并动用社会资源,才能促进生物医学技术与方法充分发挥作用,提高卫生事业的效益和效果。卫生服务研究对象和内容的不断扩展以及研究成果的不断涌现和应用,对改进卫生服务日益发挥着重要作用,是适应医学模式转变和卫生服务社会化的必然趋势。

我国是一个人口众多的发展中国家,卫生资源有限。在社会主义市场经济体制下,如何控制医疗费用上涨速度,如何提高医疗保险覆盖面和承受能力,如何用较少的投入取得更多的健康结果并兼顾卫生服务的效率与公平,提高总体人群的健康水平等,是我们必须研究的问题。卫生服务研究从公平(equity)、效益(efficiency)和效果(effectiveness)3个维度来论述卫生服务应该实现的理想境界。公平是从社会、资源分配、服务供给和健康状况4个方面衡量卫生服务公平程度的基本内涵;效益是指卫生机构通过有效配置资源以较少投入取得较大产出量,使有限卫生资源取得较大经济效益;效果衡量人群接受卫生服务以后对健康状况改善的程度。由于卫生服务研究将卫生资源的投入量直接与提高人群的健康状况相连接,因此研究结果对于提高卫生事业的社会效益与经济效益具有特别重要的意义。当今国际社会在卫生服务研究领域中较为普遍关注的三个问题是:①提高卫生服务的普及程度和居民接受卫生服务的能力,即保证卫生服务利用的社会公平性。近年来卫生服务的公平性已引起越来越多的关注。②控制医药费用,提高卫生服务的社会效益和经济效益。③改进卫生服务质量,提高居民健康水平和服务质量。因此公平、效益和质量成为当前卫生改革的主旋律,也是卫生服务研究寻求回答的永恒主题。

我国大多数地区的疾病谱和死因谱已经发生改变。传染病、寄生虫病和地方病不再是主要死亡威胁,慢性非传染性疾病已经成为威胁生产、生活和生命的最主要疾病。与此相应,医学模式已经从生物医学模式转变为生物-心理-社会医学模式。为了适应医学模式的转变和医学科学技术现代化的要求,积极开展生物医学、行为心理科学和社会医学研究,是控制慢性非传染性疾病,进一步提高人群健康状况的重要措施。卫生服务研究的基本原理、内容和方法适用于生物医学、行为心理学及社会医学范畴,因此,卫生服务研究的兴起是适应医学模式转变的必然趋势。

任何一个国家和地区的卫生资源总是有限的,要使有限的卫生资源产生最佳的卫生服务,得出最佳的社会效益和经济效益,使有限的人力物力发挥充分的作用,是所有国家卫生服务研究努力追求的目标。WHO专家委员会提出卫生服务研究应实现下列目的:

(1) 促进多学科、多部门协作,强调应用社会科学知识;

(2) 改进医疗卫生系统工作,提高卫生事业的效益及效果;

(3) 帮助促进生物医学知识应用于卫生系统领域,使生物医学知识发挥充分的作用;

(4) 广泛采用比较的方法进行调查研究;

(5) 提供制定卫生计划及决策的基本程序和方法;

(6) 从长远观点看,卫生服务研究为实现人人享受卫生保健的目标,加强国家卫生系统的职能,有助于制定卫生政策、策略和措施。

综上所述,进行卫生服务研究的根本目的是为了合理组织卫生事业,以有限的卫生人力、物力、财力、技术和信息等资源尽可能满足广大居民的卫生服务需要,从而保护和提高居民的健康水平,改善社会卫生状况。卫生服务研究从宏观和微观两个方面,广泛采用比较的方法,侧重研究卫生服务需要、卫生资源供给、卫生服务利用三者之间的制约关系,分析人群卫生服务需要量和利用率水平及其影响因素,从而为各级卫生决策部门提供合理配置、有效使用卫生资源,科学组织卫生服务,制定卫生方针、计划、策略、政策等方面提供依据。

二、卫生服务研究的分类

(一)卫生系统研究

系统是由互相作用、互相依存的若干要素所组合而成的,具有特定功能的,并处于一定环境之中的有机集合体。卫生系统研究可以将人群卫生服务需要和提供作为一个系统过程,采用系统分析的基本原理和方法,研究人群卫生服务需要、卫生资源投入及卫生服务利用水平及其联系,综合分析人群卫生服务需要是否得到满足,卫生资源配置是否适度,卫生服务利用程度是否充分等等,从而提出卫生服务的方向和重点、合理分配与使用卫生资源的原则和方法。此外,还可以将卫生服务投入量、服务过程、产出量以及效果作为一个系统来考察,或从卫生服务的组织、结构及其功能等方面进行系统研究。

(二)卫生工作研究

卫生工作研究包括工作计划、组织、指导、实施、监督、激励和评价等方面,可分为工作开发研究和目标评价研究两类。工作开发研究是通过对工作过程进行评价的方法来评价卫生服务计划的进展和工作成效,探讨新技术、新方法的应用和推广。目标评价研究是通过比较实际目标与预期计划目标的接近程度,了解计划目标的执行和完成情况。

(三)医疗预防效果评价

卫生服务研究可以促进生物医学成就应用于卫生领域,如临床试验疗效考核,新技术方法推广应用对居民健康的影响,预防措施效果评价,以及居民在利用这些新技术、新方法方面存在差异的评价等。

(四)行为医学研究

研究行为心理因素对卫生服务的影响,如研究健康者与患者的行为心理特征,医务人员行医行为,医患关系,医护关系,干群关系,个人、家庭、社区和卫生机构之间的协调、利益分配等等。

三、卫生服务研究的内容

当今世界各国的卫生服务研究内容都是根据国情和主要卫生服务问题提出来的。在我国,20世纪80年代以来以市场为导向的经济体制改革,广泛而深刻地改变了我国的社会经济环境,使原来建立在高度集中的计划经济与管理体制之上的卫生服务体系和健康保障制度发生了一系列显著的变化,提出了许多亟待研究的问题和配套改革的任务,同时拓展了我国卫生服务研究的领域。根据WHO专家委员会提出的卫生服务研究的内容,联系我国的具体情况并结合我国20年来的实践经验,我国卫生服务研究的内容包括以下几个方面。

(一)社会因素对卫生系统的影响

社会因素对卫生系统有重要影响,一个国家卫生系统的组织形式取决于历史传统、社会制度、国家的组织结构以及所处的社会经济发展阶段;教育、农业、交通、住房和社会福利等与卫生系统有密切关系;发展卫生人力取决于学校招生规模,建设医院受资金、劳力、材料以及药物供应及其生产能力的制约等;因此卫生部门提供服务的数量和质量,很大程度上受科学技术、医疗保健制度及付费方式的影响。社会各方面关心卫生部门开展治疗、预防工作和卫生服务研究情况,将卫生系统纳入社会系统之内,从宏观上探讨社会系统与卫生系统的关系,探讨卫生系统内部各个部门之间的相互协调,藉以提高卫生事业的社会效益。

(二)评价人群的卫生服务需要

了解人群卫生服务需要(包括认识到的卫生服务需要和未认识到的卫生服务需要)的性质、程度及影响因素是卫生服务研究的重要课题。长期以来,死亡率被认为是衡量医疗需要量的重要指标,而近来人们的注意力逐渐转向患病率指标,它有利于更加准确地界定人群的卫生服务需要量。对疾病进行定量研究的基础上提出卫生服务需要量,需要通过专门调查才能实现。有代表性的抽样调查是卫生服务研究的一种常用方法,通过抽样调查询问一定时期内疾病发生的频率及有关因素,如年龄、性别、文化、职业、经济状况、医疗保健制度、个人行为和生活方式(如吸烟、饮酒)、家庭卫生设施及居住面积等与患病率的关系,为资源配置和改善卫生服务指明方向和重点。

(三)合理分配和使用卫生资源

卫生计划的基本任务是密切联系人群的卫生服务需要,合理分配和使用卫生资源。卫生资源主要有卫生人力、财力、物力(机构、装备、供应)以及技术和信息等。

1. 卫生人力。在整个卫生资源中,人力资源是最宝贵的资源,需要长期培养才能使用,而且人力的计划、训练和管理要比其他资源的管理复杂得多。卫生人力的数量及分布是世界范围内人力发展研究中最受关注的问题。一个国家和地区内卫生人力的数量和分布是制定卫生计划的基础,卫生人力和人口数之比是研究地区人力分布最基本的指标。怎样培养足够数量和合格人员以满足日益发展的需要,怎样合理分配和使用卫生人员,使有限的人力最大限度地发挥作用,这是研究卫生人力中应该解决的问题。

2. 卫生经费。卫生经费研究包括研究卫生经费的来源与卫生筹资方式,卫生投入的类别与构成比例,卫生总费用与人均卫生费用,卫生费用的增长与控制等。

3. 卫生机构。制定卫生计划,必须研究卫生机构的合理设置,研究疾病预防和其他各种医疗设施的配置等。一个国家或地区内,每千人口病床数是衡量卫生资源的重要指标,医院的性质是首先要研究的问题,公立、私立、企业、慈善性质的医疗机构是4种主要的形式,医院的数量及分布是值得重视的问题。卫生服务研究可以从纵向和横向两方面研究卫生机构在系统内的变化。纵向研究主要研究各级卫生机构的分工及联系,如三级医疗卫生工作网。横向研究侧重各类不同性质医疗机构之间的分工和协调,如医院、门诊部、卫生防疫站、妇幼保健所、专业防治站所等;一个机构内部各科室之间分工及协调,如内科、外科、妇产科、儿科以及与各辅助科室之间分工和协调。

4. 装备和供应。在缺乏总体计划的情况下,购置大型现代化仪器设备往往会造成重复和浪费。由于盲目购置大型仪器而缺乏操作和维修人才,或因缺乏配套条件而造成仪器不能正常工作,或虽能工作但工作量严重不足的例子比比皆是。为了避免浪费,确保大型装备充分利用,应该制定大型仪器(如CT和核磁共振等)技术装备计划。药品来源与分配是一个值得重视的问题,卫生服务研究可以对一个国家或地区内使用技术装备、药品使用是否适宜、合理等作出评价。

5. 知识与技术。世界各国通过书籍和杂志传播医药卫生知识,但是在出版、分配和销售过程中存在不少薄弱环节。研究知识传播过程中的缺陷,有利于推广新的知识和技术,提高人群的健康知识水平和自我保健能力。

(四)卫生系统的组织结构与功能

一个国家或地区卫生系统的组织结构与功能是历史演变形式的产物。以往根据具体任务建立的组织结构与功能,并不一定与新时期的总计划和总任务相适应,需要根据新的社会经济环境和新的任务进行改革。如何审时度势、因地制宜地建立健全卫生服务体系和网络,提出协调的方法和手段,以及在提供卫生服务的内容、性质、范围及层次方面,有大量值得研究的课题。比如,第一级、第二级、第三级卫生保健之间的分工与联系;全科与专科医疗之间,门诊与住院之间,医疗与预防服务之间,各级不同性质的卫生组织或机构之间的协调发展等等。理顺卫生系统内部、外部这些纵向和横向的关系,有助于提高卫生服务系统的工作效率。

(五)卫生系统的经济分析

分析卫生系统的经济活动是制定卫生计划的基础。对卫生系统的经费进行定量研究关系到卫生服务的全局,因为经费是开展卫生服务活动的必要条件。任何一个社会,卫生经费与其他部门之间必然产生竞争,因此,卫生计划部门必须详细了解其他部门的经费来源,了解卫生部门各种经费来源的数量、分配、使用和组成,这是卫生计划制定者、决策者不可缺少的基础信息和数据。

(六)卫生服务效果评价

人群健康状况是评价卫生服务效果的最终指标。对卫生系统工作的成绩,特别是对健康状况的变化进行评价是特别困难的任务,因为卫生服务的结果往往与社会及自然因素综合在一起发生作用。当然这并不意味着工作结果的评价是高不可攀的,特别是对单项卫生工作如白喉预防接种及计划生育效果的评价,只要考核白喉发病率和死亡率以及计划生育接受率的变化即可得出结论。当工作范围扩大时,如对急诊室、初级卫生保健及妇幼卫生工作进行结果评价,其情况要复杂多了,往往需要通过建立综合评价指标体系,才能作出科学评价。

四、卫生服务研究的方法

(一)描述性研究

描述性研究(descriptive study)阐明卫生服务或健康状况的社会人群分布,了解分布的趋势及其规律,可以为制定适宜的卫生对策提供科学依据。描述性研究可从下列3个方面进行。

1. 从时间上考察卫生服务的发展速度、变动规律,预测卫生事业发展的趋势。如通过系统回顾分析建国以来卫生服务的变化,总结卫生事业的成绩和发展速度,根据WHO提出的"人人享有卫生保健"的战略目标,提出应进一步达到的目标、指标和采取的措施。

2. 比较不同国家或地区卫生服务状况及水平。通过国家间、省市及地区间卫生服务的比较,了解不同国家或地区间卫生服务的状况、水平和差距,指出差距和发展方向。

3. 按卫生部门不同专业系统分门别类地研究卫生事业的特点,评价卫生服务的效果及效益。例如1981年上海县所进行的卫生服务描述性研究,分析了上海县的医疗保健制度、乡村医生、健康状况、结核病和血吸虫病防治、计划免疫和传染病控制、妇幼保健和计划生育、环境和营养、儿童生长发育、卫生费用和卫生服务利用等,并将这些结果纳入一个系统内加以考察分析,从而对全县卫生服务的结果、影响、效果及效益有一个清楚的认识。对这些专业的描述性研究,一般是利用现成的登记报告资料,有时为了弥补常规收集资料的局限性,或验证常规登记报告资料的可靠性,或收集用常规方法不能提供的重要信息,需要采用家庭卫生服务询问抽样调查的方法,收集有关人群健康状况、医疗需要量、卫生资源及卫生服务利用资料,这样的研究方法称之为横断面研究。这类调查多属回顾性调查的范畴。

(二)分析性研究

研究影响卫生服务的因素称为分析性研究(analytical study)。如全国城乡卫生服务抽样调查研究慢性病患病率及两周患病率与年龄、性别、居住地区、职业、文化、医疗保健制度、人均收入、人均住房面积、饮水类型、卫生设施和吸烟行为等因素的关系,可采用单因素或多因素的分析方法,阐明哪些因素对疾病有重要作用。流行病学研究中的队列研究和病例对照研究,同样可以在卫生服务分析性研究中得到广泛应用。

(三)实验性研究

以社区人群作为实验观察的对象,考察卫生服务和防治对策的效果,进行干预性的实验研究是广泛应用的一种实证方法。缺氟地区在饮水中加氟预防龋齿、缺碘地区在食盐中加碘预防地方性甲状腺肿等,都是干预研究取得成效的典范。对于已经明确的诱发疾病的危险因素,采取社会措施加以控制,可以明显减少疾病的发生。例如美国1968~1978年间,全社会广泛采取改变饮食结构和饮食习惯、戒烟和重视参加体育活动等3项有效的干预措施,使心血管疾病死亡率下降20%多。

(四)理论研究

应用数学模型从理论上阐明卫生服务与有关因素的联系及规律性。数学模型是一种定量研究方法,主要阐述各变量间的函数关系。结合当地过去和现在的具体情况,通过建立数学模型预测将来,或按照既定的目标,通过建立数学模型预测本地区实现计划目标的进程或控制指标。如建立人口预测模型,病床、卫生人员需要量模型及疾病分布概率模型等。

(五)系统分析法

系统分析是一种运用系统思想分析问题和解决问题的方法。运用系统分析技术,综合分析卫生系统内部各要素之间的互相联系,提供若干个备选方案,进行可行性评价和最优化选择。由于卫生服务系统是一个复杂的系统,特别是在卫生计划和评价研究方面,系统分析方法已得到广泛应用。

(六)综合评价法

1976年WHO提出了卫生服务综合评价模式,即研究人群健康状况、医疗需要量、卫生资源、卫生服务利用的指标体系及其相互关系,评价卫生服务的效果和效益,为合理配置卫生资源提供依据。2000年WHO提出了综合评价卫生系统绩效的模式,运用健康水平、健康在人群中的分布、反应性水平、反应性在人群中的分布以及筹资的公平性5个指数并通过加权计算来综合评价191个成员国的卫生系统绩效。

(七)投入产出分析法

投入产出法主要用来研究卫生服务投入量(卫生资源)和产出量(卫生服务利用量)之间的关系,以评价卫生资源配置或使用的效益和效果。由此而衍生的成本效益分析(cost benefit analysis)、成本效果分析(cost effectiveness analysis)和成本效用分析(cost utility analysis)等方法已经在卫生服务研究领域内得到广泛应用。

需要指出的是,上述方法是现代卫生服务研究中常用的方法,是社会医学、流行病学、卫生管理学和人口学领域内常用的基本方法,均可根据实际情况运用于卫生服务研究领域。

五、卫生服务研究的进展

WHO通过对英国、美国、加拿大、荷兰、阿根廷、芬兰、前南斯拉夫等7个国家12个地区1 500万居民近10年的卫生服务抽样调查,于1976年提出了卫生服务综合评价模式。从此以后,许多发达国家都在开展卫生服务研究。20世纪80年代初期,我国开始从国外引进卫生服务研究内容和方法,经过消化吸收,结合我国卫生服务的实际,卫生服务研究已经取得了很大进展,研究结果对推动我国卫生事业现代化管理和科学化决策,发挥了重要作用。1981年中美两国科学家在科技合作项目中对上海县卫生服务进行了描述性研究,系统考察了上海县卫生服务,并将某些有代表性的、综合性的居民健康和社会卫生状况指标与美国华盛顿进行了对比分析。研究结果表明:①上海县居民健康主要指标,如总死亡率、婴儿死亡率、围产期死亡率、主要死因构成及平均期望寿命等,已经接近于发达国家水平;②上海县与美国华盛顿的社会经济状况及卫生资源存在巨大差别,但在居民健康指标方面比较接近,说明上海县卫生服务的宏观效益和效果是明显的;③上海县居民主要健康指标30多年的变动历程,在美国发生同样变化大致经历了60年,说明上海县卫生服务的发展速度非常迅速。上海县卫生服务研究开创了中国卫生服务研究先例,其研究经验以及所采用的快速评估技术与方法,尤其是家庭健康询问调查的方法,具有十分重要的示范作用。我国卫生服务研究的发展主要表现在以下几方面。

(一)上海县卫生服务研究的经验迅速得到推广应用

20世纪80年代中期以来,我国相继在约200个市、县进行过城乡居民卫生服务调查。卫生部医政司在1985年采用整群分层的抽样方法,组织了全国农村卫生服务调查,对9省45个县28万农民进行家庭健康询问调查;1986年医政司组织了城市医疗服务调查,对9省27个市9.66万城市人口进行医疗服务调查。1993年卫生部卫生统计信息中心组织了第一次全国卫生服务总调查,对全国92个县市21.6万城乡居民进行家庭健康询问调查,同时还对城乡三级医疗机构卫生资源和服务利用状况进行抽样调查,从卫生服务供给和需求双方探讨供需平衡的程度以及卫生资源的利用效率等。间隔5年,于1998年组织了第二次全国卫生服务总调查;2003年进行了第三次全国卫生服务总调查,在进行家庭健康询问调查的同时,采取了一些定性调查的方法,对部分关键人群进行了定性调查。

这些调查研究,收集了大量城乡居民健康状况、医疗需要量及卫生服务利用信息,为制定区域卫生规则,推动卫生事业现代化、科学化管理发挥了重要的作用。

(二) 卫生服务研究范围、内容和对象进一步拓展

我国卫生服务研究覆盖面从农村开始逐步向工厂、城乡结合部、流动人口、少数民族地区扩展,研究范围则从医疗服务供给及需求开始逐步扩大到预防、保健领域,如卫生部卫生防疫司组织的"卫生防疫供需及对策研究"、妇幼司在儿童基金会资助下组织的"妇幼卫生服务及经费研究"、中医局组织的"中医需求及服务利用研究"、部队总后卫生部组织的"部队指战员的卫生服务供给及需求调查"等,都是卫生服务研究范围扩大的实例。研究对象首先是对总人口进行卫生服务研究,以后扩大到对特殊人群进行调查,如老人、儿童、妇女、伤残以及产业工人等。调查内容除针对一般医疗需求及供给进行研究外,还针对特殊人群存在的特殊卫生问题进行深入调查研究,如目前针对社会弱势群体的医疗需求、利用及其影响因素、医疗救助等的方面的调查研究。家庭健康询问调查的内容和方法,已经在以往20年中得到广泛应用。

(三) 卫生服务调查研究方法向多样化发展

研究方法从初始阶段的描述性研究向分析性研究、实验性(干预性)研究发展,使获得的结论更具说服力、科学性和有效性,将卫生服务研究推向一个新阶段,主要体现在以下方面:首先是采用家庭询问调查和卫生机构调查相结合的方法,将接受卫生服务的对象和提供卫生服务的机构纳入一个系统加以分析研究,可以了解人群健康需要满足的程度,分析不能满足的原因,提出改善卫生系统功能的对策,提高卫生服务的效益。这是卫生服务研究方法的一个重要发展。其次是将常规登记收集信息的方法与抽样询问调查相结合,形成我国卫生信息系统两条腿并行发展的框架。第三是我国家庭健康询问调查从一次性横断面调查发展为重复性健康询问调查,从单纯的回顾性健康询问调查转向时间序列前瞻性调查等,克服了一次性横断面调查的一些固有缺陷,从而能够动态、连续监测人群中行为危险因素的变化趋势。

第二节 卫生服务需要、需求与利用

通过收集相关资料,研究居民健康状况、卫生服务需要(求)量、利用量和卫生资源配置及其相互之间的联系,分析需要(求)量、利用量的满足程度及其影响因素,是合理组织卫生服务,评价卫生系统工作效率和潜力,解决卫生服务供需矛盾,提高卫生事业社会效益和经济效益的常用的、有效的方法与手段,也是科学制定健康促进规划和卫生资源配置计划不可缺少的内容和重要依据。

一、几个基本概念

1. 健康(health)。随着社会经济发展、科学技术进步、居民生活及文化水平提高,人们对健康和疾病的认识在不断深化和发展。世界卫生组织宪章中对健康所下的定义:健康是指身体、心理和社会适应能力的健全状态,而不仅仅是指没有疾病或身体虚弱。

2. 卫生服务要求(want of health services)。反映居民要求预防保健、增进健康、摆脱疾病、减少致残的主观愿望,不完全是由自身的实际健康状况所决定的。居民的卫生服务要求可以从两方面来体现:一是公众对政府卫生、环保等相关部门和机构的希望、要求和建议等;二是在专门组织的健康问询调查中,收集居民的卫生服务要求。

3. 卫生服务需要(need of health services)。主要取决于居民的自身健康状况,是依据人们的实际健康状况与上述"理想健康状态"之间存在差距而提出的对医疗、预防、保健、康复等服务的客观需要,包括个人觉察到的需要(perceived need)和由医疗卫生专业人员判定的需要,以及个人未认识到的需要。只有当一个人觉察到有卫生服务需要时,才有可能去寻求利用卫生服务。例如,某个人实际存在健康问题或患有疾病但尚未被察觉,就不会有寻求卫生服务的行为发生,这种情况对健康极为不利。发现未觉察到的卫生服务需要最有效的方法是进行人群健康筛检(screening),以确定哪些是已经发现了的需要,哪些是还没有被觉察到的潜在需要(potential need),这无论对于医疗服务还是预防保健工作都有积极的意义。

4. 卫生服务需求(demand of health services)。即从经济和价值观念出发,在一定时期内、一定价格水平上人们愿意而且有能力消费的卫生服务量。可见需求的产生有两个条件:一是人们愿意购买,二是购买者有支付能力。如果只有购买的愿望而没有支付能力,或者有支付能力而无购买愿望,都不能产生有效的需求。比如有人生病,有卫生保健的需要;但因没钱,看不起病而未就医,则无法转化为卫生服务需求;或者有支付能力,但由于健康意识较差而未就医,同样也不构成卫生服务需求。需求一般可分为以下两类:一是由需要转化而来的需求,二是没有需要的需求,通常是由不良的就医和行医两种行为造成的。

5. 卫生服务利用(utilization of health services)。即需求者实际利用卫生服务的数量(有效需求量),是人群卫生服务需要量和卫生资源供给量相互制约的结果,可以直接反映卫生系统为人群健康提供卫生服务的数量和工作效率,间接反映卫生系统通过卫生服务对居民健康状况的影响,但不能直接用于评价卫生服务的效果。

6. 卫生服务需要、需求、利用之间的关系。卫生服务需求是由需要转化而来的,理论上讲,人们的卫生服务需要如果都能转化为需求,需求就有可能通过对卫生服务的实际利用得到满足,但是现实情况并非如此。一方面,由于种种主观和客观原因,并不是人们所有的卫生服务需要都能转化为需求。需要能否转化为需求,除了与居民本身是否觉察到有某种或某些卫生服务需要外,还与其收入水平、社会地位、享有的健康保障制度、交通便利程度、风俗习惯以及卫生机构提供的服务类型和质量等多种因素有关。例如,一个病人由于收入低、支付不起医药费用而看不起病,或者虽有支付能力,但由于交通不便、医疗卫生人员服务态度差、质量差等原因不愿意去看病而得不到所需的服务,需要就难以转化为需求。在我国农村地区,尤其是在一些"老、少、边、穷"地区,大量的卫生服务需要还不能或难以转化为需求。另一方面,由于卫生资源有限、配置不合理,以及存在服务质量差、效率低、资源浪费的现象,无论是由需要转化而来的需求,还是没有需要的需求,都难以得到完全满足。实际满足与否及其满足程度取决于卫生服务的供给量,当供给量大于需求量(供大于求)时,需求将会得到满足;但供大于求又往往会导致卫生资源利用不足,如人员、床位、仪器设备等的闲置,利用效率低下。当供给量小于需求量(供不应求)时,需求不可能得到全部满足,就会出现等待就诊、住院未能得到应有的服务等现象。

二、卫生服务需要

(一)卫生服务需要量的测量与分析

卫生服务需要是居民实际健康状况的客观反映。通常,可以通过对人群健康状况的测量与分析来掌握人群的卫生服务需要,包括需要量的水平、范围和类型等。反映人群健康状况的指标很多,包括疾病指标、死亡及其构成指标、残疾指标、营养与生长发育指标、心理指标、社会指标,以及由这些指标派生出来的一些指标。目前,常用疾病指标和死亡指标来反映人群的卫生服务需要。在死亡指标中,婴儿死亡率、孕产妇死亡率和平均期望寿命是综合反映社会发展水平、居民健康水平及医疗卫生保健水平的敏感指标,因而常用这3项指标反映某个国家或地区居民的卫生服务需要量水平。此外,死因顺位及构成也是反映居民卫生服务需要量的重要指标。

与疾病指标相比,死亡指标比较稳定、可靠,资料也比较容易通过常规登记报告或死因监测系统收集,并且可获得连续性资料。但是,死亡是疾病或损伤对健康的影响达到最严重时的结局,因而用死亡指标反映居民健康问题不太敏感,还需要结合疾病指标进行分析,特别是在了解人群对医疗、预防、护理、康复、健康教育与咨询等卫生服务需要中消耗资源最多的医疗服务需要时,疾病指标就显得更为重要。

反映居民医疗服务需要量和疾病负担的指标主要由疾病的频率(度)和严重程度两类指标组成,通常需通过调查得到,如家庭健康询问抽样调查。

1. 疾病频率(度)指标。卫生服务研究所定义的"患病"是从居民的卫生服务需要角度考虑的,并非严格意义上的"患病",主要依据被调查者的自身感受和经培训的调查员的客观判断综合确定。常用的指标有以下几种。

(1) 两周患病率(two weeks prevalence)＝调查前2周内患病人(次)数/调查人数×100%(或1 000‰)。

我国卫生服务总调查将"患病"的概念定义为:①自觉身体不适,去医疗卫生单位就诊、治疗;②自觉身体不适,未去医疗卫生单位诊治,但采取了自服药物或一些辅助疗法,如推拿、按摩等;③自觉身体不适,未去就诊治疗,也未采取任何自服药物或辅助疗法,但因身体不适休工、休学或卧床1天及以上者。上述3种情况有其一者为"患病"。

(2) 慢性病患病率(chronic illness prevalence)＝前半年内患慢性病人(次)数/调查人数×100%(或1 000‰)。

"慢性病"的概念被定义为:①被调查者在调查的前半年内,经过医务人员明确诊断有慢性病;②半年以前经医生诊断患有慢性病,在调查的前半年内时有发作,并采取了治疗措施,如服药、理疗等。两者有其一者为患"慢性病"。

(3) 健康者占总人口百分比,即每百名调查人口中健康者所占的百分比。健康者是指在调查期间无急慢性疾病、外伤和心理障碍,无因病卧床及正常活动受限制者,无眼病和牙病等。

2. 疾病严重程度指标。

(1) 两周卧床率＝前2周内卧床人(次)数/调查人数×100%(或1 000‰)。

(2) 两周活动受限率＝前2周内活动受限人(次)数/调查人数×100%(或1 000‰)。

(3) 两周休工（学）率＝前 2 周内因病休工（学）人（次）数/调查人数×100%（或 1 000‰）。

(4) 两周患病天数＝前 2 周内患病总天数/调查人数。

类似指标还有失能率、残障率，以及两周卧床天数、休工天数、休学天数等。对于预防保健的需要量，通常可用传染病的发病率来反映。传染病发病率高的地区对预防保健的需要量高，反之则低。传染病发病资料一般可以通过疾病登记卡获得。

3. 卫生服务需要量的分析。表 13-1 列出了我国 1985 年农村、1986 年城市以及 1993 年和 1998 年两次全国性卫生服务抽样调查中的患病指标。与 20 世纪 80 年代中期相比，90 年代我国城市和农村的两周患病率、慢性病患病率、人均年患病天数都有不同程度的增加，而且城市高于农村，反映城乡居民对医疗服务的需要量有所增加，城市居民医疗服务需要量相对较高，可能与人口逐渐老龄化、城市化，经济条件和文化水平改善，居民健康意识增强有关。农村居民人均年休工、休学、卧床天数高于 80 年代中期，而 1998 年城市居民这 3 项指标则低于 80 年代中期。

表 13-1 我国城乡居民医疗服务需要量

指标	1998 年		1993 年		1985 年	1986 年
	农村	城市	农村	城市	农村	城市
两周患病率(%)	13.7	18.7	12.8	17.5	6.9	10.5
慢性病患病率(%)	11.8	27.3	13.1	28.6	8.6	23.6
人均年患病天数	29.3	42.8	25.7	38.9	13.0	25.0
人均年休工天数	9.0	4.0	6.8	4.5	5.4	5.0
人均年休学天数	2.5	1.8	2.1	3.0	1.2	2.0
人均年卧床天数	3.1	2.5	3.2	3.2	2.4	3.0

(二) 卫生服务需要指标的应用

1. 测量目标人群的卫生服务需要量。假设两周内一次性横断面抽样调查的结果对全年有代表性，通过采用两周指标平均值乘 26（以一年 52 周计），就可得出全年每人每年患病、休工（学）及卧床人数或天数，因病伤门诊和住院人次数，以及医药费用等。由于疾病与就诊指标存在明显的季节性变动，用 2 周抽样调查结果来推算居民全年疾病发生的频率、严重程度会存在一定的偏差。如果能够在 1 年内抽样调查若干次或采用连续性抽样调查方法，1 年内由调查员连续进行资料收集，计算出的居民卫生服务需要量和利用量指标，就能更准确地测算全年目标人群卫生服务需要量和利用量的水平及其变动规律。

2. 计算因病造成的间接经济损失。每人每年因病伤休工天数乘以人均产值或利税，再乘以该地区总人口数，可以得出因病休工而引起的间接经济损失量。

3. 为合理配置卫生资源提供依据。根据患病人数可以估算门诊服务需要量，根据因病伤休工及卧床人数可以推测需住院人数，为分析医疗服务需要量提供依据。人群患病率、休工率及卧床率指标不仅可以计算医疗服务需要量，还可以进一步计算病床需要量和医务人员需要量,作为设置病床、配备人员和分配经费的依据。

需要指出的是,现阶段在制定卫生计划时应同时考虑需要和需求,要对不同地区、不同时期、不同领域以及不同类型和层次的卫生服务区别对待,既要保证城乡居民获得基本的卫生保健服务,满足他们的基本需要,以体现社会公平,又要适当地引入市场机制,提高卫生资源的配置效率,兼顾需求。

(三)影响卫生服务需要量的因素

卫生服务需要量是人群健康的客观反映,凡是影响人群健康状况的各种因素,都直接或直接地影响人群医疗服务需要量,主要有下列影响因素。

1. 人口数量、年龄及性别构成。在其他因素不变的情况下,服务人口数越多,卫生服务需要量和利用量越大。儿童及老年人的患病率高,尤其是45岁以后,随年龄增加而患病率增加;由于女性有月经期、孕期、产期、哺乳期和更年期等特殊需要,患病率、就诊率要多于男性。

2. 社会经济因素。在社会生活中,不论是政治制度、经济状况、文化教育水平,还是居住生活条件等,都可能影响居民的健康状况,造成不同的卫生服务需要。几次卫生服务调查结果都显示,经济较发达地区居民的卫生服务利用明显高于西部贫困地区,城市居民的几项主要卫生服务需要量和利用量指标都高于农村居民。

3. 卫生服务质量。提高服务质量可以缩短医疗时间,提高治愈率,进而减少对卫生服务的需要和利用;预防保健是决定卫生服务需要量的重要因素,积极开展预防保健服务的成效在短期内可能不会明显改变人群总的卫生服务需要量,但从长远的观点看,预防保健工作奏效了,疾病减少或消灭了,势必会减少卫生服务需要量和利用量。

4. 行为心理因素。行为心理因素对疾病的发生、发展及转归有明显作用,如吸烟、饮酒、不良的饮食习惯和各种不良的心理刺激等;住院、就诊方面的需要也受这类因素的影响。

5. 气候及地理条件。许多疾病的好发往往具有明显的季节性或地域性。夏、秋季易发消化系统疾病,冬、春季多发呼吸系统疾病和心脑血管疾病;克山病、甲状腺肿、血吸虫病、龋齿等地方病和寄生虫病也只有在特定的气候和地理条件下易于发生,这些现象表明在不同气候和地理条件下,居民的卫生服务需要量也有所不同。

6. 婚姻与家庭。有配偶者对医疗服务的需要少于独身、鳏寡及离婚者;配偶的存在可以减少住院次数或缩短住院时间;有时家庭的护理照料可以代替一部分住院治疗。

三、卫生服务利用

分析卫生服务利用程度,是评价卫生服务的社会效益和经济效益的常用方法。我国卫生服务利用的资料主要来源于常规的卫生工作登记及报表。这类资料一般易于收集、长期积累、系统观察,但由于一个地区的居民常常在不同的地点接受卫生服务,仅仅根据卫生部门登记报告资料不易判断人群利用卫生服务的全貌。对家庭进行抽样询问调查,可以比较全面地了解与掌握人群健康和卫生服务利用的状况。卫生服务利用可分为门诊服务利用、住院服务利用、预防保健服务及康复服务利用等几个方面。

(一)门诊服务利用

掌握居民就诊的水平、流向和特点,分析其影响因素,可以为合理组织门诊服务提供重要依据。居民门诊服务利用的指标主要有两周就诊率、两周就诊人次数或年人均就诊次数(可根据两周就诊人次数推算得到,这是估计门诊需求量的重要指标)、患者就诊率及患者未就诊率(反映就诊状况的负向指标)等,以此反映居民对门诊服务的需求水平和满足程度。

(1) 两周就诊率＝前2周内就诊人(次)数/调查人数×100%(或1 000‰)。

(2) 两周患者就诊率＝前2周内患者就诊人(次)数/2周患者总例数×100%。

(3) 两周患者未就诊率＝前2周内患者未就诊人数/2周患者总例数×100%。

(二) 住院服务利用

反映住院服务利用的指标主要有住院率、住院天数及未住院率,可用于了解居民对住院服务的利用程度,还可以进一步分析住院原因、住院医疗机构、科别、辅助诊断利用、病房陪住率以及需住院而未住院的原因等,从而作为确定医疗卫生机构布局、制定相应的病床发展及卫生人力规划的依据。

(1) 住院率＝调查前1年内住院人(次)数/调查人数×100%(或1 000‰)。

(2) 人均住院天数＝总住院天数/总住院人(次)数。

(3) 未住院率＝需住院而未住院患者数/需住院患者数×100%。

表13-2列出了全国几次城乡卫生服务抽样调查有关居民医疗服务利用量的结果,通过比较可以发现:①20世纪90年代我国城乡居民门诊医疗服务利用量较80年代中期有所增加,农村居民尤为明显。②城市居民两周患者未就诊率高于农村,且呈增高趋势。③农村居民年住院率维持在3.1%左右,城市则略呈下降趋势。农村每千人口年住院天数明显少于城市,且呈下降态势。④无论农村还是城市,90年代调查人群中需住院而未住院的比例均较80年代中期明显增加,城市则呈递增趋势。

表13-2 我国城乡居民医疗服务利用量

指标	1998年		1993年		1985年	1986年
	农村	城市	农村	城市	农村	城市
两周就诊率(%)	16.5	16.2	16.0	19.9	10.1	14.7
两周未就诊率(%)	33.2	49.9	33.7	42.4	22.9	26.6
年住院率(%)	3.1	4.8	3.1	5.0	3.1	5.1
每千人口每年住院天数	391.0	1 091.0	428.0	1 502.0	469.0	688.0
需住院而未住院率(%)	35.5	29.5	40.6	26.2	23.7	16.4

患者未就诊原因中,有相当比例的患者买药采取了自我医疗,其他原因是自感病情轻、经济困难、无时间、交通不便、服务态度差、无有效医疗措施等。未住院原因分析结果表明,城乡居民需住院者由于经济困难而未能住院的比例明显增高,城市已由1993年的40%增加到1998年的63%,农村则由59%上升到65%。

经济状况、医疗保障制度等是影响卫生服务利用的重要因素。

(三) 预防保健服务利用

预防保健服务,包括计划免疫、健康教育、传染病控制、妇幼保健等。与医疗服务相比,测量预防保健服务利用比较复杂、困难。预防服务利用常常发生在现场,资料登记收集有一定困难。有些预防服务利用率低,且又有一定季节性,对少数人群进行一次性横断面调查,常常不易获得满意的结果。采取卫生机构登记报告和家庭询问调查相结合的方法收集资料,可通过比较居民实际接受的服务与按计划目标应提供的服务量进行测量与评价。例如1名产妇应接受8次产前检查,结合某地区孕产妇实际接受的产前检查次数,可以评价这一地区围产期保健工作的质量。

表 13-3 我国城乡居民预防服务利用量

指标	1998 年		1993 年	
	农村	城市	农村	城市
产前检查率(%)	78.6	86.6	60.3	95.6
平均产前检查次数	3.2	6.4	3.9	6.4
住院分娩率(%)	43.9	93.5	8.5	61.7
在家分娩率(%)	55.9	6.5	76.6	10.7
产后访视率(%)	50.2	61.4	48.3	39.6
平均产后访视次数	1.3	1.5	2.9	2.5
婚前检查率(%)	—	—	14.1	49.2
妇女病查治率(%)	—	—	16.4	47.7

家庭健康询问调查中有关预防保健服务的利用,通常询问一定时期内接受服务的种类和数量。如果服务项目是在全年内经常开展的工作,如计划生育、妇女保健、儿童保健、健康教育、家庭访视等,以询问2周(或1个月或半年)的结果来推算全年是可行的。预防接种、妇女病普查和某些传染病防治等只发生在一年中特定的若干月份,这时应询问在一年或几年内接受服务的次数,而不宜询问在某个短时期内接受服务的次数,这一点在调查设计时应引起注意。

第三节 卫生资源

卫生资源是指在一定社会经济条件下,社会对卫生部门提供人力、物力、财力的总称,主要包括人员、经费、装备、设施、知识、技术、信息和药品等。一个国家和地区拥有卫生资源的数量,是衡量这一国家和地区经济实力、文化状况和卫生水平的客观标准。一个国家拥有的卫生资源总是有限的,社会可能提供的卫生资源与实际需要总是存在一定的差距,研究卫生资源的潜力是卫生服务研究的一项基本任务。

一、卫生人力资源

卫生人力资源是卫生资源中最重要且最具活力的一种,是制定与实现国家卫生发展计划的组成部分。卫生人力是指经过专业培训、在卫生系统工作、提供卫生服务的人员,包含已经在卫生服务岗位上工作的人员和正在接受训练的人员。卫生人力资源研究主要研究卫生人员的数量、结构和分布。卫生人力资源的开发则包括人力资源的规划、培训和管理三个方面。

(一)数量

卫生人员的数量可用绝对数和相对数表示。绝对数表示卫生人力实际拥有量。为了表达不同时期、不同地区卫生人力的水平,通常用相对数来表示,如用每千人口医师数或每名医师服务人口数来表示。

(二)结构

人力结构可以反映卫生人力的质量,说明人力资源的合理性。卫生人力作为一个人才群,合理结构应包括三个方面。

1. 年龄结构。年龄是衡量人员工作能力、技能和效率的综合指标。合理的年龄结构有助于发挥不同年龄层次人员的长处,保持卫生人力的延续性和稳定性。

2. 专业结构。不同专业人员提供不同的服务。我国卫生专门人才中,医学专业占70%左右,中医中药专业占15%,药学专业占5%,预防医学专业占4%左右;口腔、儿科、营养、检验、放射卫生、生物医学工程及卫生管理的高级人才严重不足,护理专业人员缺乏。我国医生与护士的比例为1:0.42,而大多数国家医护之比为1:2;我国护士与人口数之比为1:1 750,多数发达国家为1:(140~320)。

3. 职称结构。职称反映一定的技术水平。在一个人群中,只有一种类型人才,即使水平很高,效率也不一定很好。不同职称人员应有合适的比例。我国高、中、初三级卫生技术人员的比例为1:1.7:1,而世界卫生组织在中等发达国家制定的标准为1:3:1。

(三)分布

从卫生人员的地理分布来看,发达国家与发展中国家之间卫生人力不平衡状况严重存在。发达国家每10万人口有1 000名卫生技术人员,而发展中国家只有200名。在一个国家内部,卫生技术人员的地理分布也存在不平衡现象,大多数国家集中在城市,广大农村普遍缺少卫生技术人员。我国农村人口占75%以上,卫生技术人员只占总数的52%。

二、卫生人力规划

卫生人力规划是对未来卫生人力需要量、供应量以及拥有量进行预测,以求卫生人力供求关系的平衡。卫生人力供应不是临时准备就可以得到的,而是长期培养的结果,因此卫生人力规划显得更加重要。

(一)卫生人力的需求

卫生人力需求是从社会和经济发展、人口数量及结构变化、医学模式转变、卫生服务利用率及劳动生产率等多种因素出发,研究卫生部门在目标年间需要的人力规模。主要预测方法有以下几种。

1. 健康需要法。为了保护人群健康,应该接受哪些服务项目,根据服务的数量计算卫生人力需要量。如1名产妇需要接受8次产前检查,则每1 000名产妇中应配有1名产科医师、3名助产士和4名卫生员,才能满足围产期保健的基本需要。

2. 健康需求法。健康需求法是建立在有效需求即卫生服务的实际利用上,是根据过去和现在的实际服务需求量,并考虑到未来一定时期内影响需求量的各种因素,计算出来的服务需求量,再推算出卫生人力需求量。

3. 服务目标法。制定了服务产出量目标,卫生人力需要量即可得出。如已知1名医师1年内能提供5 000人次门诊,则根据门诊总量,即可计算出需要多少名医师。

4. 人口比值法。人口比值法可用于人力需要量预测,方法简单易行,只要掌握了预测人口数及卫生人力与人口的比值,就可计算出目标年度卫生人力需要量。

5. 趋势外推法。这是一种最简单而常用的预测方法。根据卫生人力发展连续性的规律,把过去和现在的情况延伸到将来,按外推的结果进行预测。本法对未来发展的各种因素仍按过去的规律演变,方法粗糙但简单实用。

此外,还有专家评价法、数学模型法等。应该指出:各种卫生人力预测方法都可以得出一定的结果,预测结果取决于选择的方法。不同方法具有不同的假设条件,选用不同的工作量标准。

(二)卫生人力供给

卫生人力供给是卫生服务的基础。卫生人力规划要求卫生人力的需求和供给取得平衡。卫生人力供给包括三个部分:现有卫生人力拥有量、未来卫生人力增加量及流失量。

(三)卫生人力管理

合理管理和使用卫生人力是发展卫生事业的关键。卫生人力管理主要包括:①制定卫生人力管理政策和规范;②调节卫生人力需要或需求;③卫生人力的监督和指导;④卫生人力的激励;⑤卫生人力的使用和评价。

三、卫生费用

研究卫生服务领域内经济活动的特征及规律,对合理分配卫生经费、提高卫生服务的经济效益有重要意义。

卫生费用有广义和狭义两种概念。广义的卫生费用是指一定时期内为保护人群健康直接和间接消耗的社会资源,包括一切人力、物力和财力的消耗,以货币来计算;狭义的卫生费用是指在一定时期内为提供卫生服务直接消耗的经济资源。通常所讲的卫生费用是指狭义的卫生费用,是卫生费用研究的主要对象。

卫生费用研究的内容包括:卫生服务过程中需要多少资金,卫生费用的构成和特点,卫生费用的分配和使用是否公平合理,健康需要、卫生资源和卫生服务利用之间是否平衡,以及费用的来源和去向,影响费用的因素及变动趋势,卫生费用增长的原因等。

(一)卫生费用的来源

在我国,卫生费用来源于国家、集体和个人。如国家预算拨款的卫生事业费;工矿企业从福利基金按工资总额一定比例用于劳保医疗的费用,农村集体公益金中提取的合作医疗费;公费劳保职工支付的门诊挂号费和某些药品费,健康保险和合作医疗者按一定比例由患者支付的医药费,企事业职工家属支付的医药费,自费病人就诊支付的医药费等。

(二)卫生费用分类

卫生费用可分为直接卫生费用和间接卫生费用两类。直接卫生费用是指利用卫生服务而支付的费用,包括病人看病支付的各种服务费、化验费、药费及材料费等;间接卫生费用包括因病误工的工资、车旅费、营养费、照顾病人的误工费等。间接费用不是卫生费用研究的重点,但在进行费用效益分析时,为了全面衡量因病伤造成的社会经济损失,必须全面计算直接费用和间接费用。只有这样,才能对卫生服务的投入与产出作出全面的评价。从卫生服务角度,还可将卫生费用分为医疗服务费、卫生防疫费、妇幼卫生费、医学教育费及科学研究费等。

(三)卫生费用评价指标

1. 卫生费用占国民生产总值百分比。该指标说明卫生费用的数量是否适应当地经济发展水平及人民群众卫生保健需要,以及一个国家或地区在多大程度上提供了必要的资源来保证卫生事业与社会经济协调发展。20世纪90年代以来,发达国家卫生费用占国民生产总值的比例一般在7%以上,个别发达国家,如美国、加拿大和瑞典等超过10%。我国卫生费用总额在逐年增加,但卫生费用占国民生活总值的比例,20世纪90年代以前一直在3%~3.5%之间徘徊,仅相当于发达国家50年代初的水平;进入90年代以后,该比值开始上升,达到4%,1996年为4.21%,1998年为4.68%。从总体趋势看,我国卫生总费用占GDP比重处于上升态势。

2. 人均卫生费用。说明一个国家或地区卫生费用的人均水平,也反映卫生资源在不同地区、不同人群间的分配是否合理。性别、年龄、文化及医疗保健制度等因素对人均卫生费用有重要影响。

3. 对卫生部门的投资比例。反映卫生费用在各级卫生机构中分配是否合理。

4. 门诊和住院费用构成。反映医疗机构内部费用分配和使用特征。小医院药费所占比重较大;大医院诊治病人病情复杂,使用辅助手段和昂贵的检查仪器,辅助检查的费用较多。医疗机构级别越高,辅助检查费用比重偏大,药费比重相对较小。

5. 医疗、卫生防疫和妇幼卫生费用的比例。这是卫生部门在费用分配时应该首先考虑的比例。医疗服务提供维护健康和康复服务,是利用最频繁、消耗卫生资源最多的一项服务。我国卫生系统80%左右的人力和费用使用在医疗服务系统。从卫生服务对健康的作用来看,预防保健的重要性不容忽视。确定医疗、预防和保健服务三者之间费用分配的合适比例,不仅要考虑人群需要、服务利用,还要结合社会经济发展及文化传统等因素综合考虑。

(四)卫生费用增长原因分析

卫生费用增长不仅是我国也是其他国家存在的普遍现象,而且出现的不合理增长趋势越来越明显。引起卫生费用增长的原因有以下几方面。

1. 人口老龄化。我国人口面临迅速老龄化的局面,60岁以上的老年人口增长速度很快,2000年我国已成为老年型国家。老年人群是健康方面的脆弱人群,我国1998年国家卫生服务调查资料显示,60岁以上的老年人患病率、就诊率及住院率相对较高,卫生保健需要也较高。该年龄段人口患慢性非传染性疾病的人数多,这些疾病病程长、费用高,加剧了卫生费用的上涨。

2. 物价上涨、通货膨胀。各国的研究均证实了通货膨胀对卫生费用的影响。由于国家通货膨胀因素的影响,物价普遍上涨,导致了能源、运输材料及其他卫生用品价格的上扬,加速了卫生费用的上升。

3. 人口增长。由于人口绝对数的增加,即使在人均费用不变的情况下,卫生总费用也会随之而上升。

4. 高新技术的应用。随着科学技术的进步与发展,卫生领域中新设备、新药物不断增加,许多以前被认为不可治愈的疾病通过采用高新技术和创新药物而得以治愈,从而卫生费用也上升很快。

5. 疾病谱的明显变化。社会经济的发展,使得目前慢性非传染性疾病占主导地位,且发病率不断上升,如心脑血管疾病、糖尿病、恶性肿瘤等,这些疾病一般具有病程长、难治愈、治疗费用高的特点,这些疾病的日益增加导致卫生费用的上升。

6. 卫生保健需求和健康意识的提高。随着国民经济的增长及收入的提高,人们的保健意识也不断增强,对卫生服务消费观念也发生了改变,对卫生服务呈现多层次的需求,对提供的卫生服务质量要求也有所提高。

7. 支付机制的不完善。由于卫生服务提供本身所具有的特殊性,加上支付制度的不完善,使得供方诱导需求行为发生,导致病人住院天数的延长和就诊次数的增加等。

以上影响卫生费用上涨的因素中,有些是相对可控制的,如费用支付机制,而另外一些是相对不可控,如人口的老龄化和疾病谱的改变等;卫生费用上升的趋势是客观存在的,关键是如何抑制费用的不合理上升部分,而又不损害其合理增长的成分。

第四节 卫生服务的综合评价

一、卫生服务评价及综合评价的概念和意义

卫生服务评价是评价研究的一个分支,也是卫生服务研究的一部分。卫生服务评价就是对卫生资源结构、卫生服务过程和卫生服务的结果进行评价。进行卫生服务评价工作的目的是了解卫生服务的社会需要和需求,探讨影响居民健康和寻求卫生服务的障碍因素,使人们更好地理解卫生问题,更有效地配置与使用现有的卫生资源,更合理地组织卫生保健服务,加强实施过程的监控和目标管理,提高卫生服务的效率、效益与效果,阐明卫生服务工作的进展和成效,改进与完善各项卫生服务计划,调整卫生政策以适应复杂和多变的形势。总之,评价的主要目的在于提供计划、管理及决策的合理依据,从而为人群提供效率更高、效果更好、公正平等的卫生服务,改善社会卫生状况和提高人群健康水平。评价工作内容主要包括以下六个方面:适宜程度、足够程度、进度、效率、效果与影响。

综合评价是将反映评价对象特征的多项指标进行系统加工、有机汇集,从整体上认识评价对象的优劣;或将多个单项评价指标组合成一个包含多个成分的综合指标,藉以反映评价对象的全貌。卫生服务综合评价是指围绕特定的评价目标、评价对象和评价阶段,对卫生服务的进展、成效和价值进行评判估量的过程。卫生服务的对象是社会人群、社会卫生状况和人群健康水平得到改善与提高的程度,是评价卫生服务社会效益和经济效益的最终尺度。而社会效益和经济效益的大小,不仅受到卫生资源的投入、提供服务数量和质量的高低等因素的制约,还受到社会、经济、文化、自然条件等因素直接或间接的影响。处于不同的社会经济发展阶段,人们对卫生服务的需求不同,卫生资源投入和服务水平也存

在差异,因而,对一项涉及面极广的卫生服务项目进行系统评价时,需审时度势、因地制宜地根据国情、地情,或项目本身关于卫生服务的发展计划、目标以及评价工作所处的阶段,运用多学科的适宜技术与方法,对其进行多方位、多层次、多环节、多因素的综合评价,即从卫生服务的社会需要、卫生资源投入、提供的服务量及其效率、产生的社会效益和经济效益等方面作出评价,才能比较全面地反映卫生服务的成效及其影响。

二、卫生服务综合评价的范围与内容

随着卫生事业管理的发展,20世纪70年代以来,卫生服务评价在国内外日益受到重视,并开展了这方面的研究与应用。理念上,卫生服务综合评价是多方面的,可以从不同的角度着眼,既可应用于对一个国家或地区总的卫生发展计划(或项目)、实施及结果的宏观评价,也可应用于对某个乡镇实施农村合作医疗的运作机制的微观评价;既可以是定量评价,也可以是定性评价,但应尽可能采用定量评价或定量与定性相结合的评价方法,以增强评价结果的说服力。由于评价性质、目的、角度、层次、侧重点等方面的不同,国内外至今尚未对卫生服务综合评价的范围、内容和指标体系形成广泛的共识。但是,对于一项关于卫生服务的综合评价工作来说,若不与有关反映居民健康的结果指标相联系,其局限性也是显而易见的。

派克(Parker)根据系统分析的观点,构筑了卫生服务的系统模式,并从系统的每一个要素的特征以及各个要素间的相互关系出发,提出可从人群卫生服务需要量、资源投入量、服务产出量、工作过程、结果、效益、效果等7个方面进行评价。劳埃姆(Roemer)根据卫生服务的内容,建议从8个方面进行评价:①项目目标评价;②医疗服务需要量评价;③卫生服务利用接受能力评价;④卫生资源评价;⑤工作活动和态度评价;⑥工作过程评价;⑦结果与效果评价;⑧费用与效益评价。萨盖持(Sackett)根据卫生服务研究的对象,在《预防医学与公共卫生》一书中,提出卫生服务评价应围绕卫生服务是否有效,公众能否利用到有效的卫生服务,提供服务的数量和质量是否充分、可靠,费用是否低廉等4个方面进行评价。

【案例】

卫生服务

卫生服务利用应以适度为佳,过度利用则造成资源浪费、医药费用上涨,利用不足又使人群医疗卫生服务需要(求)量得不到满足。卫生服务研究的目的不仅要了解居民利用卫生服务的数量和质量,还要研究卫生服务需要、卫生资源和卫生服务利用三者之间的关系,分析"供求矛盾"的现况及其变动趋势,以此作为宏观调控、配置卫生资源的决策依据。1976年世界卫生组织根据对美国、加拿大、阿根廷、英国、荷兰、芬兰、南斯拉夫等7国12个地区1 500万居民近10年的卫生服务抽样调查结果,进行了卫生服务综合评价,并提出了综合评价模式(见表13-4)。这种综合评价模式的基本思路是将人群健康需要、卫生服务利用和卫生资源3个方面有机联系起来,以人群健康需要量、卫生服务利用量及资源投入量3类指标的平均数作为划分高低的标准,组成8类组合,以此对一个国家或地区的卫生服务状况进行综合评价,为制定卫生服务发展规划、合理配置卫生资源提供参考依据。

表 13-4 卫生服务综合评价模式

卫生服务利用	高需要		低需要	
	高资源	低资源	高资源	低资源
高	A 型(平衡型) 资源分配适宜	B 型 资源利用率	E 型 过度利用	F 型 资源利用率高
低	C 型 资源利用率低	D 型 资源投入低	G 型 资源投入过度	H 型(平衡型) 资源分配适宜

A 型:资源充足,利用良好,人群卫生服务需要量大,三者之间保持平衡。

B 型:人群卫生服务需求量大,卫生资源不足,卫生服务利用率高,低资源与高需要不相适应。由于资源利用紧张,通过提高利用率保持平衡,但不能持久,应向 A 型转化。

C 型:人群卫生服务需要量大,卫生资源充分,卫生服务利用率低,需研究卫生服务利用的障碍因素,提高卫生服务的效益。

D 型:资源投入不足、利用率低,不能充分满足人群卫生服务需要量。应该增加投资、提高服务利用率,以适应人群卫生服务需要。

E 型:资源充分,人群卫生服务需要低,卫生服务利用充分。由于资源充分,个别人群过度利用卫生服务,浪费卫生资源。

F 型:低资源投入,高服务利用,是服务效益良好的标志,但是低资源与人群的低卫生服务需要相适应。

G 型:人群卫生服务需要量低,资源充分,卫生服务利用低,卫生资源投入过度、应向 H 型转化。

H 型:人群卫生服务需要量低,资源不足,服务利用率低,三者在低水平状态下保持平衡。

思考 1. 卫生服务研究的主要研究方法与内容有哪些?

思考 2. 试述卫生服务需要、需求、利用的含义及其内在联系。

思考 3. 表达卫生服务需要和利用的指标有哪些?

思考 4. 简要描述卫生服务综合评价模式。

Chapter 13　Health Services Research

Section 1　Summary

　　The health services research has been a booming discipline of the 20th century since its development in 1980 in the health field of China and has become an important discipline of the social medicine and health management. The health services are the set of the processes that the health department provides, such as medical, preventive, health care, rehabilitation by adopting some methods and approaches. The health services are faced with different problems due to the different levels of social and economic development, culture background, health services system, medical security system, lifestyle and many other factors. So in different countries, the definition of health service research is ambiguous. The consultant committee of WHO (World Health Organization) put forward that the health services research systematically explore and analyze all kinds of factors that affect the health service utilization, put emphases to study correlation between the coverage, health accessibility, medical demand, health resource and the impact of these factors on the health system. Commonly, we think that the health service research studies the health services organization, implementation as well as the factors affected and the relationship between them and the inhabitants' health status, explores the approach of improving the function of health system and increasing the use benefits of the health resource from the health services provider, to the consumer, and to third party (such as the medical insurance agent) and the correlation between them. The category of health services research includes theory study, development study, health service plan, analysis evaluation and policy analysis, offers the warrants for formulating health policy. The embodied research contents cover the health services plan, organization, management, implementation, control, evaluation, services utilization and expenditure, benefit, effect analysis, etc. The basic procedure is composed of the three loops: planning, implementation and evaluation that link up each other forming a cycle.

1. The objective and significance of health services research

　　Under the circumstances of medical model transformation, the socialization and modernization of heath services, only to depend on the biomedical achievements, advanced disease treatment and preventive technology can't ensure that it can acquire the satisfactory prevention and cure effect and improve the health level of population. For the purpose of taking sufficient advantage of biomedical technology and method, and to enhance the benefit and effect of health service use, the following steps must be taken: adjustment and improvement of the organization structure, function, work style and approach of health system to adopt the plans corresponding to health service plan, managing the techniques of implementation and evaluation, to allot and use the health resource reasonably and put the social resource to use. The extension of object and content of health services research constantly, the teeming and application of these research outcomes play an important role in ameliorating health services, which is an inevitable trend for adapting the medical model transformation and socialization of health services.

China is a developing country holding large number of people and the health resources are limited. In the market economy system of socialism, we must study the following issues: the ways to control the speed of medical expenditure, the ways to increase the coverage of the medical insurance and enhance the enduring capacity, the ways to use the less input to acquire more health output, at the same time, to give attention to the efficiency and equity of health services, and improving the health level of the whole population, etc. The ideal scenario in health services research may be achieved through the following three dimensions: equity, efficiency, effectiveness. Equity measures the basic connotation of the health service degree according the following four aspects: society, collected resources, services provided and health status. Efficiency implies the use of the less input to achieve more output by effectively allocating resources and making the limited health resources to produce more economic benefit. Effectiveness measures the ameliorative extent of the population health after they accept the health services. Because the health services research is directly related to the input of health resources for improving the population health status, the research result plays an important role in improving the social benefit and economic benefit of health cause. Nowadays, we should pay more attention to three problems in the health services research: ①To enhance all the pervading extents of health services and to cap the inhabitants to accept the health services, namely to ensure the social equity of the health services utilization, lately, the equity if health services have achieved more and more attention. ②To control medical expenditure, enhance the social benefit and economic benefit of health cause. ③To improve the health services quality and enhance the public health status and service quality. Thus, the equity, efficiency and quality have become the main theme for health reform currently and also the permanent theme for which the health services researches seek.

The disease spectrum and cause of death have changed in most of the regions in our country. The communicable diseases, parasitic diseases and endemic diseases have no longer been the leading death threats, and the chronic and non-communicable diseases have become the most leading disease to threaten people's production, living and life.

Corresponding to these situations, the medical model has transformed from biomedical model to the bio-psycho-social medical model. To adapt to the transformation of the medical model and requirement of the modernization of medical science and technology, to develop biomedicine actively, behavioral and psychological science and social medicine research are the important measure to control chronic non-communicable disease, and to constantly increase the population health status. The basic principle, contents and methods of health services research adapt the category of biomedicine, behavioral and psychological science and social medicine. Thus, the springing up of health services research is the inevitable trend to adapt to the transformation of medical model.

The health resources of any country or region are always definite, namely, to make the limited health services resources produce the optimal health services, and make the limited manpower produce the optimal social and economic benefits, and to use the material resources well. These are the objectives that all countries try hard to pursue. WHO expert committee put forward the following aims and obliged that they should be realized by the health services research: ①To promote the multi-discipline and multi-section coloration, to apply the social science knowledge. ②To improve work of medical system, enhance the benefit and effectiveness of health cause. ③To help to apply the knowledge of biomedicine in the health system, and take full advantage of the biomedicine. ④To adopt the comparative method widely to carry out the survey study. ⑤To provide the basic procedures and means for formulating health plan and making decisions. ⑥From the long term views, health services research helps to realize the objective of health for all, strengthen the function of national health system, formulate the health policy, and take the strategic measures.

According to the above views, the ultimate objective of carrying out health services research is to organize health system reasonably, to use the limited health manpower, material resources, money, technique and information resources, etc. to meet the health services need of vast people and to further protect and improve the health level of inhabitants, and to improve the social health status. From the macro- and micro-aspects, health services research widely adopted the comparative methods to emphasize particularly on studying conditions of relationship between health services need, health resources supply and health services utilization, to analyze quantity of health service need of population, utilization rate and the effect factors, to offer warranty for the all levels health decision-making department to rationally allocate and effectively use the health resources, to organize health services scientifically and formulate health guide line, plan, strategy and policy and other aspects.

2. Sorts of health services research

(1) Health system research

The system is aggregately comprised of the umpteen key elements that react and depend on each other, and hold special function in a certainty setting. Health system research may put the population health need and supply in a systematic process, adopting the basic principle and methods of system analysis to study population health services need, health resources input, health services utilization rate as well as the relationship between them, to comprehensively analyze whether the population health services need is met, the health resources allocation is moderate enough, the health services utilization is sufficient, is undue or shortage and so on, thereby, to put forward the direction and emphasis, the principle and methods to allocate and use health resources rationally. Furthermore, the health system research can put the quantity of health services input, services proceeding, output and effectiveness as a system to review, or conduct the system research from the health organization, structure and function.

(2) Health work research

The health work research includes work plan, organization, guidance, implementation, supervision, inspiration and evaluation, etc. It can categorize the job exploitation research and objective evaluation. Job exploitation researches assess the progress of health services plan and work effect by appraising the work proceeding, exploring application and generalization of the new techniques and methods. The objective evaluation finds out the situation of the plan implementations and achievements by comparing the factual objective with the prospective objective.

(3) The medical and preventive effectiveness assessments

Health services research can help the accomplishment of application of biomedicine in the health field, such as assessing the effect of treatment during the clinical trial, the impact produced on inhabitant's health by the new technology or methods, the assessment of effectiveness of the preventive measure as well as assessing the differences existing when the inhabitants utilize the newly techniques and methods.

(4) Behavioral medical research

To study the effect on the health services brought about by the behavioral and psychological factors, such as the behavioral and psychological character of healthy behaviors and sickness, the physician's practice behavior, the doctor and patient relationship, doctor and nurse relationship, cadre and mass relationship, the collaboration and interest allocated between the individual, family, community and health organization.

3. Contents of health services research

Nowadays, the contents of health services research are brought forward according to the situation and the main health problems faced by every country in the world. Since the 1980s, the market-oriented economy system reform has deeply and widely changed our country's social and economic environment, the diversified health services being created and health insurance system established based on the highly centralized planned economy and management system bringing out a series of remarkable changes. On one hand, this situation brought forward many problems waiting urgently to be studied and to be reformed, while, at the same time, it opened up the field of health services research in our country. Based on the contents of health services research put forward by the WHO expert committee, related to our country's ideographic setting and combination of the practice experience achieved in 20 years, the contents of health services research include the following aspects:

(1) The impact produced by social factors on the health system

The social factors have an important impact on the health system. The health system of a state lies on the history, tradition, social system, state's organization structure as well as the social and economic development stage, the education, agriculture, traffic, housing and social well-being, etc. They all have close relation with health system, development of the health manpower depending on the scale of the school recruiting students. Constructing a hospital is restricted by the capital, work force, material, drug supply and production capacity, etc. The quantity and quality of the health services are provided by the health section depending on the scientific technique, medical care system and payment style. Aspects of society are all concerned for the health section to carry out the treatment, preventive work and health services research, put the health system well-fitted in the social system, explore the relationship between the social system and health system from the macro angle as well as with the mutual coordination between the each department of the interior health system, thus, to enhance the social benefit of health cause.

(2) To estimate the health services need of population

It is an important task to know properly the extent and the affecting factor of health services that the population need (include the cognitive and un-cognitive health services need). For a long time, mortality rate has been considered an important indicator to scale the medical need. Later, the researchers began to put the attention to the illness prevalence, which can be in favor of determining the quantity of health services need more correctly. If we put forward the quantity of health services need based on the quantitative research for the disease, it needs the special survey to make it come true. The representative sampling survey is the method which is often being used in the health services research, by the sampling survey to ask the illness frequency in a definite time and related factor, such as age, sex, culture, occupation, economic status, medical care system, individual behavior and lifestyle (smoking, drinking), the family sanitation facility and dwelling area, etc, then to analyze the correlation between these factors and illness prevalence. This research will help us to point out the bearing and emphases of allocating resources and improving health services.

(3) To allocate and utilize the health resources rationally

The basic task of health plan is to allocate and utilize the health resources based on the health services need of population. The health resources mostly include health manpower, financial, material resources (institution, equipment, supply), technique and information, etc.

1) Health manpower

Manpower resource is the most valuable among the health resources, need to spend long time on training, then can be used. So planning, training and management of the manpower are more complicated than other resources. People put most attention to the quantity and distribution of the health manpower in the manpower development research around the world. The quantity and distribution of a state or region's health manpower is the foundation to formulate the health plan, and the ration of health manpower for the population is the basic indicator to study the regional health manpower distribution. The following problems should be resolved by the health services research: the ways to train enough and eligible personnel to meet the increasing need, the rational ways of the allocation and the use of the health manpower, and the ways to make good use of the limited health manpower.

2) Health expenditure

Health expenditure research includes the source of health expenditure, the health financing mode, the sort and proportion of investments in health, total expenditure on health and total health expenditure per person, health expenditure increasing and controlling, etc.

3) Health institution

If we want to formulate the health planning, we must study the rational setup of health institutions, the allocation of disease prevention and other medical establishments. In a state or a region, the quantity of sickbed per thousand is an important indicator to measure the health resources. The property of hospital is the first problem to be studied. The public, the private, the enterprise and the charity are the dominating form of medical organizations. The quantity and distribution of the hospital should be paid attention to. The health services research can study the changes in the system in the form of the portrait and landscape orientation. The longitudinal research mainly studies the division of the work and relationship of all levels of health organization, and the transverse research emphasizes particularly on studying the division of the work and coordination between different forms of medical organizations, such as the hospital, clinic, epidemic prevention post, etc. as well as the division of work and coordination between all levels of sections in an organization, such as internal medicine, surgery and so on.

4) Equipment and supply

Due to the lack of proper planning, purchase of the large modern apparatus and equipments often leads to the waste. It often happens when the apparatus cannot work because of the lack of the operating and maintenance staff or lack of matching conditions and when the workload is seriously insufficient during the apparatus operation. For the sake of avoiding waste and making full use of the large equipment, we need to formulate plan of large modern apparatus and equipments (such as CT), and the source and distribution of drug should be paid more attention to. Health services research can work out the evaluation about the fitting and rationality of the equipment, as well as the use of drug for a state or a region.

5) Knowledge and technique

All of the states in the world spread the medical and sanitation knowledge by books and journals, but there are still many weaknesses existing in the processes of publishing, distributing and selling. Studying the weakness of the knowledge spreading process can help to generalize the new knowledge and technique, and enhance the health knowledge level and self-caring ability of population.

(4) The organization structure and function of health system

The organization structure and function of health system is the production of the history for a state or a region. The organization structure and function established according to the special task during the different periods can't always adapt to the plan and task of the new phase, and needs to be reformed based on the new social and economic setting and new task. There are many problems worth studying: the ways to set up the health system and network and put forward the coordinating methods and means considering the prevailing situation. Clarifying the longitudinal and transverse division of work and relationship existing in the interior and exterior of health system can help to enhance the efficiency and potential of the health system.

(5) The economy analysis of health system

To analyze the economic activity of health system is the foundation to formulate health plan, and to carry out the quantitative study of the health system expenditure relates to the whole health system, because expenditure is the necessary condition for developing health services. In any society, health section must compete the expenditure with other sections. So, the health planning section must know in detail the expenditure source of other sections, the quantity, distribution, using and composing of all kinds of resources in the health section. It is the necessary basic information and data for the health planning formulator and the decision-making.

(6) Effective evaluation of health services

The health status of population is the final indicator to assess the health services effectiveness. It is a very difficult task to assess the achievement of health system and especially assess the change of health status because the health services are related to social and natural factors creating the impact on health status. Certainly, it is not predictable that the effective evaluation can't be carried out.

4. Research methods of health services

(1) Descriptive study

Descriptive study illustrates the social population distribution of health services or health status, knows the trend and law of its distribution, and puts forward scientific warranty for formulating health plan.

1) To review the tempo and change law of health services from time angle, forecast the trend of health cause development. For example, by reviewing systematically the health services change since 1949, to sum up the achievement and tempo of health cause, to put forward the objective, indicator and measures based on the health for all.

2) To compare the health services status and level of different states or regions: by comparing the health services between states or regions, to know the health services status, level and gap of the different states or regions, to point out the gap and direction of development.

3) To study the health cause character according to different specialty systems and evaluate the effectiveness and benefit of health service: in 1981, the health descriptive study carried out in Shanghai county analyzed the medical care system, village doctor, health status, tuberculosis and schistosome prevention and cure, planning immunity, communicative disease control, family planning, health expenditure, health services utilization and so on. They put the outcome into a system to analyze, based upon these facts, to have a clear understanding about the outcome, impact, effectiveness and benefit of the county health service.

(2) Analytical study

To study the factors affecting the health services includes analytical study. The health services sampling survey in urban and rural areas of the whole country studies the relationship between the two weeks prevalence, chronic illness prevalence and age, sex, dwelling area, occupation, culture, medical insurance system and so on. It can adopt single or multi-factor analysis methods to illustrate which factor plays an important role in the disease occurrence. The cohort study and case-control study of the epidemiology can also be widely applied in the analytical study of health services.

(3) Experiment study

To put the community population as the experiment subjects and to study the effect of the health services and preventive strategy, to carry out the intervention trial study is a demonstration method applied widely. To add the fluoride in the region lacking fluoride to prevent tooth decay, and to add the iodine in the region where there is shortage of iodine to prevent endemic struma are all the paragon that have been achieved by intervention. There are risk factors that have been testified to induce the disease; to adopt social measure to control these factors can reduce the illness prevalence obviously.

(4) Theory study

Application of mathematical model illustrates the relationship between health services and other pertinent factor and law from the theory. The mathematical model is a quantitative method, which mainly expounds the functional relationship between every variable. Combining the past and present situation, construction of the mathematical model can predict the future, or constructed mathematical model forecast the course of the plan objective according to established objective. For example, to construct population forecast model, needed quantity of sickbed and health manpower forecast model and so on.

(5) System analysis

System analysis is the method to analyze problem and resolve problem by adopting system idea. By applying the system analysis technique, we can analyze synthetically the mutual relationship between the interior key factors of the health system, put forward several optional schemes, and carry out the feasibility evaluation and optimizing selection. Because the health services system is a complicated system, especially in the research of health planning and assessing, the system analysis has been applied widely.

(6) Synthetic appraise

WHO put forward the comprehensive evaluation model of health services in 1976, namely to evaluate the health services effectiveness and benefit by studying the indicator system of population health status, medical need quantity, health resources, health services utilization and the mutual relationship between them, to further provide the gist for rationally allocating the health resources. In 2000, WHO put forward the comprehensive evaluation model of health system performance, to adopt the five indicators: the overall level of health, the distribution of health in the population, the overall level of responsiveness, the distribution of responsiveness, the fairness in financial contribution and further calculated by weighing the five indicators to assess the health system performance of 191 WHO member states.

(7) Input and output analysis

Input and output analysis methods mainly study the relationship between input quantity (health resources) and output quantity (health services utilization) and further evaluate the benefit and effectiveness of health resources allocation and utilization. After that, the cost benefit analysis, cost effectiveness analysis and cost utility analysis are derived from it and these methods have been widely applied in the field of health services research.

5. The evolvement of health services research

In 1976, according to the result of sampling survey about health services conducted in the 7 states including UK, USA, Canada, Holland, Argentina, Finland, former Yugoslavia and 12 regions, WHO carried out the comprehensive evaluation of health services among 15 million inhabitants during 10 years and put forward comprehensive evaluation model. Since then, many developed countries started carrying out health services research. At the initial stage in the 1980s, our country began to introduce the contents and methods of health services from overseas, and the health services research has made great progress by the assimilating, absorbing and combining our country's fact. The finding of the study played an important role to drive our country's health system modernized and started to take scientific decision-making. In 1981, the scientists of the China and America cooperated to carry out health services descriptive study in the Shanghai county. They investigated systematically the health services of shanghai county, compared some representative and comprehensive indicators of inhabitants health and social health status with the indicator of Washington, America. The finding of the study indicated that: ① the main inhabitants health indicators of Shanghai county, such as crude mortality, infant mortality rate, perinatal mortality, constitution of main cause of death, life expectancy, all have been close to level of developed country; ② there exists a huge gap between the Shanghai county and Washington in the social and economic status as well as health resources, but the inhabitants health indicator is close. This finding indicated that the macro benefit and effectiveness of health service in Shanghai county were obvious; ③ the changing course of inhabitants main health indicator in Shanghai county is 30 years, while that in America is 60 years. It indicates that the tempo of Shanghai's health services was very speedy. The health services research in Shanghai county inaugurated a leading card of health services research in our country, its study experience and adopted rapid assessment technique and methods especially the methods of family health survey played a demonstrated role. The development course of health services research embodied the following aspects:

(1) The experience of Shanghai county's health services research had been generalized and applied rapidly

Since the metaphase of the 1980s, there have been two hundred cities and counties to carry out inhabitants' health services research. In 1985, Medical Department of Health Ministry adopted the cluster stratified sampling method to organize the health services survey in rural areas of the whole country, carrying out the household health survey in the 9 provinces, and 45 counties, altogether 280 thousand peasants. In 1986, Medical Department of Health Ministry organized the urban medical services survey, carried out in 9 provinces, 27 cities, altogether 96.6 thousand persons. In 1993, the Health Statistics Information Center of Health Ministry organized the first health services overall survey in the whole country, carried out the family health survey in 92 cities and counties, altogether 216 thousand inhabitants, at the same time, carried out the sampling survey of the health resources and health services utilization of the urban and rural third class medical institutions, to explore the balance level of supply and demand, the utilization efficiency of health resources from the respect of health supply and demand. After five years, the Health Statistics Information Center again organized the second health services overall survey in the whole country. In 2003, the Health Statistics Information Center again organized the third health services overall survey in the whole country, carried out the household health survey, at the same time, adopted some qualitative methods.

These survey study had collected a lot of information about the inhabitants health status, medical need quantity and health services utilization, and the information played an important role in formulating district health layout, forcing the health system to modernize and have the scientific management.

(2) The scopes, contents and objects of health services research have been enlarged constantly

Our country's health services research began in the rural. The coverage of study enlarged step by step to rural, factory, combined spot of urban and rural floating population, religion of minority. The study scope firstly began from the medical service supply and demand, subsequently, expanded to the field of prevention and care. The research firstly put the general population as objects, subsequently, expanded the objects to special group to carry out survey, such as elder, children, women and handicapped and industrialist, etc. Besides studying the general medical demand and resources supply, the research contents have also involved the special health problem for special group to carry out deep survey. At present, to study the medical demand, utilization, affected factor and medical salvation has been the hotspot in the field of health services research. The contents and methods of family health survey have been applied widely during the past 20 years.

(3) Developing diversified health services research

The research methods developed from descriptive study in the early phase to analysis, trial (interventional) study, and the transformation made the study conclusion more persuasive, scientific and valid, made the health services research to a new phase. These changes embodied mainly the following aspects: the first was to combine the family health survey with health organization survey and put the subjects who received health services and organizations who provided health services to a system to analyze, to know the meeting level of the population health need, to analyze the cause that led to the unmet need, to put forward the countermeasure about improving health system function and enhance the health services benefit. This transformation is the new development of health services research methods. The second combined the routine information collection with sampling survey and shaped the framework such that the two means of collecting information developed jointly. The third national family health survey had developed from the one-off cross-sectional survey to the repeating health survey, from the simple retrospective health survey to the time-serial prospective survey, etc. These methods overcame some connatural shortcoming of the one-off cross-section survey and could monitor the trend of change in the behavioral risk factor in the group both dynamically and continuously.

Section 2 Need, Demand and Utilization of Health Services

By collecting interrelated data, we can study the inhabitant health status, health services need (demand) quantity, utilization quantity, health resources collocating and the relation between them, analyze the content degree and affecting factor of need (demand) quantity and utilization quantity. It is the common use and effectual approach and means for organizing the health services in reason, evaluating the work efficiency and potential of health system, resolving the contradiction between provider and the need, increasing the social benefit and economic benefit of health cause. At the same time, it is the necessary content and important gist for formulating the health promotion program and plan of collocating health resources.

1. Several basic conceptions

(1) Health

With the social and economic advancement, the advancement of science and technology, the improving of inhabitant life and culture, people's understanding of health and disease has been deepened and developed constantly. The definition of health put forward by WHO in the charter is the sanity state of physically, psychologically and the socially adapting capaurban, not only without disease or physical weakness.

(2) Want of health services

It reflects the subjective wish of preventive care, health promotion, cast off disease, deformity reduction, and cannot be determined completely by the individual's actual health status. The inhabitants's want of health services can be embodied from two aspects: the first is the wish, requirement and advice put forward by public to governing department of health, environment and other pertinent section or institution, and the second is the health requirement collected from the inhabitants in the special organizing health survey.

(3) Need of health services

Need of health services mainly depends on the inhabitants' individual health status, is the objective need of medicine, prevention, care and rehabilitation services put forward according to the gap between the actual health status and above-mentioned ideal health status, includes the perceived need by the individual and the need judged by the medical professional and the need that can't be perceived by the individual. Only if a person has perceived the health services need, he will be likely to seek to use health service. For example, the person has existing health problems or suffers from disease, but he can't perceive. In this situation, the seeking of health services can't happen, it adverse health more. The most effective method which can find the unperceived need is population screening, which can determine the needs which have been found and the potential need which can't be perceived. It has the active meaning whether to medical services or to preventive care work.

(4) Demand of health services

From the angle of economy and value, demand of the health services implies the health services quantity that people want and have the capacity to consume during definite time and at definite price level. There are two conditions for the demand engendering: the first is the willing to buy, the second is the capacity of payment. If people only have desire but no payment capacity, or have the payment capacity but no desire, this situation cannot represent the effective demand. For example, if one person falls ill and has the need of health services, but, because he has no money and can't see a doctor, in this situation, the health need can't transform the health demand, or if the person has the payment capacity, but due to lack of health consciousness can't see a doctor, the health need can't transform the health demand. Commonly, the health need is of two kinds: the first is the demand transformed by the health need, the second is the demand transformed by no health need and leads to this phenomenon growth by diseased seeing a doctor practicing medicine.

(5) Utilization of health services

The quantity of health services (namely the effective quantity of demand) utilized really by the demander is result of the mutual restriction between the quantity of population health services need and the quantity of health resources supply. The health services utilization can reflect directly the health services quantity and work efficiency provided by the health system for the population health and reflect indirectly the effect for inhabitant health status brought about by the health services provided by the health system, but, it can't be employed directly to evaluate the effect of health services.

(6) The relationship among health service need, demand and utilization

The health services demand is transformed from the health services need. In theory, if the health services need of population can all transform into demand, the need would be likely to be met by using health services. But the realistic status is not always so. On one hand, due to the reason of subject and object, all of the health services need of population can't transform into demand completely. Also if the need transform into demand, and the inhabitants have perceived some kinds of health services need, they should also be concerned with the factors, such as income level, social status, the health insurance system, convenient level of transportation, custom and habit, the services types and quality provided by the health organization. For example, a patient is unwilling to see doctor and can't obtain the needed services due to the low income, un-convenient transportation, poor services attitude of the physician and poor quality. So, the need can't transform into demand. On the other hand, whether the demand transformed by need or the demand should do not exist in fact are difficult to meet because of the limited resources, un-rational allocation, the poor quality, low efficiency and the resources wasting. The actual meeting and meeting level of the demand depend on the quantity of supply. When the quantity of supply exceeds the quantity of demand, the demand will be met, but, it can lead to the insufficiency of utilizing the health resources, such as the leaving unused of personnel, bed, apparatus and low utilization rate. When the quantity of supply is less than the quantity of demand, the demand cannot entirely be met, and it leads to waiting to see doctor and can't obtain the services that should be obtained.

2. Need of health service

(1) The measuring and analyzing of need of health services

The need of health service is the objective reflection of inhabitants' actual health status. Commonly, we can grasp the population's need of health services by measuring and analyzing the population's health status, which includes the quantity scale, scope and types of need. There are many indicators to reflect the population's health status, including illness indicator, death as well as constitution indicator, deformity indicator, nutrition and growth indicator, mentality indicator, social indicator and other indicator derived from these indicator; at present, to use the disease indicator and death indicator usually reflects population' health status. Among the death indicator, the infant mortality rate, maternal mortality rate and life expectancy are the sensitive indicator to reflect the social development level, population's health status and medical care level comprehensively. As a result, three indicators are often used to reflect the inhabitants' health need quantity of some country or region. Besides the indicator mentioned above, the rank order of cause of death as well as constitution are also the important indicator to reflect the inhabitants' health need quantity.

Compared to the disease indicator, the death indicator is relatively stable and reliable. These data can be easy to collect by the routine enrolling report or from death monitoring system, and can obtain the continuous data. But, the death is the most serious outcome of the disease or trauma. As a result, to use the death indicator to reflect the inhabitants' health problem is not sensitive, and it needs to combine the sickness indicator to analyze, especially when we want to know the need that consumes the maximum health resources among these needs about medical, preventive, nursing, rehabilitation, health education and consultation, etc. The disease indicator is the most important.

The indicator reflecting the inhabitants' medical need quantity and disease loading includes two kinds of indicator: The frequency level and serious level of disease, these indicators can be obtained by survey such as family health sampling survey.

1) The indicator of disease frequency (rate)

The definition of sickness in health services research considered from the inhabitants' health services need, not strictly means sickness. It is determined by the informant's self cognition or the trained investigator's objective judgment. The indicators in common use are the following:

①Two weeks prevalence equal to the number of sickness person or counts during two weeks before the time of carrying out survey/the number of people surveyed×100% or 1,000‰.

The health services general survey in our country defined the sickness as: A. the physical discomfort and to go the medical unit to see doctor or be treated; B. the physical discomfort and not to go the medical unit to see doctor or be treated; but, to adopt dosing or other assistant treatment by self, such as massage; C. the physical discomfort and not to go to the medical unit to see doctor or be treated; and not to adopt dosing or other assistant treatment by self, but stopping to work, suspending one's schooling or taking bed rest for more than one day due to the physical discomfort. The people having any one of the above-mentioned situations are considered to be sick.

②Chronic illness prevalence equal to the number of person suffereing from chronic disease during half of year before the time of carrying out survey/the number of people surveyed×100% or 1,000‰.

The definition of chronic disease is that: A. the person suffers from the chronic disease diagnosed definitely by the physician within the recent half year before the survey; B. the person suffers from the chronic disease diagnosed definitely by the physician half year before, the disease often outbreaks within the recent half year before the survey and the person surveyed adopted treatment measure such as dosing, physical therapy etc. Any one of the two should be taken as chronic disease.

③The percentage of the health person number accounts for total population: The healthy person is with no urgent or chronic disease, injury, psychological handicap and so on.

2) The indicator of disease seriousness level

①Two weeks person with bed volume equal to the number of sick person or counts for sickbed within recent two weeks before this survey/the number of people surveyed×100% or 1,000‰.

②Two weeks volume of actives limitation equal to the number of actives limitation persons or counts within recent two weeks before this survey/the number of people surveyed×100% or 1,000‰.

③Two weeks volume of lost working days equal to number of person with lost working days within recent two weeks before this survey/the number of people surveyed ×100% or 1,000‰.

④Two weeks sick days equal to the total of sick days within recent two weeks before this survey/the number of people surveyed.

For the need quantity of preventive care, we often use the incidence of communicable disease to reflect it. The need quantity of preventive care is high in the high incidence of communicable disease region. The data of communicable disease can be obtained from the disease registers card.

3) The analysis of need quantity of health services

Table 13-1 lists the sickness indicator of the health services sampling survey in 1985 (rural), 1986(urban), 1993(rural and urban) and 1998((rural and urban). Compared with the metaphase of the 1980s, the two weeks prevalence, chronic illness prevalence, average number days of sickness per year per person all increased to a different extent in the 1990s in our country's urban and rural area, and the urban's is higher than rural's, which reflected that the medical services need quantity of the residents in our country's urban and rural area increased, and the medical services need quantity of the urban residents is relatively higher. This may be related with aged population, urbanization, the economic condition and improving education level, as well as strengthened health consciousness of individual.

Table 13-1 the inhabitants' medical services need quantity in our country's urban and rural areas

indicator	1998		1993		1985	1986
	Rural	Urban	Rural	Urban	Rural	Urban
two weeks prevalence(%)	13.7	18.7	12.8	17.5	6.9	10.5
chronic illness prevalence(%)	11.8	27.3	13.1	28.6	8.6	23.6
average number days of sickness per year per person	29.3	42.8	25.7	38.9	13.0	25.0
average number of days of stopping work per year per person	9.0	4.0	6.8	4.5	5.4	5.0
average number of days of suspending one's schooling per year per person	2.5	1.8	2.1	3.0	1.2	2.0
average number of days of keeping the bed per year per person	3.1	2.5	3.2	3.2	2.4	3.0

(2) The application of need of health services

1) To scale the health service need quantity of objective population

On the assumption of the result of once cross-sectional sampling survey within two weeks as representative of the whole year, we can deduce the number of sickness per year per person and volume of lost working days or with bed days and medical expenditures by the average of two weeks indictors multiplied by 26. Because the indicator of illness and consultation bear the character of seasonal changes, obviously, it will bias to certain extent to calculate the frequency and severity level of the inhabitants' whole year disease by using the result of cross-sectional sampling survey. If we can carry out several or continuous sampling survey and the investigation continuously collecting the data within one year, then the quantity of residents' health services need and indicators of utilization calculated based on these results will give exactly the whole year health services quantity, utilization quantity and altering law of the objective population.

2) To calculate the indirect economy loss due to the disease

We can calculate the indirect economy loss quantity by multiplying the lost working days due to disease per year per person by average of production value per person by the total population.

3) To provide the warrant for allocating health service rationally

We can estimate the outpatient service need quantity based on the illness of person, the number of persons needing hospital admission and on the number of persons losing work with bed rest due to disease, and all these results can provide the warranty for analyzing the medical health services. The indicators of two weeks volume of lost working days and persons with two weeks' bed rest can not only calculate the medical services need, but also further calculate the sickbed need quantity and medical manpower need quantity. These outcomes can become the warranty of setting up sickbed, staffing the personnel and distributing expenditure.

It is necessary to point out that during the formulation of health plan the need and demand in the existing stage must be considered, distinctively treat the health services of different regions, periods, fields, category and stratum, not only to ensure the inhabitants obtain the basic health care services and meet their basic need, embody the social equity, but also to introduce market mechanism duly to enhance the allocation efficiency of health resources and give attention to the demand.

(3) The factors affecting the quantity of need of health services

The quantity of health services need is the actual reflection of population health status. Any factor that affects the population health status all directly or indirectly affects the quantity of population's health services need, and the primary affected factors are as follows:

1) The quantity of population, age and sex constitution

In the constancy of other factors, the larger the quantity of population served, the higher the quantity of the health services need and utilization. The illness prevalence of children and elderly is high, especially the person whose age exceeds 45, and their illness prevalence increases along with the age increasing. Because the female have the menses, pregnant period, menopause, etc., the illness prevalence of the female is higher than that of male.

2) Social and economic factor

In the social life, whether the political system, economic status, culture and education level, or the inhabitancy and life condition, all can affect inhabitants' health status and lead to the different health service need. The research result of several health services general surveys all indicated that the inhabitants' health services utilization rate in the developed region is higher than that in western poverty-ridden regions obviously, and several primary indicators about the inhabitants' health services need quantity and utilization quantity in the urban areas were higher than those in the rural areas.

3) Quality of health services

Improved health service quality can shorten the treatment time, enhance the cure rate, and further reduce the quantity of health service need and utilization. The preventive care is the deciding factor to determine the quantity of health services need, although the effect achieved by actively developing preventive care cannot obviously change the total quantity of population's health services need in a short time. However, from the long term view, if the preventive care bears fruit, the disease will be reduced or annihilated, and certainly will reduce the quantity of health services need and utilization.

4) Behavioral and psychological factors

The behavioral and psychological factors play an important role in the disease occurrence, developing and relapsing, such as smoking, drinking, ill dietetic habits and other ill psychological stimulants, etc.. The need of being in hospital and seeing doctor is also affected by these kinds of factors.

5) The climatic and geographical condition

The occurrence of lots of diseases bears obviously the character of season and terrain. Digestive system diseases happen easily in summer and autumn, respiration system diseases occur in winter and spring, the following diseases like goiter, schistosome, decayed tooth and parasite only occur in the special climate and geography. These phenomena indicate that in the different climate and geography conditions, the inhabitants' health services needs are also different.

6) Marriage and family

The medical services quantity of person who has spouse is less than the bachelordom, widow and divorcee; the existence of spouse can reduce the number of being in hospital and shorten the time of being in hospital. Sometimes, the nursing and caring of family can replace a part of treatment in hospital.

3. Utilization of health services

Analyzing the level of health services utilization is the common method in use to evaluate the social and economic benefit. The data of health services utilization in our country is mainly rooted in the routine health work registers and reports. These kinds of data can be easily collected, accumulated for a long term and observed systematically, but, we can't easily judge the panorama of the population utilizing health services only by relying on the routine health work registers and reports, because an inhabitant often goes to different places `to accept the health service. We can relatively understand and grasp the population health and health services utilization status by carrying out sampling family health survey. The health services utilization includes utilization of outpatient health services, utilization of inpatient health service, preventive care and rehabilitation utilization and other utilization.

(1) Utilization of outpatient health services

Grasping the level, flowing and character of consultation and analyzing the affected factors can provide an important warranty for organizing rational consultation services. The main indicators of inhabitants' outpatient health services are: persons with physician contact within two weeks, patients with physician contact within two weeks, the average counts of consultation per year per person and patients without physician contact within two weeks and so on. These indicators can reflect the level of outpatient services demand and meeting degree.

①Persons with physician contact within two weeks equal to the number of persons with physician contact within recent two weeks before this survey/the number of people surveyed×100% or 1,000‰.

②Patients with physician contact within two weeks equal to the number of patients with physician contact within recent two weeks before this survey/the total of patient within two weeks ×100%.

③Patients without physician contact within two weeks equal to the number of patients without physician contact within recent two weeks before this survey/the total of patient within two weeks×100%.

(2) Utilization of inpatient health service

The indicators reflecting inpatient health service utilization involve persons with hospital admission within twelve months, average volume of hospital days, persons without hospital admission within twelve months. These indicators can be used to know the level of utilization of inpatient health service, to further analyze the cause of in-hospital and should have but without hospital admission, level of hospital and so on, to provide warranty for determining the health organization layout, formulating sickbed and health manpower plan.

①Persons with hospital admission within twelve months equal to the number of persons with hospital admission within twelve months before this survey/the number of people surveyed×100% or 1,000‰.

②Average volume hospital days equal to the total of hospital days/total of the number of persons with hospital admission.

③Persons without hospital admission within twelve months equal to the number of persons should have but without hospital admission/the number of persons should have hospital admission×100%.

Table 13-2 lists the result of inhabitant's medical health utilization quantity of the several health services sampling surveys in our country's urban and rural areas, to find out:①Comparing with the 1980s, the quantity of inpatients medical services utilization increased within the 1990s in our country's urban and rural areas, especially in the rural areas; ②Patients without physician contact within two weeks of urban inhabitants are higher than those of the rural inhabitants, and take on the increasing trend; ③Persons with hospital admission within twelve months kept in the around 3.1% in ruralarea,the same indicator in urban area taken on decreasing trend; ④The proportion of person obliged to be admitted but without hospital admission within twelve months increased both in the urban and rural areas.

Table 13-2 the quantity of inhabitants' medical services utilization in our country's urban and rural areas

indicator	1998		1993		1985	1986
	Rural	Urban	Rural	Urban	Rural	Urban
Persons with physician contact within two weeks(%)	16.5	16.2	6.0	19.9	10.1	14.7
Patients without physician contact within two weeks(%)	33.2	49.9	33.7	42.4	22.9	26.6
Persons with hospital admission within twelve months(%)	3.1	4.8	3.1	5.0	3.1	5.1
Average volume hospital days per year per one thousand persons	391.0	1,091.0	428.0	1,502.0	469.0	688.0
Person should have but without hospital admission within twelve months (%)	35.5	29.5	40.6	26.2	23.7	16.4

Among the reasons for not being admitted despite the necessity, the self-treatment by the patient buying the necessary drugs accounts for the large of proportion, other reasons are as follows: unnecessary, economic hardships, limitation of time, inconvenience of traffic, poor services attitude and on the effective medical treatment and so on. The result of cause analysis indicated that the proportion for necessary hospital admission but without hospital admission increased because of the economic hardships, the proportion in urban areas increased from 40% in 1993 to 63% in 1998, and the proportion in rural areas increased from 59% in 1993 to 65% in 1998.

The economic status, medical insurance system, etc. are the important factors affecting the health services utilization.

(3) Preventive care

The measurement of preventive care utilization, such as planning immunization, health education, communicable disease control and maternal and childcare, etc. Is relatively complex and difficult to compare with medical service utilization. The preventive services utilization frequently happens on the spot. It is difficult to collect the data by registers. Some preventive services utilization rate is low, and holds the seasonal character, and we can't often obtain the satisfactory outcome by carrying out one cross-sectional survey for few group. We can collect data by adopting the methods of combining the health institution register report and household survey. We can carry out the measure and evaluation by comparing the services quantity actually received by the residents with the service quantity that should be provided according to the planning objective. For example, a pregnant woman should receive 8 prenatal examinations; we can evaluate the quality of perinatal care based on the actual number of prenatal examination the pregnant woman received.

Table 13-3 The quantity of inhabitants' preventive services utilization in our country's urban and rural area

indicator	1998		1993	
	rural	urban	rural	urban
Prenatal examining rate(%)	78.6	86.6	60.3	95.6
Average number of prenatal examination	3.2	6.4	3.9	6.4
Delivery in hospital rate(%)	43.9	93.5	8.5	61.7
Delivery in home rate(%)	55.9	6.5	76.6	10.7
Postnatal visiting rate(%)	50.2	61.4	48.3	39.6
Average number of postnatal visiting	1.3	1.5	2.9	2.5
Pre-marry examination rate(%)	—	—	14.1	49.2
Female disease checking and treating rate(%)	—	—	16.4	47.7

About the preventive care services utilization in family health survey, it is often necessary to ask the category and quantity of the services the inhabitants received during some period. If these services items are often developed in the whole years, such as family planning, maternal and child health care, health education, etc., it will be feasible to use the result obtained by applying two weeks' (or one month or half years) to calculate the whole year result. We should ask the number of accepted services about the planning immunizations, maternal screening and other communicable disease prevention and cure in a year or several years, but not ask the number of accepted services within a short time, because these items only happen several months within a year, and this should be paid attention to when we carry out the survey design.

Section 3 Health Resources

Health resources are the integrated title of the manpower, material resources and finance provided by society for the health development in the prevailing social and economic condition, and mainly include personnel, outlay, furniture, establishment, knowledge, technique, information and media materials and so on. The quantity of health resources held by the country is the objective criterion to measure economic strength, culture status and health level. The health resources that a country holds are always limited, and there always exists some gap between the health resources that can be provided and the health resources that are needed. To study the potential of health resources is a basic task of health services research.

1. Health manpower resources

Health manpower resource is a kind of the most important and most activated health resources, and it is a complementary part to formulate and to realize the national health development plan. Health manpower is the personnel that receive the professional training, work in the health system and provide health services, including the personnel that have worked in the health services post and are being trained. The health manpower research mainly studies the quantity, structure and distribution of health personnel. The exploitation of health manpower comprises of manpower program, training and management.

(1) Quantity

Relative number and absolute number can denote the quantity of health personnel. For the sake of expressing the level of health manpower in the different periods or different regions, the relative number can be often used, such as the physician number per 1,000 or the number of population per physician.

(2) Structure

The manpower structure can reflect the quality of health manpower and illustrate the rationale of manpower. As a group of persons with ability, the rational structure of health manpower should include the following three aspects:

①Age structure: Age is a synthetic indicator to measure the work capacity, skill and efficiency of staff. The rational age structure can help the strongpoint of each age level bring out good play, and keep the continuity and stability of health manpower.

②Specialty structure: Different professionals provide different services. Among the professionals in our country, the modern medical specialty account for about 70%, Chinese traditional medical specialty account for 15%, pharmaceutics specialty account for 5%, preventive medical specialty account for 4%, the high-grade professional of ENT, pediatrics, nutrition, laboratory, biomedicine and health management are in serious shortage. The proportion of doctor by nurse is 1 : 0.42 in our country, and that the proportion of doctor by nurse is 1 : 2 in most developed countries, proportion of nurse by population is 1 : 1,750, the proportion is 1 : (140 – 320) in developed countries.

③The structure of title of a technical post: Title of a technical post reflects a certain extent of technique level. If there is only one kind of professional in a colony, and the level of the professional is high, the efficiency cannot always be high. There should be right proportion in different titles of a technical post of staff. The proportion of high by middle by primary of title of a technical post is 1 : 1.7 : 1, the standard proportion put forward by WHO should be 1 : 3 : 1 in midline developed countries.

(3) Distribution

From the geographic distribution of health manpower, there exists a serious imbalance in the developed and undeveloped countries about the health manpower. The developed country holds 1,000 health technical personnel per 100 thousand people, whereas the developing country only holds two hundred. In any country, there also exists imbalance in the geographic distribution of health manpower. The staff concentrate in the large cites in most countries, while shortage of health technical personnel is a universal phenomenon in rural areas. The rural population accounts for above 75% in our country, and the quantity of health technical personnel only accounts for 52%.

2. Health manpower program

The health manpower programming means predicting the amount of health manpower demands, supply and possession in the future, in order to be balanced between the demands and supply of health manpower. Health manpower programming seems more important since the health manpower supply cannot be acquired temporarily, but is the result of long-term cultivation.

(1) The demands of health manpower

The demands of health manpower refer to the research of the requisite manpower scales of health departments in target years on the basis of the developments of society and economy, the change of people's structure and amount, the transition of medical model, the utility rate of health services, and the labor product rate, etc. The cardinal estimating methods include:

①The method of health need in order to promote peoples health, which services items should be accepted, the needed number of health manpower and so on can be calculated by the amounts of services. For example, 1 pregnant woman needs 8 antepartum exams, so the basic demands of perinatal care can not be satisfactory unless there is 1 obstetrician, 3 accoucheuses and 4 health attendants per 1,000 pregnant women.

②The method of health demands: The method of health demands calculate the service demand amounts and the health manpower demands amounts on the basis of actual utilities of effective demand namely health services and based on the actual service demand accounts of the past and present and consider the various factors that effect the demand amounts in certain period.

③The method of service-target: The health manpower need amount can not be acquired unless the service output objective is made. For example, if 1 doctor can see 5,000 outpatients in 1 year, then the amount of doctor can be calculated by the total amounts of outpatients.

④Population ratio method: The population ratio method can be used to predict the amounts of manpower needed. The method is simple and the needed number of health manpower of objective year can be calculated if the ratio between the population and the ratio between health manpower and population is acquired.

⑤Trend extrapolation: It is a simplest and frequently used prediction method. It can be predicted by the result of extrapolation based on the continuity law of health manpower development and extend the condition of past and now to the future. The method evolves the various factors influencing the future development on the basis of past law. It is simple and practiced, though it seems rough.

In addition, there are experts' evaluation methods, mathematics model method, etc. And the things that should be pointed out are that various health manpower prediction methods can get certain outcome, and the prediction outcome depends on the selected method. The different method has the different assumption term, and different workload standard selected.

(2) The supply of health manpower

The supply of health manpower is the basis of health services. Health manpower programming needs the balance of demand and supply. The health manpower supplies include three parts: the current possession amounts of health manpower, the additional number of future health manpower and the amounts of loss.

(3) Health manpower management

Reasonable management and use of health manpower is the key to developing the effective health care. Health manpower management includes:

①The establishment of health manpower management policy and norm;

②The adjustment of health manpower demand or need;

③The monitoring and guidance of health manpower;

④The encouragement of health manpower;
⑤The use and evaluation of health manpower.

3. Health expenditure

It is important for the reasonable allocation of health expenses and the improvement of economic profit of health service to research the character and law of economic activities in the field of health services.

Health expenses contain two concepts with broad and narrow meanings. The broad meaning refers to the wasting social resources directly and indirectly in order to protect the population health in a certain period. It contains the total waste of manpower, material resources and financial capacity, and it is calculated by money. The narrow meaning refers to the wasting economic resources directly in order to supply the health services in a certain period.

The health expenses usually referred to are the narrow health expenses; they are the main targets of health expenses research.

The contents of health expenses research conclude; the amounts of fund in the course of health services, the constitution and character of health expenses, whether the allocation and use of health expenses is fair and reasonable, and whether the relation among the health need, health resources and health services utility is balanced. It also researches the source and output of expenses, the factors, which influence the expenses and their varying trend, the reason of increase of health expenses.

(1) The source of the health expenses

The health expenses are from the nation, collective and individuals in our country, such as health care financial allocated by the national budget, expenses used to labor insurance by certain proportion from gross payroll by industrial and mining establishments, the co-operation expenses from collective public welfare fund in villages. Some outpatient service registered fee and medicine fee by public expense labor insurance workers, the medicine fee paid by the people with health insurance and co-operation by certain proportion, the medicine fee paid by the family members of workers in business, the medicine fee paid by the patients at their own expenses, etc.

(2) The classification of health expenses

The health expenses can be classified into direct health expenses and indirect health expenses.

Direct health expenses, paid by the using of health service, include the various services fee, assay fee, medicine fee and material fee paid by patients, etc. Indirect health expenses include the wages delaying the work, the traveling fare, nourishment fee, and the delayed fee by caring the patients, etc. The direct expenses are not the keystones of health research, but the input and output of health services cannot be evaluated entirely unless the direct expenses and the indirect expenses are calculated completely in order to weigh comprehensively the social economic loss caused by illness and injury when we analyze the expense effectiveness. And the health expenses can be divided into medical services fee, health epidemic prevention fee, women and children fee, medical education fee and scientific research fee, etc. from the angle of health services.

(3) The evaluation index of health expenses

①The percentage of health expenses out of gross national products This index explains that whether the quantities of health expenses are suitable of the economic development level and the people's health care needs in local community, and shows the degree of resources provided by nation or local authority to insure the harmonizing developments between the health care and social economy. The developed countries' proportion of health expenses out of GNP is usually above 7% since the 1990s, and in some developed countries, such as the United States, Canada and Sweden, the proportion is above 10%. The amounts of health expenses are increasing year by year, but the proportion of health expenses out of GNP was lingering between the 3% - 5% before the 1990s, which was equal to the level of developed countries in the 1950s. The proportion began to ascend since the 1990s, and reached 4%. It is 4.21% in 1996 and 4.68% in 1998. The proportion of health expenses out of GNP is in the state of ascension if we observe the total trend.

②The health expenses per person This index explains the average level of people in one country or district, and shows whether the allocation of health resources to different districts and population is reasonable. The factors, such as sex, age, culture and medical care system, etc., have the important influence on average health expenses.

③The proportion of the investment to health departments It reflects whether the allocation of health expenses to health organization is reasonable.

④The constitution of out-patient service and hospitalization It reflects the expenses allocation and use characters inside medical organization. The medicine fee has a comparatively large proportion in small hospitals. The aiding checking fee, however, has the large proportion in big hospitals as a result of the complexity of patients' state of illness and the use of aiding instruments and expensive checking apparatus. The higher the level of medicine organization is, the larger proportion of aiding checking fee and smaller proportion of medicine fee.

⑤The proportion of medicine, health epidemic prevention and women and children health expenses It is the proportion that should be noticed first by health departments before allotting expenses.

Medical services offer the services of health maintenance and recovery, and these services use health resources most frequently and waste them most; the 80% of manpower and expenses are used in medical services system in the health system in China.

The importance of prevention and care should not be neglected seeing from the function of health services to health. The determination of appropriate proportion of expenses allocation among medicine, prevention and care services should be considered synthetically combining the social economic development and cultural tradition besides the population need and services utility.

(4) Reason analysis of increasing health expenses

The increasing of health expenses is a universal phenomenon in our country and all over the world. And the trend of unreasonable increasing seems more and more obvious. The reasons causing the increase of health expenses include:

①The trend of population aging: The population in our country is facing the situation of rapid aging, the old-age population above 60 have a rapid increasing rate, and our country has become an aging country since 2000. The old-age crowd is the frail population in health aspect, according to the research data of national health services in 1998. The prevalence rate, the rate of seeing doctor and the admission rate of the old are comparatively high, and their needs of health care are high, too. The people in this age phase are vulnerable to have the chronic and non-infectious diseases, which have a long course of diseases and a high expense, and aggravate the soar of health expenses.

②Price rising and inflation: The research in various countries validates the inflation's influence on health expenses. The price soar of energy sources, carriage material and other health necessities accelerate the ascending of health expenses with the influence of inflation and universal soar of price.

③The population increasing: The total health expenses will mount up with the increasing of population absolute number, even on the unchangeable condition of average expenses.

④The application of the advanced and new technique is another reason of the soar of health expenses. The health expenses increased rapidly because some incurable diseases were cured by advanced and new technique with the improvement and development of science and technique and the adding of new equipment and new medicines in the field of health.

⑤The obvious variety of the disease spectrum: The chronic and non-infectious diseases are in the dominant places and their incidence rate is rising constantly. These diseases, such as of heart and brain blood vessel, diabetes, malignancy, usually have the characters such as long course of diseases, difficult to cure, and high treatment fee, and the increasing of these diseases results in the soar of health expenses.

⑥The advance of health care demands and health consciousness: People's health care consciousness was strengthened and the consumption concept of health services were changed with the economic development and the increased income, and people's demands to health services appeared multi-layer and needed the advanced quality of health services.

⑦The imperfection of payment mechanism: The prolonging of the day in hospitals and the increasing frequency of seeing doctors occurs with the occurrence of inducing demands behaviors because of the particularity of health services themselves and the imperfection of payment systems. Among the factors which influence the soar of health expenses, some can be controlled comparatively, such as expenses payment mechanism, others cannot be controlled, such as the aging of population and the changing of diseases spectrum. The trend of health expenses' soar is objective existence; the ways to control the part of unreasonable soar of expenses and not harming the part of reasonable increase is the key.

Section 4 The Synthetic Evaluation of Health Service

1. The concept and significance of health service evaluation and synthetic evaluation

Health service evaluation, which is a branch of evaluation research, is also a part of health service research as well. It means the evaluation on health resources construction, health service process and outcome. It aims to realize the social need and demand of health service, find out the obstacle factors for residents' health and their search of health service so as to make people realize health problem, more effectively allocate and utilize the present health resources, more reasonably organize health care service, improve the control over application process and target management, advance the health service efficiency, benefit and effectiveness, illuminate the headway and result of health service work, reform and improve the health service planning of any item, and adjust health policy to adapt to complex and changing situation. In a word, its cardinal aim lies in offering the reasonable basis of plan, management and decision, thus to provide more efficient, more effective and fair and equal health service, improve social health condition and advance the crowd health level. The cardinal characteristic of evaluation contents includes six aspect: proper degree, enough degree, progress, efficiency, effect and influence.

Synthetic evaluation will get a systematic process and organic collection of all kinds of index that reflect the features of evaluation object and so realize the quality of evaluation object, or get a composite index made up of every constitution out of many single-item evaluation indexes to reflect the panorama of evaluation object. Health service synthetic evaluation means a process of judgment and estimation on health service development, effect and value around particular evaluation target, evaluation object and evaluation stage. The aimed object of health service is social population, and the final scale to evaluate the social and economic benefit of health service is the degree to which the social health service and population health level are improved and advanced. However, the social and economic benefit is affected not only by the input of health resources, quantity and quality of the provided services, but also by social, economic, cultural, natural situation directly or indirectly. People's demand of health service varies in different social and economic development stages, so do the health resources input and service level. Therefore, when making a systematic evaluation of health service item that involves various factors, we should consider the situation and adjust measures to local conditions to utilize the proper technology and method of multi-subjects and thus make a synthetic evaluation of multi-direction, multi-level, multi-link and multi-factor. Namely, as long as we make the evaluation from various aspects of health service such as social need, health resources input, service quantity and efficiency provided, the generated social and economic benefit, we can better reflect health service's effect and influence.

2. The scope and contents of health service synthetic evaluation

Along with the development of health care management, health service evaluation has received more and more attention since the 1970s, and some relative study and application was put into effect. In principle, health service evaluation can go from various aspects and points of view, and it can apply not only in the macro-evaluation on a national or regional general health development planning (or item), application and outcome but also in the micro-evaluation on rural cooperative medical care's application system of some town; it can serve as a quantitative one and qualitative one as well. But we should introduce quantitative evaluation or combination method of quantitative evaluation and qualitative evaluation as much as possible to enhance the persuasion of evaluation outcome. Because of the difference in evaluation property, purpose, angle, level and emphasis, the extensively uniform realization of health service, synthetic evaluation has not come into being with regard to its scope, content and index system. However, as the synthetic evaluation work of health service, if not combined with some relative outcome index that reflects the resident's health, its limits are self-evident.

Parker constructed the systematic model of health service according to the principle of systematic analysis. Considering the feature of each element and their correlation, we can make evaluation from 7 aspects as follows: the population's need quantity of health service, the resources input, the service output, work process, outcome, benefit, effect. Roemer, according to the contents of health service, suggests making evaluation from 8 aspects: ①item target evaluation; ②medical treatment service need evaluation; ③health service utilization acceptance ability evaluation; ④health resources evaluation; ⑤work activity and attitude evaluation; ⑥work process evaluation; ⑦outcome and effect evaluation; ⑧expenses and benefit evaluation. In the book *Preventive Medicine and Public Health*, Sackett, according to the research object of health service, suggested that health service evaluation should go around such 4 aspects as if the health service is valid, if the public can utilize the valid health service, if the quantity and quality of provided service is sufficient and credible, if the expenses are low.

Case Example

Health Services

It is good to utilize health service reasonably. To use health services unduly will lead to squander health resources and increasing of medical expenditure, and the deficiency of utilization can't meet the population's health services need (or demand). The purpose of health services research is not only to know the quantity and quality that inhabitants utilized, but also to study the relationship among the health services need, health resources and health services utilization, to analyze the existing situation and changing trend of supply and demand contradiction based on these research finding, providing the decision-making warranty for regulating and allocating health resources. In 1976, according to the result of sampling survey about health services conducted in the 7 states: USA, Canada, Argentina, UK, Holland, Finland, Yugoslavia and 12 regions, altogether 15 million inhabitants during 10 years, WHO carried out the comprehensive evaluation of health services and put forward comprehensive evaluation model (see to table 13-4). The basic idea of this kind of comprehensive evaluation model is to relate the population health need, health services utilization and health resources together and make the average of the three kinds of indicator: quantity of health need, health services utilization and resources input as the criterion to judge the performance. There are 8 kinds of compounding based on this, to evaluate a state's or region's health services situation comprehensively and provide the referenced warranty for formulating health services development programming and allocating health resources rationally.

Table 13-4 the comprehensive evaluation model of health services

Health services	High need		Low need	
	high resource	low resource	high resource	low resource
high	Type A (balance) The allotting of resources is fitting	Type B High rate of resources utilization	Type E Use in excess	Type F High utilization rate of resources
low	Type C Low utilization rate of resources	Type D Low investing in the health resources	Type G The resources investing is excessive	Type H (balance) The allotting of resources is fitting

Type A: The resource is sufficient, is to be utilized well. The population health services need is large and need to keep balance between three.

Type B: The population health services need is large, the resource is insufficient, and the rate of health services utilization is high. It is not adapted between the low resource and high need. Due to the strain of resources utilization, this can be kept in balance by increasing the rate of utilization, but, this state cannot be permanent and should be transform in to type A.

Type C: The population health services need is large, the resource is sufficient, and the rate of health services utilization is low. It is necessary to study the factor that handicap ped people use the health services and improve the benefit of health services.

Type D: The investment of resources is deficient, the utilization rate is low, and it can't meet the health services need quantity of the population. It should adapt to the health services need of population by adding investment and increasing the rate of utilization.

Type E: The resource is sufficient; the population health services need is low and the health services have been used well. Due to the sufficient resources, it leads to some people to use the health services unduly and squander the health resources.

Type F: Low resources investing, high health services using, it is the symbol of good health services benefit, but the low resources adapt the low population need of health services.

Type G: The population health services need is low, the resource is sufficient and the utilization rate of health services is low. It indicates that the investment to health resources is excessive and should transform to the type H.

Type H: The population health services need is low, the invested quantity of resources is deficient, and the utilization rate is low, to keep balance between the three situations in the low level.

The subject of consideration and discussion:

1. What are the main research methods and contents of health services research?

2. To narrate the meaning of need of health services, demand and utilization as well as the relationship between them.

3. What are the indicators of the health care need and utilization?

4. To describe briefly the comprehensive evaluation model of health services.

第十四章 社区卫生服务

随着经济的发展、社会的进步,传统的生物医学模式已为生物-心理-社会医学模式所取代,人们对健康和疾病的认识日益深化,健康的内涵也在扩大,从生理健康到生理、心理和社会健康,以疾病为中心、以个体为对象的医疗卫生服务模式越来越不适应社会发展的需要。社会医学提出的"四个扩大"正在逐步得到社会的认可,健康优先、预防优先的发展策略以及人人享有基本卫生保健的战略,孕育了以健康为中心、以群体为对象的新型的卫生服务模式——社区卫生服务。当前,我国的卫生事业面临着许多新的问题,如:随着人口老龄化的进程加快,老年病、慢性非传染性疾病的防治成为日益迫切的问题;随着医学模式的转变及人人享有卫生保健战略的实施,人们对卫生服务的要求越来越高;随着高科技检测、治疗手段的应用,医疗费用不断上涨,但对改善人类总体健康状况却收效甚微,成本与效益严重失衡;随着医学专科的不断分化,对疑难重症的解决不断有所突破,但医患关系淡漠却成为越来越普遍的问题。在应对这些问题方面,社区卫生服务具有无可比拟的优势。从20世纪80年代末至今,经过引进、宣传、交流、研究和试点等一系列实践之后,社区卫生服务在我国得到了政府的大力提倡和支持。1997年《中共中央、国务院关于卫生改革与发展的决定》明确提出发展社区卫生服务以来,不少城市积极试点探索,既取得了一定成效,同时也暴露出了一些问题。为了解决社区卫生服务试点中遇到的具体问题,1999年和2002年卫生部等10部委又分别下发了《关于发展城市社区卫生服务的若干意见》和《关于加快发展城市社区卫生服务的意见》,进一步促进了社区卫生服务的发展。

第一节 社区卫生服务的概念与特点

一、社区卫生服务概念

(一)社区

社区是指一定地域内,按一定的社会制度和社会关系组织起来的、具有共同人口特征的地域生活共同体。社区是社会有机体组成部分,是宏观社会的缩影。

社区一般具有五个构成要素：一定的社会关系为基础组织起来的，进行共同生活的人群；人们赖以从事社会活动的具有一定界限的地域；一整套相对完备的生活服务设施；特有的文化背景、生活方式的认同；一定的生活制度和管理机构。

(二)社区卫生服务

社区卫生服务是社区建设的重要组成部分，是在政府领导、社区参与、上级卫生机构指导下，以基层卫生机构为主体，全科医生为骨干，合理使用社区资源和适宜技术，以人的健康为中心、家庭为单位、社区为范围、需求为导向，以妇女、儿童、老年人、慢性病人、残疾人等为重点，以解决社区主要卫生问题、满足基本社区服务需求为目的，融预防、医疗、保健、康复、健康教育、计划生育技术服务等为一体的，有效、经济、方便、综合、连续的基层卫生服务。

社区卫生服务的对象是社区内的全体人群，主要包括：①病人，包括各种慢性病病人、需要急救的病人、常见病病人等。②各种弱势人群，如儿童、妇女、老年人、残疾人等。③高危人群，即具有危险因素的人群，其患病率高于普通人群。如具有吸毒、酗酒等不良嗜好的人群，从事危险职业的人群，高危家庭中的成员等。④亚健康人群，即没有明显的疾患，但呈现不同程度的体力、反应能力、适应能力等下降的人群。⑤健康人群，这里的健康是指躯体上、心理上和社会适应方面都具有完好状态。社区卫生服务以健康人群为服务对象，充分体现了预防为先的特点。

二、社区卫生服务的特点

社区卫生服务是推行以社区为定向的基层医疗，即在社区中同时发展初级卫生保健和社区医学的有关项目，并将两者有机地结合到基层医疗实践中。其具有以下特点。

1. 系统性。社区卫生服务的实施是一项系统工程，包括医疗卫生保健的提供者——卫生部门与工、农、教育、社会福利等有关部门，也包括卫生服务的接受者——医疗卫生服务的受益者，两者相互联系、相互影响，构成了一个整体目标明确、层次分明、相互关联的系统。而社区卫生服务本身是医疗卫生工作的一个子系统，同时又是社区服务工作的一个子系统。

2. 人性化。社区卫生服务强调"以人为本"，突出"生命至上"的宗旨，它把病人看做有个性、有感情的人，而不是疾病的载体，其照顾的目的不仅仅限于寻找病理问题，而要为患者提供精神的、文化的和感情的服务；要把尊重人、关爱人、方便人、服务人贯穿于社区卫生服务的全过程。因此，医患之间有着一种很亲密的关系。

3. 连续性。社区卫生服务贯穿于人生的各个阶段，从围产期保健、婴幼儿保健、儿童期保健、青年保健、中老年保健等一直到濒死病人的临终关怀，充分体现了其"从摇篮到坟墓"的连续服务过程。

4. 个体化。社区卫生服务是从社区及家庭的背景上去考察和解决个人的健康和疾病问题。对病人的看法，首先是人，而后才是疾病，从生理、心理、环境和社会诸多方面去考虑解决病人的问题。

5. 综合性。这一特性简明地体现了全科医学的"全方位或全主体"：就服务对象而言，不分年龄，性别和疾病类型；就服务的内容而言，包括医疗、预防保健、康复和健康教育;就服务层面而言,包括个人、家庭和社区;就服务项目而言,包括生理、心理和社会文化各个方面。

6. 一体化。社区卫生服务是集医疗、预防、保健、康复、健康教育、计划生育技术指导等为一体的综合服务。它强调预防为先,并尽量在社区内解决群众的基本医疗需求。

7. 协调性。社区卫生服务是协调各有关部门,动用社会、社区有关部门以及家庭的各种资源,通过会诊、转诊等协调性措施,调用其他医疗保健体系共同完成对社区居民的医疗保健服务,因而它体现了一种协调性服务。

8. 可及性。可及性服务包括方便可靠的基本医疗设施、固定的医疗关系、有效的预约系统、下班后和节假日的服务、地理位置上接近、病情熟悉、医患关系亲密、经济上可接受等。

三、发展社区卫生服务的意义

1. 提供基本卫生服务,满足人民群众日益增长的卫生服务需求,提高人民健康水平的重要保障。社区卫生服务覆盖广泛、方便群众,能使广大群众获得基本卫生服务,也有利于满足人民群众日益增长的多样化卫生服务需求。社区卫生服务强调预防为主、防治结合,有利于将预防保健落实到社区、家庭和个人,提高人群健康水平。

2. 深化卫生改革,建立与社会主义市场经济相适应的城市卫生服务体系的重要基础。社区卫生服务可以将广大居民的多数基本健康问题解决在基层。积极发展社区卫生服务,有利于调整城市卫生服务体系的结构、功能、布局,提高效率,降低成本,形成以社区卫生服务机构为基础,大中型医院为医疗中心,预防、保健、健康教育等机构为预防、保健中心,适应社会主义初级阶段国情和社会主义市场经济体制的城市卫生服务体系新格局。

3. 建立城镇职工基本医疗保险制度的迫切要求。社区卫生服务可以为参保职工就近诊治一般常见病、多发病、慢性病,帮助参保职工合理利用大医院服务,并通过健康教育、预防保健,增进职工健康,减少发病,既保证基本医疗,又降低成本,符合"低水平、广覆盖"原则,对职工基本医疗保险制度长久稳定运行起重要支撑作用。

4. 有利于加强社会主义精神文明建设,密切党群、干群关系,维护社会稳定。社区卫生服务通过多种形式的服务为群众排忧解难,使社区卫生人员与广大居民建立起新型医患关系,有利于加强社会主义精神文明建设。积极开展社区卫生服务是为人民办好事、办实事的德政民心工程,充分体现全心全意为人民服务宗旨,有利于密切党群干群关系,维护社会稳定,促进国家长治久安。

第二节 社区卫生服务的功能

根据卫生部等10部委《关于发展城市社区卫生服务的若干意见》,社区卫生服务应具有"六位一体"的功能,"六位"是指健康教育、社区预防、社区保健、社区治疗、社区康复、计划生育指导;"一体"是指社区卫生服务站(中心)提供综合、连续的服务。

一、健康教育

健康教育是指通过信息传播和行为干预,促使人们自愿采取有利于健康的行为和生活方式,消除或减轻影响健康的危险因素,预防疾病、促进健康和提高生活质量。

健康教育需要把对整个人群的普遍预防和对高危人群的重点预防结合起来,既要开展面向全人群的健康教育,指导居民纠正不良的行为生活方式,又要明确健康教育的重点对象,消除高危人群的危险因素。此外,健康教育还应配合上级部门对免疫接种、无偿献血、生殖健康、社会病预防等进行宣传和教育工作。

健康教育应具有科学性、针对性、启发性、直观性、灵活性,不能简单说教,应尽量引起群众的兴趣,最终实现"知——信——行"的改变,即通过健康知识的传播,使人们形成正确的健康观念,从而改变不良行为生活方式。

二、社区预防

(一)社区卫生诊断

社区卫生诊断是了解特定时间和特定范围内的人群中的健康状况以及疾病与相关健康影响因素的关系。社区卫生诊断可在街道办事处、居民委员会等社区管理部门组织领导以及卫生行政部门的指导下,了解社区居民的健康状况以及影响居民健康的主要危险因素,了解居民的基本卫生服务需求,针对社区主要健康问题,制定和实施社区卫生工作计划。

(二)疾病预防

这里的预防主要是对常见病和多发病、传染病、地方性疾病、寄生虫病、职业病、慢性非传染性疾病以及精神性疾病等的预防。主要措施包括:①开展计划免疫等预防接种工作。②严格执行法定传染病登记与报告制度。③当有传染病流行时,配合有关部门处理疫情,控制和消灭传染病的发生和蔓延。④开展传染病、地方病、寄生虫病的社区防治。⑤做好对职业病的诊断、登记和报告工作。⑥对慢性病人群进行监测,做好健康指导和行为干预工作。⑦开展精神卫生宣传和教育工作。⑧对精神性疾病患者及时发现,及早治疗,对康复期精神疾病患者进行有效监护。

三、社区保健

(一)特殊人群保健

特殊人群保健主要是对妇女、儿童及老年人群的保健。妇女保健主要包括围产期保健、产前保健、产后保健、更年期保健以及常见妇科疾病的筛查等。儿童保健主要包括新生儿保健、婴幼儿保健、学龄前期保健、学龄期保健以及意外伤害的预防等。老年人群保健主要包括了解老年人的健康状况、指导老年人进行自我保健以及防止意外伤害、自杀等的发生。

(二)心理健康保健

社区卫生服务应做好社区居民的心理保健工作,对有心理问题的居民应及时进行心理疏导,增强心理健康,使社区居民具有良好的心理素质。此外,应加强特殊时期的心理保健工作,如非典型肺炎流行时期,进行心理宣传和指导,减轻心理恐慌,促进居民的心理健康,对战胜"非典"具有重要意义。

四、社区治疗

社区治疗主要包括四个方面的内容:①提供一般常见病、多发病和诊断明确的慢性病的医疗服务。②恰当处理疑难病症,对不能确诊的病例应及时做好转诊工作。③做好对危、急、重症病人的现场救护工作。④提供家庭出诊、家庭护理、家庭病床等家庭医疗服务。

五、社区康复

根据 WHO 的定义,社区康复是指在城乡社区,调动和协调有关部门及包括康复对象和家庭成员在内的全体人员参与,充分开发和利用社区资源,在医疗康复的基础上,实现全面康复。全面康复包括四个层次,即医学康复、教育康复、职业康复和社会康复。

医疗康复是应用医学技术,进行功能诊断、治疗、训练和预防等,从而达到慢性病人、残疾人和老年人身心康复的目的。

教育康复是在康复医学的指导下,对康复对象进行道德教育、文化教育、职业技术教育和普通教育,对智力、视力、听力及语言障碍者进行特殊教育,为康复对象参与社会生活,适应社会需要创造条件。

职业康复是通过对康复对象进行就业咨询、职业能力测试、岗前职业教育、就业安置等,使康复对象解决就业问题。

社会康复是通过社会和康复对象自身的共同努力,维护康复对象的尊严和权利,创造条件使康复对象在教育、婚姻、住房、娱乐等生活方面与正常人享有平等的待遇,充分参与社会生活,实现自身价值。

六、计划生育指导

计划生育指导的目的是促使人们做到优生优育,提高民族素质。可采取以下措施:①婚前检查。对直系血亲或三代内旁系血亲者应禁止其结婚。对患有性病、精神病以及患有某种法定传染病并在规定隔离期内者,应尽量劝阻其结婚。某些遗传病患者可以结婚,但应劝阻其生育。②在夫妻双方知情和选择的前提下,指导夫妻双方避孕、节育。③提供避孕药具及相关咨询。通过宣传教育,提高对婚育知识的理解。

第三节 社区卫生服务的组织与运作

一、社区卫生服务的组织

目前,我国社区卫生服务的组织形式多种多样,但其内容都是一致的,最终都是为了实现社区卫生服务的功能。因此,尽管各地社区卫生服务组织形式不一,但一般都遵循以下原则。

1. 政府领导，多部门参与。社区卫生服务的组织应在政府领导下进行，有关部门都应给以支持。各级政府要成立社区卫生服务协调组织，卫生、财政、物价、劳动与社会保障、民政、人事等有关部门应各尽其职，完善有关配套政策和措施，及时协调解决社区卫生服务发展过程中遇到的问题和困难。

2. 合理设置社区卫生服务机构的布局。社区卫生服务机构的设置应根据该地区的人口密度、卫生需求、地理位置等合理布局。有的专家提出，社区卫生服务半径以0.7～1.0千米为宜，而且应注意与社区医院和其他医疗机构应保持一定距离。

3. 合理配备医疗人员。在我国目前全科医师缺乏的情况下，应满足社区人员每万人至少配备2名全科医师。全科医生与社区护士的比例不低于1：2，口腔医生、康复治疗技师、社会工作者等其他技术人员按实际需求配备。

4. 基本设施配备。社区卫生服务机构业务用房、床位、基本设备、常用药品和急救药品应根据社区卫生服务的功能、居民需求配置。

5. 健全各项管理制度。主要包括医疗人员的培训、管理、考核和奖惩制度，服务差错及事故防范制度，会诊及双向转诊制度，财务、药品、设备管理制度，档案、信息资料管理制度，社区卫生服务质量管理与考核评价制度等。

二、社区卫生服务的运作

社区卫生服务不同于门诊部，其运作也不同于过去的"坐堂问诊"形式。社区卫生服务的运作是一个系统、复杂的过程，需要多个部门的配合，共同实现其服务功能。社区卫生服务的运作一般应包括以下四个步骤。

(一)进行卫生服务需求评价

这是社区卫生服务运作的前提，也是配备卫生人员、配置卫生资源的重要依据。只有了解了社区居民的卫生服务需求，才能制定出有效的卫生服务计划。一般来说，卫生服务需求评价应达到以下目的：了解社区居民的一般健康状况；了解社区居民的卫生需要和需求；确定社区内的主要卫生问题以及影响健康的主要危险因素等。

卫生服务需求的评价经常采用调查问卷的方法来收集资料，通过问卷形式一般可收集到丰富而可靠的资料。近年来，国内外不少学者将人类学、社会学等学科的定性研究方法用于社区卫生服务需求评价，取得了良好效果，常用的定性方法有观察法、访谈法等。

(二)根据调查结果，配备相应卫生资源

根据社区居民的卫生服务需求，合理筹集资金、配备社区卫生服务人员以及医疗设备等。

1. 资金筹集。社区卫生服务担负着大量的公共卫生服务项目，这些非个人受益的服务必须由政府来拨款。因此，社区卫生服务的资金筹集应以政府投入为主，兼之以社区卫生服务自身开展的医疗卫生保健等业务费用。

2. 社区卫生服务人员的配备。目前我国的全科医师较为缺乏，因而，社区卫生服务机构不可能都招收医药院校毕业的全科医师，更为快捷的方法是对基层卫生机构中学历较低但实践经验丰富的卫生人员进行培训，以适应社区卫生服务的需要。其他医护人员的上岗也都需接受全科医学和社区护理等相关知识的培训。

3. 医疗设备配备。社区卫生服务机构至少应具有以下基本设备：听诊器、体温计、血压计、血糖仪、急救箱、抢救床、氧气瓶、氧气袋、气管插管、洗胃器、康复器材、健康教育设备、药品柜、档案柜、心电图机、紫外线灯、污物桶、出诊设备、出诊交通工具、电话；备基本药物120种以上，包括常用急救药品和中成药品。

（三）根据居民需求，利用卫生资源，对居民进行服务

社区卫生服务的形式多种多样，各地可根据本社区的具体情况，采取不同的服务形式。一般社区卫生服务形式有以下几种。

1. 在社区卫生服务中心和社区卫生服务站开展工作。
2. 上门服务，通过电话预约、卫生服务小分队等形式服务上门。
3. 社区医生责任制。由一名医生专门负责几个居民区的卫生保健、健康教育、医疗服务等。
4. 医疗咨询热线服务。开通热线电话，提供各类服务包括就医指南、健康心理咨询、联系住院、建立家庭病床等服务。
5. 社区卫生服务合同制。居民与某一医疗人员签订合同，由该医生专门负责自己和家庭的卫生保健，医生则根据合同提供定期或不定期的医疗卫生服务。英国的通科医生一般就是采取这种形式提供服务。

（四）进行社区卫生服务项目评价

各种卫生保健服务的提供并是社区卫生服务的终结，社区卫生服务人员还应开展随访工作，对提供的服务进行评价。评价的目的在于：

（1）确定社区卫生服务所开展的活动的种类、数量，确定所开展的活动是否适合社区居民；

（2）确定社区卫生服务是否达到了预期目标；

（3）发现社区卫生服务运作过程中存在的问题，确定在哪一方面进一步改进；

（4）向有关领导部门提供评价报告，总结所取得的成果及不足之处，提供经验或教训。

第四节　社区卫生服务的可持续发展

一、国内外社区卫生服务发展概况

（一）国外社区卫生服务发展概况

社区卫生服务是20世纪60年代在国外首先实行的，目前许多发达国家如英国、德国、澳大利亚、美国、加拿大等的社区卫生服务均代表了世界先进水平，亚洲开展得比较好的国家是泰国、日本、新加坡等。一般认为，英国的社区卫生服务代表了今后社区卫生服务发展的方向。

综合国外社区卫生服务的发展，一般都具有以下几个共同点：

（1）政府重视。如澳大利亚政府意识到社区卫生服务是减轻财政压力的重要手段，对社区卫生服务给予较大的政策倾斜，不仅从财政上给以支持，而且重点强调对社区卫生

服务的组织和管理,以保证社区卫生服务的规范化和实施效果。

(2) 资金到位。如英国政府每年至少有40%的卫生经费用于社区卫生服务,对社区保健和基层卫生服务的投入比例相当大。

(3) 人员充足。如美国90%以上的医学院设有家庭医学系或科,有300多所医院作为家庭医生(全科医生)的进修学院。英国和德国的全科医生分别占全国医生总数的30%和40%。

(4) 转诊方便。如美国根据疾病诊断治疗分类标准(DRGs),明确规定某种疾病或手术过了一定的康复阶段或住院天数,病人必须转往社区卫生服务机构或回家接受社区卫生服务,否则,超出时间的住院费用由病人自己负担。

(5) 布局合理。如英国卫生法规定,每名全科医生的服务对象为1 800~3 200人,全科医生服务饱和的地区限制其他社区卫生服务机构的设立。对条件较差、服务不足的地区,适当提高卫生服务的报酬,鼓励全科医生开业。

(6) 利用率高。如英国的社区卫生服务占总卫生服务提供的90%,医院服务仅占10%;德国的医院一般不开设门诊部,只提供住院服务,一般的门诊服务由全科医生提供,全科医生与医院建立有转诊和其他业务合同。

(7) 重视老年保健。如日本社区卫生的核心就是老年保健。日本专门实施了针对老年人的"促进老年保健,福利十年计划",简称"黄金计划",采取各种措施加强老年人的健康保健。

(二) 我国社区卫生服务发展概况

社区卫生服务在我国已经得到了重视,1997年《中共中央、国务院关于卫生改革与发展的决定》就明确指出:"改革城市卫生服务体系,积极发展社区卫生服务,逐步形成功能合理、方便群众的卫生服务网络。"1999年卫生部等10部委印发《关于发展城市社区卫生服务的若干意见》,明确规定了社区卫生服务的基本原则、总体目标和相应配套措施。2000年10月和12月,卫生部又相继出台了《城市社区卫生服务基本工作内容(试行)》和《卫生部关于2005年城市社区卫生服务发展目标的意见》,提出了城市社区卫生服务发展的总体目标。可以说,经过近几年的努力,我国发展社区卫生服务的"国家级"的基本宏观政策已经形成。

国家的宏观政策在各地也分别得到了细化和深化。据不完全统计,截至2001年底,全国已有24个省、自治区、直辖市印发了省级社区卫生服务的基本文件。全国31个省市共建有社区卫生服务中心2 593个,社区卫生服务站9 229个,总数达到11 722个。开展社区卫生服务的城市达到308个,近90%的地级城市开展社区卫生服务工作。部分农村地区也在积极探讨发展社区卫生服务的策略和措施。

目前我国社区卫生服务发展比较好的城市有北京、上海、深圳、广州、济南等,它们以国家宏观政策为导向,结合本地实际情况,积极研究、探索发展社区卫生服务的思路,取得了不少成功的经验。如济南的社区卫生服务1996年刚刚起步,如今已在四个城区建立起覆盖全部居委会的社区卫生服务网。

学术界也积极响应国家号召,进行了许多关于社区卫生服务发展的调查研究,既发现了我国社区卫生服务实施过程中存在的一些问题,又提出了许多宝贵的意见,为我国社区卫生服务的发展提供了理论依据。

二、我国社区卫生服务发展过程中存在的问题

尽管我国社区卫生服务的发展取得了不少经验成果,但同时也暴露出了一些问题,这些问题严重制约着我国社区卫生服务的可持续发展。

1. 思想认识上存在偏差。目前我国对社区卫生服务的性质还没有明确定位,一些地方政府对发展社区卫生服务的重要性、紧迫性认识不足,组织领导和推动力度不够,有的地方甚至还没有将社区卫生服务发展提到议事日程。

2. 资金落实不到位。目前我国卫生事业经费的投入主要着力于大型医院建设上,而对社区卫生服务方面的投入不足。尽管国家一再宣传社区卫生服务的重要性,但社区卫生服务的实际发展却不尽人意。

3. 社区卫生服务人员不足。许多医学院校毕业生不愿到基层卫生单位工作,而目前对全科医师的培养又显得不足,致使基层卫生技术人员尤其是全科医生极为缺乏。

4. 功能不到位。社区卫生服务应以健康教育和社区预防为主,但实际上许多地区的社区卫生服务仍仅限于社区医疗这一功能,预防保健工作缺乏经费保障,只能靠医疗收入来补偿,从而出现防保工作无人愿做的现象。

5. 布局不合理。有的地区把社区卫生服务当成一种时髦,一哄而起,一级、二级、三级医院都在搞;有的地区的社区卫生服务站则单纯是医疗机构"伸腿设点"。这些情况致使社区卫生服务站林立,卫生资源设置重复,效率不高。

6. 居民利用少。有的居民缺乏对社区卫生服务具体内容的认知,有的居民由于费用得不到报销而不愿利用社区卫生服务,有的居民则对健康和疾病意识淡薄,宁愿把钱花费在烟酒方面,而不愿接受社区医护人员的健康服务。种种原因导致社区卫生服务利用率低下。

三、我国社区卫生服务的可持续发展

根据国外社区卫生服务发展经验,结合我国社区卫生服务发展过程中暴露出的一些问题,我国社区卫生服务的可持续发展应做到以下几点。

1. 加强政府的领导工作。社区卫生服务是"政府实行一定福利政策的社会公益事业的具体体现",必须由政府来组织实施。政府应将社区卫生服务提到日常议事日程,制定相应的法规政策及配套措施,将社区卫生服务作为社区建设的重要组成部分,纳入社区规划,建立起政府领导、部门协作、街道负责、居委会参与的社区卫生行政管理体制。

2. 给予合理的经济补偿。各级政府应设立一项用于社区卫生服务的专项基金,纳入政府年度财政预算,并明确政府补助的数量。各级卫生行政部门应调整卫生费用的支出结构,对社区卫生服务的预防保健经费一定要落实到位。此外,社区卫生服务可从别的渠道筹集资金,如接受社会团体、慈善机构等的援助,向国际有关组织争取社区卫生服务的项目贷款,等等。

3. 建立合理的社区卫生医疗人员队伍。提高社区卫生服务医护人员的待遇和工资水平,尤其要引进预防保健、健康教育等人才,并保证其生活待遇水平。应加强对全科医

师的培养,各医学院校应开设全科医学专业,培养全科医学人才,以满足社区卫生服务发展的需要。在目前全科医生较为缺乏的情况下,可对一些实践经验丰富的卫生人员进行短期培训,采用半脱产轮训方式,本着缺什么补什么的原则,就地培养,快速合成,以适应目前社区卫生服务的需要。现阶段应把这部分在职人员的培训作为重点。

4. 真正实现社区卫生服务"六位一体"的功能。社区卫生服务应以健康教育和社区预防为主,一定要体现其预防保健的功能,绝不能等同于医院的门诊部。社区卫生服务机构在资金到位的情况下,应把重点放在预防上,做好社区的公共卫生服务工作,减少社区居民的发病机会,提高居民的健康水平。

5. 合理设置社区卫生服务机构。社区卫生服务机构的设置应纳入区域卫生规划,由政府卫生行政部门统一规划布局,在政府有困难的情况下,可鼓励大、中型医院开展社区卫生服务,引导和扶持企事业单位、社会团体、个人等力量举办社区卫生服务机构。

6. 将社区卫生服务纳入基本医疗保险范围。劳动与社会保障部门应把符合要求的社区卫生服务机构作为职工基本医疗保险定点医疗机构,把符合基本医疗保险有关规定的社区卫生服务项目纳入基本医疗保险支付范围,明确规定接受社区卫生服务的费用允许报销。对参保人员在不同级别医疗机构就诊实行不同的个人支付比例,即在社区卫生服务机构就诊的自付比例要低于在大医院就诊的自付比例,以引导居民到社区卫生服务机构就诊,真正实现"小病进社区"的服务宗旨,并逐渐发展形成社区医师首诊制度。

7. 加强对社区卫生服务的宣传,引导居民建立健康的生活方式。利用广播、报纸、电视等宣传媒体向居民宣传社区卫生服务的目的、功能等,使居民对社区卫生服务有一定了解,增加对社区卫生服务的信任,从而主动到社区卫生服务机构就诊。通过健康知识的宣传,使居民增加对健康的投入,主动关注健康,寻求健康。

案例

北京市的社区卫生服务

北京市政府为了促进社区卫生服务发展,主要做了以下工作:

1. 1998年北京市13个部委局共同签署的《关于加快发展社区卫生服务的意见》描述了未来5年的设想。

2. 专门设立了全科医学培训工程,计划三年培训出1 000名全科医生。

3. 让一批二级医院和所有一级医院转换成社区卫生服务中心,把一批散布在社区的小医院门诊部或诊所改造成社区卫生服务站。

4. 北京市卫生局专门订立了一整套"准入制度",包括社区卫生服务项目、基本用药目录、医护人员的岗位管理等,规定社区卫生服务中心要经检收合格了才准许开业。

5. 市政府连续4年每年投资1 800万元进行网点建设和人员培训。各个街道办事处也加大投入。经济较差的宣武区,这几年来也投了350万元,还动员企业等渠道投了560万元。

6. 整合资源,明确分工,逐步实现"大病去医院,小病在社区"的医疗模式。北京市规定,标准的社区卫生服务站应当是医疗、预防、保健、健康教育、康复、计划生育六位一体。

现在，北京有 120 多个社区卫生服务站挂起了计划生育服务站和康复服务站的牌子。

7. 北京鼓励大型综合医院与卫生服务中心建立定点协作支持关系，或成立医疗集团，推行双向转诊制，使大医院和社区医院既相互分工又资源共享。如今，北京已成立了天坛医院、宣武医院、友谊医院等 9 个医院组成的医疗集团。社区看不了的病，社区医生开个条很快就转诊到大医院。

8. 通过管理整合，打破条块分割，北京还推进医疗机构的全行业管理，改变过去企事业单位办医院越办越萎缩的局面。由地方卫生行政部门把企业医院都统起来。例如甜水园社区卫生服务站过去是个工厂医院的门诊部，效益一直较差，实行全行业管理后，达到了社区医院的标准，工作已做得有声有色。

9. 2001 年 2 月印发的《北京市基本医疗保险规定》明确规定：包括社区卫生服务机构在内的一级医院以及家庭病床所发生的医疗费用，个人自付比例普遍分别比二级医院、三级医院低 3 个和 5 个百分点。

通过这些工作，北京市已基本建立了社区卫生服务体系。老百姓对社区卫生服务交口称赞。三里河社区 79 岁的高老说，社区卫生站每年都有一次免费体检，门诊挂号费用只收 5 角，不仅看病方便了，而且健康日历还能进行追踪指导。

老百姓尤其喜欢社区卫生服务机构开展的健康宣传活动。如每月免费赠送的健康杂志，举办的健康讲座；每年发送的健康日历，开展的健康食谱评比等等。通过健康教育，居民的健康知晓率提高了 80%。社区卫生服务机构开展的"一对一"的家庭医生服务改变了原有医患关系。病人可以选择自己的家庭医生，每年的合同费仅为 30 元。家庭医生备有所有的签约病人的健康档案，一旦病人感到身体不适，可以迅速与家庭医生联系。对于行动不便、重病在床的患者，家庭医生会出诊就医，出诊费用仅为 10 元。若病人遇到急诊情况，家庭医生也会及时联系到相关的三级医院，为病人办好入院事宜。许多卫生服务机构都为老年患者设置了专门的服务项目。如复兴卫生服务中心增添的日间住院服务，即针对老年人的生活护理。

思考 1. 结合本案例，谈谈如何进完善社区卫生服务"六位一体"的功能。

思考 2. 如何保持社区卫生服务的持续健康发展？

Chapter 14 Community Health Services

Along with the development of economy and social advancement, bio-psycho-social medical mode has taken the place of traditional biomedical model. People's understanding of health and disease has become deeper than ever. The connotation of health is extending. It has changed from physiological health to the health including physiological, mental and social health. Medical health services mode, which regards disease as center and individual as object, is less and less adapted to social evolving. "Four amplifications" that social medicine raised has been recognized by society gradually. It conceives a new mode of health service called community health that puts the strategy of health and prevention first, and recognizes that everyone should enjoy primary health care. The new mode regards health as center, and population as object. Nowadays, our country's health care faces a lot of new problems, such as aging process speeding up makes it increasingly become urgent problems to be solved that prevent and treat geriatric diseases and chronic noninfectious disease. Along with the medical mode transformation and the strategy that everyone should enjoy health care putting into practice, people's demand on health services becomes higher. Along with the application of high-tech detection and therapeutic methods, medical treatment expenses keep on rising. But this brings very little benefit on human being's health condition as a whole. The cost and benefit is out of balance seriously. Along with the continuoaly dividing of medical specialty, the solutions to the difficulty and complicated case of illness have been broken through continuoaly, but it becomes a widespread problem increasingly that the relation of doctor and patient is apathetic. In dealing with these problems, community health services have incomparable advantage. From the end of the 1980s till now, community health services have gained government's strong promotion and support in our country after a series of practicing, such as recommendation, making propaganda, interchange, research and making experiments, etc. A lot of cities are actively engaged in conduct test and exploration, since the Central Committee of the of the CPC and State Council brought up the opinion of developing community health services in *The Decision of Chinese Communist Party Central Committee* and *The State Council about Health Reform and Development*, in 1997. They achieved certain success and exposed some problems at the same time. In order to solve the specific problems, which met in community health services conduct test, Ministry of Health allied another ten ministries and commissions apart to promulgate *Several Opinions about the Development of City Community Health Services and Some Opinions about Quickening the Development of City community Health*

Services. The documents further promoted community health services development.

Section 1 Concept and Characteristics of Community Health Services

1. Concept of community health services

(1) Community

Community is a regional living federate group, which in certain district, organization based on certain socialist system and social relations, bears common population characteristic. The community is an organic constituent part of society and is a miniature of macro view of society.

Generally, community is composed of five main factors: the crowd that live together, based on certain social relation; the definite district, people engaged in social activity; a whole range of comparative complete living service facilities; special culture background and self-identity of lifestyle; certain living system and administrative setup.

(2) Community health services

The community health services are an important part of the community construction with the leadership of government, attendance of community and guidance of higher health organization, health organization of basic level as main body and general practitioner as main force, by the way reasonably utilizing the community resources and proper technology, with people's health as center, family as unit, community as scope, demand as guidance, mainly open to women, children, old man, chronics and the disabled, with the purpose of solving the major health problem of the community and meeting the basic needs of community services. It has such six functions as prevention, medicine, health care, rehabilitation, health education, technological services for family planning, and provides economical, convenient, integrated and successive services.

The subjects of community health services are all the members in community. They primarily include: ①Patients, including all kinds of chronic disease patients, the patients who demand emergency treatment, common ailment patients, etc. ②Every kind of weak momentum crowds, such as children, women, the aged, disabled, etc. ③High-risk crowd, that is to say, the crowd which have dangerous factors and higher morbidity rate than common crowd, such as the person who has unhealthy habit, for example drug addiction, alcohol abuse; the person who is engaged in dangerous work; the member of high-risk family. ④The sub-healthy crowds, that is to say, the crowds who have no obvious effects, but their physical power, reactive potency and adaptive faculty decline more or less. ⑤The healthy crowds, health means the crowds' body, mind and social adjustment being in good condition in this regard. Community health services regard healthy crowds as service subjects. This reflects the characteristics of putting prevention first adequately.

2. The characteristics of community health services

The community health service is grass-roots medical treatment, faced by community. That is to say, it develops primary health care and the item of the community medicine at the same time, and joins them together into the practice of grass-roots medical treatment.

It has the characteristics as follows:

(1) Systematicness

Putting community health services into practice is a systemic engineering. It includes sanitation departments that provide medical health care and other departments, suchas industry, agriculture, education, and social welfare. It also includes health service receivers — the beneficiaries of medical and health service. The two sides, which connect mutually and influence each other, comprise a system with definite whole aim, being well arranged and connecting each other. And the community health services itself is a subsystem of medical and health service; at the same time, it is a subsystem of community service.

(2) Pedestrianization

Community health service emphasizes the tenet of "person is the most important" and "life is the highest". It doesn't regard patients as the carrier of diseases but persons with individuality and affection. Its concern not only is limited in looking for pathologic problems, it also offers mental, cultural and emotive service. It runs through the whole process of community health service respecting person, caring person, making things convenient for person, and serving person.

Therefore, doctor and patient have a very intimate relation.

(3) Continuity

The community health services run through every stage of human life, and they include from the perinatal period health care, infant health care, child period health care, youth health care and the aged health care to the care of the dying. This adequately reflects that community health services are a continuous service of "from cradle to grave".

(4) Individualization

From the background of community and family, community health services research and solve the problems of individual health and diseases. When patients go to see the doctor, they are regarded as person first, and then as patient. Doctors think and solve patients' problems from aspects of physiology, mind, environment and society.

(5) Comprehensiveness

This characteristic briefly reflects community health services' "all-directions or whole main body", that is to say, as far as service object is concerned, community health services don't differentiate age, sex and the kind of disease; as far as service contents are concerned, community health services include medical treatment, preventive care, rehabilitation and health education; as regard to service level, it includes the individual, family and community; as far as service items are concerned, community health services include all aspects of physiology, mentality and social culture.

(6) Integration

Community health services are an omnibus services, which include medical treatment, prevention, health care, rehabilitation, health education, technical director of family planning, etc.

It emphasizes prevention first, and solves crowd's primary medical demand in community as far as possible.

(7) Harmony

The community health services moderate every department related, and use every kind of resources of society, community departments related and families. It harmonizes other health care systems to fulfill the services of medical health care together, through the measures of consultation and transfer diagnosis. So it is a harmony service.

(8) Accessibility

Accessibility means community health services has many favorable conditions such as convenient and dependable primary medical treatment facilities; permanent medical treatment relationship; effective and efficient reserving system; the service of coming off work, festival and holiday; come-at-able geographical position; knowing well the condition of patients; close relation between the doctor and patient; acceptability on economy.

3. The meaning of developing community health services

(1) Offering basic health service to satisfy the people's increasing demand of health service and to improve the level of people's health.

Community health services, which have wide coverage area and the character of convenience, offer primary health services for the people, and benefits satisfying the people's diversified demands of health services, which keeps on increasing. Community health services emphasize prevention first, combining prevention and treatment. This is benefit to carry out preventive health care in community, family and individual, and is good to increasing crowd's health level.

(2) Community health services are the important foundation of deeper health service reform, establishing city health service system, which adapts to socialist market economy.

Community health services can solve numerous primary health problems of vast residents at grass roots. Positively improving community health services will play an important role in readjusting the organization, function, layout of the urban health services system and increasing the efficiency and reducing the cost, so will it do in forming a new system of urban health services compatible with the reality of socialist primary stage and the socialist market economy, in which the community health services organization acts as the basic unit, the large and medium-size hospital as medical center, the organization of prevention, health care and health education as the center of prevention and health care.

(3) It is the urgent requirement to establish the system of basic medical treatment insurance for the town staffs and workers.

The community health services can help to guarantee receiving the treatment services of the common diseases, disease of frequent occurrence and chronic, and reasonably utilizing the services of large-sized hospital. It can also increase the employees' health and reduce their disease incidence by offering health education and prevention and health care. Therefore, it not only ensures the basic health medicine but reduces the cost, which is in accord ance with the principle of "low level but wide coverage" and of supporting importance in ensuring the lasting stable development of the basic medical insurance system for employees.

(4) It is benefit to enhance the development of socialism spirited civilization, to build closer relations between the party and crowd, cadre and crowd, to maintain social stability.

The workers of community health services build up a new relation with most of residents, through offering multiple kinds of service to solve the crowd's problems. This is benefit to enhance the socialism spirited civilization developments. Carrying out community health services positively is a project with benevolent rule and popular feelings, which does good deed and actual work for the people. It reflects the tenet of serving the people whole-heartedly and adequately, benefits to increase the relation between the party and the people and the relation between cadres and the people, supports the social stability, promotes the national long-term peace and stability.

Section 2 The Function of Community Health Services

According to the document of *Some Opinions About Developing City Community Health Services*, which was made by ten ministries and commissions, community health services should have six-in-one function. "six" refers to the six functions: health education, community prevention, community health care, community treatment, community rehabilitation and family planning conduct; "Integration" refers to offering synthetical and continuous service.

Chapter 14 Community Health Services

1. Health education

Health education means stimulating people to adopt healthy behavior and lifestyle voluntarily by information communication and behaviors intervention, which eliminate or lessen unhealthy dangerous factors and prevent diseases, promote health and improve life quality.

The health education needs to link up the general prevention of the whole crowds and the stress prevention of high-risk crowds. It develops the health education faced by the whole crowds, instructs the resident rectifying their bad behavior and lifestyle, while making clear the emphasis object of health education, eliminating unhealthy factors lying in the high-risk crowds.

In addition, health education should cooperate with the higher departments' propagandizing and education of vaccination, voluntary blood donation, generating health activities, and prevention of social diseases, etc.

The health education should have scientific spirit, aim spirit, suggestive spirit, directive spirit and flexible spirit, and can't in brief preach, should as far as possible cause the crowd's interest, at last achieve the target of change of "knowledge-belief-behaviour", namely, let people form the right conceptual of health through the health knowledge's spreading, then change their bad behaviour lifestyle.

2. Community prevention

(1) Community health diagnosis. Community health diagnosis is to understand the health condition of the crowd in a certain time and area, the relationship between diseases and health and related influence factors as well.

In order to solve the primary problems in community, it is necessary to make and carry out the working plan of community health, community health diagnosis, understand the residents' health condition and the main dangerous factors which affect residents' health, and understand residents' primary demand of health service, under the guidance of health administrative departments and the leadership of community regulatory agency such as sub-district office and resident committee.

(2) Disease prevention

Prevention aims primarily to common ailments, frequently occurring diseases, infectious diseases, endemic diseases, parasitical diseases, professional sickness, chronic noninfectious diseases and mental diseases, etc.

The primary measure includes:

①Waging the work of preventive inoculation, such as planed immunity.

②The legal infectious disease's registering and reporting system should be carried out strictly.

③When infectious diseases become prevalent, we should cooperate with the related departments to deal with the epidemic situation, control and eradicate the infectious diseases' occurrence and spread.

④Carry out community prevention of infectious diseases, endemic diseases, and parasitic diseases.

⑤Do well diagnosing, registering and reporting work of occupational diseases.

⑥Monitor the patients of chronic diseases, do the work of health guidance and behavior interference well.

⑦Mental health propaganda and education work should be carried out.

⑧Mental patients should be discovered and treated in time, and the mental patients who are in the period of rehabilitation should have effective custody.

3. Community health care

(1) The special crowds' health care

Women, children and the aged are the primary subjects of the health care. Women health care primarily includes the perinatal period health care, antenatal care, postpartum care, climacteric care and screening of common gynopathy. Children health care primarily includes neonates care, infant health care, preschooler period health care, school age period health care and prevention of unexpected injury, etc. The aged health care primarily includes knowing the health condition of the aged, guiding the aged carrying out health care of by themselves and preventing the occurrence of accident and suicide, etc.

(2) Mental health care

The community health services should do a good work of mental health care, make the residents who have mental problems get mental guidance in time and improve their mental health, make community residents have good mental quality. In addition, it should improve mental health care work in special period. For example, in the prevalent period of SARS, it has important meaning to conquer SARS that community health services carries out mental propagandizing and guiding, alleviates mental panic, promotes resident's mental health

4. Community treatment

There are four primary contents. Community treatment includes:

(1) Providing the medical services to common diseases, frequently occurring diseases and the chronic diseases that have been diagnosed clearly.

(2) Treating the difficult and complicated disorders appropriately, doing well the work of reference of the patients who can't be diagnosed doubtlessly.

(3) Doing well the work of spot rescue to dangerous patients, emergency patients

and serious patients.

(4) Providing the family medical treatment, which includes visiting patients at home, family nursing, family sickbed, etc.

5. The community rehabilitation

According to the definition of WHO, community rehabilitation is implementing complete rehabilitation on the basis of medical rehabilitation in the city and town's community, through mobilizing and harmonizing the related departments, all the members the families, exploiting and utilizing community resource adequately. What is called all-round rehabilitation includes four levels, namely medical rehabilitation, educational rehabilitation, and social rehabilitation.

Medical rehabilitation is that community health services apply medical technique, carry out functional diagnosis, treatment, training and prevention to reach the aim of making chronic disease patient, disabled persons and the aged achieve psychosomatic rehabilitation.

Educational rehabilitation is to make condition for rehabilitation objects taking part in social living and adapting to social demand. Community health services carry out moral education, cultural education, vocational technical education and common education to rehabilitation objects, carry out special education to the mentally disabled, eyesight, audition and language, under the guidance of rehabilitation medicine.

Occupational rehabilitation is solving the problem of rehabilitation subjects' employment through vocational consultation, occupational ability test, vocational education before work and installation, etc.

Social rehabilitation is that community health services, through the society and rehabilitation subjects' endeavor together, maintain rehabilitation objects' dignity and rights, create advantageous condition to make rehabilitation objects enjoy equal treatment in social living, such as education, marriage, housing and amusement, and make rehabilitation objects take part in social living adequately and achieve their self-worth.

6. Family planning conduct

The purpose of family planning conduct is urging people to attain prepotency and well raising, then increasing the quality of the race. It can adopt measures as follows:

(1) Premarital check. Lineal relatives or collateral relatives by blood within three generations should be forbidden to marry. Patients, who are afflicted with STD (sexually transmitted diseases), mental diseases and certain kind of legal infectious diseases in prescript period of quarantine, should be dissuaded from getting married. Some patients of hereditary diseases can get married, but should be dissuaded from bearing children.

(2) Under the premise of knowing and selecting, the husband and wife are guided to

contraceptives and execute birth control. (3) Providing prophylactic and correlative consultation service. The husband and wife's comprehension about the knowledge of marriage and bearing children can be increased, through propaganda and education.

Section 3 The Organization and Operation of Community Health Services

1. The organization of the community health services

There are various organization forms of community health services in China at present, but they have the same contents despite of their different forms. Their ultimate aim is to achieve the function of community health services.

Therefore, although there are various organization forms of community health services in different districts they usually follow the principles as follows:

(1) Led by government and joined by many departments. Community health services should be led by government and supported by other related departments. The local governments should establish and coordinate organization of community health services, and the departments of health, finance, commodities price, labor and society security, civil administration, personnel, etc, ought to fulfill their duties to consummate the policy and measures concerned and to harmonize and solve the problems and difficulties in the course of community health services' development.

(2) The layout of community health services organization should be set reasonably. The establishment of community health services organization should be set according to local population density, health demand, geography, etc. Some expert suggests that the radius within 0.7 – 1.0 kilometer is appropriate to community health services, and certain distance between community hospitals and other medical organizations should be kept.

(3) Medical personnel should be staffed reasonably. Two general practitioners should be staffed among per 10,000 people on the condition that the general practitioners are scanty in China at present. And the proportion of general practitioners to community nurses should not be lower than 1 : 2. Other technical personnel such as stomatologic doctors, rehabilitation treatment doctors and social workers are supposed to be prepared according to actual need.

(4) The equipment of basic facilities. The operational housing, bed, basic equipments, frequently-used drugs and first-aid drugs of community health services organization should be equipped according to the function of community health services and the demand of residents.

(5) Improving all kinds of management system. The improvement of management

system primarily includes the systems of training, management, check and rewards and punishments to the medical personnel; the preventive system of service mistake and accidents; the system of consultation and double-direction transfer reference; the management system of finance, drugs and equipments; the management system of files and informational data; the system of quality management and check evaluation of community health services, etc.

2. The operation of community health services

The community health services are different from clinic, and their operations differ from the previous forms of "doctoring in room". The operation of community health services is a systematic and complicated process, which needs the cooperation of many departments to realize its function. It generally includes four steps as follows:

(1) evaluating the demand of health services

It is a premise of operation of community health services and an important basis of allotting health personnel and deploying health resources. An efficient health services plan cannot be established unless the health services demand of residents in community is acquainted. The evaluation of health services demand, generally speaking, is supposed to realize the purposes as follows: understand the general health conditions and health demand and need of residents in community; make sure the cardinal health problems and main risk factors which influence health, etc.

The evaluation of health services demand usually adopts the method of questionnaire to collect data, and through this method generally can collect the abundant and incredible data. In recent years, some scholars at home and abroad adopted qualitative research methods which are used in anthropology and sociology, etc., to appraise community health services demand and obtain the good effect; the frequently used qualitative research methods include observational method and interview method, etc.

(2) equipping corresponding health resources according to the inquisition consequence

Personnel and medical equipments for community health services should be financed and prepared according to health services demand of community residents.

①Financing. Community health services assume a large quantity of public health services, which are supposed to be allocated funds by governments. Therefore, the financing of community health services should mainly be by the way of governments input, and secondly by the operation expenses carried by community health services themselves.

②Staffing the community health services. Community health services organization cannot all recruit general practitioners graduating from medical colleges, for the general practitioners are still scanty in China at present, and the more efficient method is to train the medical personnel with low academic qualification and plenty to experiences in basic level health organization to meet the demand of community health services. The employment of other medical or nursing personnel also need the knowledge of training concerned, such as general medicine or community nursing, etc.

③Equipping armamentarium. The community health services organization should have at least the basic equipments as follows: Stethoscope, clinical thermometer, blood pressure meter, blood sugar meter, first-aid kit, rescue bed, oxygen bottle, oxygen bag, trachea cannula, stomach pump, rehabilitation device, health education equipments, drugs cabinet, file cabinet, cardiogram machine, ultraviolet ray light, filth bucket, equipments and vehicles for visiting patients at home, telephone; Basic drugs above 120 kinds, including frequently used first-aid drugs and Chinese medicinal preparation.

(3) supplying services for residents using health resources according to their demand

Each local community should adopt various servicing forms according to local actual conditions in view of the variety of community health services.

The forms of community health services generally include several kinds as follows:

①Working at community health services centers or community health services stations.

②Service at home by the forms of telephone appointment and health services in small groups, etc.

③Community doctors responsibility system. One doctor is in special charge of health cares, health education, medical services of several residential quarters.

④The hot-line services for medical consultation. The hot-line telephone should be open to supply various services such as hospitalizing guide, health mental consultation, connecting to hospitalization, establishing family sickbed, etc.

⑤The contract system of community health services. Residents can contact with some medical personnel who specially preside over themselves and their family's health care, and the doctor supplies medical health services periodically or non-periodically according to contact. General practitioners in England usually supply services by this form.

(4) evaluating the items of community health services

The offering of various health care services is not the end of community health services; the community health services personnel should carry out follow-up work to evaluate the offered services.

The purpose of evaluation is:

①Making certain the categories, quantity of activities waged by community health services, and making sure whether the activities are appropriate to residents in community;

②Ensuring the community health services come to the expected target;

③Discovering problems in the course of operation of community health services and ascertaining which facet needs to be improved;

④Offering evaluation reports to leading departments concerned, and summing up the acquired success and deficiency to supply experiences or lessons.

Section 4 The Sustainable Development of Community Health Services

1. The general situation of community health services at home and abroad

(1) The general situation of foreign community health services

Community health services were first put into practice at abroad in the 1960's, and nowadays the community health services in many developed countries such as Britain, Germany, Australia, the United States, Canada, and some Asian countries represent the world advanced level; in Asia, community health services developed well in Thailand, Japan, Singapore, etc. Community health services in Britain, generally considered, represent the direction of development of community health services in the future.

The development of overseas community health services generally bears some common characters as follows:

①The consideration of government. For example, Australian government is aware that community health services are important ways to alleviate financial pressure, so they give community health services a great policy support, not only supporting it in finance, but also emphasizing the organization and management to community health services to guarantee the standardization and actualized effect of community health services.

②The offer of funds. For example, British government inputs at least 40% of health outlay to community health services every year. It is a great proportion of input to community care and gross-root health services.

③The plentitude of personnel. For instance, in above 90% of medical colleges in the United States are departments of family medicine, and in about 300 hospitals are postgraduate colleges for family practitioners or general practitioners. General practitioners in England and Germany accounted respectively for 30% and 40% of the total amount of national doctors.

④The convenience of transfer to another hospital. The United States, for example, prescribes definitely that the patients must transfer to community health services organization or go home to receive community health services when some diseases or operations have reached certain recovering stage or hospitalization days. Otherwise, the expenses beyond fixed time in hospital should be paid by patients themselves, according to diagnosis related groups (DRGs).

⑤ The reasonable layout. English health status ruled that one general practitioner serve people within 1800 – 3200, and the community health services are restricted to be established in the area with a saturated services. And the rewards of health services are increased to encourage general practitioners to practice in the area with bad conditions and scanty services.

⑥ The high utilization rate. The community health services in England account for about 90% of all the health services supplies, and the hospital services account only for 10%. The hospitals in Germany generally do not set up outpatient departments, but only provide hospitalization services, and the general practitioners who contract with hospitals at transfer diagnosis and other professional works offer the general outpatient services.

⑦ Paying attention to senile cares. For example, the center of community health in Japan is senile cares. Japan exclusively carried out the "the decade welfare plan to promotion of senile cares" which was called for short "gold plan" aiming at the aged. They take various measures to improve senile health cares.

(2) The general situation of the development of community health services in our country

The community health services are valued in China. *The Decision of Chinese Communist Party Central Committee and The State Council about Health Reform and Development* in 1997 has already pointed out definitely that "Reform health services systems in cities, develop actively community health services, and form gradually the health services network with the reasonable function and convenience for the masses." The ten Ministries and Commissions including Ministry of Health printed and distributed *Several Opinions about the Development of City Community Health Services* in 1999 which make clear the essential principle, overall target and corresponding counterpart measures of community health services. In October and December, 2000, the Ministry of Health went on to publish *The Basic Work Contents of Community Health Services (try out)* and *Some Opinions about Quickening the Development of City Community Health Services*, which brought out overall object about development of community health services. It can be said that the "national-level" basic macro-policy about developing community health services in China has been formed after several years' endeavors.

And the national macro-policy has been applied carefully and deeply in many districts. About 24 provinces, autonomous regions or municipalities directly under the central government have printed and distributed province-level basic documents about community health services by the end of 2001, according to incomplete statistics. The 31 provinces, autonomous regions or municipalities in China established totally 2,593 community health services centers and 9,229 community health services stations, and the sum reached 11,722. The cities that develop community health services amount to 308, and about 90% of the municipalities carry out community health services working. A part of villages are also probing into the policies and measures actively as to the development of community health services.

The cities in China whose community health services develop well at present mainly include Beijing, Shanghai, Shenzhen, Guangzhou, Ji'nan, etc. These cities research and probe into the methods of developing community health services actively under the guide of national macro-policy and considering their local actual conditions, and they have got many successful experiences. The community health services in Jinan, for example, have established the community health services net covering the total residents committees in four city zones since the beginning in 1996.

The academic circles, enthusiastically responding to national policy, carried out many surveys and researches about the development of community health services in academic concern, discovering some problems in the course of implementing community health services and bringing forward many valuable opinions, which offer the theoretical base for the development of community health services in our country.

2. The problems in the process of the development in domestic community health services

In spite of a few experiences obtained during the development of Chinese community health services, there are still some underlying problems, which roughly restrict its sustainable development.

(1) The deviation of the thought. At present, owing to the lack of the clear definition of the property of community health services, some local governments fail to understand the importance, urgency of community health services and effectively organize, lead and push it, with some regions even not putting it on the agenda.

(2) Without the arrival of the funds. At present, our country inputs the health budget primarily on the establishment of large hospital, but pays less attention to community health services. Although China again and again publicized the importance of community health services, its development is dissatisfactory.

(3) There is the lack of community health services personnel. The graduate students of many medical colleges are reluctant to work in grass-roots health unit. There is scarce education of the general doctors. This leads to the lack of the health technical personnel, particularly the general practitioners.

(4) Its function does not show perfectly. More attention should paid to health edu-

cation and community prevention of community health services, but actually just to community medical treatment in many regions, and the funds of preventive health care work are not guaranteed and only compensated by the medical treatment income, which all result in the phenomenon that nobody wish to take on the prevention and health care work.

(5) Unreasonable layout. Taking community health services as a kind of fashion, the hospitals at all levels in some regions rush headlong into mass action, including that of first level, second level, third level. In some regions, the community health services station is purely the outspread part of the medical treatment organization. These circumstances mentioned above lead to the great numbers of the community health services station, the repetitive establishment of the health resources and the efficiency is not high.

(6) Few residents make use of it. Some residents do not understand the concrete contents of community health services, some are reluctant to take advantage of it because the expenses can not compensated, and some lack the clear understanding of health and disease. So they would rather spend money on cigarette and wine than make use of the health service of the community medical personnel. All kinds of reasons cause the low utilization of community health services.

3. The sustainable development of our country's community health services

In light of the experience according to the foreign community health services and considering some problems exposed in the process of the development of our country's community health services, the following should be attained:

(1) Enhancing the leading work of government

Community health services indicates "the concrete embodiment of a social and public-spirited business carried out by the government with certain welfare policy now". So it must be organized into practice by the government. Government should put the community health services on the agenda of usual matter, establish relevant law and policy and complementary measures, take the community health services as the main part of the community development and bring it into the community programming and establish an executive administration system for community health with the guidance of government, cooperation of the various sections, responsibility of the street, attendance of the reside committee.

(2) Giving it the reasonable economic compensation

The governments at all levels should establish a special fund used for the community health services, bring it into the annual financial budget of government, and fix on the clear amount of government subsidy. The health executive of all levels should readjust the expenditure construction of the health expenses, and ensure the preventive health care budget community health services in its place. In addition, we can raise the funds from other ways, such as accepting the assistance of social group and charitable institution, striving for the item loan of community health services from relevant international organization, etc.

(3) Establishing a reasonable group of community health medical personnel. Increase the treatment and wages of the community health personnel, specially introduce the talent of the prevention and health care and health education and guarantee their treatment. We should enhance the education of general practitioners, and general medicine should be set up in each medicine college to exclusively educate the general practitioners. To solve the problem of lack of general practitioner, we can offer short-term training to some health personnel with practical skills, with the rotating form, the principle of supplying the lack, and train them right on the spot and attain fast efficiency, to adapt to the current demand of community health services. In present stage, we should pay more attention to the training of this part of personnel on the job.

(4) Actually fulfiling the function of community health services, "integrative whole of six functions". Health education and community prevention are the major part of the community health services. So the function of prevention and health care must show, and it must not act like the hospital's out-patient department. On the condition of the arrival of the funds, the community health services organization should take the prevention as the emphasis and complete the work about community health services, reduce the disease incidence of the community resident, and increase the resident's health level.

(5) Reasonably establishing the organization of community health services. The establishment of community health services organization should come on the coverage of the district health programming, and be systematically planned and laid out by government and health executive. If the government has difficulty, we can encourage the large- and medium-sized hospital to develop community health services, and lead and support the enterprise and government unit, social group, individual and other power to hold the community health services organization.

(6) Making community health services run under the coverage of the basic medical insurance. The section of labor and social guarantee should make the community health services organization of conformity become the fixed-point medical treatment organization of basic medical insurance for employees, and the service item of conformity under the coverage of the payment of basic medical insurance, with the clear provision that the expenses on the community health services can be sent in account. Different proportions of individual payment are taken for those insured to the medical organization of different levels, namely, the proportion of individual payment to the community health services organization is lower than that to that of the big hospital. According to the aim that leads residents to the community health services organization and really realizing "those with small illness to the community", a first-diagnosis system by community doctor will

gradually come in forth.

(7) Enhancing the publicity of community health services, guide the resident to establish healthy lifestyle. Make use of such medium as broadcast, newspaper, television to publicize the purpose and function and so on of community health services, in order to make the resident get certain understanding of community health services and enhance their trust in community health services and see a doctor to community health services organization on their own. By publicizing the health knowledge, we can make the resident increase input on health and actively concern and look after health.

Case Example

Community health serices in Beijing

In order to promote the development of community health services, Beijing Municipality has primarily done some work as follows:

1. In 1998, thirteen departments in Beijing signed together the file *Some Opinions about Quickening the Development of Community Health Services*, which described the assumption in the coming 5 years.

2. Established specially the training project of general practitioner, intending to train 1,000 general practitioners in three years.

3. Switched some gradetwo hospitals and all grade one hospitals to community health services center and transformed a batch of small hospital out-patient departments or clinics which scattered in community into the community health services station.

4. The bureau of public health of Beijing made specially a whole set of "admittance system", including the community health services items, basic medical catalogue, the post management of medical personnel, etc., and ordered that community health services center could not practice until checked.

5. Municipality invested 18 million Yuan to net construction and personnel training per year for four years on end. And each district also increased input. Xuanwu District, whose economy was poor, invested 3.5 million Yuan in recent years and mobilized the business enterprises to invest 5.6 million Yuan.

6. Integrated resources and divided the work definitely to realize gradually the medical model of "serious diseases in the hospital and ailments in community". Beijing prescribed that the standard community health services should offer such services as medical treatment, prevention, health care, health education, rehabilitation, and technical director of family planning. At present, more than 120 community health services stations in Beijing have set up the brand of family planning services and rehabilitation services.

7. Encouraged the large polyclinics and health service centers to establish the fixed cooperation and supporting relation, or to unite to medical group, carrying out the system of double-direction transfer diagnosis and making the polyclinics and community hospitals divide the work and share the resources. For the moment, Beijing has already established nine medical groups, such as Tiantan Hospital, Xuanwu Hospital, Youyi Hospital, etc. By signing community doctors will transfer the patients who cannot be diagnosed or cured in community to polyclinic quickly.

8. Broke the situation of respective partition through the management integration, advanced industry-wide management in medical institute, and changed the situation that enterprises units set up hospitals but became more and more terrible in the past. The local health administrative departments, however, control all the enterprise hospitals. Tianshuiyuan community health services station is a policlinic of factory hospital in the past whose benefits were always bad; at present, it has reached the standard of community hospital after carrying out industry-wide management and done their work very well.

9. The *Primary Medical Insurance Rule in Beijing* printed in February, 2001, prescribed definitely that individual medical expenses spending on grade-one and family sickbed including the community health services organization are lower, 3% and 5% respectively, than grade two hospitals and grade three hospitals.

Beijing has set up primarily community health services system by these works. Civilians all applaud community health services. Mr. Gao, who aged 79 and lived in Sanlihe community, said that community health station offered free medical examination every year, and that the register fare in ambulant clinic was only 0.5 Yuan, which was very convenient for seeing a doctor. What's more, the health calendar can make trace for guiding the patients.

Residents especially are fond of health propaganda carried out by community health services organizations, such as the free presentation of health magazine and the course of health lectures per month, the given health calendars and healthy cookbook appraising through comparison every year, etc. The residents' understanding rate about health has added by 80% through health education. The "one-to-one" family doctor service, carried out by community health services organizations, changed the relation between doctors and patients formerly. Patients can choose their own family doctors, and the contract fee is only 30 Yuan every year. Family doctors have all health files of the patients who contact with them, and the patients can contact with their family doctors quickly once they feel uncomfortable. And the family doctors will visit the patients whose activities are difficult or the patients who were ill at their home, and the fare for visiting is only 10

Yuan. When patients encounter emergency, family doctors will contact the related grade three hospitals in time, and finish the hospitalization procedures. Many health service organizations set specialized service item for the old. For example, the daytime hospitalization services added by Fuxing Health Service Center are aiming at the life nursing of the old.

Discussion:

1. Please discuss how to perfect the "six-in-one" function of community health services combining with this case.

2. Think: how to keep the sustainable and healthily development of community health services?

第十五章 社会保障制度

第一节 社会保障制度概述

一、社会保障的定义及特点

"社会保障"(social security)一词首先使用于1935年美国"新政"中的《社会保障法》。国际劳工组织于1944年在美国费城召开的第26届国际劳工大会上发表了著名的《费城宣言》,提出要"扩大社会保障措施"。从此,社会保障这个概念逐渐被广泛使用。

一般说来,社会保障是以国家政府为主体,依据法律规定,对国民收入进行再分配,为社会成员暂时或永久失去劳动能力及因为各种原因造成生活困难时,提供维持最低生活水准,保证基本生活的制度。

社会保障具有以下五个特点:强制性、社会性、福利性、互济性和不可逆性。

1. 强制性。社会保障的强制性集中表现在强制参加和强制缴纳两方面,即每一位社会成员只要符合社会保障的有关法律规定,都必须参加社会保障并受其保障;凡符合有关社会保障税法或社会保险基金统筹法令、法规的缴纳条件的个人和团体,都必须按要求纳税和交费,否则将追究其法律责任。

2. 社会性。社会保障作为强制性、普遍性的社会"安全网",是现代大生产的产物,是典型的社会行为。社会保障的保障对象不是社会的少数人,而是全体社会成员。社会保障制度的覆盖面愈大,其抵御风险的能力愈强,这就是人们所说的"大数法则"。

3. 福利性。社会保障的各环节不以赢利为目的,它不仅无偿地对被保障人给予资金给付,而且提供社会服务。而保障的个人一般不直接交付全部保障费用,由实施的社会保障部门统一筹集经费,既有政府财政的部分,也有企业和个人缴纳的部分,还包括社会各方面的捐赠。

4. 互济性。社会保障有以丰补歉、同舟共济的特点,即通过所有成员的互助共济实现对少数遭遇风险成员的收入损失等的补偿。

5. 不可逆性。众所周知,社会保障的给付带有特别强的不可逆性,或曰刚性。一旦将社会保障水平确定在一个较高的水准之上,要将其降下来是十分困难的。西欧大多数国家推行的高保障、高福利制度,如今暴露出越来越多的弊端。20世纪80年代以来,这些国家为减轻政府财政压力,陆续进行了社会保障改革,以期削减保障项目和福利开支。但所有这些改革最后终因民众的强烈反对而搁浅。社会保障的不可逆性,要求社会保障的水平必须与社会生产力的发展水平相适应,否则就会产生一系列的社会和经济问题。

二、社会保障制度的内容

社会保障制度的内容在划分方法和项目设置上各国有所不同,一般来说,主要包括社会保险、社会救济、社会福利、社会优抚和社会互助。其中,社会保险是社会保障的核心部分,社会福利是社会保障的最高层次,社会救济是社会保障最基础、最底线的部分。

(一)社会保险

社会保险是国家通过立法,对劳动者在暂时或永久丧失劳动能力,或虽有劳动能力而无收入来源的情况下,给予一定的收入补偿,使之能够维持基本生活的保障制度。社会保险主要面对劳动者,也有个别国家面对全体国民。社会保险的项目一般包括养老保险、医疗保险、工伤保险、失业保险、生育保险等,是社会保障中承担风险最多、占用资金最大的部分。社会保险是一种强制缴费制的社会保障,实行权利与义务相关的原则。一般说来,各国保险待遇水平的差别主要取决于本国社会生产力的发展水平,一国内部不同劳动者的待遇水平也因为个人贡献和缴费等情况不同而有差异。

(二)社会救济

社会救济是国家和社会对无力维持最低生活的社会成员给予救助的社会保障制度。社会救济分为贫困救济和灾害救济,前者救济那些没有劳动能力又无依无靠的孤儿、残疾人、老人等没有生活来源者和虽有劳动能力但收入低于法定最低生活标准的人,后者救济那些因遭受洪水、地震等自然灾害或战争等社会灾害而暂时无法维持基本生活的人。社会救济保障的是公民的基本生存,是社会保障的"最后一道防线"。

(三)社会福利

社会福利的概念有广义和狭义之分。广义社会福利主要包括政府提供的文化教育、公共卫生、公共娱乐、市政建设、家庭补充津贴、教育津贴、住房津贴等公共福利事业,目的是提高整个社会的福利水平;狭义的社会福利主要包括老人、儿童、妇女、青少年、残疾人等特殊人群的福利,目的是对需要社会特别关怀的人群提供必要的政府和社会援助,改善他们的生活。社会福利不仅是保障公民的最低生活需要,更多的是保障人民的生活随着生产力的发展而得到改善,不仅是物质上的改善,也有精神、文化上的改善。

(四)社会优抚

社会优抚主要包括向烈属、军属、复员退伍军人、残废军人提供抚恤金、优待金、补助金以及举办荣誉军人疗养院和光荣院、安置复员转业军人、为军队离退休干部提供服务等,目的是安定军心,维护国家安全。

(五)社会互助

社会互助是受到政府鼓励和支持的社会各界自愿的公益性扶弱济困活动。

三、社会保障的功能和作用

(一)社会保障的功能

1. 补偿功能。社会保障的补偿功能是指劳动者和其他社会成员在因风险暂时或永久失去收入时必须获得一定程度的经济补偿或物质帮助。社会保障的补偿功能,主要体现在社会救助和社会保险两个方面,社会保险尤为明显。社会保障主体筹集起来的社会保障资金,用于部分社会成员的损失补偿,这是保险的原理"集众多的力量,分担个别意外的损失"。

2. 稳定功能。稳定功能是社会保障的第一功能。社会保障的稳定功能是指社会保障依法对社会成员的基本生活权利予以保障,它通过国民收入再分配调节人们的物质利益关系,从而发挥社会稳定机制的作用。社会保障在西方被称为"安全网"、"社会内稳定器"。

3. 调节功能。现代社会保障作为国家实施的重要社会政策,是调节收入、缩小贫富差距、缓和社会矛盾的重要手段。采取的基本措施是,一方面以累进的方式向高收入阶层(如雇主)征收社会保险基金,另一方面以累进的方式向贫困者提供资助,收入越少的人得到的越多。另外,社会保险基金的筹集、支付及其投资活动,本身就是一种国民收入分配和再分配活动,它必然会对国民经济的运行产生调节作用。

(二)社会保障的作用

社会保障的作用,是社会保障功能的具体表现,是社会保障功能发挥出来的效果。如今,社会保障对于我国社会经济持续发展的作用越来越大,主要表现在:第一,社会保障制度的建立和实施,为我国新时期劳动、人事制度的改革创造了重要条件,从而加快了我国劳动力资源的合理流动和优化配置。第二,劳动者有了社会保障,解除了后顾之忧,生产积极性必然得到激发,从而有利于劳动生产力的提高和全社会的经济增长。第三,社会保障有利于控制人口的过快增长和缓解人口老龄化的压力。中国有"养儿防老"的传统观念,这就不可避免地造成了人口的过快增长。社会保障制度的建立和完善可以较好地解决老年人口的生活保障问题。这一目标的实现,必然会淡化传统的养老观念,从而提高人们实行计划生育的自觉性。第四,社会保障体现了人与人之间的互助共济行为,体现了权利和义务相结合的关系,从而推进了精神文明的建设。第五,社会保障制度的建立,增进了人的平等,维护了社会公正。如实施城镇居民最低生活保障制度,使那些不能达到当地最低生活保障线标准的城镇居民能够在社会中继续生存下去。

第二节 中国城镇职工医疗保险制度改革

一、国外医疗保险模式

医疗保险是随着工业革命而产生的。当时工人们为了规避疾病的风险,在行会中产生了"保险基金",即工人交纳一定的费用,类似储蓄,当他们生病时再使用这笔储蓄款。世界上第一个国家医疗保险是于1893年由德国实施的。当时的首相俾斯麦出于政治考虑而推出了这项政策,即《疾病社会保险法案》。1911年,英国建立了国家卫生计划。1980年,几乎所有的发达国家都建立了覆盖所有公民的医疗保险,如英国的国家卫生服务(national health service,NHS)、加拿大的全民保险计划(universal insurance plan)等等。迄今为止,国外医疗保险制度历经百余年的发展与演变,目前其模式主要有四种类型。

(一) 商业医疗保险

以美国为代表。保险以市场为导向,自由买卖,自愿投保,自由选择。保险是依仗投保人群分担疾病风险,医疗保险公司充当了供需双方之外的第三方。由于供需双方都追求效用极大化,容易造成费用膨胀,也会刺激医疗技术的发展,促进新技术和新药的利用。在保险市场中存在着各种"逆选择"(adverse selection)和"道德损害"(normal hazard)。为了提高效率,管理型医疗保健(managed care)应运而生,成为美国医疗改革的方向。为了提高公平性,美国通过类似国家医疗保险和社会医疗保险的"医疗照顾"(medicare)和"医疗救助"(medicaid)计划,向老人、穷人和儿童提供医疗保障。

(二) 社会医疗保险

以德国、加拿大、日本等国为代表。这种模式通过国家立法,强制缴费,但具体保险的运作方式不求统一,国家自行管理或委托保险机构实施管理,管理层次多,管理难度大。在德国,全国有1 214个疾病基金负责筹集保险金和通过医师协会支付医疗提供者,它们是非政府、非营利机构。筹资均来自雇主、雇员,按工资或收入的一定比例提取,筹资稳定,共济程度高。超过政府确定的工资上限的部分高薪人群参加私人保险。政府在医疗保险的筹资、组织和管理中起重要作用。

(三) 国家医疗保险

以英国(国家卫生服务)为代表。通过税收筹资,变"费"为"税",法律的约束性更强。政府直接参与医疗服务的筹资、计划、管理、分配与提供,通过拨款补偿供方,免费消费,覆盖全体居民,福利程度高。这种体系计划性强,卫生总费用上涨相对较慢,但缺乏市场机制,效率低下,另外,国家财政负担很重,而纳税人和筹资者甚至矛盾激化。1991年,英国引入"内部市场"的竞争机制,一部分持有资金的通科医生可以代表病人的利益,通过转诊向医院购买服务,医院和医务人员以及通科医生之间形成了竞争。

(四) 储蓄性医疗保险

以新加坡为代表。它有保险储蓄(medisure)、健保双全(medishield)(补偿大病保险)和保健基金(medifund)(贫苦居民医疗救助)等不同计划。所谓保险储蓄,是全国性强制储蓄计划,按工资总额的一定比例缴费,不同年龄的储蓄缴费率为工资收入的6%～8%不等。这些保险费大部分进入了个人的医疗储蓄账户,可以支付本人和亲人的住院开销和某些大病门诊治疗。每个人年轻时为年老储蓄资金,为子女和家庭积累资金,每个家庭、一代和几代人之间,以足够长的时间连续分担疾病风险。付费有顶限、每日提款限额,一般只支付基本医疗服务费等。雇主和雇员的储蓄为医疗基金,政府负担轻,但社会共济程度差。

二、中国城镇职工医疗保险制度改革的背景:公费、劳保医疗保障制度

中国传统医疗制度主要由机关事业单位的公费医疗、城镇国有集体企业的劳保医疗

和农村合作医疗三部分组成。其主体部分是面向城镇职工的公费医疗与劳保医疗。

职工医疗保障制度创立于20世纪50年代初期,有两大组成部分:一是公费医疗,主要对象为机关、事业单位工作人员,革命伤残军人和大学生,其经费来源于各级财政拨款。二是劳保医疗,主要对象是国有企业职工,部分集体企业参照执行,其经费在企业按工资总额的一定比例提取的福利费中列支。劳保医疗经费在不同企业之间没有调剂,属于典型的"企业自我保障"类型。在当时经济条件下,中国的职工医疗保障制度对于保障职工基本医疗、促进经济发展、维护社会稳定都发挥了重要的作用。

随着经济的发展和改革的深入,特别是在建立社会主义市场经济体制的新形势下,这种制度存在的缺陷日益突出。主要表现为:

一是"多",即国家和单位对职工医疗费用包揽过多,职工缺乏自我保障意识,财政和企业不堪重负,反过来使群众的基本医疗服务得不到有效的保障。

二是"快",即对医患双方缺乏有效的制约机制,医疗费用增长过快、浪费严重,一些职工缺乏节约医疗费意识,"小病大养"、"一人看病,全家吃药"的现象在一些单位不同程度地存在。

三是"低",即管理和服务的社会化程度低。在不同地区、不同所有制、不同行业和不同单位之间,职工享受的医疗待遇差异过大,苦乐不均,还有相当一部分职工得不到基本的医疗保障。在一些生产经营状况不好的企业里,许多职工医疗费一年只有几十元钱,不少单位职工医疗费长期得不到报销,医疗费拖欠现象比较严重。

四是"窄",即医疗保障的覆盖面窄。改革开放以后发展起来的外商投资企业、股份制企业、私营企业的职工和个体工商户,很多没有参加社会医疗保障,这些企业的职工得不到有效的基本医疗保障。

推行城镇医疗保险制度改革,是实现国有企业改革和发展目标的迫切需要。当前,国有企业职工很多人不愿去非公有制单位就业,除了就业观念方面的问题外,社会保障没有覆盖到这些单位、职工有后顾之忧也是一个重要原因。因此,建立覆盖城镇所有单位和职工的医疗保险制度,有利于转变职工就业观念,拓宽就业渠道,加快国有企业改革进程。

进行职工医疗保险制度改革,是建立社会主义市场经济体制的必然要求。在实行社会主义市场经济的条件下,政府必须通过建立养老、医疗和失业保险制度,来分散和化解由市场竞争带来的风险,维护社会公平和稳定。经过多年改革探索,我国已初步建立了全国统一的企业职工基本养老保险制度、国有企业下岗职工基本生活保障和失业保险制度,城市居民最低生活保障制度已在全国400多个城市建立,但城镇职工医疗保险制度改革相对滞后。只有加快这项改革,建立健全社会保险体系,才能加快建立社会主义市场经济体制的进程。

三、中国城镇职工医疗保险制度改革的任务、基本思路和应遵循的原则

针对公费、劳保医疗制度存在的问题,1994年底,江苏镇江和江西九江开始的医疗保险改革试点(俗称"两江方案")正式拉开了职工医疗保障制度改革的序幕。1996年底,医改试点城市扩大到57个。1998年底,根据《国务院关于建立城镇职工基本医疗保险制度的决定》,职工医疗保险改革在全国范围内推开。该决定为各地建立适合本地特点的具

体实施方案规定了基本原则和运作框架,大大推进了城镇职工基本医疗保险制度改革的进程。2000年2月,国务院办公厅又转发了国务院体改办等八部委局《关于城镇医疗卫生体制改革的指导意见》,强调职工基本医疗保险制度、城镇医疗卫生体制、药品生产流通体制"三项改革"要配套联动,促使医疗保险制度改革取得突破性的进展。到目前,各省市区的城镇职工基本医疗保险制度已基本建立。

按照建立社会主义市场经济体制的需要和配套推进国有企业改革的要求,根据我国社会主义初级阶段的基本国情,《决定》提出改革的任务是要在全国范围内建立与社会主义初级阶段生产力水平相适应的,符合社会主义市场经济体制要求,充分考虑财政、企业和个人承受能力,切实保障职工基本医疗需求的基本医疗保险制度。与公费、劳保医疗制度相比较,改革要实现四个转变:一是保障方式从单位保障向社会保险转变,二是保障范围从国有单位逐步向城镇全体劳动者转变,三是费用负担从单位负担向单位和个人双方负担转变,四是保障责任从无限责任向基本保障转变。

建立城镇职工基本医疗保险制度的基本思路是"基本保障、广泛覆盖、双方负担、统账结合、多层保障"。"基本保障"是指基本医疗保险的水平要和我国社会主义初级阶段的生产力发展水平相适应,相应的筹资水平要根据目前我国财政和企业的承受能力确定,只能保障职工的基本医疗需求;"广泛覆盖"是指基本医疗保险要覆盖城镇所有用人单位和职工,不论是国有单位,还是非国有单位,不论是效益好的企业,还是效益差的企业,都要参加基本医疗保险;"双方负担"是指改变过去职工医疗费由国家和企业包揽,个人不承担医疗保险责任的状况,实行基本医疗保险费用由单位和个人共同合理负担;"统账结合"是指基本医疗保险实行社会统筹和个人账户相结合,建立医疗保险统筹基金和个人账户,并明确各自的支付范围,统筹基金主要支付大额医疗费用,个人账户主要支付小额医疗费用;"多层保障"是指为解决基本医疗保险之外的医疗费用,满足不同层次的医疗需求,在建立基本医疗保险的同时,同步建立和发展多种形式的补充医疗保险,逐步建立多层次医疗保障体系。

按照这一基本思路,在建立城镇职工基本医疗保险制度的过程中,应遵循四条原则:一是基本医疗保险的水平要与社会主义初级阶段生产力发展水平相适应;二是城镇所有用人单位及其职工都要参加基本医疗保险,实行属地管理;三是基本医疗保险费由用人单位和职工双方共同负担;四是基本医疗保险基金实行社会统筹和个人账户相结合。

四、目前职工医疗保险制度改革中应注意的问题

(一)关于属地原则和"条""块"矛盾问题

医保方案实行属地原则,本意是打破计划经济体制下"条""块"分割现象,更好地实现社会公平。但在实际操作中,由于地区经济发展极不平衡,属地化管理仍有很大阻力。实行费改税、政事分开不失为好的举措。

(二)关于"社会统筹"与"个人账户"的结合

在试点实践中,对"统账结合"的具体操作方式,曾发生过"通道式"和"板块式"的争议。而"个人账户"对于促进个人"纵向"积累、防范疾病风险的功能尚未体现,因而"统账结合"的必要性与可行性面临挑战。

(三)关于"基本"与"补充"的关系

职工基本医疗保险制度主要体现社会保障的共济性与公平性,还难以适应广大职工群众医疗需求的差异性与层次性,因而在推进基本医疗保险制度建设的同时,需要加快补充医疗保险的配套,这样可以部分缓解属地管理原则下"同地不同级"、"同地不同业"的"条""块"矛盾与行业矛盾,还可以进一步发挥补充性调节职业收入与福利分配的功能。

(四)关于特困人群的医疗保障

城镇贫困人群比例近些年有扩大趋势。其主要构成部分有:年迈或多病,已丧失劳动能力,又无子女亲友供养者;产业结构调整过程中下岗、失业的原劳动者;农村盲目流入城市、缺乏适宜的劳动技能的农民;残疾人或严重慢性病患者等。对于特困人群的医疗保障,建议从"供"、"需"两方面双管齐下。如举办"平民医院"、减免或缓收医疗费用、动员社会公益性筹资捐赠、将特困者纳入社区综合卫生服务对象等。

第三节 中国农村合作医疗制度

一、农村合作医疗制度的由来及其发展

根据1979年底的《农村合作医疗章程(试行草案)》,农村合作医疗是指"人民公社社员依靠集体力量,在自愿互助的基础上建立起来的一种社会主义性质的医疗制度,是社员群众的集体福利事业"。

一般认为,合作医疗制度源于20世纪40年代的陕甘宁边区的医疗合作社,属于社区医疗保险的性质,其基本做法为:村民采取集资方式支付医疗费用,共同承担疾病风险。新中国建立后,在合作化时期合作医疗制度进一步发展,成为由集体公益金支付主要部分、农民个人支付一小部分,共同分担风险的社区医疗保险制度。该制度依托新建成的县、乡、村三级医疗预防保健网,资金由乡村两级管理。在70年代,该制度与农村三级医疗保健网、赤脚医生一起成为农村医疗的"三大法宝",并受到世界卫生组织专家的称赞。到农村生产责任制改革之前的1978年,全国农村合作医疗覆盖率达到80%~90%。80年代初农村实行联产承包责任制以后,全国大多数地方集体经济逐渐解体,农村合作医疗制度失去了经济后盾,加上制度本身设计中的不合理,致使这项制度崩溃了。1989年,全国只有4.8%的行政村依然在实行这项制度。到了90年代,农民的医疗问题再次引起政府的重视,农村合作医疗再次被摆上议事日程。但是,根据卫生部制定的《2000年"人人享有卫生保健"最低限标准(以县为单位)》,到2000年农村集资医疗保健制度的覆盖率(以县为单位)应当达到50%~60%,而实际情况并不乐观。到1998年合作医疗人口覆盖率只有6.61%,村级覆盖率也只达到13%。

二、合作医疗的形式

各地农村合作医疗改革中出现了多种形式,如合作形式、管理形式、补偿形式,按照不同的形式有不同的分类。

1. 按合作形式分类:①合医不合药。合作医疗参加者就诊的四费(挂号、注射、处治、

出诊)全免或某些检验、检查收费按比例减免,而药费全部自费。②合药不合医。合作医疗参加者就诊的医疗费全部自费,药费按比例减免。③合医又合药。合作医疗参加者就诊的医疗费和药费均按比例减免。

2. 按管理形式分类:①村办村管。以行政村为单位举办合作医疗,由本村居民及企事业单位职工参加,村民委员会与合作医疗管理小组负责管理、筹集、使用资金。②村办乡管。村成立合作医疗管理小组,乡成立合作医疗管理委员会下设办公室,根据各村的经济水平、农民承受能力、医疗预防保健服务项目与数量,确定每人每年的筹资金额,由各村委会和合作医疗管理小组负责收集,汇总到乡合作医疗办公室,以村为核算单位,设立专项账户,统一管理、使用资金。③乡办乡管。这是合作医疗较理想的管理形式。以乡为单位兴办合作医疗,由乡合作医疗管理委员会统一组织筹集资金,各村委员会与合作医疗管理小组负责收集,然后汇总到乡合作医疗管理办公室,全乡统一核算、使用、管理资金,分村决算,各村年终结余资金留存下一年度滚动使用,超支部分由下一年度筹资补足,或在特定情况下由乡统筹资金协助解决。真正体现了"互助共济、风险分担"的合作精神。④乡办县统筹医疗保险。以乡为单位兴办合作医疗,由县统一筹集大病保险资金。由于是全县统筹,每人每年缴纳的金额不会很高,但对参加者医疗费补偿较高,更体现"合作互助、风险分担"的精神。这种管理形式符合"大病频率低,支付费用高;小病频率高,支付费用低"的规律,是向社会医疗保障过渡的最佳形式。

3. 按补偿形式分类:①福利型。参加者就诊的门诊医药费按比例补偿,住院医药费不补偿,所以又称"保小不保大"。②风险型。参加者住院医药费按比例补偿,门诊医药费不补偿,又称"保大不保小"。③福利风险型。参加者就诊的门诊医药费和住院医药费均按比例补偿,又称"保小又保大"。④合作医疗健康保险。这种形式的合作医疗所提供的服务和费用补偿不仅包括医疗,而且包括预防、保健、环境卫生等项目,如儿童计划免疫、妇女产期保健、计划生育、地方病疫情监测、饮食及饮水卫生、粪便管理、健康教育等。它既"保小",又"保大",为农村合作医疗的发展提供了一个新模式。

三、构建新型农村合作医疗制度

(一)新型农村合作医疗制度出台的背景

1. 体现医疗筹资公平性的需要。2001年世界卫生组织卫生工作报告对卫生筹资的公平性在全世界191个国家和地区,将中国排在第188位。尽管中国对卫生筹资公平性系数计算方法有异议,但我国农村医药消费水平远远低于城市,是不可争议的事实。根据卫生部制定的《2000年"人人享有卫生保健"最低限标准(以县为单位)》,到2000年农村集资医疗保健制度的覆盖率(以县为单位)应当达到50%~60%,而实际情况并不乐观。到1998年合作医疗人口覆盖率只有6.61%,村级覆盖率也只达到13%。2001年全国城镇居民人均医疗保健支出343.28元,而农村居民人均医疗保健支出仅为96.61元,相差3.5倍还多。

2. 满足农民提高健康水平的需要。20世纪80年代以来,尽管经济和收入水平提高较快,但无论生命指标还是健康指标,农村均低于全国平均水平。2001年,全国人口平均期望寿命为71.8岁,农村人口平均期望寿命为69.55岁;全国婴儿死亡率和孕产妇死亡率分别为33.2‰和53/10^5,而农村分别为33.8‰和60/10^5。

3. 解决因病致贫、因病返贫问题的需要。实行家庭联产承包责任制以后,农民的生活条件有所改善,但仅能维持一般消费支出的可支配收入,无力承担疾病医药费的风险。因此,达到温饱型的农民,一旦遇到家庭成员患大病、重病,就会导致因病重新变成困难户。新型合作医疗制度,通过互助互济形式,就可解决因大病发生的大额医药费问题,从制度上防止农民因病致贫。

4. 符合农村卫生投入对象和方式转移的需要。建国以来,我国对农村卫生投入一直投向供方——乡镇卫生院。近几年来,由于乡镇卫生院人浮于事,管理不善,其政府卫生投入几乎用在超编人员的费用上,农民在经济方面并没有得到实惠。新型农村合作医疗制度实行后将卫生投入直接投给需方——农民,不仅会提高资金使用效益,切实把资金用在农民健康保健方面,也会促进乡镇卫生院精简人员、加强管理、提高服务质量。

(二)建立新型农村合作医疗制度的目标和原则

建立新型农村合作医疗制度是新时期农村卫生工作的重要内容,是实践"三个代表"重要思想的具体体现,对提高农民健康水平、促进农村经济发展、维护社会稳定具有重大意义。

2003年1月《关于建立新型农村合作医疗制度的意见》提出:新型农村合作医疗制度是由政府组织、引导、支持,农民自愿参加,个人、集体和政府多方筹资,以大病统筹为主的农民医疗互助共济制度。

从2003年起,各省、自治区、直辖市至少要选择2～3个县(市)先行试点,取得经验后逐步推开。到2010年,实现在全国建立基本覆盖农村居民的新型农村合作医疗制度的目标,减轻农民因疾病带来的经济负担,提高农民健康水平。

建立新型农村合作医疗制度要遵循以下原则:①自愿参加,多方筹资。农民以家庭为单位自愿参加新型农村合作医疗,遵守有关规章制度,按时足额缴纳合作医疗经费;乡(镇)、村集体要给予资金扶持;中央和地方各级财政每年要安排一定专项资金予以支持。②以收定支,保障适度。新型农村合作医疗制度要坚持以收定支、收支平衡的原则,既保证这项制度持续有效运行,又使农民能够享有最基本的医疗服务。③先行试点,逐步推广。建立新型农村合作医疗制度必须从实际出发,通过试点总结经验,不断完善,稳步发展。要随着农村社会经济的发展和农民收入的增加,逐步提高新型农村合作医疗制度的社会化程度和抗风险能力。

第四节 工伤和生育保险制度

一、工伤保险制度

工伤保险是劳动者在生产劳动和工作中遭受意外伤害或因长期接触职业性有毒有害物质引起的职业病伤害后,由国家或社会给予负伤、致残、死亡者本人及其家属提供物质帮助的一种社会保障制度。它具有工伤补偿、工伤预防和职业康复三项职能。

中国的工伤保险制度是新中国成立初期建立起来的,分为干部和企业职工两大类。1950年,内务部制定《革命工作人员伤亡褒恤暂行条例》,建立了国家机关和事业单位职工的工伤保险制度。1951年政务院公布了《中华人民共和国劳动保险条例》,1953年进行了修订,颁布了《劳动保险条例实施细则》,从而建立起企业职工工伤保险制度。随着社会经济的发展,以"单位保险"为主要特征的工伤保险制度越来越显示出其存在的问题,主要是实施范围窄、待遇偏低、社会共济性差、工伤认定及评残的标准和程序不健全。

按照党的十四届三中全会决定关于"普遍建立企业工伤保险制度"的要求以及《劳动法》第9章有关社会保险的规定,劳动部在总结试点经验和借鉴外国经验的基础上,于1996年8月颁布实施《企业职工工伤保险试行办法》,有力地推动了工伤保险制度的改革进程,把我国工伤保障制度从"企业保险"转向了"社会保险"。《试行办法》规定:我国企业工伤保险覆盖范围包括各种所有制的各类企业及其劳动者,工伤保险基金实行地市级统筹,工伤保险待遇包括医疗康复待遇、伤残待遇和死亡待遇三部分。我国机关事业单位的工伤保险实行因工伤残抚恤制度,管理办法和待遇标准都与企业工伤保险不同。

各地在改革过程中存在的主要问题是参保率不高,不少省份的职工参保率不足50%,主要原因是一些地方的工伤保险不包括乡镇企业,此外外商投资企业和私营企业参保率也较低。

2003年4月27日,国务院总理温家宝签署第375号国务院令,颁布《工伤保险条例》。此条例自2004年1月1日起施行。《工伤保险条例》具有以下特点:

第一,扩展了工伤保险制度的适用范围。从权利主体的角度看,凡是中华人民共和国境内的各类企业的职工和个体工商户的雇工,均享有工伤保险待遇权利。而不管劳动者与用人单位是否订立书面劳动合同,不管劳动者的用工形式如何,不管劳动者的用工期限长短,也不管劳动者的身份是什么。

从义务主体角度看,凡在中华人民共和国境内的各类企业、有雇工的个体工商户,都有义务参加工伤保险,为本单位全部职工缴纳工伤保险费。"各类企业"涵盖投资者所有制性质和企业组织方式各不相同的各类企业,既包括个体工商户、农村集体所有制企业、城镇集体所有制企业、私营企业,也包括股份有限公司(含上市公司)、有限责任公司、个人独资企业、合伙企业,以及其他民办的企业化经营的事业单位。

第二,解决了工伤保险费的缴纳主体问题。条例规定,用人单位应当按时缴纳工伤保险费,职工个人不缴纳工伤保险费。

第三,解决了工伤保险基金的来源和安全性问题。条例规定,工伤保险基金由用人单位缴纳的工伤保险费、工伤保险基金的利息和依法纳入工伤保险基金的其他资金构成。工伤保险基金存入社会保障基金财政专户,用于工伤保险待遇、劳动能力鉴定以及法律、法规规定的用于工伤保险的其他费用的支付。任何单位或者个人不得将工伤保险基金用于投资运营、兴建或者改建办公场所、发放奖金,或者挪作其他用途。

在工伤认定方面,《工伤保险条例》作出了以下规定:

条例规定,在上下班途中,受到机动车事故伤害的职工应当认定为工伤。

职工有下列六种情形之一,也应认定为工伤:在工作时间和工作场所内,因工作原因受到事故伤害的;工作时间前后在工作场所内,从事与工作有关的预备性或者收尾性工作受到事故伤害的;在工作时间和工作场所内,因履行工作职责受到暴力等意外伤害的;患职业病的;因工外出期间,由于工作原因受到伤害或者发生事故下落不明的;法律、行政法规规定应当认定为工伤的其他情形。

条例还规定,职工有下列情形之一的视同工伤:在工作时间和工作岗位,突发疾病死亡或者在48小时内经抢救无效死亡的;在抢险救灾等维护国家利益、公共利益活动中受到伤害的;职工原在军队服役,因战、因公负伤致残,已取得革命伤残军人证,到用人单位后旧伤复发的。

但劳动者违反《治安管理处罚条例》受伤,酗酒醉酒后导致自己受伤或自残自杀等,不属于工伤保险的保护范围。

二、生育保险制度

生育保险是指通过国家立法,对怀孕、分娩女职工及时给予物质帮助的一项社会保险政策,以保障女职工生育期间的生活和基本医疗保健需要,帮助她们恢复劳动能力,重返工作岗位。

中国生育保险制度创建于20世纪50年代初期,由企业生育保险和机关、事业单位生育保险两项制度组成。1951年2月26日颁布的《中华人民共和国劳动保险条例》,对职工的生育保险制度作出了规定。

中国生育保险制度对维护孕产女职工的特殊合法权益,促进就业平等的实现,提高妇女地位和妇女的社会劳动参与率都起了重要作用。但是随着改革和发展的深入,传统生育保险制度的弊端也逐步暴露出来。主要是:企业之间生育保险负担畸轻畸重,影响女性就业;女职工生育期间应享受的保险待遇难以保证;生育保险待遇偏低。

1988年,我国开始生育保险制度改革,在总结30多年实践经验的基础上,国家颁发了《女职工劳动保护规定》,将产假从56天延长到90天。1994年,劳动部颁布了《企业职工生育保险试行办法》,要求各地按属地原则组织开展生育保险费用社会统筹。1995年我国政府颁布《中国妇女发展纲要》,对生育保险改革的实施范围、覆盖方式及时间进度作了更明确的政策规定。

我国现行生育保险制度的覆盖范围是城镇企业及其职工,即国有企业、股份制企业、城镇集体企业、私营企业、外商投资企业及其职工,实行市(地)或县级范围统筹,属地管理,参加统筹的企业按规定比例缴费,具体比例由各地政府确定,最高不超过企业工资总额的1%,个人不缴费。参保职工享受生育津贴和生育医疗服务。生育津贴按照本企业上年度职工月平均工资计发,支付期限一般为三个月。一些地区将奖励假期生育津贴也纳入了生育保险范围。生育医疗待遇贯穿妊娠、分娩全过程,女职工生育期间的检查费、接生费、手术费、住院费和药费、生育出院后因生育引起疾病的医疗费由生育基金支付,女职工流产也享受有关生育保险待遇。

我国现行生育保险制度存在的主要问题是:覆盖面较窄,全国还有不少城市没有实行企业职工生育费用社会统筹,多数地区的机关、事业单位没有开展生育保险制度改革;待遇标准不规范,不少地区没有将产前检查、流产等纳入生育保险范围,生育津贴的计发标准也不统一;社会化管理水平较低,多数地区将女职工生育津贴和生育医疗费按照定额标准返还企业,再由企业自付给职工。有的企业还有克扣女职工生育津贴的情况。

> [案例]

吉林农安县合隆镇的合作医疗制度

吉林农安县是吉林比较富裕的县,每村都有集体经济收入,据估计有些村每年的集体经济收入可达50万~60万元。该县原有的合作医疗于1983年停止。1999年由县里统一安排实行农村合作医疗,具体方式由乡镇自主选择。该镇采取合医部分合药的方式,这也是多数其他乡镇采取的方式。

在机构方面,设立镇合作医疗管理委员会,由镇党委书记担任主任。管委会下设办公室,设在镇卫生院,主管的党委副书记担任主任,由院长担任副主任。合作医疗运作至2000年,目前已经停止。

合作医疗的执行方式:首先对乡村医生进行了清理,收费由镇里强制进行,以户为单位加入,每人10元/年。但一些老百姓对此不理解,并进行了抵制。而一些村与镇里讨价还价,执行了5元/(人·年)的不同标准,截至1999年末,仅筹集资金14万多元,仅占应筹集金额的20%多一点。而来自政府的筹资也出现了问题,镇里原拟投入公益金每人2元没有兑现,而县财政补贴每人5角钱的承诺,也没有兑现。

由于出现了不同的筹资标准,乡里相应设立了不同的报销标准:

对于每年缴纳10元的农民,他们在村卫生所看病无须缴纳诊费,药费可以报销15%,村医生由村里发工资。到乡卫生院看病,看病不花钱,报销25%药费,而检查费,如心电图、B超、X光、化验、血常规等均免费。转诊的报销比例在10%~15%之间,最高不超过1 000元。缴纳5元的农民,所有费用减半处理。

院长有权审批金额在100元以内的报销单,而金额在100元以上的由主管书记审批。

在实行了一年的合作医疗以后,县里没有兑现承诺,也没有再强调建立合作医疗制度,镇里也不再投入人力物力。尽管制度运行尚属良好,资金仍有节余,老百姓也开始接受这种制度,但这里恢复合作医疗的行动"无疾而终"。

思考1. 合作医疗制度实施的难点在哪里?

思考2. 如何促进合作医疗制度的可持续发展?

Chapter 15   The Social Security System

Section 1   The Outline of a Social Security System

1. The definition and feature of a social security system

The word "Social Security" was first introduced in *Social Security Law* during American New Deal in 1935. At the 26th session of international labor conference convoked in Philadelphia, USA, in 1944, International Labor Organization delivered the famous *Declaration in Philadelphia*, bringing forward "expanding social security". From then on, the concept was gradually put into more extensive usage.

Generally speaking, social security is the system, in which national government plays the dominant role and, according to the law, affords the lowest standard of living by the sub-allotment of national revenue to the social members who temporarily or permanently lose the ability to labor and who are in living difficulty for various reasons, so as to guarantee their basic living.

Social Security bears five main features as follows: enforceability, sociality, welfare, reciprocity and irreversibility.

(1) Enforceability

This focuses on the compulsory attendance and the compulsory payment which each social member must participate in and accept its safeguard; Individuals and parties who should do their duties to conform to the relevant tax law of Social Security or qualify for the insurance fund financing law and code must pay taxes and pay for it. Otherwise, they will be charged with legal duty.

(2) Sociality

As a compulsive and widespread social "safe net", Social Security is the outcome of modern large-scale production and is a typical social behavior.

What it will safeguard are all the social members, not only the minority.

The larger the number of those involved, the greater the ability of it to resist risk, which is so-called "majority law".

(3) Welfare

Each link of social security does not aim at making profit. It will not only make gratis payment but also provide social services for those who are guaranteed. Premium is not all from the guaranteed, and finance raising is not the exclusive responsibility of the social security section. Part will come from government finance, part from what corporation and individual pay, and part from the social endowment.

(4) Reciprocity

One feature of Social Security is "to fill the deficit with surplus, and to help others in the same boat", that is, to make up for the loss that the minority encounter with the mutual assistance among all participants.

(5) Irreversibility

The payment of social security has strong irreversibility, which is also called rigidity. It is difficult to lower the level of social security once it is fixed on at a high level. The system of high guarantee and high welfare promoted by most western European countries now shows more and more limitations. Since the 1980s, these countries in succession have reformed social security system to cut down the insurance item and welfare expenditure to alleviate the pressure on government public finance. But all these reforms finally run aground because of people's strong opposition. The irreversibility, or rigidity, requests that the level of social security should accord with that of social productivity. Otherwise, a series of social and economic problems will inevitably arise.

2. The institutional contents of a social security system

The classification method and the item establishment vary among different countries. By any large, they include social insurance, social relief, social welfare, preferential job placement for ex-servicemen and social mutual aid, among which social insurance is the nuclear part, social welfare is the tallest level, and social relief is the most fundamental part and lowest require ment.

(1) Social insurance

Social insurance is the system in which nations legislate to deliver certain income to those who temporarily or permanently lose the ability to work and those who have no income source though with the ability to work, so as to ensure them basic living standards. It is chiefly open to workers, but also to all citizens in some countries. Social insurance generally includes old-age insurance, medical insurance, work-related insurance, unemployment insurance and maternity insurance. Social insurance is the very part of social security that undertakes the largest risk and takes up the biggest part of the funds. One of its marked features is compulsory payment and it adheres to the principle of right relative to duty. Generally speaking, a country's social insurance level primarily lies in its development level of social productivity. In some countries, different workers have different treatment levels on account of different individual contribution and payment.

(2) Social relief

Social relief is a social security system in which the nation and society give relief to those members who have no ability to maintain basic living standards. It includes poverty relief and disaster relief. The former is provided for those who are helpless and without the ability to labor thus gain no living sources, such as orphans, the disables, old men and so on, and for those whose income is lower than the legal lowest living standard despite the ability to labor; the latter is provided for those who cannot temporarily maintain basic living standards because of social disaster like war and of natural disaster such as flood, earthquake, etc. Social relief guarantees an individual fundamental subsistence, and it is "the final defense line" of social security.

(3) Social welfare

The concept of social welfare contains the broad one and the narrow one. The former primarily includes the public welfare work provided by government, such as culture and education, public health, public amusement, municipal construction, family subsidy, education subsidy, housing subsidy and so on, aiming at increasing the welfare level of the whole society. The latter is primarily open to a special group including the aged, children, women, teenagers, the disabled and so on, aiming at improving their life by the provision of necessary governmental and social assistance. Social welfare not only guarantees the citizen's subsistence, but more chiefly guarantees the improvement of people's life along with that of the productivity, not only material improvement, but also the mental and cultural improvement.

(4) Preferential job placement for ex-servicemen

This primarily includes offering pension, special treatment money, and subsidy to the family of a martyr, family of a soldier, deactivated veteran and disabled soldier, setting up the honored soldier's sanatoria, installing the deactivated and demobilized soldier of the army, and providing service for the retired cadres, aiming at stabilizing military heart and upholding national security.

(5) Social mutual aid

This activity is encouraged and supported by governments, in which all levels of society volunteer to help the weak and the poor.

3. The function and effect of social security

(1) The function of social security

①Compensation. Compensation means workers and other social members will receive certain financial compensation and material help when they suffer from risk and thus temporarily or permanently lose their income. The function of social security mainly reflects on social relief and social insurance, the latter being particularly distinct. The funds raised by the main body of social security will be used to compensate the loss of part of social members, according to the insurance principle "gathering the numerous power to share the individual unexpected loss".

②Stability. Stability is the primary function of social security. It guarantees the basic living rights of social members by laws and harmonizes relationship among people's material interests by sub-allotting the national revenue thus functioning as the social stability mechanism. In the west, social security is called "safety net" and "stability regulator inside the society".

③ Regulation function. Modern social security, as the cardinal social policy performed by a nation, is a very important method to regulate the income, reduce the gap between the poor and the rich and alleviate social conflict. Basic measures are adopted as follows: on one hand, to collect the insurance funds in a progressive way from the high income level, such as employers; on the other hand, to offer a stake in a progressive way to the poor, and the less he earns, the more he gets. In addition, the raising, payment and investment of the social insurance funds itself is an allotment and sub-allotment of national revenue which will consequentially regulate the function of the national economy.

(2) The effect of social security

The effect of social security is the concrete performance of social security's function and the impact exert on which by the social security. Nowadays, social security plays a more and more important role on the sustainable development of our country's social economy. Its effert reflects the following aspects Firstly, the establishment and implement of social security system creates cardinal terms for the labor and personnel reform during the new period, and thus quickens the reasonable mobility and optimizes collocation of our country's labor force resources. Secondly, the workers, who have the social security, relieved of the future troubles, their enthusiasm must be inspired by social security and it further enhances the labor's productivity and increases social economy. Thirdly, social security will be in favor of controlling the excessive increase in population and alleviate the pressure of the aged. In China, there has been a traditional idea "give birth to a son against old age", which inevitably leads to the population explosion. To establish and perfect a social security system will more preferably guarantee the aged living conditions of the aged, to realize the objective inevitably would weaken that traditional idea of providing for the aged and stimulate people's consciousness to abide by the family planning policy. Fourthly, social security embodies the interpersonal mutual assistance and the combination of right and duty and will advance the development of a spiritual civilization. Fifthly, the establishment of a social security enhances the equality among the human beings and maintains the social equity. For instance, to implement the system of subsistence allowances for the urban poor can help those who are under the lowest living level of local living standard to continue their life.

Section 2 The Reform of the Medical Insurance System for Urban Workers in China

1. Foreign model of a medical insurance

Medical insurance came into being during the Industrial Revolution, when "insurance fund" was produced to avoid risk of disease, that is, workers handed in some money which was similar to saving, and used it when they got disease. The first national medical insurance of the world was introduced in Germany in 1893, when prime minister Bismarck pushed *Disease Social Insurance Bill* for political reason. In 1911, UK established a national health plan. In 1980, almost all developed countries established a nation-wide medical insurance plan, such as *National Health Service* (*NHS*) in UK, *Canadian Universal Insurance Plan*, etc. Up to the day, through more than 100 years, foreign medical insurance system is now offered in four main types:

(1) Insurance of business medical

The United States follows the orientated on market, the allowed free trade, the voluntary insurance and the free choice. The insurance relies on insured groups to share the risk of disease with the medical insurance company acting as the third party. Both the provider and the demander pursue the maximization of utility, which will easily result in the expenses inflation while stimulating the development of the medical technique and promoting the application of new technique and new medicine. There are various kinds of "adverse selection" and "normal hazard" in the insurance market. To increase efficiency, managed care has been advised as the direction of the medical reform in the United States. For the sake of the equity, the United States produces Medicare and Medicaid, similar to national medical insurance and social medical insurance, to guarantee services to the old, the poor and children.

(2) Social medical insurance

In Germany, Canada and Japan that are the representatives of this mode, compulsory payment is demanded according to laws. The concrete form varies, and the nation by itself manages or entrusts the insurance organization to manage, which thus results in too many management levels to manage with difficulty. In Germany, there are 1,214 disease funds, as non-government and unprofitable agency to be responsible for gathering the insurance funds and paying the provider of medical treatment via the doctor's association. The funds come from the employer and employee, raised in proportion to their wages or income, money-raising stable, mutual aid degree high. Part of the good-money crowds whose wages are over the upper limit fixed on by government should participate in the private insurance. Government plays a significant role in money financing, organization and management of social insurance.

(3) National medical insurance

In UK (NHS) that is the representative of this mode, the funds are raised by tax, turning "fee" into "tax". So the restriction of laws becomes stronger. The government directly participates in the money-raising, plan, managing, allotting and offering of the medical service, and compensates the provider via appropriation. This type of medical insurance is characteristic of free consumption, nationwide coverage and high welfare degree. In this system, the total health expense correspondingly rises slowly owing to the strong plan, but efficiency is low owing to the lack of market mechanism. In addition, the national fiscal burden is very heavy, while the contradiction between taxpayer and money-raiser is sharpening. In 1991, "internal market", as a competition mechanism, was introduced into UK, in which part of general practitioners who held the funds could represent the benefits of the patient and purchase the service from the hospital via trans-diagnosis, which led to the competition between hospital, medical staffs and general practitioner.

(4) Savings medical insurance

In Singapore, Savings Medical Insurance includes Medisure, Medishield (paying only for large medical expenses) and Medifund (medical assistance for the poor resident). The so-called savings insurance indicates a national compulsory saving plan, in which the premium is paid in certain proportion to the total wages, 6% – 8% according to the different age. A large part of the premium enters the individual medical savings account, later used to pay for his or his relatives' hospitalization expense and the ambulatory treatment of some serious diseases. Every young person saves the funds against his old age and for his sons and daughters and other family members. Thus, there will be a long period enough to continuously share the disease risk in families and generations. There is a maximum limit and a dally maximum of the payment, generally used for the basic medical service. The employer and employee's savings act as medical funds. So there exists light government burden but bad mutual assistance.

2. The background of the reform of the medical insurance system for the urban workers in China: public welfare of medical care and labor insurance medical care

The traditional medical system in China mainly consists of public welfare of medical care in government and institutional agency, labor insurance medical care of the state-owned and collective enterprises in urban areas, and cooperative medical care in rural areas, among which the former two are the main part.

The medical insurance system in urban areas was founded in the early 1950s and consisted of two main parts: one is public welfare of medical care, mainly opening to the government employees, the revolutionary wounded and handicapped soldier and university man, the fund of which was from financial appropriation. The other is labor insurance medical care, mainly opening to the employees of state-owned enterprises and those of some collective enterprises, the fund of which was from these enterprise's welfare fees collected in certain proportion to total amount of wages. The fund cannot be co-used between different enterprises, so it belongs to the typical "enterprise's self-security". At that time, the medical insurance system for urban workers played an important role in guaranteeing the basic medical treatment of the employees, promoting economic development and maintaining social stability.

However, with the development of economy and reform, especially in the new condition of establishing the socialist market economy, the limitation of the system is increasingly obvious as follows:

Firstly, "excessiveness", namely, the nation and unit take on the fee-for-service so excessive that the employees lack the consciousness to guarantee themselves, and finance and business enterprise cannot bear the heavy burden, which in turn results in basic medical service not being validly guaranteed.

Secondly, "quickness", namely, there is no valid disciplinary mechanism between doctor and patient, so fee-for-service rises much quickly, waste is serious, some employees lack the consciousness to economize the fee-for-service, and there exists the phenomenon "much money for small illness" and "one person sees a doctor, the whole family take medicine" in some units to different degrees.

Thirdly, "low", namely, the socialization degree of management and service is low. Medical treatment varies significantly in different regions, systems, trades and units, and there are a considerable number of employees who cannot get the basic health insurance. In some poor enterprises, many employees get only 10 RMB per year as their fee-for-service. Not a few units cannot afford fee-for-service over a long time, and the default is also serious.

Fourthly, "narrow", namely, the coverage is narrow. Many employees working in overseas-funded enterprises, the joint-stock companies, the private enterprises and many individual households, did not participate in social medical insurance, thus could not get valid basic medical treatment.

To reform the medical insurance system in urban areas is the urgent demand of attaining the goal of the state-owned enterprise reform. At present, many workers in state-owned enterprise are reluctant to go to non-public units, not only on account of their mentality about employment, but also because that social security does not cover these units, which leads to their worries about the future. Therefore, to establish the medical insurance system covering all the units and employees in urban areas will be beneficial to changing the employees' idea of employment, opening up more avenues for employment, and quickening the reform of state-owned enterprises.

To reform the medical insurance system for urban workers is also the inevitable request of establishing the socialist market economy. Under socialist market economy, the government must scatter the risk caused by market competition by establishing old-age insurance, medical insurance and unemployment insurance to maintain social stability and social equity. After years of reform, our country now has initially established the unified national basic old-age pension insurance system, basic living allowances for laid-off workers from state-owned enterprises, and unemployment insurance system. System of subsistence allowances for the urban poor has been established in over 400 cities. However, the reform of the medical insurance system in urban areas lags relatively. So, we shall do nothing but quicken it and establish and improve social insurance system to advance the establishment of socialist market economy.

3. The task, basic outline and principle of the reform of the medicial insurance system for the urban workers in China

To solve the above problems, the experimental reform of medical insurance, which began in Zhenjiang, Jiangsu Province, and Jiujiang, Jiangxi Province at the end of 1994, was extended to 57 cities by the end of 1996 (called "the two Jiangs' Projects" and formally pulling open the prelude of this reform). At the end of 1998, according to *The State Council's Decision on Establishing the Basic Medical Insurance System for Urban Workers*, the reform was applied throughout China. The Decision formulates the basic principle and operation frame for each region to establish the local characteristic program and enormously pushes forward this reform. In February, 2000, the State Council Office transmitted *The Guiding Opinion on Reforming the Urban Medical Health System* constituted by 8 bureaus including System Reform Office of the State Council, and emphasizing that the three reforms — the basic medical insurance system for urban workers, the urban health care system, and the drug production and distribution system — must be in harmony with each other to ensure a breakthrough progress of the medical insurance system. Up to now, the basic medical insurance system for urban workers has already basically been established in each province and region.

According to the demand of establishing the socialist market economy, the request of systematically advancing the reform of state-owned enterprises, and our basic situation in the primary stage of socialism, The Decision brings up the mission of this reform: to establish such a basic medical insurance system throughout the country that adapts to the productivity level of the primary stage of socialism, meets the needs of the socialist market economy, sufficiently takes into account the endurance capacity of finance, enterprise and individual, and assuredly guarantees the basic medical health of the workers. Compared with the original public welfare of medical care and labor insurance medical care, the current reform exhibits four changes: first, from unit security to social insurance with regard to security mode; second, from the state-owned unit gradually to all the town workers with regard to the security coverage; third, from the burden of only the unit to that of both unit and individual with regard to the expenses support; fourth, from the unlimited responsibility to the fundamental security with regard to the security responsibility.

The basic outline of this reform is "basic security, extensive coverage, the both parties' responsibility, integrated discount combined with individuals, multilevel security". "Basic security" means that the level of basic medical insurance has to adapt to that of the productivity in the primary stage of socialism, that the money-raising level has to be fixed on according to the current endurance capacity of our finance and enterprises, and that it only guarantees the basic medical service of the workers. "Extensive coverage" means that it should cover all the town units and their workers, regardless of state-owned unit or non-state-owned one, good business benefit or bad one. "Both parties' responsibility" demands that the employees' fee-for-service should be undertaken by both unit and individual, no longer only by state and enterprise. "Integrated discount combined with individual one" demands that social integrated funds and individual discount should be established and given respective payment scope, the former used to pay for the big fee-for-service, the latter for the small one. "Multilevel security" demands that, to meet the medical demand at different levels and deal with the expenditures other than what basic medical insurance can pay, the complementary medical insurance of various forms should be established and advanced along with the establishment of basic medical insurance, which will gradually lead to the establishment of a multilevel security system.

According to this outline, in the process of establishing the basic medical insurance for urban workers, we should stick to four principles as follows: Firstly, the level of the basic medical insurance must be compatible with that of productivity of the primary stage of socialism. Secondly, all the urban units and their workers must participate in the basic medical insurance, adhering to principle of territory. Thirdly, the basic premium is born by both the unit and its workers. Fourthly, the basic medical insurance fund comes from both the social integrated fund and individual discount.

4. The current problems of this reform

(1) Concerning the principle of territory and the contradiction between "strip" and "block"

The original purpose of carrying out the principle of territory in the program of medical insurance is to reverse the situation that central government and local ones compartmentalized their work in the planned economy, and to better realize social equity. But in practice, there are still many obstacles in carrying out the resident management because of the economical imbalance between regions. Transforming administrative fees into taxes and separating the functions of government from those of institutions are good ways we should take.

(2) Concerning "integrated discount combined with individual one"

In the practice of experimental reforms, there once existed the argument about which operation mode we should take, "channel model" or "block model". On the other hand, "individual discount" has not showed its function of increasing personal fore-and-aft accumulation and preventing risk of disease. So the necessity and feasibility of "integrated discount combined with individual one" is in question.

(3) Concerning the relation of "basic medical insurance" with "complementary medical insurance"

The basic medical insurance for urban workers primarily reflects the mutual assistance and equity of social security, but it fails to meet people's different and multilevel demands. Therefore, along with advancing the reform of basic medical insurance, we should also quicken the reform of complementary medical insurance so as to alleviate the contradiction between "strip" and "block", such as "the same region, the different rank", "the same rank, the different work", and trades contradiction in the principle of resident administration, and further complementarily adjust the occupational income and the distribution of welfare.

(4) Concerning the medical security for the neediest urban crowd

In these years, there has been an expansion trend of poor urban crowd, which is mainly composed of those who are old or of many diseases, have already lost the ability to labor, and also have no sons and daughters to support them; those previous labors who come off sentry duty and out of work in the process of the readjustment of the industrial structure; those farmers who blindly swarm into the city and lack of proper labor skill; and those disabled or of serious chronics. As to this crowd, there is a suggestion that we perfect the medical security by perfecting both the provider and the demander. For example, holding "civilian's hospital", reducing or later charging the fee-for-service, mobilizing the social financing and donation, and providing the community health service for the neediest.

Section 3 The Rural Cooperative Medical Care in China

1. Origin and development of the rural cooperative medical care

According to *The Rural Cooperative Medical Care Constitution (Proposed Draft)* issued at the end of the year 1979, the rural cooperative medical care indicates that it is a socialist medical system on the basis of voluntarily mutual assistance, established by members of People's Commune with the strength of the collectivity, and it is a collective welfare of the masses.

Generally speaking, the rural cooperative medical care system originated from the medical cooperative society of the 1940s in west border areas like Shanxi province, Gansu province, Ningxia municipality, and it belonged to a kind of community medical insurance, in which villagers pay the fee-for-service by raising fund to share the risk of disease. After the foundation of New China, it made further headway in the cooperation period, and became a community medical insurance system, with collective public welfare fund accounting for the main part and farmer for the small part, thus the two parties together bearing the risk of disease. This system relied on the three-level health care net by county, township and village, with its funds managed by township and village. In the 1970s, the rural cooperative medical care, the rural three-level health care net, and barefoot doctor were called "three great magic weapons" of the rural medical care praised by the experts of WHO. In 1978, the household production contract system being introduced, the coverage rate of the rural cooperative medical care throughout China even reached 80-90 percent. Afterwards, collective economy gradually disintegrate in most regions, thus resulting in the lack of economical backing. Its design was not reasonable, and theseled to the collapse of the rural cooperative medical care. In 1989, only 4.8 percent of administrative villages of the whole China still continued this system. In the 1990s, the medical problem of the farmer was again taken into account by the government, so the rural cooperative medical care was again put on the agenda. According to The Lowest Standard of "Health Care for Everyone by 2000" (Regarding County as the Unit) established by Ministry of Health, the coverage rate of rural fund raising medical system (regarding county as the unit) should arrive at 50 – 60 percent by 2000. But it was not the case. In 1998, the population coverage rate of cooperative medical care was only 6.61 percent, the village coverage rate only 13 percent.

2. The form of the cooperative medical care

The local forms vary much, such as the cooperative form, management form, compensated form, according to which there are different classifications.

(1) The classification according to cooperative form: ①the free cure but not free medicine: The participant is free of four kinds of fee-for-service (registered fee, injection fee, treatment fee, fee for visiting-a-patient-at-home), and some fee for examinations and checks is reduced or remitted in certain proportion; but medicine fee is self-provided. ②the free medicine but not free cure: All the fee-for-service of the participants are self-provided, but medicine fee is reduced or remitted in certain proportion. ③ both free cure and free medicine: Both the fee-for-service and the medicine fee are reduced or remitted in certain proportion.

(2) Classification according to management form: ①held and managed by village: It is held by administrative village as the unit, covering the village resident and employees of enterprise and institutional unit, with its fund being managed, gathered and used by the village committee and cooperative medical management group. ②held by village and managed by town: The village establishes cooperative medical care management group, and the town establishes cooperative medical care management committee to which the cooperative medical management office is affiliated to fix on the amount of money-raising per man per year, in the light of the village's economic level, the endurance capacity of the farmer, the items and amount of medical and preventive service. The fund is collected by the village committee and cooperative medical management group to cooperative medical management office in the town, which regards village as accounting unit, establishes segregated account to collectively manage and use the fund. ③held and managed by town, which is a more perfect form. Town as the unit holds it; the town cooperative medical care management committee is in charge of organizing money-raising; the village committee and cooperative medical management group is in charge of collecting fund to the town cooperative medical care management office. The whole town collectively checks, uses and manages funds, settling it in terms of each village. The annual balance fund of each village is kept for the next year and like this, and the overbalance fund will be complemented by the next year's or by the town's fund. By this way, the cooperative spirit, "share the risk by mutual aid" is reflected. ④held by town and raised by county: The town as the unit holds it; country unifies to collect the funds of big disease insurance, thus, the amount of per man per year is not very large. However, this form more highly compensates the fee-for-service of the participant, which even more embody the spirit of "mutual aid, risk sharing". This form, according to the law that "the frequency of big disease is low, but the expenses is high; the frequency of small illness is high, but the expenses is low", is the best transitional form to social medical security.

(3) The classification according to compensation form: ①welfare type: Among the participants, the out-patient's medical and medicine fee is compensated in some proportion, but the in-patient's is not compensated. Therefore, this form is also called "protect small not big". ②risk type: Among the participants, the in-patient's medical and medicine fee is compensated in some proportion, but the out-patient's is not compensated. Therefore, this form is also called "protect big not small". ③welfare-risk type: Among the participants, both the in-patient's and the out-patient's medical and medicine fee is compensated in some proportion. Therefore, this form is also called "protect big and small". ④cooperative medical care health insurance: This kind of cooperative medical care offers compensation of service and expenses to not only the treatment but to such items as prevention, protection, sanitation, which, in details, include planned im-

munity for children, perinatal care for women, family planning, endemic disease monitoring, sanitation of food and water, control of feces, and health education. So, it compensates not only the "small illness", but also the "big disease", as a new mode of the rural cooperative medical care.

3. To outline a new rural cooperative medical care system

(1) The background

①The establishment of this new system is the demand of embodying medical financing equity

In 2001, in the report on the health work of the World Health Organization, China was ranked in the 188th place in terms of health financing equity, among 199 nations and regions of the whole world. Although China disagrees with WHO about the calculation method of equity coefficient of the health fund-raising, it is an undebatable fact that our rural consumption level of treatment and medicine is far below the urban one. According to *The Lowest Standard of "Health Care for Everyone by 2000" (regarding county as the unit)* established by Ministry of Health, the coverage rate of rural fund raising medical system (regarding county as the unit) should arrive at 50 – 60 percent till 2000, but it was not the case. In 1998, the population coverage rate of cooperative medical care was only 6.61 percent, and the village coverage rate was only 13 percent. In 2001, as for national town residents, the per capita health expenditure of urban residents is 343.28 yuan, and that for rural residents is only 96.61 yuan, 3.5 times down that of the urban.

②It is the demand of enhancing the health level of the farmers

Since the 1980s, not only life index but also health index of the countryside has been lower than that of the whole nation, though its level of economy and income increased more quickly. In 2001, the expectancy life of national population was 71.80 years old, in contrast to that of the rural population which was 69.55 years old. And as such, infant mortality rate and maternal mortality rate of the whole nation is respectively 33.2/1,000 and 53/100,000, in contrast, respectively 33.8/1,000 and 60/100,000 in the countryside.

③It's the demand of preventing the farmers from getting into or turning into poverty by disease

After carrying out the household production contract system, the living conditions of the farmers have been for sure improved, but they can only sustain the general consumption and cannot take on the risk of fee-for-service. Therefore, for the farmer who has been able to dress warmly and eat fully, medical care system, by the mutual aid with each other, can resolve the big fee-for-service of serious disease, and thus prevent the farmer from getting into poverty.

④It's the demand of transferring the object and the way of medical devotion

Since the foundation of the New China, the government has devoted the health devotion to the provider, the township health center, which, in the last few years, was overstaffed, and badly managed. Therefore, the health devotion of government is almost used on the overstaffed personnel, and the farmer did not get the real financial benefit. Since the new rural cooperative medical care system was put into practice, directly devoting the health devotion to the demander, farmer, will increase the funds-using benefit, and practically devote the funds on the farmer's health. At the same time, it will also urge the township health center to reduce the personnel, improve management, and enhance the service quality.

(2) The target and the principle of establishing the new rural cooperative medical care system

Establishing the new rural cooperative medical care system is the significant content of rural health work in new times, and is the concrete embodiment of practicing the cardinal thought of "three representatives", and it plays a significant role in enhancing the farmer's health level, thus advancing rural economic development and maintaining social stability.

In 2003, *The Proposal on Establishing A New Rural Cooperative Medical Care System* provides that the new rural cooperative medical care system is organized, guided and supported by government and is a rural medical mutual aid system, in which the farmer voluntarily participates, with funds raised from individual, collectivity and government.

From 2003, each province, autonomous region and municipality directly under the Central Government should select at least 2 - 3 counties(cities) as experimental units and later gradually spread them with their experiences. By 2010, we should realize the target of this new system by and large covering the whole nation, to alleviate the farmer's financial burden caused by the disease and improve the farmer's health level.

The following principles should be stick to: ① voluntarily participating, raising funds through a variety of channels. Regarding family as unit, the farmer can voluntarily go to the new system, abiding by related regulation and paying cooperative medical funds in full and on time. The county (town), village collectivity should provide them with the funds supports. Each level finance of the center authority and local government should all set up special funds to support them. ②deciding on the expenditure according to income, providing the moderate security. The new system should adhere to the principle of "deciding on the expenditure by income, balancing the expenditure and income", which will ensure that this system runs efficiently and sustainablly and that the farmer receives the most basic medical service. ③carrying out experimental reform in advance, and gradually expanding it later. To establish this system, we must sum up new experience from practice, continualy perfect and steadily develop it. Also, with the development of the rural economy and the increase of farmer's income, we should gradually enhance its socialized degree and ability to withstand risks.

Section 4 Industrial Injury and Maternity Insurance System

1. The work related insurance system

The work-related insurance is a system in which the nation or the society offers material help to those workers injured, disabled and losing their lives and their family, after they suffer from unexpected accidents or the occupational diseases because of (which result from) a long-term contact with the occupational poisonous and harmful material during labor and work. It has three functions: compensating the industrial injury, preventing the industrial injury and enabling the worker to return to his occupation.

China's work-related insurance system was established shortly after the establishment of the People's Republic of China, and was divided into two types: one is for the cadre, the other for the workers of enterprises. In 1950, Domestic Affairs Ministry established *The Temporary Rregulation of Praising and Comforting and Compensating The Injured and Dead Revolutionary Worker*, which marked the establishment of work-related insurance system for the government employees. In 1951, Governmental Affairs Ministry announced *Labor Insurance Regulation of the People's Republic of China*, which, in 1953, was amended into *The Detailed Enforcement Regulations on The Application of labor Insurance*, which marked the establishment of work-related insurance system for the workers of enterprises. With the development of social economy, the work-related system with characteristic of "unit insurance" more and more exploded its problems. They are, in the main, as follows: narrow implementation area, low treatment, bad social mutual aids, unsound standard and procedure of recognizing the industrial injury and assessing the disability.

According to the request of the Third Plenary Session of the Fourteenth Central Committee about "widely establishing the work-related insurance system for enterprises' workers" and to the regulation relevant to social insurance in Chapter 9 of *Labor Law*, Labor Department, on the basis of summing up the experimental experience and using foreign experience for reference, put into practice *Proposed Regulation on Work-related Insurance System for Enterprises' Employees* in August, 1996, which effectively pushed the reform of the work-related insurance system and transferred it from "unit insurance" to "social insurance". *Proposed Regulation* provides: Chinese work-related insurance for enterprise covers the enterprises of different ownership and their workers;

its funds are raised unifiedly(collectively) by region or city; the treatment includes three parts: recovery treatment, wound and disability treatment and death treatment. The management way and treatment standard of the work-related insurance for Chinese government units is a system of comforting and compensating the wounded and disabled for work reason, different from that for enterprise.

The critical problem in the process of this reform is that the participation rate is low, even under 50 percent in many provinces, mainly because the country(township) enterprise in many places is excluded. In addition, the rate of enterprise of outside investment and the private enterprise is much lower.

On April 27th, 2003, the State Department (China) Premier Wen Jiabao signed the No. 375 order of the State Department, and announced *The Regulation of The Work-related Insurance*, which will come into operation on January 1, 2004. Its features are, in the main, as follows:

Firstly, it expands the coverage of the work-related insurance system.

As the holder of rights, workers in various enterprises in China and employees in individual households possess the right of work-related insurance, regardless of whether the written labor contract is signed or not, the work form, the length of work term, and the worker's identity.

As the subject of a duty, all the domestic enterprises of various types and the individual households employing employees are liable to participate in the work-related insurance, and pay the premium for their workers. The "enterprises of various types" cover the enterprises of different ownership and different modes of organization, not only the individual household, the enterprise of the rural collective ownership, the enterprise of urban collective ownership, private enterprise, but also the incorporated company (containing the quoted company), the company with limited liability, sole corporation, partnership business, and other institutional unit run by the local people in the form of corporation.

Secondly, the payment principal of the work-related premium is recognized.

Regulation provides that the unit should pay the work-related premium on time, and that the workers need not pay it.

Thirdly, the source and safety of the fund of the work-related insurance is ensured.

Regulation provides that the fund of the work-related insurance is composed of the work-related premium paid by unit, the interest of the fund of the work-related insurance and other funds under the coverage of the funds of the work-related insurance according to the law. The fund is deposited into the special account of the funds of social security, used for the treatment of the work-related insurance, the checkup of labor ability, and other expenses provided by laws and code. Any unit or individual must not use the funds of the work-related insurance to invest and run, set up or rebuild the official place, provide bonus, or make other purposes.

The Regulation of The Work-related Insurance provides the regulations as follows on recognizing the industrial injury:

Regulation provides that the workers injured by motor vehicles on the way to work or going home from work should come under the coverage of the industrial injury.

The workers under the following six situations should also come under the coverage of the industrial injury: those suffering from accident for the work reason at work time and in work place; those suffering from accident in work place before or after work time when being engaged in relevant preparatory work or ending work; those suffering from unexpected accident such as violence in performing work duties at work time and in work place; those who get the occupational disease; those for the work reason injured or with whereabouts unknown because of accident when on a business trip; and other situation under the coverage of the industrial injury, according to the law and administrative regulation.

The regulation also provides that the workers under the following situations should come under the coverage of the industrial injury: those who, at work time in work place, suffer from sudden death because of disease or from death though given an emergency treatment within 48 hours; those injured in defending national interest and public benefits such as fighting emergency and disaster; those disabled or wounded because of the war or the work when in military services and having already obtained the revolutionary wounded and disabled certificate, relapse after arriving at the unit.

However, the workers who are injured because of disobeying *Security Administration Punishment Regulation*, and who are injured or commit suicide because of excessive drinking, should not come under the coverage of the industrial injury.

2. The maternity insurance system

Maternity insurance is a social insurance policy that by legislation in time offers material help to the pregnant and natal women workers to guarantee their basic life and basic medical care, help them recover labor ability and return to the work post.

This system was produced in the early 1950s, consisting of two sub-systems, one for the enterprises, the other for the government unit. *The Labor Insurance Regulation of the People's Republic of China* delivered on February 26, 1951, provided some related regulations on the maternity insurance for the employees.

At that time, this system was of great importance in defending the special legal rights of the maternal women workers, promoting the employment equality, increasing the women's status and labor attendance. But, with the thorough reform and development, the limitations of this traditional system gradually appeared. They are as follows: the great difference in the burden of the maternity insurance between different enterprises, which affects female employment; women workers' benefits in a child-bearing period were hardly guaranteed; the low benefits of the maternity insurance.

Since 1988, the reform of the maternity insurance system has been started. Summing up the experience of more than 30 years, China issued *The Labored Protection Regulation for Women Workers*, prolonging the maternity leave from 56 days to 90 days. In 1994, the Labor Department promulgated *The Proposed Regulation of Maternity Insurance for The Workers of Enterprise*, requesting that every local government must develop the social money-raising of the maternity premiums according to the principle of territory. In 1995, *The Development Outline of Chinese Women* was issued, which makes more definite provisions about the implementation scope, coverage form and rate of progress of this reform.

The current maternal insurance of China is open to the urban enterprises and their workers, including state-owned enterprises, joint-stock enterprises, enterprises of urban collective ownership, private enterprises, and enterprises of foreign investment. Its fund is raised by the municipal city according to the principle of territory, with the participant enterprise paying the premium in the fixed proportion, which is fixed on by the local government, and of which the top limit is not over the 1 percent of the total wages of the enterprise, the workers not being required to pay premiums. The participant workers enjoy the maternity subsidy and the medical service in the child-bearing period. The maternity subsidy is provided according to the average wages per month of employees in the last year, and its payment period is often three months. In some regions, the incentive holidays as a maternity subsidy also come into the coverage of the maternity insurance. The benefits of the maternity service are provided through the whole process of pregnancy and delivery. Such fee is provided from the maternity funds as the check fee, delivery fee, operation fee, hospitalization fee and the medicine fee in the child-bearing period and the fee-for-service of the disease due to bearing after leaving hospital. The abortive worker can also enjoy the relevant benefits of the maternity insurance.

The key problems that exist in the current system are the narrow coverage, namely, in the whole country, there are still a few cities that do not have the social unified planning of the funds of the maternity insurance, and the government units in most regions have not carried out this reform; the treatment standard is not normative. For example, in most regions, such items as the antenatal check and abortion do not come under the coverage of the maternity insurance, and the provision standard of the benefits in these regions is not uniform; the relatively low level of socialization management means in most regions the maternity subsidy and the medical treatment fee provided to enterprises, then enterprises offer to workers, and there are some enterprises skimping the maternity subsidy for the women workers.

Chapter 15　The Social Security System

Case Example

The Cooperative Medical Care System of Helong Town, Nong'an County, Jilin Province

Nong'an county is relatively wealthy in Jilin, of which each village has collective economic income, by estimation, 500,000 – 600,000 yuan per year in some villages. The original cooperative medical care of this county ceased in 1983. In 1999, the new system was planned by the county government uniformly, whose concrete form was revised by its town. Helong, following the example of other town, adopted the form of "joint cure and partly joint medicine".

As for the organization, the town cooperative medical management committee was established, with the town party clerk acting as its director. The management office which was affiliated to the committee was established in the town health center, with the vice-secretary of the town party branch in charge serving as its director and the head of the health center serving as its vice-director. This system lasted till 2000 and is not now in existence.

Mode of execution: Screened the village doctor, and the town charged the fee, door as the unit, 10 Yuan per man a year. Some ordinary people did not understand this measure, and rejected it. Meanwhile, some villages, bargained with the town and charged 5 Yuan per man a year. Therefore, up to the end of 1999, only about 140 thousand Yuan was collected, accounting for only 20 percent of the desired amount. At the same time, the money-raising from the government suffered from setbacks, and the plan that town provided 2 Yuan to each man and county complemented half a Yuan per man was not implemented.

Owing to the different standards of the money-raising, the town government established different standards of reimbursement:

For the farmers who paid 10 Yuan a year, they did not need to pay the diagnosis fee when seeing a doctor in the village health center, with the medicine fee being reimbursed by 15 percent. The village doctor got wages from the village. Should they go to the town health center to see a doctor, these farmers were free of diagnosis fee, check fee, such as electrocardiogram, B-ultra, X-rays, laboratory examinations, and the routine examination of the blood, with medicine fee being reimbursed by 25 percent. The trans-diagnosis fee was reimbursed by 10 – 5 percent, and the top was not over 1000 dollars. As to the farmers who paid 5 yuan, half of their expenses was reduced.

The expense account that was not over 100 yuan was examined and approved by the director, and over 100 yuan by the.

After a year, the county did not fulfill its promises, and did not emphasize again establishing the cooperative medical care system; the town either no longer devoted the manpower and material resources to it. Therefore, although this system was in good function, the funds still had surplus, and common people began to accept this system, the cooperative medical care has not been restored till now.

Discussion:

    1. What is the difficulty in implementing the cooperative medical care system?

    2. How to promote the sustainable development of the cooperative medical care system?

参考文献
References

1. 龚幼龙主编.社会医学.北京:人民卫生出版社,2000
2. 何廷尉主编.社会医学理论与实践.成都:四川科学技术出版社,1991
3. 张拓红主编.社会医学.北京:北京医科大学出版社,2002
4. 世界卫生组织第五十五届世界卫生大会报告
5. 刘雪林,等.对传染病再度肆虐的反思.医学与哲学杂志,2003,24(5):17~20
6. 郭继志,等主编.新编社会医学.北京:中医古籍出版社,1998
7. 顾杏元,龚幼龙主编.社会医学.上海:上海医科大学出版社,1990
8. 张方振主编.社会医学基本理论与方法.北京:人民卫生出版社,1995
9. 周达生,戴梅竞编著.现代社会病.上海:上海中医学院出版社,1993
10. 卢祖洵主编.社会医学.北京:科学出版社,2003
11. 翟书涛编著.选择死亡.北京:北京出版社,2001
12. Emile Durkheim 编著.自杀论.钟旭辉,等译.杭州:浙江人民出版社,1988
13. 肖迅.自杀与精神障碍的关系.临床精神医学杂志,1998,8(3):165
14. 答旦.对诱发自杀行为的社会因素初探(上).临床精神医学杂志,1997,7(3):166
15. 贾丛山主编.社会医学概论.乌鲁木齐:新疆科技卫生出版社,1995
16. 胡怀明主编.社会医学.北京:人民军医出版社,1998
17. 蒋泽先,李钰荣编著.生命的透支.南昌:江西人民出版社,1998
18. 李绍六著.成瘾性.北京:中国社会出版社,1997
19. 姜佐宁主编.海洛因成瘾与现代治疗.北京:科学出版社,1995
20. 姜佐宁主编.药物成瘾的临床与治疗.北京:人民卫生出版社,1997
21. 张晓磊编著.维护你的心——远离网络伤害.北京:中国纺织出版社,2002
22. 师建国主编.成瘾医学.北京:科学出版社,2002
23. 万崇华,等.海洛因依赖者戒毒期生存质量变化的影响因素分析.中国公共卫生,1998,14(4):244~246
24. 冯正仪.社区护理干预对提高糖尿病患者生活质量的影响.中华护理杂志,1998,33(5):251~253
25. 丁小强.尿毒症透析患者生活质量及其影响因素.中国行为医学科学,1998,7(4):285~287
26. 黄敬享主编.健康教育学.上海:上海医科大学出版社,1997
27. 中国农村初级卫生保健发展纲要(2001~2010年)

28 中共中央、国务院关于卫生改革与发展的决定

29 胡鞍钢. 透视 SARS 健康与发展. 北京：清华大学出版社，2003

30 郑杭生主编. 社会医学新编. 北京：中国人民大学出版社，1989

31 梁万年主编. 社区卫生服务管理. 北京：人民卫生出版社，2002

32 董先雨主编. 社区卫生服务与管理. 北京：华夏出版社，2000

33 卢祖洵，金生国主编. 国外社区卫生服务. 北京：人民卫生出版社，2001

34 卫生部，教育部，等 10 部委. 关于发展城市社区卫生服务的若干意见. 1999

35 卫生部，等 11 部委. 关于加快发展城市社区卫生服务的意见. 2002

36 梁沂滨，王菱. 看病就在家门口. 经济日报，2000-09-25

37 张彦，陈红霞. 社会保障概论. 南京：南京大学出版社，1999

38 宋晓梧. 中国社会保障制度改革. 北京：清华大学出版，2001

39 孙光德，董克用. 社会保障概论. 北京：中国人民大学出版社，2000

40 沈文虎，李致中，等. 农村合作医疗管理模式的应用. 广西预防医学，1999，5(3)：170~172

41 中国医疗保险制度改革政策与管理. 北京：中国劳动和社会保障出版社，1999

42 龚幼龙，冯学山. 卫生服务研究. 上海：复旦大学出版社，2002

43 李鲁主编. 社会医学. 北京：人民卫生出版社，2003

44 何清涟. 现代化的陷阱——当代中国的经济社会问题. 北京：今日中国出版社，1998

45 Barr M L. Determinants of quality of life changes among long-term cardiac transplant survivors: results from longitudinal data. J Heart Lung Transplant, 2003, 22(10):1157-1167

46 Little D J, Kuban D A. Quality-of-life questionnaire results 2 and 3 years after radiotherapy for prostate cancer in a randomized dose-escalation study. Urology. 2003, 62(4):707-713

47 Yamamoto D. A comparison between electrocautery and scalpel plus scissor in breast conserving surgery. Oncol Rep. 2003, 10(6):1729-1732

48 Uliukin I. Quality of life of mothers having nosocomially HIV-infected children in Russia. Disabil Rehabil. 2003, 25(20):1147-1152

49 Dianne Hales. An Invitation to Health. The Benjamin/Cummings Publishing Company, Inc, 1994